Adaptation Biology and Medicine

Volume 4: Current Concepts

SERIES EDITORS: **P.K. Singal and N. Takeda**

Adaptation Biology and Medicine

Volume 4: Current Concepts

EDITORS

A. Hargens

N. Takeda

P.K. Singal

Narosa Publishing House

New Delhi Chennai Mumbai Kolkata

SERIES EDITORS: **P.K. Singal and N. Takeda**

EDITORS

A. Hargens
Department of Orthopaedics
University of California, San Diego 350
Dickinson Street, 8894 San Diego, CA 92103-8894 USA

N. Takeda
Department of Internal Medicine
Aoto Hospital, Jikei University School of Medicine
Tokyo, Japan

P.K. Singal
Institute of Cardiovascular Sciences
St. Boniface General Hospital Research Center
Department of Physiology Faculty of Medicine
University of Manitoba Winnipeg, Canada

NAROSA PUBLISHING HOUSE PVT. LTD.

22 Daryaganj, Delhi Medical Association Road, New Delhi 110 002
35-36 Greams Road, Thousand Lights, Chennai 600 006
306 Shiv Centre, D.B.C. Sector 17, K.U. Bazar P.O., Navi Mumbai 400 705
2F-2G Shivam Chambers, 53 Syed Amir Ali Avenue, Kolkata 700 019

www.narosa.com

ISBN 81-7319-571-4

Published by N.K. Mehra for Narosa Publishing House, 22 Daryaganj, Delhi Medical Association Road, New Delhi 110 002 and printed at Rajkamal Press, Delhi, India

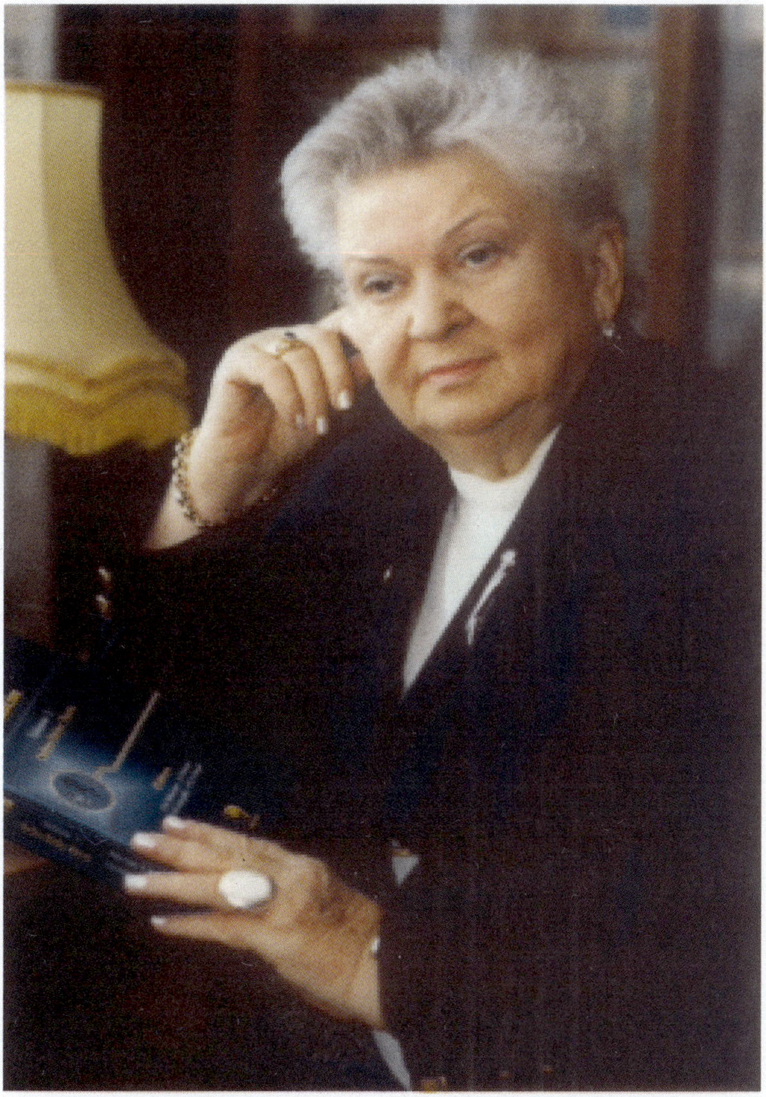

Prof. Ludmila Lukyanova, M.D., Moscow, Russia

Ludmila Lukyanova is one of the founding members of the International Society for Adaptive Medicine and has been an important member of the Executive Committee. She is Professor of Biophysics, Corresponding Member of the Russian Academy of Medical Sciences, Chairman of the Inter-Departmental Scientific Council on Problems of Hypoxia (Russia), Head of the Department of Bioenergetics. Prof. Lukyanova is engaged in the study of bioenergetics of Hypoxia as well as in the applied medical aspects related to the development of new biotechnologies for the creation of hypoxia therapeutics. She has been a constant participant of the World Congress of the ISAM and will chair the 8th World Congress in 2006 to be held in Russia. Her scientific leadership and active interest in the well being of the Society is commendable and is highly appreciated.

Preface

International Society for Adaptive Medicine (ISAM) was established in 1990 in Freiberg (Germany) to increase awareness as well as understanding of adaptive changes in human body organs in response to exercise, environmental factors, disease conditions, work related stress and drug treatments. In recent decades, it has been shown that gradual adaptation to repeat exposures to these "body stresses" increases the resistance of the organism not only to that specific condition but also to other potentially harmful challenges. Such protective cross effects have stimulated the development of a new scientific era of adaptive medicine. The Society aims at not only the study of basic mechanisms of adaptation but also their applications for the treatment and prophylaxis of diseases. Another aim of the Society is to understand failed adaptations or maladaptations that may precede disease.

At present, the Society is comprised of members worldwide and its meetings bring together clinicians, scientists and engineers who constitute a unique international forum with a vibrant atmosphere. The Society also sponsors regional symposia as well as World Congresses around the world. The Seventh World Congress of the ISAM was held in San Diego, USA during August 20-23, 2003. The previous World Congresses of the Society were held in Freiberg, Moscow, Tokyo, Chandigarh, Framingham and Lyon. The Congress in San Diego brought together basic and clinical scientists who shared a common interest in discussing the current concepts for adaptation of different body systems in physiological and pathophysiological states and application of this knowledge in therapeutic approaches. More than 200 participants from abroad and USA also highlighted major and rapidly expanding areas of adaptive medicine that are relevant to the understanding of biology of the adaptive processes. Another important feature of the Congress was presentation of the awards to students and young investigators.

The present book is based on papers selected from the invited symposia speakers as well as poster presentations. Although the entire book is one continuous discussion of issues as well as data dealing with the subcellular basis of adaptive responses and their potential applications in different therapies, it has been divided into three sections for an easy reading. Section A. **Understanding Adaptation**, comprised of eight chapters, highlights the mechanisms of adaptations in different biological systems. These initial papers are followed by eight chapters in Section B on **Biological Applications of Adaptation** and Section C, **Inducing Adaptations**, in the remaining nine papers, discusses enhancement of subcellular adaptation.

The book would be of great interest to biologists and clinicians interested in the overexpression of good adaptive responses and underexpression or blunting of maladaptive changes in improving the health of populous.

A. Hargens, *San Diego*
N. Takeda, *Tokyo*
P. K. Singal, *Winnipeg*

Acknowledgments

The Congress in San Diego was a resounding success with respect to the high quality scientific program and active participation by new members of our Society. Ample time was provided for informal exchanges among delegates in an array of carefully planned social events. All this was made possible by the efforts of many volunteers, financial support from different private and government organizations as well as the organizational skills of all the members of the local organizing team. Grants from the U.S. Army Medical Research and Material Command (DAMD17-03-1-0503) and NASA Headquarters Bioastronautics Research Division through Goddard Flight Center (NNGO4GB54G) are gratefully acknowledged. We would also like to thank the following for their time and outstanding efforts in the organization of the various aspects of this Congress as well as publication of these proceedings: Patrik Danaher, Rynda Clark, Jill Collier, Cheryle Genovese, Jason Harris, Maureen Helinski, Linda Johnson, Brandon Macias, Lisa Rhodes and Kathy Smith (San Diego); and Jennifer Fowler and Dr. Thomas P. Thomas (Winnipeg).

A. Hargens, *San Diego*
N. Takeda, *Tokyo*
P. K. Singal, *Winnipeg*

Contents

Biological Applications of Adaptation

Inducing Adaptation

Contributing Authors

H. T. Abul
Department of Pharmacy
Faculty of Medicine
Kuwait University, Kuwait

E. M. Ali Emadi
Department of Medical Laboratory Sciences
Faculty of Allied Health Sciences
University of Kuwait, Kuwait

M. A. Al-Jarallah
Ministry of Health
State of Health
Sulaibikhat, Kuwait

M. B. Anand-Srivastava
Department of Physiology and Groupe de recherche sur le système nerveux autonome
Faculty of Medicine
University of Montreal
Montreal, Quebec, Canada

Yu V. Arkhipenko
Moscow State University
Moscow, Russia

J. E. Baker
Division of Pediatric Surgery
Medical College of Wisconsin
Milwaukee, WI 53226 USA

R. E. Ballard
Life Science Division
NASA Ames Research Center
Moffett Field, CA 94035-1000 USA

J. X. Bao
Department of Aerospace Physiology
Fourth Military Medical University
Xi'an 710032, P. R. China

Y. N. Bhambhani
Faculty of Rehabilitation Medicine University of Alberta
Edmonton, AB T6G 2P6, Canada

A. A. Bludov
Russian Peoples' Friendship University
Podolskoye sh., 8/5. Moscow. 113093. Russia

A. Ya. Chizov
Russian Peoples' Friendship University
Podolskoye sh., 8/5. Moscow. 113093. Russia

F. M. Clarke
School of Biomolecular and Biomedical Science
Faculty of Science and Technology
Griffith University, Australia

N. S. Dhalla
Institute of Cardiovascular Sciences
St. Boniface General Hospital Research Center
Department of Physiology
Faculty of Medicine
University of Manitoba
Winnipeg, Canada

V. Elimban
Institute of Cardiovascular Sciences
St. Boniface General Hospital Research Center
Department of Physiology
Faculty of Medicine
University of Manitoba
Winnipeg, Canada

F. Furuyama
Department of Neurophysiology Brain Science
Nagoya City University Graduate School of Medicine
Nagoya 467-8601, Japan

N. K. Ganguly
Director General ICMR
New Delhi, India

A.V. Goryacheva
Institute of General Pathology and Pathophysiology
Baltijskaya 8, Moscow 125315, Russia

S. K. Gupta
Institute of Cardiovascular Sciences
St. Boniface General Hospital Research Center
Department of Physiology
Faculty of Medicine
University of Manitoba
Winnipeg, Canada

H. T. Hammel
Medical Sciences
Indiana University School of Medicine
Bloomington, IN 47405, USA

A. R. Hargens
Department of Orthopaedics
University of California, San Diego
350 Dickinson Street, 8894 San Diego, CA 92103-8894 USA

H. Katano
Division of Ophthalmology and Visual Science
Faculty of Medicine
Tottori University
Yonago 683-8503, Japan

J. Jiang
Central Institute for Electron Microscopic Researches
Nippon Medical School
Sendagi, Bunkyo-ku, Tokyo, Japan

K. Kaur
Institute of Cardiovascular Sciences
St. Boniface General Hospital Research Center
Department of Physiology
Faculty of Medicine
University of Manitoba
Winnipeg, Canada

Y. Kawai
Division of Adaptation Physiology
Faculty of Medicine
Tottori University
Yonago 683-8503, Japan

S. Kimura
Department of Orthopaedics
University of California, San Diego
350 Dickinson Street, 8894 San Diego, CA 92103-8894 USA

I. P. Khomenko
Institute of General Pathology and Pathophysiology
Baltijskaya 8, Moscow 125315, Russia

H. Kohzuki
Department of Food and Nutrition
Okayama Gakin University
Okayama, Japan

S. V. Kruglov
Institute of General Pathology and Pathophysiology
Baltijskaya 8, Moscow 125315, Russia

R. C. Kukreja
Division of Cardiology
Department of Internal Medicine
Virginia Commonwealth University
Richmond, VA 23298-0281, USA

D. Kumar
Institute of Cardiovascular Sciences
St. Boniface General Hospital Research Center
Department of Physiology
Faculty of Medicine
University of Manitoba
Winnipeg, Canada

A. Kuroshima
Department of Physiology
Asahikawa Medical College
Asahikawa 078-8510 Japan

G. Lappas
Department of Physiology and Groupe de recherche sur le système nerveux autonome
Faculty of Medicine
University of Montreal
Montreal, Quebec, Canada

H. B. Lillywhite
Department of Zoology
The University of Florida
Gainesville, Florida 32611-8525 USA

D. T. Lincoln
Department of Medical Laboratory Sciences
Faculty of Allied Health Sciences
University of Kuwait, Kuwait

H. Lou
Institute of Cardiovascular Sciences
St. Boniface General Hospital Research Center
Faculty of Medicine
University of Manitoba
Winnipeg, Canada

L. D. Lukyanova
Head of the Department of Bioenergetics and Hypoxia Problems.
Institute of General Pathology and Pathophysiology of Russian Acad. Med. Sci.
Moscow

R. V. Maikala
Liberty Mutual Research Institute for Safety
Hopkinton, MA 01748, USA

I. Yu. Malyshev
Institute of General Pathology and Pathophysiology
Baltijskaya 8, Moscow 125315, Russia

E. B. Manukhina
Institute of General Pathology and Pathophysiology
Baltijskaya 8, Moscow 125315, Russia

S. Yu. Mashina
Institute of General Pathology and Pathophysiology
Baltijskaya 8, Moscow 125315, Russia

F. Z. Meerson
Institute of General Pathology and Pathophysiology
Baltijskaya 8, Moscow 125315, Russia

Q. J. Meng
Department of Aerospace Physiology, Fourth Military Medical University
Xi'an 710032, P. R. China

M. Mozzaffari
Department of Oral Biology and Maxillofacial Pathology
Medical College of Georgia
School of Dentistry
Augusta, Georgia

M. S. Nijjar
Institute of Cardiovascular Sciences
St. Boniface General Hospital Research Center
Department of Physiology
Faculty of Medicine
University of Manitoba
Winnipeg, Canada

H. Nishino
Department of Neurophysiology Brain Science, Nagoya City University Graduate School of Medicine
Nagoya 467-8601, Japan

K. Okuyama
Clinical Research Laboratory of IHT
2-21-15 Shimouma Setagaya-ku Tokyo, Japan

J. J. Pedley
Life Science Division
NASA Ames Research Center
Moffett Field, CA 94035-1000 USA

D. A. Pokidyshev
Institute of General Pathology and Pathophysiology
Baltijskaya 8, Moscow 125315, Russia

E. V. Popkova
Institute of General Pathology and Pathophysiology
Baltijskaya 8, Moscow 125315, Russia

V. I. Potievskaya
Institute of General Pathology and Pathophysiology
Baltijskaya 8, Moscow 125315, Russia

K. A. Pritchard Jr.
Division of Pediatric Surgery
Medical College of Wisconsin
Milwaukee, WI 53226 USA

M. G. Pshennikova
Institute of General Pathology and Pathophysiology
Baltijskaya 8, Moscow 125315, Russia

P. Rafiee
Division of Pediatric Surgery
Medical College of Wisconsin
Milwaukee, WI 53226 USA

C. Ricci
University of South Alabama, College of Medicine
Department of Pharmacology
Mobile, Alabama

T. G. Sazontova
Institute of General Pathology and Pathophysiology
Russian Academy of Medical Sciences

S. W. Schaffer
University of South Alabama
College of Medicine
Department of Pharmacology
Mobile, Alabama

Y. Shi
Division of Pediatric Surgery
Medical College of Wisconsin
Milwaukee, WI 53226 USA

O. Shido
Department of Physiology
Shimane Medical University
Izumo 689-8501 Japan

P. K. Singal
Institute of Cardiovascular Sciences
St. Boniface General Hospital Research Center
Department of Physiology
Faculty of Medicine
University of Manitoba
Winnipeg, Canada

V. Solodushko
University of South Alabama
College of Medicine
Department of Pharmacology
Mobile, Alabama

K.F. Tonissen
School of Biomolecular and Biomedical Science
Faculty of Science and Technology
Griffith University, Australia

J. S. Tweddell
Division of Cardiothoracic Surgery
Medical College of Wisconsin
Milwaukee, WI 53226 USA, and
Section of Cardiothoracic Surgery Children's Hospital of Wisconsin
Milwaukee, WI 53226 USA

T. Ueno
Department of Orthopaedics
University of California, San Diego
350 Dickinson Street, 8894 San Diego, CA 92103-8894 USA

I. B. Ushakov
State Scientific Research Testing Institute of Military Medicine
Moscow, Russia

M. A. Vlasova
Institute of General Pathology and Pathophysiology
Baltijskaya 8, Moscow 125315, Russia

D. E. Watenpaugh
Naval Submarine Medical Research Laboratory
Groton, CT 06349

F. A. C. Wiegant
Utrecht University
Utrecht, The Netherlands

L. Xi
Division of Cardiology
Department of Internal Medicine
Virginia Commonwealth University
Richmond, VA 23298-0281, USA

T. Yahata
Department of Nursing
Nayoro City College
Nayoro 096-8641 Japan

O. M. Zelenina
Institute of General Pathology and Pathophysiology
Baltijskaya 8, Moscow 125315, Russia

L. F. Zhang
Department of Aerospace Physiology
Fourth Military Medical University
Xi'an 710032, P. R. China

W. Zhang
Institute of Cardiovascular Sciences
St. Boniface General Hospital Research Center
Department of Physiology
Faculty of Medicine
University of Manitoba
Winnipeg, Canada

Adaptation Biology and Medicine (Volume 4: Current Concepts)
Editors: A. Hargens, N. Takeda and P.K. Singal

1. Novel Approaches to the Understanding of Molecular Mechanisms of Adaptation

Lukyanova L.D.

Head of the Department of Bioenergetics and Hypoxia Problems.
Inst. Of General Pathology and Pathophysiology of Russian Acad. Med. Sci., Moscow.

Special literature of recent 5-6 years have extensively discussed mechanisms of cell oxygen sensitivity, regularities of developing the response to oxygen deficiency and realization of adaptive responses. The following issues are discussed most of all:

= whether a cell is capable for differential gradual changes in environmental oxygen;

= what serves as the intracellular sensor of oxygen and whether a universal oxygen sensor exists;

= whether the mitochondrial respiratory chain is able to serve as an oxygen sensor and regulator of adaptive responses, taking into account that cellular ATP depletion is a key feature of hypoxia;

= what is the role of reactive oxygen species in formation of compensatory and adaptive responses of cell to changes in environmental oxygen.

In this process, the following possible oxygen sensors are under discussion:

= mitochondrial respiratory chain;

= intracellular metal-containing oxidases;

= free radical processes;

= role of gene metabolism in cell sensitivity and adaptation to hypoxia.

The question on whether a cell is capable for differentiate gradual changes in external oxygen has a long-standing prehistory. Warburg [59] was the first to study this problem in the beginning of the previous century, but he failed to identify the relationship between cell system respiration and oxygen concentration for methodical reasons. Ten years later, however, Tang showed that this relationship does exist and is described with a hyperbole [57]. Much later the data were confirmed by Bander and Kiesee, who established that the dependence of oxygen consumption rate on oxygen tension (VO_2/pO_2) is subject to the Michaelis-Menten kinetics [3]. In 1982 we demonstrated that the VO_2/pO_2 ratio is a net result of diverse intracellular oxidase functioning and that hyperbolic VO_2/pO_2 relationship reflects contribution of various mitochondrial substrates [44].

This is due to the fact that the oxygen affinity of intracellular oxidases as evaluated by the value of oxidase K_M for O_2 can vary by several orders of magnitude (Table 1). For example, monoaminoxidase $K_M(O_2)$ is equal to 10^{-3} – 10^{-3} M, while cytochrome oxidase $K_M(O_2)$ is equal to 10^{-6} – 10^{-8} M.

Therefore inactivation of these enzymes will occur at different oxygen values, which should undoubtedly affect the VO_2/pO_2 curve.

Table 1. Kм(O_2) for some oxidases (by [44]).

Enzymes	Intracellular Localisation	Kм(O_2), M
Cytochrome oxidase	mitochondria	$10^{-8} - 10^{-7}$
Cytochrome P-450-dependent reactions	endoplasmic reticulum	$10^{-6} - 10^{-5}$
Aldehyde oxidase	cytosol	2×10^{-6}
Lipid peroxidation	membranes	3×10^{-5}
Microsomal oxidase	endoplasmic reticulum	2×10^{-5}
Xanthine oxidase	cytosol	$2.5 \times 10^{-5} - 2.5 \times 10^{-4}$
Monoamine oxidase	mitochondria	$5.5 \times 10^{-3} - 2 \times 10^{-4}$
Glycolate oxidase	peoxisome	4×10^{-4}

Indeed, in isolated hepatocytes, the hyperbolic VO_2/pO_2 ratio is indistinct during activation of oxidases with a low oxygen affinity, that is, with high Kм(O_2) values, in this instance glyoxylate oxidase. In contrast, the VO_2/pO_2 ratio recovers in the presence of succinate, a mitochondrial substrate stimulating the oxidase activity of mitochondrial respiratory chain. The dependence is slightly attenuated in the presence of both succinate and glycolate, and becomes completely linear in the presence of KCN, a cytochrome oxidase inhibitor (Fig.1).

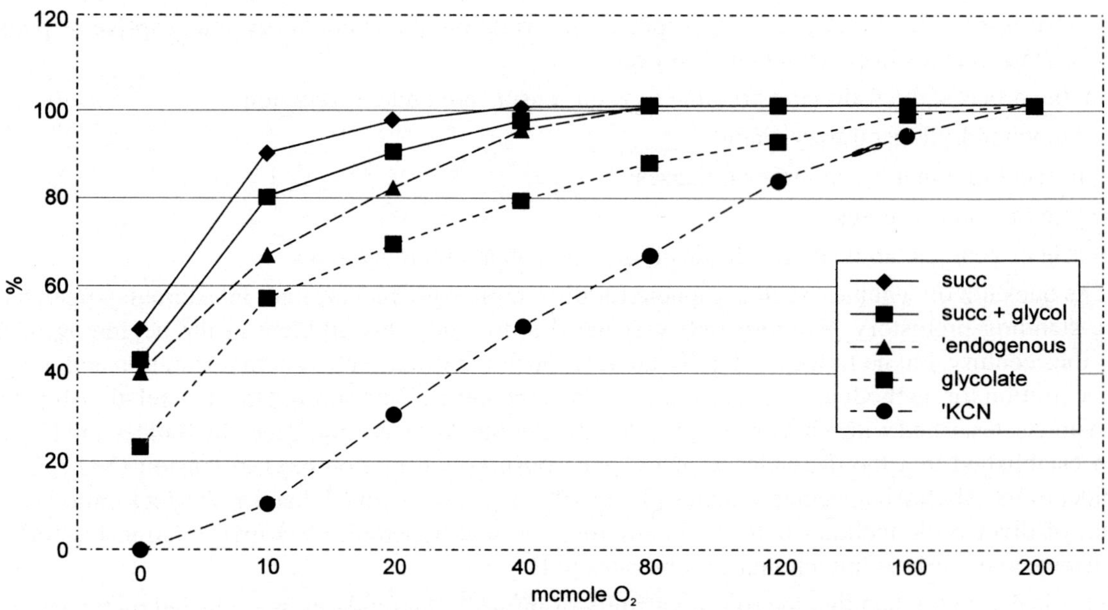

Fig. 1. Dependence of respiratory rate on [O_2] in isolated hepatocytes oxidizing substrates of diverse oxidases. 1–succinate: 2–succinate + glycolate; 3–endogenous substrates; 4–glycolate; 5–KCN

These data lead to three following conclusions:

1. Obviously a cell isolated from central and humoral influences can differentiate gradual changes in environmental oxygen and respond with respiratory changes.
2. Intracellular oxidases participate in regulation of cell oxygen sensitivity. Therefore cell possesses not a single metabolic system but multiple ones that serve as oxygen sensors.
3. The hyperbolic dependence of VO_2/pO_2 reflects the contribution of oxidation of various metabolic substrates stimulating activity of the respiratory chain oxidase that possesses a maximum oxygen affinity.

Considering the nature of cell oxygen sensor, it is necessary to remind that the critical event characteristic of hypoxia is ATP depletion. Earlier we have shown that the ATP/$[O_2]$ ratio as well as the VO_2/pO_2 ratio approaches the hyperbolic relationship [40,43]. Moreover it was demonstrated that changes in adenylate pool parameters are the earliest predictors of hypoxia.

Diagram on Figure 2 summarizes regularities typical of this process. It is seen that the cell energy deficiency develops as a phase process and is determined by intensity and duration of the hypoxic exposure. Based on changes in various parameters of the adenylate pool we have isolated at least three areas of oxygen concentrations corresponding to three different functional and metabolic states of the cell:

(1) Area of a disbalance developing in the adenine nucleotide pool (which is next to area of persisting homeostatic balance between different components of the adenylate pool). This disbalance correlates with the decreased regulatory role of ATP/ADP ratio and the enhanced regulatory role of ATP/ADP ratio and the enhanced regulatory role of ATP/AMP ratio.

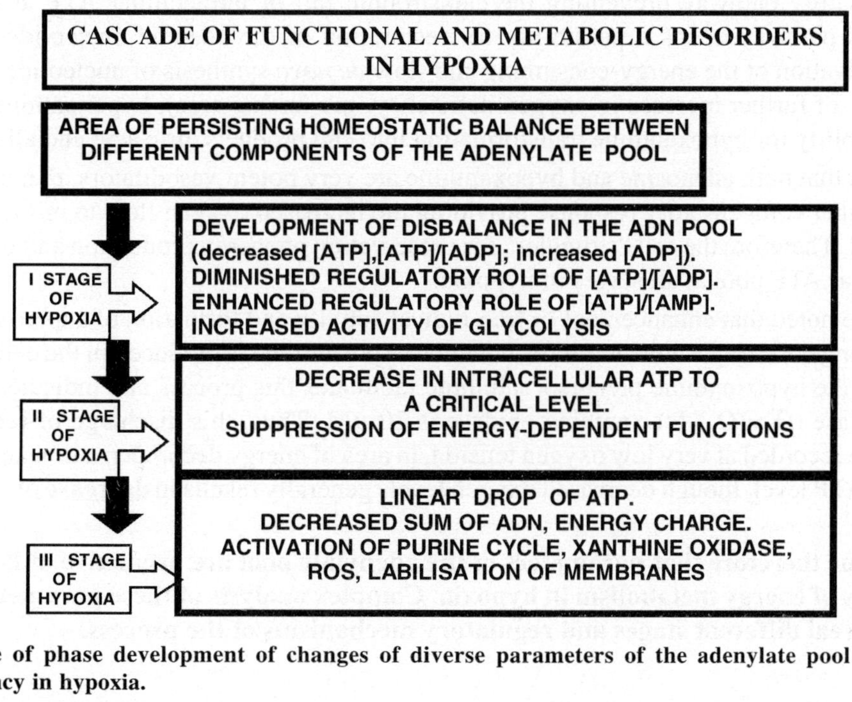

Fig. 2. Scheme of phase development of changes of diverse parameters of the adenylate pool and of energy deficiency in hypoxia.

(2) Area of intracelluar ATP decreasing to a critical level and suppression of energy-dependent functions.

(3) Area of rough disorders in energy metabolism. This is the area of linear decrease in intracellular ATP, reduction of total adenylate pool values and energy charge, which reflects intensification of adenine nucleotide degradation.

In this connection, two aspects should be emphasized.

At the early stage of hypoxia, compensatory activation of glycolysis correlates with the increased regulatory role of ATP/AMP ratio, which is fully explainable from the biochemical standpoint. In this period, glycolysis considerably affects the nature of ATP/[O_2] relationship stabilizing the intracellular level of ATP. However in the area of ATP linear decline, even hyperactivation of glycolysis cannot prevent this process [4, 43].

Therefore **glycolysis takes part in stabilization of the intracellular ATP level only at initial stages of hypoxia**. The more severe oxygen deficiency the lesser effect of glycolysis on this process despite glycolysis hyperactivity. This suggests that disturbances in the adenine nucleotide pool in this period are associated with the suppressed aerobic component of ATP synthesis.

It is necessary to dwell specially upon the process of adenine nucleotide degradation. The question on whether this process exists *in vivo* remains open in bioenergetics science as yet. We have shown that degradation of adenine nucleotides indeed occurs in hepatocytes [43]. However it takes place in the area of very low oxygen concentrations (in the area of energy decompensation and linear fall of intracellular ATP level) and goes through several stages, which are different in high-resistance (HR) and low-resistance (LR) animals. At first adenosine and purine cycles including reactions of adenine transformation into adenosine and AMP become activated. Activation of these cycles can be regarded as a compensatory pathway preventing the catastrophic fall of intracellular ATP at late stages of hypoxia. This pathway opens a possibility for restoration of the adenine nucleotide pool without additional activation of the energy-consuming and slow *de novo* synthesis of nucleotides. And only in the conditions of further increase in oxygen deficiency (pre-anoxic area), hypoxanthine is formed to create a possibility for hypoxanthine transformation into end products, uric acid and allantoin [43].

It is known that both adenosine and hypoxanthine are very potent vasodilators, that is, their effects represent another compensatory response providing the increased oxygen flow to mitochondria at the systemic level. Therefore the cell "struggles" for preservation of energy production and maintenance of the intracellular ATP pool at all stages of hypoxia.

It should be noted that enhancement of free-radical activity and formation of superoxide anion can occur in the range of oxygen concentration, at which hypoxanthine is produced in the cell (6-2 $\mu M\ O_2$). Formation of the hypoxanthine precursor xanthine facilitates this process and indicates activation of xanthine oxidase (($K_M(O_2)$ for xanthine oxidase is 10 μM. Thus, this discharge of reactive oxygen species can be recorded at very low oxygen tension, in area of energy decompensation and linear fall of intracellular ATP level, though decreased oxygen levels generally results in **decrease** of radical oxygen activity.

It is obvious therefore that parameters of the adenylate pool are predictive of both early and late disorders of energy metabolism in hypoxia. Complex analysis of these parameters and their ratios can reveal different stages and regulatory mechanisms of the process.

Studies of E.I. Maevsky have shown that ATP synthesis is possible also in the anaerobic conditions [47] and that there are several metabolic pathways, besides glycolysis and aerobic oxidation in the respiratory chain, which provide this process for about 40 first minutes of anoxia.

Analysis of [ATP]/[O_2]a plots allowed us to introduce the notion of **critical oxygen concentration** for ATP, that is, the concentration, below which the subsequent decrease in intracellular ATP resulted in suppression of energy-dependent functions (Fig.3). This process took a start, when intracellular ATP decreased only by 10-15% of the value typical for the region of homeostatic balance, and displayed a pronounced sigmoid pattern. This why when ATP fell by only 25-30% a complete suppression of energy-dependent processes was observed [15,16,40,43].

In this connection it becomes clear that **this is just the decrease in intracellular ATP below its critical concentration that underlies multiple systemic and organ disorders characteristic of hypoxia. Therefore the tactis and strategy for protection or recovery of cell functions disturbed by hypoxia should be aimed at preservaion of ATP values above the critical level rather than maintenance of intracellular ATP in general.**

Studying the dependence of disorders in key functional and metabolic systems on oxygen levels have allowed a conclusion that the following sequence occurs in the cascade of hypoxia-induced metabolic disturbances: decrease in intracellular ATP below the critical level → suppression of energy-dependent functions (including electrogenic, contractile, ion-transport, detoxication, anabolic processes, etc.) → activation of adenine nucleotide degradation processes → activation of xanthine oxidase and free radical processes → disturbance of membrane permeability → loss of cell viability.

Therefore it is of basic importance that changes in adenine nucleotide pool begin in the area of oxygen concentrations an order of magnitude exceeding those inducing changes in permeability and viability of cells. Furthermore changes in energy metabolism precede enhancement of free radical activity and selective permeability of cell membranes. This is indicative of the fact that reactive oxygen species can hardly claim for the role of oxygen sensors at early stages of hypoxia.

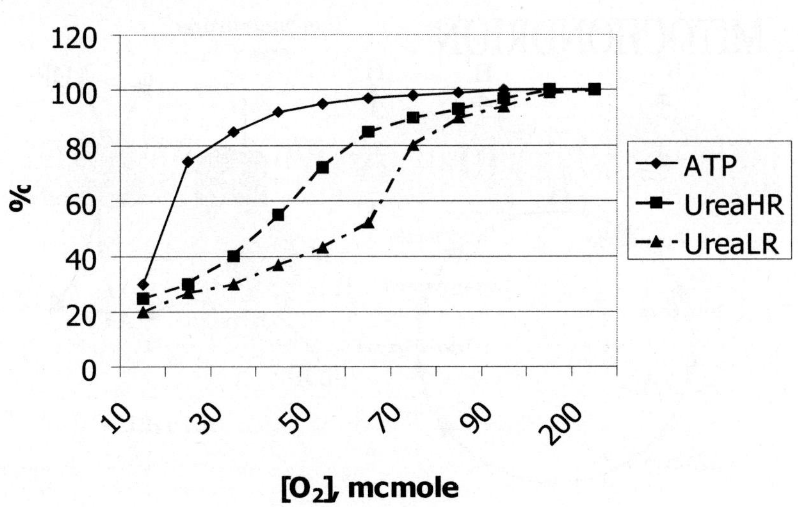

Fig. 3. Dependence of intracellular ATP concentration and energy-dependent functions (urea synthesis) on [O_2] in hepatocytes of high- (HR) and low-resistance (LR) rats.

A very important conclusion follows from the above-said: **in studying functional and metabolic disturbances induced by oxygen insufficiency, it is necessary to take into account the phase pattern of cell response to oxygen shortage. Of special importance are early stages of the disorders, when cell regulatory mechanism aimed at prevention of ATP loss are preserved and involved. Therefore modeling of acute hypoxia (pre-anoxic or anoxic states) associated with already irreversible changes induced by loss of these mechanisms cannot provide an objective information about trigger mechanisms of the process as a whole.**

According to the above-said it is reasonable to consider the role of respiratory chain enzymes in development of energy deficiency in hypoxia.

Mitochondrial electron transport chain, the major source of ATP in cells, consists of five multi-enzyme oxidative phosphorylation complexes located on mitochondrial inner membrane (Fig.4). Complexes I-IV are oxidoreductases, which participate in the transfer of reduction equivalents from NAD- and FAD-dependent substrates to oxygen and create an electrochemical proton gradient across the mitochondrial inner membrane. Complex V (F_0F_1-ATPase) uses this proton gradient for synthesis of ATP. All complexes occur in spatial sequences optimizing the electron transfer efficiency while minimizing the possibilities for the single-electron "leakage" to oxygen, that would generate oxy-radicals. The system is finely balanced: damage to any complex both reduces the ATP yield and aggravates the inevitable leakage of oxy-radicals from the system.

At present it is proven experimentally that phase disturbances of the adenine nucleotide pool leading to energy deficiency result from a number of successive changes in activities of various mitochondrial enzyme complexes [32-40]. The latter changes depend on severity and/or duration of the hypoxic exposure and predetermine the phase pattern of the entire process. Changes in the electron transport function of the respiratory chain begin at its substrate (NADH-dependent) site and are due to functional disturbances of the mitochondrial enzyme Complex I. The decreased oxygen level initially potentiates and then suppresses activity of the complex (activation-inhibition of the NADH-dependent pathway of

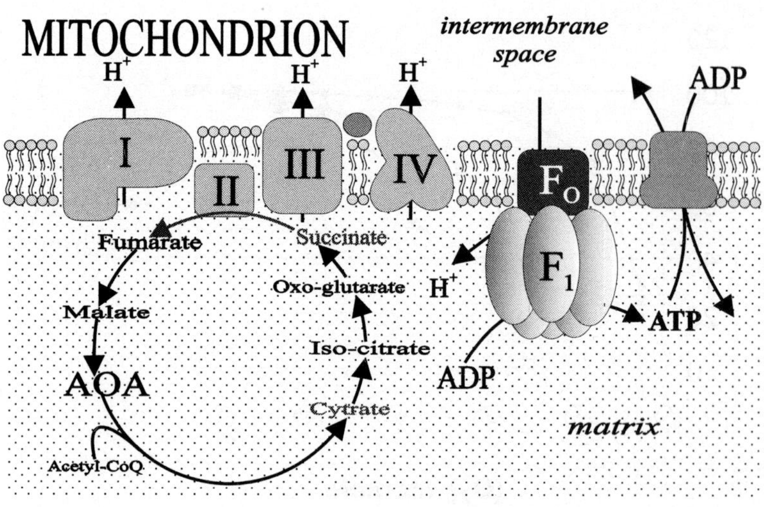

Fig. 4. Structural scheme of mitochondrial respiratory chain enzyme complexes within the mitochondrial inner membrane.

substrate oxidation in the tricarbonic acid cycle, the major supplier of reduction equivalents to the respiratory chain). This process is generally associated with recruitment of compensatory pathways for oxidation of substrates supplying reduction equivalents to the cytochrome site, specifically to Complexes III and IV, among which special role belongs to activation of complex II (enhancement of the succinate oxidation pathway) (compensatory stage of tissue or bionergetic hypoxia).

In increasing severity and/or duration of hypoxic exposure, the disorders of respiratory chain electron transport function successively spread at first to Complex III (site of cytochromes ***b-c***) (decompensation stage) and then to Complex IV (cytochrome oxidase), which is inactivated only at very low po_2 values (terminal stage of bionergetic hypoxia) due to its kinetic properties (very high oxygen affinity) (Fig 5).

Therefore **the inadequate oxygen supply to tissues and organs in hypoxia results in dysfunction of the mitochondrial apparatus evident as phase changes in activities of mitochondrial enzyme complexes and ensuing suppression of aerobic energy synthesis, energy-dependent functions and cell metabolism.**

Appropriateness of the above ideas on causes and phase pattern of energy metabolism disorders in hypoxia is supported by multiple experimental evidence that inhibition of Complex I indeed passes ahead of inactivation of the other mitochondrial enzymes [10,18, 32-43, 45, 48, 54, 55, 61] and is associated with changes in functions and content of incorporated iron-sulfur centers [5,11].

I would like to underline again the exclusive importance of activating the succinate oxidase pathway in the conditions of limited performance of Complex I. This is an alternative pathway, which takes up the function of providing electrons to the cytochrome region of respiratory chain in these conditions to maintain ATP production at the expense of working Complexes III and IV. Therefore activation of this pathway in the conditions of oxygen shortage is an urgent compensatory mechanism used by the cell for ATP production. This process is reversible. When the environmental level of oxygen is normalized,

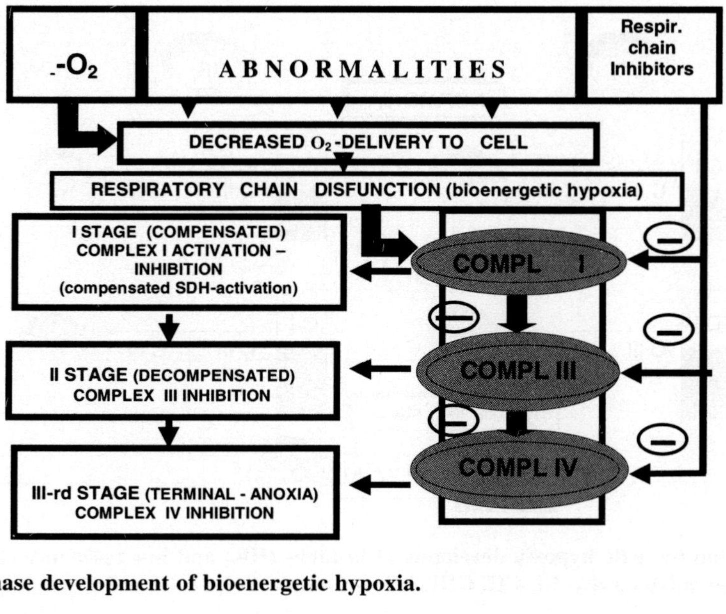

Fig. 5. Scheme of phase development of bioenergetic hypoxia.

the activity of Complex I also becomes recovered. Peter Hochachka was one of the firsts who has found and described this pathway in some swimming animals. Functional relevance of this pathway in hypoxia was substantiated by studies of M.N. Kondrashova [28-30]. By now the possibility of involvement of such compensatory mechanism at early stages of hypoxia has been demonstrated on various mitochondrial and organ models [32-36, 39-42, 47]. Furthermore its role in development of individual organism resistance has been established.

For instance, we showed that inhibition of NAD-dependent oxidation pathway and activation of the succinate oxidase pathway related with Roberts cycle activity really occurred in the brain cortex of LR rats at the initial stage of hypoxia. In contrast, the brain of HR rats, in which the NAD-dependent oxidation pathway basically predominated, displayed enhancement of precisely this pathway with only a slight activation of succinate oxidase oxidation. Increasing the severity of hypoxia resulted in suppression of all respiratory chain enzymes (Fig.6) [10, 18, 32-34, 37 –40].

As distinct from the brain, the succinate oxidase pathway of substrate oxidation normally prevails in the myocardium of high-resistance rats while the NADH-oxidase oxidation pathway prevails in the myocardium of low-resistance rats. This predetermines different resistance of the heart to hypoxia in thesse two types of rats (Fig.7) [32, 34, 39].

At the late stage of hypoxia, the electron transfer through the cytochrome region of respiratory chain (Complex III) becomes to be restricted, which may be due to labilization of membranes and release of cytochrome *c* and free coenzyme Q from the inner mitochondrial membrane. Theoretically, the cytochrome oxidase activity and ability for oxidative phosphorylation would be still preserved in these conditions due to performance of Complex IV. Nevertheless the restricted delivery of electrons from the respiratory chain substrate region through Complex III results in limitation of this process and decrease in intracellular ATP.

Thus **in the conditions of reduced oxygen delivery to cells, the mitochondrial respiratory chain is involved in the process as a single functional and metabolic unit which performs thereby as a**

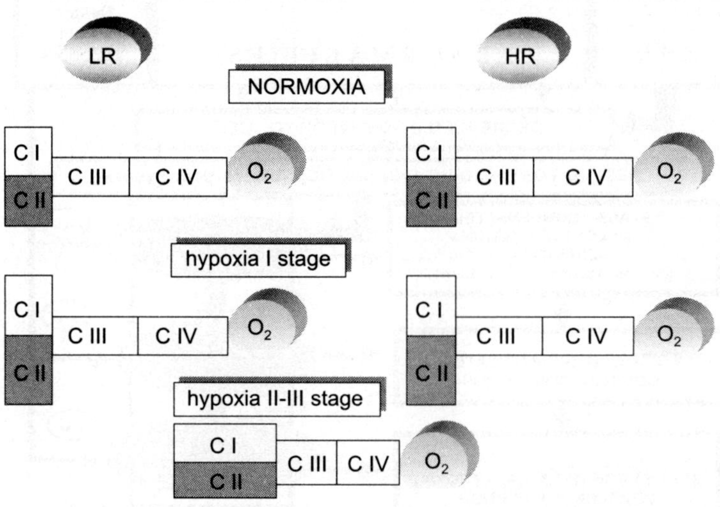

Fig. 6. Peculiarity of bioenergetic hypoxia development in high- (HR) and low-resistance (LR) rat brain during hypoxia of progressive servity. CI, CII, CIII, CIV – Complexes I, II, III and IV respectively.

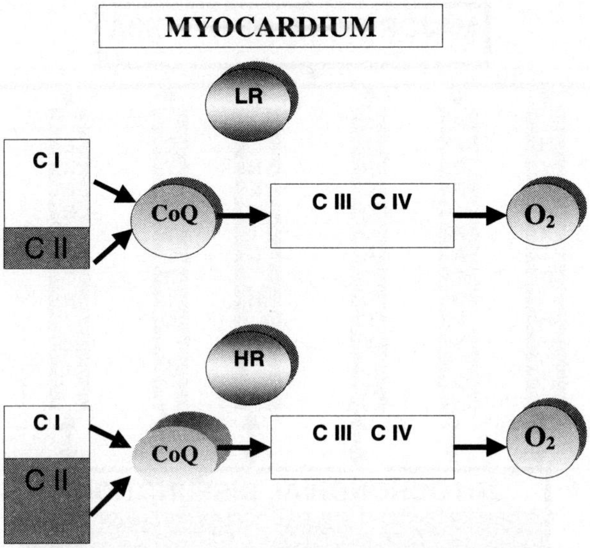

Fig. 7. Basal differences in activity of myocardium Complexes I and II from high- and low-resistance rats (HR and LR respectively).

regulator and modulator of oxygen consumption and rate of delivery from the extracellular medium to mitochondria.

This is just this process termed by us **bioenergetic hypoxia** that can play a role of intracellular trigger system signaling of changes in extracellular oxygen and initiating a cascade of functional and metabolic intracellular responses to oxygen shortage at the systemic level.

The described disturbances of mitochondrial bioenergetic functions in hypoxia can be detected by both direct effect of oxygen on isolated cells and at the systemic level, via activation of the sympathetico-adrenal system and the cascade of functional disorders typical for this process, and secondarily leading to mitochondrial cytopathies and energy-releted disorders (Fig.8) [1, 15-16, 18, 39-43].

Moreover a growing body of data shows that energy metabolism is subject to hormonal control. Studying these relationships acquires a special importance in hypoxia. Receptor systems and neurotransmitters can be responsible for recruitment of compensatory metabolic responses modulating and regulating energy metabolism in these conditions [27, 30].

Thereby, there exists a complex regulatory system of interactions between the systemic response of the organism to hypoxia, which develops as a stress reaction, and the changes occurrings in the cell and leading to bioenergetic disturbances. However the end result in this instance is also mitochondrial dysfunction, which develops according to the above scheme and results in suppression of energy-dependent functions.

Thus, **the organism response to O_2 deficiency reflects a complex multifunctional cell response, which is coordinated by neurohumoral mechanisms. In this process, energy metabolism acts as a trigger within the hierarchy of intracellular processes whereas the disturbed function of mitochondrial enzyme complexes is a basis mechanism in any type of hypoxia.**

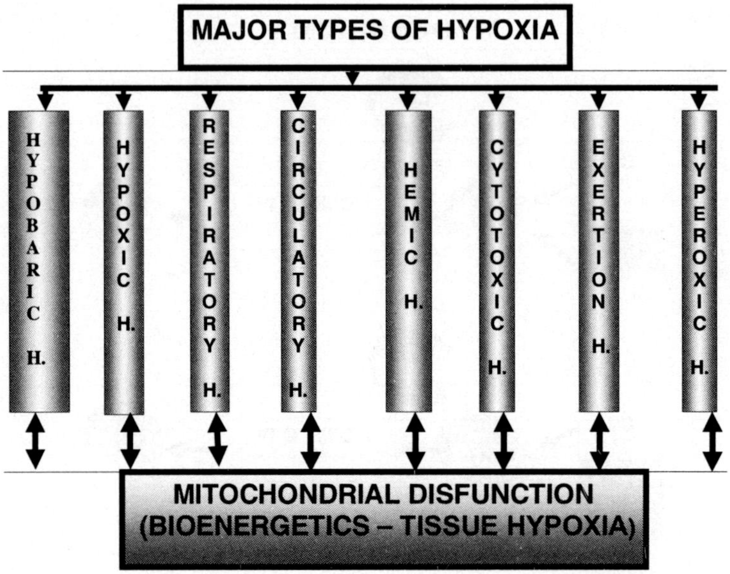

Fig. 8. Mitochondrial dysfunctions as a basis mechanism in different types of hypoxia.

This is well seen on Fig. 9, which demonstrates that bioenergetic hypoxia occupies a special place among different forms of hypoxia **being their constituent.**

Moreover it is obvious already now that mitochondrial dysfunction is an obligatory component of any pathology and can be considered as a **typical pathological process** [40]. A great deal of information has appeared in recent years, which confirms the conclusion that disorders of Complex I are included in pathogenesis of various diseases as an obligatory component. Phenotypic and genotypic defects of Complex I function has been established in all types of hypoxia and ischemia, stress, chronic alcohol consumption, cancer, traumatic shock, Parkinson's disease, fatal infantile lactocidosis, neurological and mental diseases, cerebral palsies, myocardiopathies, myopathies, encephalopathies, physical intolerance, optical neuropathy, I type diabetes mellitus, connective tissue diseases, tuberous sclerosis, hereditary forms of nanism, endotoxicoses, etc [9, 12, 20, 31, 40-42, 45, 48, 51, 53-55, 61].

It became also clear that genetically predetermined differences between HR and LR animal tissues in the oxidative capacity of respiratory chain NAD-dependent region reflect peculiarities of kinetic parameters of NADH-ubiquinone oxidoreductase, the major enzyme of Complex I. For instance, the maximum activity (Vmax) and KM (NADH) values of this enzyme were significantly lower in the brain of LR rats as compared to HR animals (Table 2) [17 – 19, 32-40]. Similar though less pronounced differences in kinetic parameters are characteristic of brain cytochrome oxidase in intact HR and LR animals. It means that these enzymes are more rapidly saturated with substrates (NADH or cytochrome *c)* and they more slowly oxidize the substrates in the brain of LR rats. This may be the reason for lower activity and more rapid inactivation of, for example, the NAD-oxidase oxidation of substrates in the brain of LR animals.

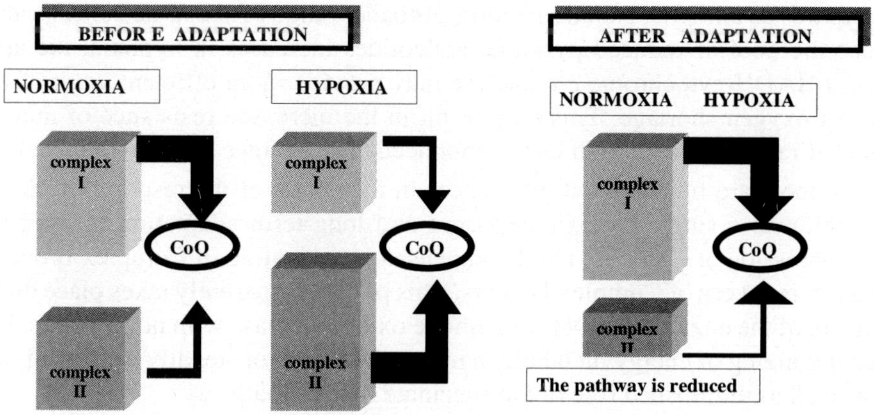

Fig. 9. Relative Contribution of NADH-oxidase and succinate-oxidase pathways before (A) and after (B) adaptation to hypoxia.

Table 2. Kinetic characteristics of some mitochondrial enzymes in the brain of HR and LR rats nonadapted and adapted to hypoxia

Enzymes	Parameters	HR	LR	HR/LR	HRad	HRad/HRc	LRad	LRad/LRc	HRad/LRad
NADH-rotenon-sensitive ox-red	Vmax Km (NADH)	0.143 13.30	0.061 2.9	2.34** 4.60***	0.100 5.40	0.70** 0.41***	0.167 14.30	2.73** 4.93***	0.60** 0.38***
Succ-ox-red	Vmax Km (succ)	0.11 32.00	0.10 116.0	1.10 1.14	0.11 135.00	1.0 1.02	0.12 116.00	1.20 1.00	0.92 1.16
COX ox-red	Vmax Km (cyt. C)	0.77 3.33	0.67 1.67	1.15 2.00**	1.06 2.38	1.38* 0.77*	1.11 3.33	1.66* 1.78**	0.95 0.85

The same kinetic features of the enzyme underlie the lower oxidative efficiency of NADH-cytochrome *c* reductase in the brain of LR rats at the low values of $NAD^+/NADH$ ratio characteristic of hypoxia. Due to these kinetic peculiarities, the limitation of NAD-oxidase pathway occurs earlier and is more pronounced in the brain of LR than HR animals. Therefore while the NADH-oxidase pathway is the limiting step in the brain of both HR and LR animals at early stages of hypoxia, the extent of hypoxia suppression is different in these animals. This fact predetermines the dissimilar nature of subsequent energy production disorders.

At the same time, energy metabolism is a key factor determining the formation of genetically consolidated individual resistance of the organism.

Peculiarities of Complex I functioning play a special role in the conditions of adaptation to hypoxia. In the brain of HR rats adapted to hypoxia, Vmax and KM for NADH-cytochrome *c* reductase decreased while in the brain of LR rats these parameters manifold increased and became significantly higher than in the brain of HR rats (Table.2.). Therefore activity of this enzyme increased and its affinity to substrate (NADH) decreased in the brain of LR rats during adaptation [17-19, 37-40, 43]. Physiological relevance of such transformation may be that in hypoxia-adapted LR animals, the enzyme acquires an ability to function within a broader range of substrate concentrations and at higher rates. Since the pool of reduced pyridine nucleotides increases in hypoxia, the appearance of new properties in HADH-cytochrome *c* reductase may provide more efficient work of the enzyme in the conditions of oxygen shortage. This may result in the increased resistance of mitochondria to acute hypoxia in LR rats. Similar though less pronounced changes take place with cytochrome oxidase.

Therefore there are fundamental differences in formation of the response of the respiratory chain substrate region to a single hypoxic exposure and long-term adaptation to hypoxia. In the former instance, suppression of Complex I and compensatory activation of Complex II occur (Fig.10). In the latter instance, recovery of Complex I occurs. This process apparently takes place due to appearance of a new isoform of the enzyme NADH-ubiquinone oxidoreductase with new chemical properties, which provide economizing of energy metabolism in the conditions of steadily decreased oxygen level in the medium as well as diminished role of the succinate oxidase pathway.

The above facts indicate **that the mitochondrial respiratory chain performs as an intracellular oxygen sensor.** In this process, the trigger mechanism participating in this process in Complex I, in particular its major enzyme NADH-ubiquinone oxidoreductase rather than cytochrome oxidase, which comes into contact with oxygen. **NADH-ubiquinone oxidoreductase is responsible also for initiation of urgent compensatory responses of energy metabolism aimed at maintaining the**

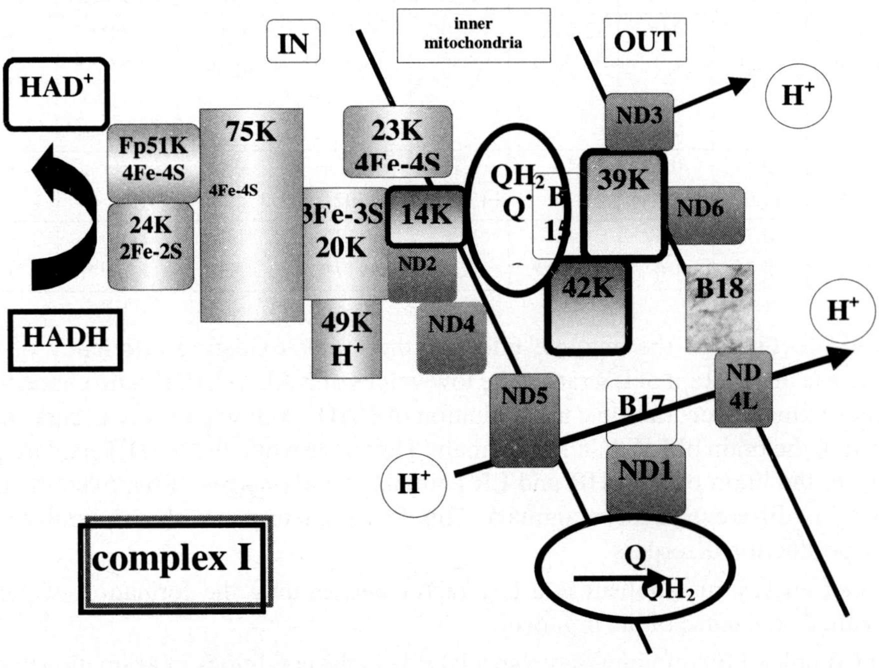

Fig. 10. Complex I of mitochondrial respiratory chain [by 54].
The complex is depicted as an elbow shaped assembly with one arm facing into the matrix and the other arm being associated with inner membrane. The subunits considered to be involved in the transport of electrons are the 51 K flavoprotein containing a 4Fe-4S center, with the 24K, 75 R, 23 K, and 20 K iron sulfur proteins. Two quinone reduction sites are postulated. The mt-DNA-encoded subunits are all part of the membrane arm of the complex and some of them are possibly involved in proton pumping functions.

physiological level of ATP in the cell and for the individual organism sensitivity to oxygen deficiency and formation of adaptive responses under the action of hypoxic factor.

In this connection it is reasonable to dwell on peculiarities of Complex I structure and to discuss what might be the cause of its inactivation.

The mammalian multi-subunit Complex I (NADH-ubiquinone oxidoreductase) serves as a principal entry point of electrons into the enzymic transport chain and to reduce ubiquinone with NADH as the electron donor. This complex appears to contain at least 41 distinct proteins [5.4]. it is not known how many of them are involved in the electron transport coupled to vectorial proton movements. The proteins of Complex I are traditionally divided into flavoprotein, iron protein and hydrophobic protein fractions [11, 24, 54]. Mitochorndria of higher animals haves seven mitochondrially encoded proteins in Complex I that are associated with the inner mitochondrial membrane and constitute a part of hydrophobic protein fractions [46].

Little is known about the physiological regulation of Complex I. Electrons pass through the FMN center located in a 51 kDa protein, then through the 4Fe-4s center the same protein, then through the 2Fe-2S center in a 24 kDa protein, the 4Fe-4S center in a 75 kDa protein and then probably through iron-sulfur centers in 20 kDa and 23 kDa subunits (Fig. 10) [8, 53, 54]. The final electron acceptor is ubiquinone although there is evidence that at least two quinone acceptance loci exist with different sensitivity to quinone analogue inhibitors [20, 58]. The mechanism of reaction, by which electron transfer is coupled to vectorial proton translocation, is not clear [8]. There is evidence that the semiquinone radical is produced within Complex I being its integral subunit [56].

The current prevailing concept is that suppression of Complex I results from redox transformations of iron-containing protein centers in the Complex associated with activation of free radical processes. Two major sources of ROS are under discussion: 1) the respiratory chain itself and 2) various intracellular oxidases and oxygenases. It is known that reactive oxygen species (ROS) are oxygen-containing molecular entities which are more potent and effective oxidizing agents than molecular oxygen itself. Recently ROS have been considered as important intracellular signaling molecules, which may act as mediators or second messengers in many cell functions. It has been known for some time that free radicals, especially the superoxide ion O_2^-, are generated by respiratory chain activity. Indeed, it has been estimated that the fate of 1-4% of all electrons passing down the electron transport chain is to be diverted into the formation of superoxide radicals [8]

Complex I is a major source of ROS in mitochondria. Superoxide itself probably arises from interaction between molecular oxygen and a species of semiquinone (UQ_{10}), which is a natural intermediate in one-electron reduction events during electron transport through Complexes I and III [7]. Little is known about the processes involved in this generation of superoxide, though it is reasonable to guess that it occurs at the juxtaposition of an electron carrier such as at FeS protein and a site of quinone reduction within the respiratory chain complexes [6]. Semiquinone radicals generated in the vicinity of the TYKY 23 kDa Fes protein would be the prime candidates as electron donors for superoxide formation.

Removal of free radicals generated in the course of normal electron transport is obligatory if cellular damage is to be avoided. Superoxide is removed by the enzyme Mn^{2+} superoxide dismutase, which is mitochondrial, and $Cu^{2+}Zn^{2+}$ superoxide dismutase, which is extramitochondrial and also exists in an extracellular form [12, 49]. Both superoxide dismutases produce hydrogen peroxide which, unlike superoxide, is probably diffusible across biological membranes and is reasonably stable. Thus hydrogen peroxide produced both inside and outside the inner mitochondrial membrane can be removed by the activity of either catalase or glutathione peroxidase. Dependence on the latter enzyme may then be linked to the availability of glutathione.

The two compartments are depicted as the inside of the mitochondrial matrix space and the space outside the mitochondrial matrix. When superoxide production exceeds the capacity of MnSOD to remove it, damage to FeS centers may result in release of free iron. More severe damage to DNA, lipids and proteins can occur if hydrogen per oxide is not removed and forms hydroxy1 radicals by the Fenton reaction. Furthermore, hydrogen peroxide is believed to promote channel activity and to stimulate K^+ channels. Evidence exists for the participation of hydrogen peroxide-dependent regulation of prostaglandin production and soluble guanylate cyclase activity resulting from the metabolism of peroxide by cyclooxygenase and catalase, respectively, in pO_2-elicited signaling mechanisms that regulate force generation in vascular wall [60].

At the same time, literature discusses also contribution of other intracellular oxidases containing proteins that have naturally undergone redox transformation during generation of ROS and their subsequent interaction with iron-containing proteins of Complex I. Since $K_M(O_2)$ values for these oxidases are 2 to 4 orders of magnitude higher than for cytochrome oxidase, suppression of their activity can occur even at a relatively modest decrease in surrounding oxygen. In this process, formation and accumulation of oxygen reduction intermeadiates become possible. These intermediates, in their turn, can provide changes in physico-chemical characteristics of membrane lipids, in particular, their microvicosity and density up to alterations of conformational mobility and functional activity of membrane bound proteins, carrier proteins, receptors, enzymes, ion channels, surface charge values, etc.

The following candidates are considered as primary regulators of signal transduction: plasma membrane NAD (P)H oxidase, NADH oxidase of the outer mitochondrial membrane not linked to the respiratory chain, microsomal NAD(P)H oxidase whose activity is controlled by the redox state of cytosolic NAD(P)H, and an number of cytosolic oxidases [2,11,14, 50, 52, 60].

A possible candidate for the role of ROS sources in the cell under hypoxia may also be monoaminoxidase (MAO), an enzyme localized on the outer mitochondrial membrane. It is known that hypoxia alters the substrate specificity of type A MAO; hypoxia decreases MAO activity and affinity to specific substrates. This process is associated with accumulation of serotonin and norepinerphrine, deamination of di- and polyamines, histamine, AMP, aminosugars as structural components of membrane, and discoordination of mediator system performance [22]. These events provide generation of ROS including hydrogen peroxide (H_2O_2), which can interact with iron-containing proteins of Complex I by the above-described mechanism of signal transduction due to relatively modest remoteness of the proteins from the mitochondrial respiratory chain. MAO possesses a low affinity to oxygen; the value of $K_M(O_2)$ for MAO is equal to 5×10^{-3} M, therefore the enzyme has to be inactivated at relatively small decreases in environmental oxygen. This is why signal effects of MAO associated with ROS generation can manifest themselves at relatively small decreases of oxygen tension in the medium.

As mentioned above, free radicals can be generated by the cytosolic enzyme xanthine oxidase, which is actiated by proteolytic conversion of xanthine hydrogenase in the conditions of high reduction in cell. However since one of reaction substrates is represented by the adenine nucleotide product hypoxanthine, the reaction can apparently occur only at very low oxygen tension (terminal stage of hypoxia, the period of energy decompensation).

Appreciating promising studies on relevance of ROS for signal transduction processes, it should be nevertheless recognized that their role as signaling mechanisms can be considered today as proved for only late stages of hypoxia (pre-anoxic period) and postichemic (reperfusion) state. Data on the role of ROS at early stages of hypoxia, when dysfuction of mitochondrial enzymes begins and disbalance of the adenylate pool appears, are completely absent. Taking into account the above evidence that the broad-range decrease in surrounding oxygen more than does not initiate the free-radical activity but, in contrast, inhibits it to the point of pre-anoxic region, when a ROS outburst occurs, the concept of the role of ROS as universal oxygen sensors is hardly acceptable.

A special place among signal transduction processes belongs to nitric oxides, primarily peroxynitrite. It is known that concentration of nitric oxide and peroxynitrite increases in many pathophysiological condition. The recent findings that mitochondria of carotid body contain a specific NO synthase isoform, which produces significant amounts of NO for regulation of their own respiration, suggest that NO may be important for regulation of mitochondrial energy metabolism and oxygen sensing in the carotid body [21, 23]. In this process, NO has a dual effect on carotid chemoreception depending on the oxygen and NO levels. During hypoxia, NO performs predominantly as an inhibitory modulator of carotid chemoreception, while in normoxia NO potentiates chemosensory discharges. The excitatory effect produced by no is likely mediated by an impairment of mitochondrial electron transport and oxidative phosphorylation, which is expected to increase the chemosensory activity [25, 26]. It is also known that NO and peroxynitrite are capable of reversibly and irreversibly raising the cytochrome oxidase KM for oxygen [13].

I would like to dwell on one more question.

It is known that cell response to hypoxia involves oxygen-sensitive control of physiologically important genes. Acute hypoxia stimulates specific gene induction, which enhances oxygen delivery. These genes include erythropoietin, which promotes erythropoiesis and increases red blood cell mass; transferrin, which provides iron transport and sustained erythropoiesis; nitric oxide synthase (inducible and endothelial isoforms), endothelin-1, adrenomedullin, heme oxygenase 1, which facilitates recovery of vascular tone and vasodilation to increase blood supply; vascular endothelial growth factor and placental growth factor, which stimulate angiogenesis and increase the density of vascular network.

Hypoxia-activated genes are controlled by transcription factors, primarily HIF-1. Hypoxia-inducible heterodimeric transcription factor-1 (HIF-1) is considered to be a global regulator of oxygen homeostasis [1, 9, 62] because:

= It is expressed in a wide variety of cells, if not all.

= Functionally critical HIF-1 DNA binding sites (Hypoxia Response Elements) are present in control regions of many hypoxia-regulated genes.

= Hypoxia-inducible genes are expressed in non-epo producing cells.

= HIF – 1 activation of hypoxia-regulated genes shares the properties of epo activation.

= Phosphorylation activates HIF-1

It was established that HIF-1 is involved in the hypoxia-sensitive gene transcription via activation of HIF-1α and HIF-1β expression. However this complicated multi-step process is triggered only at decreases in oxygen to very low values and is evident at least one hour after the exposure. Therefore the immediate cell response to changes in environmental oxygen, which is realized within minutes or even seconds, is controlled by some other mechanism. Taking into account that literature discusses possible role of these proteins as oxygen sensors, it should be apparently suggested that their expression is a trigger mechanism for development of long-term adaptive responses and can underlie formation of new enzyme isoforms with new kinetic properties in the conditions of prolonged application of hypoxia. This would be particularly true for enzymes of the mitochondrial respiratory chain including NADH-ubiquinone oxidoreductase.

Summarizing the above-said we can make the following conclusions.

1. A complexly arranged tissue-specific regulatory system exists, which takes part in oxygen sensing of cell. The trigger mechanism of this sensing apparently involves oxidases, among which mitochondrial NADH-oxidase of the respiratory chain plays the key role.
2. Urgent cell responses to gradual changes in external oxygen concentration are under the control of respiratory chain enzymes. Transformation of these enzymes, primarily of Complex I, forms phase changes in intracellular ATP and other components of the adenylate pool to determine the phase nature of disorders in other functional and metabolic parameters under hypoxia.
3. In gradual changes of oxygen level, mitochondrial dysfunction represents a fundamental molecular mechanism of any type of hypoxia and a typical pathological process incorporated into any pathological process as an obligatory component.
4. ROS are apparently included into the mechanism of signal transduction in acute forms of oxygen insufficiency and participate in formation of long-term adaptation mechanisms. However their role in suppression of mitochondrial enzyme Complex I at slight changes of environmental oxygen concentrations (early stages of hypoxia) remains unclear.
5. Specific hypoxia-induced proteins participate in mechanisms for long-term adaptation of cell function to hypoxia and can apparently provide survival of cell function to withstand anoxia.

References

1. ***Agani F.H., Pichule P., Chavez C., LaManna J.C.*** Inhibitors of mitochondrial complex I attenuate the accumulation of hypoxia-inducible factor-1 during hypoxia in Hep3B cells. Compar. Biochem. Physiol. – Part A. V 132, Issue 1, 2002 p. 107-109.
2. ***Amor Y., Chevion M., Levine A.*** Anoxia pretreatment protects soybean cells against H_2O_2– induced cell death: possible involvement of peroxidases and of alternative oxidase. FEBS Let. 2000. V.477. Issue 3, pp. 175-180.
3. ***Bänder J., Kiesee F.*** Die Wierkung Sauerstoffubertragenden. – Arch. Exp. Und Pathol. Pharm. 1955, Bd.224, S. 312-317.
4. ***Belousova V.V., Dudchenko A.M., Lukyanova L.D.*** Role of glycolysis in maintaining the energy-synthesizing function in hepatocytes from rats adapted and non-adapted thypoxia at different O_2concentrations. Bull. Exp. Biol. Med., 1995, 119: 1: 23-27.
5. ***Beregoskaya N.N.*** In: Bioenergetic damages in pathology and pathways of its correction. 1993, Moscow, pp. 11-20.
6. ***Beyer B.*** An analysis of the role of coenzyme Q in free radical generation and as an oxidant. Biochem. Cell. Biol. 70(1991) 343-390

7. ***Boveris A., B. Chance.*** Mitochondrial production of superoxide radical and hydrogen peroxide. In: M. Revich, R. Coburn, S. Lahiti, B. Chance (Eds), Tissue Hypoxia and Ischemia, Plenum Press, New York, 1977, pp. 67-82.
8. ***Brandt U.*** Proton translocation by membrane-bound NADH-ubiquinone oxidoreductaise (complex I) through redox-gated ligand conduction. Bioch. Biophys. Acta. 1997. v. 1318.pp. 79-91.
9. ***Chandel. N. S., Schumacker P.T.*** Cells depleted of mitochondrial DNA(ρ^0) yield insight into physiological mechanisms. FEBS Lett. 1999, v 454 pp. 173-176.
10. ***Chernobaeva G.N., Belousova V.V., Vlasova I.G., Lukyanova L.D.*** Brain bioenergetic parameters in rats with different resistance to hypoxia. Bull. Exp. Biol. Med., 1993, 115: 3: 251-254.
11. ***Chomyn A., S.D. Patel, M.W.J. Cleeter, C.I. Ragan, G. Attardi.*** – The site of synthesis of the iron-sulfur subunits of the flavoprotein and iron protein factions of human NADH dehydrogenase. – J. Biol. Chem.. 1988, 31, pp. 16395-16400.
12. ***Ciafoloni E., E. Ricci, S. Shanske.*** MELAS: Clinical features, biochemistry and molecular genetics. Ann. Neurol. 31(1992) 391-398.
13. ***Cooper Ch., Davies N.*** Effects of nitric oxidase and peroxynitrite on the cytochrome oxidase Km for oxygen: implications to mitochondrial pathology. BBA – Bioenergetics. V.59. Issue 2-3. 2000. pp 390-396.
14. ***Di Lisa F., Ziegler M.*** Pathophysiological revelance of mitochondria in NAD+ metabolism. FEBS Letters 2001, 492, pp.4-8
15. ***Dudchenko A.M., Belousova V.V., Lukyanova L.D.*** Relationships of energy-consuming and energy-synthesizing reactions in rat hepatocytes at different O_2 concentrations. Bull. Exp.Biol. Med., 1992, 114: 12: 588-590.
16. ***Dudchenko A.M., Belousova V.V., Lukyanova L.D.*** Effect of O_2 concentrations at the ATP level in isolated hepatocytes of adapted and non-adapted to hypoxia rats. Bull. Exp. Biol. Med., 1994, 118: 12: 1268-1272.
17. ***Dudchenko A.M., Belousova V.V., Lukyanova L.D.*** Effects of adaptation to periodic hypoxia on the brain respiratory chain kinetic parameters. Bull. Exp. Biol. Med., 1996, 121: 3: 252-255.
18. ***Dudchenko A.M., Chernobaeva G.N., Belousova V.V., et al.*** Bioenergetic parameters of rat brain with different resistance to hypoxia. Bull. Exp. Biol. Med., 1993, 15: 3: 251-254.
19. ***Dudchenko A.M., Lukyanova L.D.*** Effects of adaptation to periodic hypoxia on the cytochrome content in rat brain and liver. Bull. Exp. Bio. Med., 1996, 121: 3: 232-235.
20. ***Genova M.I., C. Casteluccio, R. Fato, G. Parenti-Castelli, M. Merlo-Pich, G. Formiggini, C. Bovina, M. Marchetti, G. Lenaz.*** Major changes in Complex I activity in mitochondria from aged rats may not be detected by direct assay of NADH-coenzyme Q reductase. Biochem. J. 1995, 311, pp. 105-109.
21. ***Ghafourifar P., Richter C.*** Nitric oxide synthase activity in mitochondria. FEBS letters 1997.-418: 291-296;
22. ***Goroshinskaya I.A., Neskubina I.V.*** Monoamine content in hypobaric hypoxia and the protective effect of pyrazidol. Voprosy Med. Khimii. 1999, No. 5, pp.432-439 (in Russian)
23. ***Guilivi C.*** Functional implications of nitric oxide produced by mitochondria in mitochondrial metabolism. Biochem. J. 1998, 332: 673-679).
24. ***Hatefi Y.*** The mitochondrial electron transport and oxidative phosphorylation system. Ann. Rev. Bioch.-1985.-34, pp. 1015-1027.
25. ***Henrich M., Hoffmann K., König P., at all.*** Sensory neurons respond to hypoxia with NO production associated with mitochondria. Mol Cell Neurosci. 2002. V. 20. Issue 2. pp. 307-322.
26. ***Iturriaga R., Villanueva S., Mosqueria M*** – Dual effects of nitric oxide on carotid body chemoreception.- J. Appl Physiol 2000, 89: 1005-1012.).
27. ***Kondrashova M.N. Doliba N.M.*** Polarographic observation of substrate-level phosphorylation and its stimulation by acetylcholine. FEBS Lett. 1989, 243, 153-155.

28. ***Kondrashova M.N.*** The formation and utilization of succinate in mitochondria as a control mechanism of energization and energy state of tissue. In: Chance B. (Ed.). Biological and Biochemical Oscillators, Academic Press. New York, NY, pp373-397.
29. ***Kondrashova M.N.*** The interaction of transmination and oxidation of carboxylic acids in different functional states of tissues. Biokhimiya 1991, 56, 243-310.
30. ***Kondrashova M.N.*** Succinate in medicine. Ed. Kondrashova M.N. Pushchino, Nauka, 1996, 300 P.
31. ***Kunz W.S. Kudin A.P., Vielhaber S., Blumke I., and all.*** Mithocondrial complex I deficiency in epileptic focus of patients with temporal lode epilepsy. 2000, Ann. Neurol, 48, 766-773
32. ***Lukyanova L.D.*** About regulatory mechanisms of tissue respiratory kinetics under the different conditions of hypoxia. In: 3d All-Union Conference on Adaptation. Moscow. 1982, pp. 133-135
33. ***Lukyanova L.D.*** Limiting steps of energy metabolism in brain in hypoxia. Neurochem. Intern., 1988, 13: S.I: 146.
34. ***Lukyanova L.D.*** Bioenergetic mechanisms of hypoxic states and principles of pharmacological correction. In: Pharmacological Correction of Hypoxic States. Lukyanova L.D. (ed.), Moscow, 1989, p.11-44.
35. ***Lukyanova L.D.*** Pharmacological aspects of cell bioenergetics in hypoxia. In: Cell Mechansims in Pharmacological Effects Realization. Seredenin S.B. (ed)., Moscow, 1990, p. 184-216.
36. ***Lukyanova L.D.*** Bioenergetic mechanisms of hypoxic state development and strategies for its pharmacological correction. In: Antihypoxants. Lukyanova L.D. (ed)., Moscow, 1991, pp. 5-35
37. ***Lukyanova L.D.*** Bioenergetic mechanisms of the cells adaptation to hypoxia and individual resistance of the organism. Proc. Int. Soc. Pathophysiol., Moscow, 1991, p. 249.
38. ***Lukyanova L.D.*** Molecular, metabolic and functional mechanisms of individual resistance to hypoxia. In: Adaptation Biology and Medicine, Sharma B.K., Takeda N., et al. (eds)., Narosa Publishing House New Dehli, India. 1997, V.I, P. 261-272.
39. ***Lukyanova L.*** Bioenergetic hypoxia: Definition, Mechanisms, and Methods of Correction. Bull. Exp. Biol. Med., 1997, 124: 9: 244-254.
40. ***Lukyanova L.D.*** Dysregulation of energy metabolism is a typical pathological process. – In: Dysregulation of Processes in Pathologies, Moscow, 2002, pp. 188-215
41. ***Lukyanova L.D.***Cellular mechanism responsible for beneficial effects of hypoxic therapy. In: Adaptation Biology and Medicine, Moravec, et al. (eds), , Narosa Publishing House New Dehli,. India. 2002, v.3, pp. 290-303.
42. ***Lukyanova L.D.*** Actual problems and perspectives of hypoxic states pharmacological correction. Current problems and prospects in pharmacological correction of hypoxic states.- In: Pharmacotherapy in Neurology and Psychiatry. Lectures for Practitioners at the8th Congress "Man and Drug", Moscow, 2002, p. 22-34.
43. ***Lukyanova L.D., Dudchenko A.M.*** Regulatory role of the adenylate pool in the formation of hepatocyte resistance to hypoxia. In: Adaptation Biology and Medicine, K.B. Pandolf, N. Takeda, P.K. Singal (eds.) 1999, Narosa Publishing House New Dehli, India. pp. 139-150.
44. ***Lukyanova L.D., Balmuchanov B.C., Ugolev A.T*** Oxygen-dependent processes in the cell and its function. Moscow.- Nauka.- 1982.-256 P.
45. ***Maklashinas E, Sher E., Zhou H-Z., Gray M. and all.*** Effect of anoxia/reperfusion on the reversible active/ de-active transition of comlexI in rat hear. BBA – Bioenergetics 2002, v. 1556, Issue 1pp. 6-12.
46. ***Mariottini P., A. Chomyn, M. Riley, B. Cotrell, R.F. Doolittle, G. Attardi. –*** Identification of the polypeptides encoded in the unassigned reading frames 2, 4, 41 and 5 of human mitochondrial DNA. – Proc. Natl. Acad. Sci U.S.A 83 (1986) 1563-1567.
47. ***Maevsky E.I., Rosenfeld A.C., Grishina E.V.,Kondrashova M.N. -*** Correction of metabolic acidosis by maintaining the mitochondrial function. – Pushchino. – 2001.- 155 P. (in Russian)
48. ***Mela L., Goodwin C.W., Miller L.D.*** In vivo control of mitochondrial enzyme concentrations and activity by oxygen. AM. J. Physiol., 1976, 231: 1811-1816.

49. ***Pitkanen S., B.H. Robinson,*** Mitochondrial complex I deficiency leads to increased production of superoxide radicals and induction of superoxide dismutase. J. Clin. Inves. 1996, 98, pp. 345-351.

50. ***Peers Ch., Kemp P.J.*** Acute oxygen sensingt: diverse but convergent mechanisms in airway and arterial chemoreceptors. Respiratory Research. 2001.V. 2(3), pp. 145-149.

51. ***Pitkänen S., Merante F., McLeod D.R., B.H. Robinson,*** Familial cardiomypathy with cataracts and lactic acidosis: A defect in complexes I of the mitochondrial respiratory chain. Pediatr. Res. 1996, 39, pp. 513-521

52. ***Porwol T., Eheleben W., Brand V., Acker H.*** Tissue oxygen sensor function of NADPH oxidase isoforms, an unusiual cytochrome aa_3 and reactive oxygen species. Respiration Physiology, 2001, V 128, Issue 3, pp. 331-348.

53. ***B.H. Robinson***. Lacticacidemia. Bioch. Biophys. Acta. 1994, 1182, pp.237-244.

54. ***B.H. Robinson***. Human Complex I deficiency: Clinical spectrum and involvement of oxygen free radicals in the pathogenicity of the defect. Bioch. Biophys. Acta. 1998, 1364, pp. 271-286.

55. ***Roulsin W., millard R.W.*** Canine myocardial ischemia: defect in mitochondrial electron transfer complex I.J. Mol. Cell. Cardiol. 1980, 12: 639-645.

56. ***Sardanelli A.M., Papa S et al.*** Phosphorylation of an 18 kDa subunit of bovine Heart Complex I by camp dependent kinase FEBS letters 1996, 379, pp. 299-301.

57. ***Tang P.S.*** – by Petersen C.L. at al. –The effect of energization of the apparent Michaelis-Menten constant for oxygen in mitochondrial respiration. –Biochem. J. –1974,- v. 142, PP. 247-252.

58. ***Ueno H., H. Mioshi, K. Ebusui, H. Iwamura.*** Comparison of the inhibitory action of natural rotenone and its stereoisomers with varius NADH- ubiquinone reductases. Eur. J. Biochem. 255 (1994) 411-417.92.

59. ***Warburg O.*** Uber Eisen den sauertoffubertragenden Bestandteil des Atmungsfermentes. – Biochem. Ztshcr. 1924, Bd. 152, S. 479-494.

60. ***Wolin M.S., Th. M. Burke-Wolin, K.M. Mohazzab-H.*** Role for NAD(P)H oxidases and reactive oxygen species in vascular oxygen sensing mechanisms. Respiration Physiology. V.115, Issue 2 (1999) 229-238.

61. ***Veitch K., Hombroeck A., Caucheteux D. et al.*** Global ischemia induces a biphasic response of the mitochondrial respiratory chain. Biochem. J. 1992, 281: 709-715.

62. ***Zhu H., Bunn F.*** Oxygen sensing and signaling: impact on regulation of physiologically important genes. Respiration Physiology V. 115, Issue 2 (1999) 239-247.

Adaptation Biology and Medicine (Volume 4: Current Concepts)
Editors: A. Hargens, N. Takeda and P.K. Singal

2. Responses of the Inbred FOK Rat to Ambient Heat and Cold—In pursuit of Common Mechanisms to Endure Various Stresses

Fijiya Furuyama[1], Akihiro Kuroshima[2], Takehiro Yahata[3], Osamu Shido[4], and Hitoo Nishino[1].

[1]Dept. Neurophysiol. Brain Sci., Nagoya City Univ. Grad. Sch. Med. Sci., Nagoya 467-8601, Japan; [2]Dept. Physiol., Asahikawa Med. Col., Asahikawa 078-8510, Japan; [3]Dept. Nurs., Nayoro City Col., Nayoro 096-8641, Japan; [4]Dept. Physiol., Shimane Med. Univ., Izumo 689-8501, Japan;

Introduction

Severe environmental stressors such as heat, cold or hypoxic environment induces physiological stress such as hyperthermia, hypothermia or hypoxic hypoxia in the body. An adaptive change is likely able to increase resistance to the stressor, expand areas to live comfortably, and build up health. For example, rats exposed to a moderate heat for several weeks tolerated extreme heat longer than controls (5). Two categories of adaptations are recognized: phenotypic and genotypic adaptation. Phenotypic adaptation occurs within a lifetime. Genotypic adaptation, based on gene selection over many generations, is inherited by descendants in a fixed manner when survival favors this trait under certain environment. It is a further issue whether an adaptive change to a stressor increases power of resistance to other stressor. If power of resistance to other stressor was increased, it would be suggested that common mechanisms underlay for resisting to different stressors. We had special concern with the genotypic adaptation to severe hot environment. We selected rats for generations by a standard ambient heat, and developed an inbred FOK rat (FF93) as a model with genotypic heat adaptation. Genes responsible for resistance to heat stress had widely scattered throughout the species. Considerable sum of them were collected in the genome of the FOK rats by us. General mechanisms for resistance to high temperature in the species can be studied using the FOK rat, because they were selected by phenotype.

In the present paper, we report the strategy and mechanisms of thermoregulation for enduring heat, and whether heat-selection for generations also promoted cold resistance.

Heat Resistance of the Heat-Resistant Rats

The FOK rat is the most resistant to heat among 18 existing strains which were examined by us (3). Sample tracings of the core temperature (T_c) responses to prolonged exposure to an ambient temperature (T_a) of 42.5°C (a standard heat stress protocol) are shown in Fig. 1. The order of heat

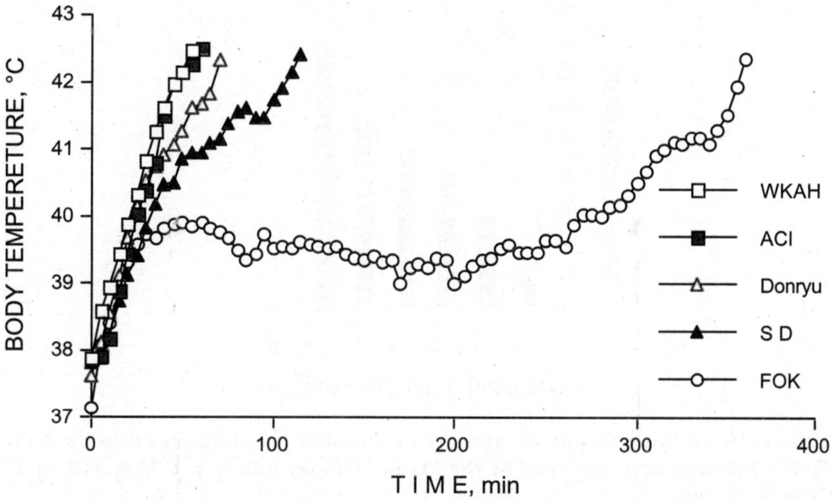

Fig. 1. Sample tracings of the T_c responses to ambient heat. One rat from each strain was exposed to a T_a (42.5°C). T_c was monitored using a telemetric system. Exposure was stopped when core temperature arrived at 42.5°C.

endurance times at this temperature was FOK >> SD > Donryu = ACI=WKAH. The sample data is coincident with the early reports (3).

Inheritance mode of heat resistance

In order to clarify how many genes contribute to heat resistance, the FOK rat was backcrossed to the Long-Evans rat which is heat-sensitive. Rats were exposed to a T_a of 42.5°C, and heat endurance time of each rat was determined. In F2 rats, the values of heat endurance time scattered in a wider range than those in F1rats. Thus, it was shown that inheritance mode of heat resistance. is polygenic inheritance.

Strategy of thermoregulation for enduring heat

The time course of T_c in response to ambient heat is a good indicator of thermoregulatory ability. In most rats, T_c continuously increases up to a final temperature, or increases with an initial convex-shaped rise followed by final rise at a standard T_a (42.5?). Somewhat heat-resistant rats respond with a triphasic pattern composed of a rapid rise of T_c followed by steady-state hyperthermia and then a further rise (3). The SD rat is one of the most heat tolerant among existent strains (3). The steady-state hyperthermic level in SD rats varies in response to ambient heat (4). It is an important issue how is the strategy of thermoregulation for enduring heat in FOK rats.

T_c of the FOK rats possesses the steady-state hyperthermia which lasts for several hours at T_as between 35.0 – 45.0°C, whereas the T_c increased rapidly in ACI rats (Fig. 2). Plateau T_c of FOK rats was constant (39.5 ± 0.7°C) for several hours over the T_a range from 37.5 to 42.5°C ($p < 0.0001$). It should be noted that the T_a. was higher than the plateau T_cs at T_a higher than 40.0°C. Evaporation is only one pathway for heat dissipation at a T_a higher than body temperature, and also a powerful pathway for heat dissipation (572.8 cal/ 1.0 g water, 43.2kJ/ mol, at 40°C).

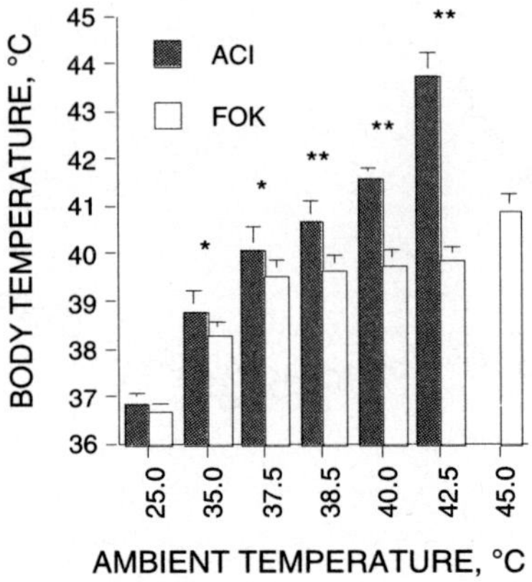

Fig. 2. T_c in ACI and FOK rats after 60 min of exposure to various T_as. Values are mean ± s.d. (N = 7). Differences T_c between the 2 strains were analyzed by the Mann-Whitney test. *: $p < 0.05$, ACI vs. FOK rats; **: $p < 0.005$, ACI vs. FOK rats.

Two general categories of adaptation have been recognized: capacity adaptation and resistance adaptation (9). Capacity adaptation allows animals to maintain their internal parameters within a normal range when exposed to varying external conditions. Resistance adaptations are those that permit a shift of internal functions (for example, the Tc), and expand the environment that can be survived. The strategy of FOK rats was to shift T_c from the normal T_c (near 37°C) to the hyperthermic level of 39.5 ± 0.7°. Thus, the strategy of rats is a case of resistance adaptation. This strategy of FOK rats is beneficial to health in two respects. *First*, the FOK rats can escape cell death caused by the multisystem disorders as a result of heatstroke, because their steady-state hyperthermic level (39.5 ± 0.7°C) is approximately 3°C lower than the upper limit (43.1-43.3°C) for stroke (3). Severe hyperthermia results in disseminated intravascular coagulation and excess of inflammatory responses (1). Hyperthermia increases blood-brain permeability, brain water content and the glial fibrillary acidic protein level in rats, and by decreases in mean arterial pressure, cerebral blood flow and myelin basic protein (10). *Second*, serious cellular disorder by aggravation of dehydration/ hyperosmolality, is delayed in FOK rats. Dehydration results from long-term evaporative cooling (5). Serious dehydration/ hyperosmolality also attenuates evaporative heat loss and the firing rate of the warm-neurons in the median preoptic nucleus (7), and therefore cause further worsening of hyperthermia. The regulated plateau (39.5 ± 07°C) is 2 – 3°C higher than the normal T_c (near 37°C) in FOK rats. Although species with sufficient sweating reduces the T_c to normal level (near 37°C), FOK rats do not. Thus, FOK rats are able to retain body fluid which would be lost if the T_c were depressed to 37.0°C.

Pathway for thermal salivation and regulation mode

Saliva spreading is crucial for expression of the steady-state hyperthermia. FOK rats spread their saliva over the entire ventral surface (3). The extent of body fluid evaporated by FOK rats amounted to approximately 14% of body weight within 5 – 6 hours at a T_a of 42.5°C (3). Which efferent pathway does control the thermal salivation? Ligation of the submandibular gland ducts abolished the heat-induced salivation of the FOK rats, whereas ligation of the parotid duct had no effect. These findings indicate that the pronounced thermal salivation is controlled by the preoptic nucleus in hypothalamus -

superior salivatory nucleus in medulla oblongata - chorda tympanyi - submandibular gland pathway, not *via* inferior salivatory nucleus..

The relationship between the saliva secretion rate and the T_c differed among the rat strains (repeated measures ANOVA: $p < 0.0001$) (Fig. 3). The saliva secretion rates in Donryu and SD rats did not increase proportionally with T_c. Conversely, the saliva secretion rates of the FOK rats increased proportionally with T_c [39.0 – 42.0°C (rho = 0.883, $p < 0.0001$)]. The increase in the salivation rate per °C was 16.21 ± 3.01 mg/100 g body weight/min in FOK rats, but only 7.64 ± 1.14 mg/100 g body weight/min in ACI rats. Thus, regulation mode of thermal salivation in FOK rats is a type of negative feedback regulation.

Role of central nervous system in the evaporative cooling

It is the next issue which plays the dominant role in potentate thermal salivation, central event or glandular event. Submandibular glands of FOK rats significantly differed from those of other rat strains. The submandibular, sublingual and lachrymal glands in the FOK rats were 1.3 - 1.5, 1.25 - 1.4 and 1.3 - 1.5 times heavier, respectively, than those in the other 3 strains, whereas the parotid gland of the FOK rats was not enlarged. Large amount of cromogranin A was released form submandibular gland of FOK rats (4). Cromogranin A stores a large number of Calcium and a part of IP3 receptor. To examine this issue, submandibular glands of the 4 strains were perfused *in vitro* by 0.5μM Ach (Table 1) (4). Salivation rates *in vitro* in the 3 control strains were high as same as those in FOK rats (Table 1). The secretion rate corresponded to those in FOK rats *in vivo* with a T_c of 40.0-41.0°C. These evidences showed that parasympathetic efferent signal from the thermoregulation center in the central nervous system plays an main role in the evaporative-cooling regulation, whereas significant changes were observed in salivary glands.

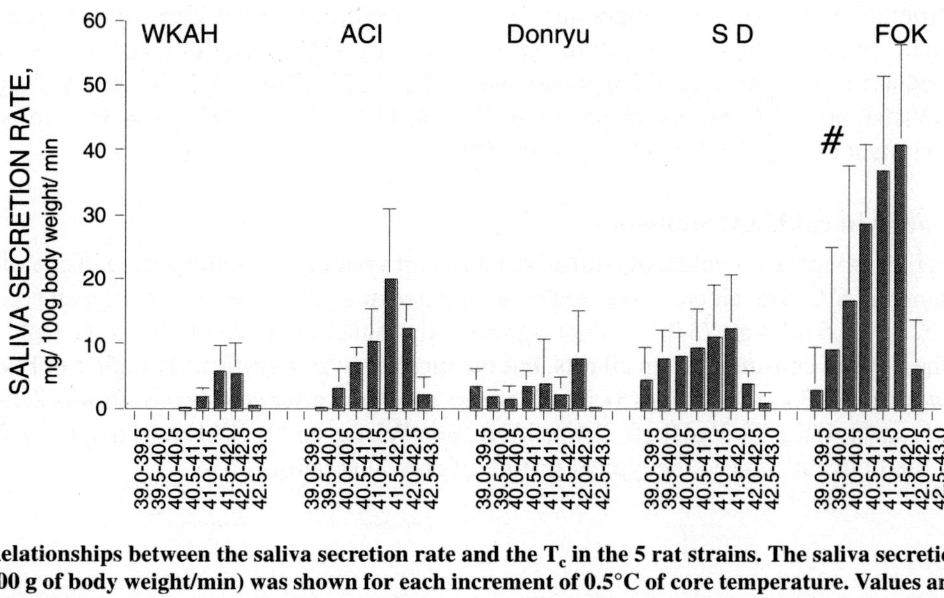

Fig. 3. Relationships between the saliva secretion rate and the T_c in the 5 rat strains. The saliva secretion rate (mg/100 g of body weight/min) was shown for each increment of 0.5°C of core temperature. Values are the means ± s. d. (N =6). #: The slope of salivation rate over T_c was significantly steeper in FOK rats than those in other strains ($p < 0.001$)(Spearman Rank correlation test).

Table 1. Strain difference in saliva secretion rate *in vitro*

	Saliva secretion rate	
Strain	mg/ g gland/ min	mg/ 100g bw/ min
ACI	116.34 ± 45.45	16.64 ± 6.60
Donryu	97.26 ± 38.16	15.96 ± 6.71
S D	119.81 ± 43.51	15.06 ± 5.41
FOK	93.04 ± 31.50	16.52 ± 5.87

Values are means and s. d. Submandibular glands were perfused by 0.5μM Ach, at 37°C. Statistically significant difference was not observed among rat strains.

Properties in Thermoneutral Zone

O_2 consumption (W/m^2 and W/kg) *in vivo* at the thermoneutral zone did not changed through heat selection for generations (11). Skin temperature also did not changed. The resting T_c of the FOK rats was significantly lower ($P < 0.05$) than those of the other rat strains, but the difference was only within 0.5°C (11, 12). These evidence suggests that whole -body metabolism and thrmoregulation in thermoneutral zone do not largely changed by heat selection for generations. Main changes resulted from heat selection for generations are supposed to be expressed in response to stressors.

Cold Resisce of the Genetically Heat-Resistant Rats

Cold resistance

It is a question whether the heat-tolerant FOK rats are resistant to cold stressor. The required capacities for cold resistance and for heat resistance are opposite, and it is thus probable that there exists a negative cross-adaptation between heat and cold tolerance (2, 6). Cold resistance of the rats was evaluated from the fall of colonic temperature under acute cold exposure. Overnight-fasted rats were sheared of hair, and the colonic temperature was measured by a thermistor during exposure to 0°C for 3 h. The decrease in T_c after 3 h cold exposure was 1.5 ± 0.17°C, 5.4 ± 0. 51°C, and 6.3 ± 0.33°C in FOK, Slc: Wistar, and WKAH rats, respectively (Fig. 4) (12). Thus, FOK rats were surprisingly the most cold-resistant among the 3 rat strains ($P < 0.001$).

Thermogenesis in cold environments

O_2 consumption *in vivo* was evaluated with an open circuit system. The temperature inside of chamber was maintained at 5°C. The air was analyzed by an oxygen analyzer. The resting oxygen consumption of FOK (1,021 ± 27.5 ml / kg0.75 / h) was not significantly higher than that of other rats. Cold exposure increased the oxygen consumption in all rats, but the increase was significantly higher in FOK than in the other two strains ($P < 0.001$) (Fig. 5). The increase at 30 min after cold exposure was 2,225 ± 51.7, 1,713 ± 52.1, and 1,485 ± 79.3 ml/kg0.75/h in FOK, Slc: Wistar, and WKAH rats, respectively (Fig. 5) (12). Thus, the FOK rat showed the typical feature of cold adaptation.

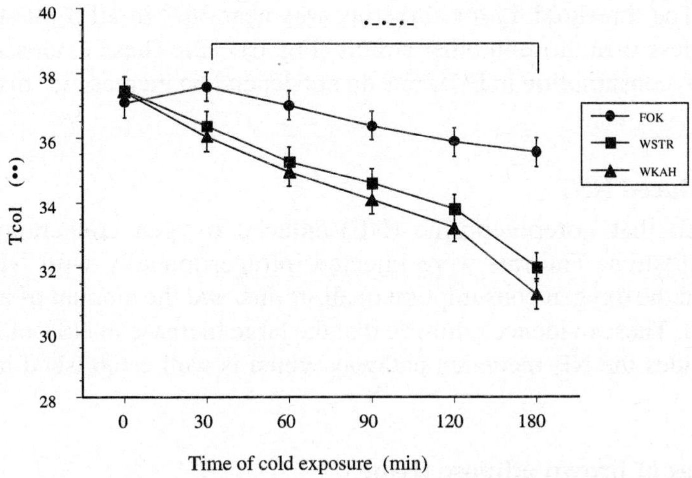

Fig. 4. Changes in colonic temperature (Tcol) of conscious rats exposed to 0°C. Data are means ± s. d. Tcol: colonic temperature. *: Tc of FOK rats significantly different from those of WSTR and WKAH, P < 0.001.**

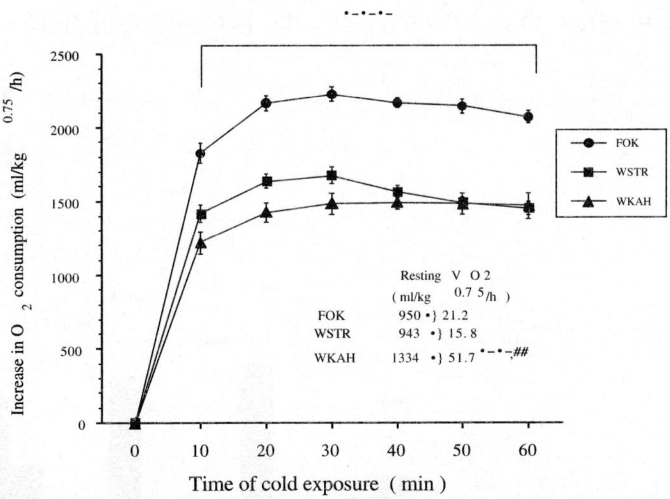

Fig. 5. Changes in oxygen consumption of conscious rats during cold exposure (5?C). ●: FOK, ■: WSTR, ▲: WKAH. Number of rats in each group was 5. ***Significantly different from WSTR and WKAH, p < 0.001. Resting VO2 was described in the figure. **Significantly different from FOK, P < 0.01. ##Significantly different from WSTR, P < 0.01.

Shivering thermogenesis

It is well established that cold-induced thermogenesis is based on shivering thermogenesis and non-shivering thermogenesis (NST). Shivering thermogenesis in FOK rats was compared with those in control rat strains (Fig. 6). Shivering activity was assessed by the amplitude of the electromyogram in urethane-anesthetized animals (1g/kg bw, ip) at 5°C for 90 min. During cold exposure, the final T_c of FOK (33.3 ± 0.21°C) was again higher than in Slc: Wistar (29.3 ± 0.20°C) and WKAH rats (30.2 ±

0.34°C) ($P < 0.01$). The threshold T_c for shivering was near 35.7 in all 3 rat strains. The shivering activity in FOK was less than those in other strains (Fig. 6) (12). These evidences showed that cold-induced increase in O_2 consumption in FOK rats do not depend on increase in shivering thermogenesis but NST.

Norepinephrine-induced NST

It is well established that norepinephrine (NE)-induced oxygen consumption is increased by phenotypic cold adaptation. The rats were injected intraperitoneally with NE (0.75 mg/kg body weight). NE increased the oxygen consumption in all strains, and the amount of increase did not differ among rat strains (12). These evidences showed that the large increase in NST of FOK rats depends on unknown factors besides the NE-mediated pathway which is well established in case of phenotypic cold adaptation.

Thermogenic indices of brown adipose tissue

Brown adipose tissue (BAT) composition was determined. DNA content measured fluorometrically was 50% higher in FOK rats than in other strains ($P < 0.05$), suggesting increase in cell number. Percentage of fat-free dry matter ($P < 0.01$) as well as the protein content ($P < 0.001$) of BAT in FOK was larger than those in other strains. Conversely, the percentage of lipid was lower in FOK as

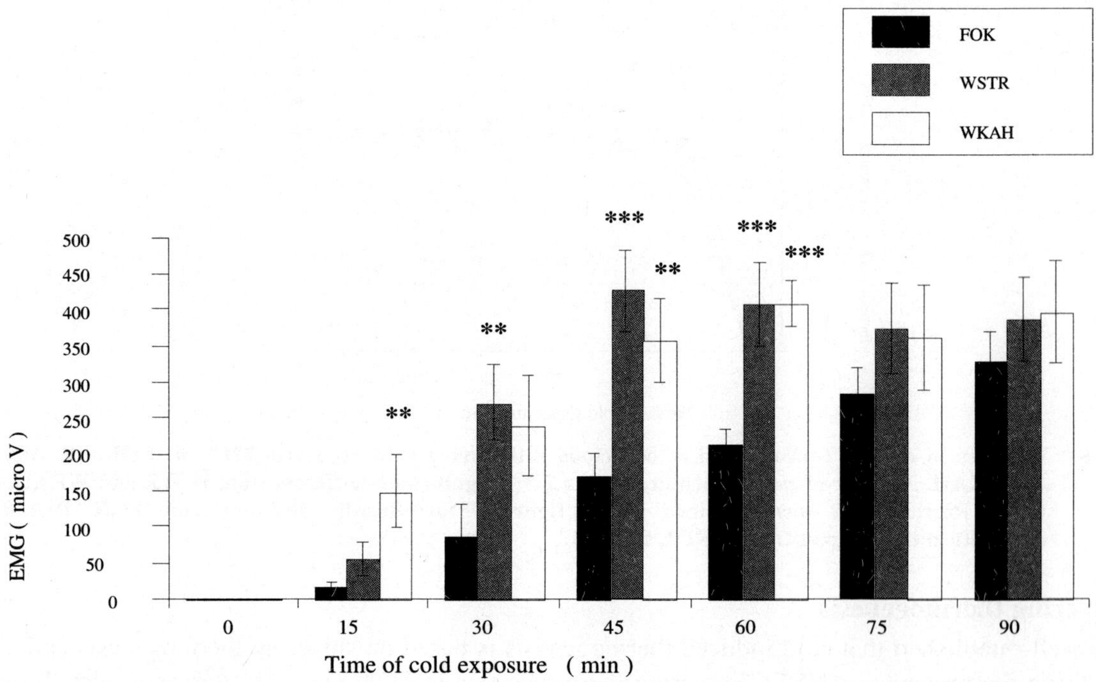

Fig. 6. Changes in amplitude of EMG as an index of shivering activity in urethane-anesthetized animals during cold exposure (5°C). Data are means ± s.d. ** and*: significantly different from FOK rats, P, 0.01 and 0.001, respectively.**

compared with that of other strains (P < 0.001), and there was no difference among the strains in the content of mitochondrial UCP1 of BAT (Table 2). It should be noted that polyunsaturated fatty acids in phospholipid fraction in BAT were higher in FOK rats than those in other rat strains (8), suggesting coincidence with phenotypic cold adaptation.

Plasma lipid profile

Overnight-fasted rats were sheared of hair and exposed to 0°C for 60 min, then blood was collected. Glycerol and free fatty acid levels were measured with F-kit glycerol, Boehringer Mannhaeim Co. Inc. and NEFA C-test Wako, respectively. The plasma levels of glycerol and free fatty acid did not differ among the rat strains at a T_a of 25°C. Although cold exposure increased markedly the plasma glycerol and free fatty acid levels (P < 0.01) in all strains, the both levels were higher in FOK than those in the other groups (P < 0.05).

Conclusion

Genes responsible for heat resistance scatters throughout the species, rats. These genes were collected by us in the genome of the FOK rat through heat selection and inbreeding. FOK rats resists heat using a negative feedback regulation for potentate evaporative heat loss. Thermoregulation center was shown to be the main site of the strain difference. The FOK rat surprisingly had became cold resistant as a result of heat selection for generations, suggesting cross-adaptation. The cold resistance depended on NST which is not mediated by increased effects of NE as the typical cold adaptation. BAT of these rats contains larger amount of polyunsaturated fatty acids. In perspectives, the FOK rat is an genetic model for enduring mechanism for many types of stresses.

References

1. Bouch AB, and Knochel JP. Heat Stroke. *N Eng J Med* 346:1978-1988, 2002
2. Fleischner JR and Sergent F. Effects of heat and cold on the albino rat: crossed resistance or crossed sensitization? J. Appl. Physiol. 114: 789-797, 1959.
3. Furuyama F and Ohara K. Genetic development of an inbred rat strain with increased resistance adaptation to a hot environment. Am J Physiol Regulatory Integrative Comp Physiol 265: R957-R962; 1993.
4. Furuyama F *et al*. Regulation mode of evaporative cooling underlying a strategy of the heat-tolerant FOK rat for enduring ambient heat. Articles in PresS. Am J Physiol Regul Integr Comp Physiol (September 11, 2003). 10.1152/ajpregu.00198.2003 (In Press).
5. Horowitz M *et al.* Heat acclimation and hypohydration: involvement of central angiotensin?receptors in thermoregulation. *Am J Physiol Regulatory Integrative Comp Physiol* 277: R47 R55, 1999.
6. Kuroshima A. *et al.* Thermal and metabolic responses of temperature-acclimated rats during cold and heat exposures. Jpn. J. Physiol. 32: 561-571, 1982.
7. Nakashima T *et al.* Osmosensitivity of preoptic thermosensitive neurons in hypothalamic slices in vitro. *Pfluger Archiv* 405: 112-117, 1985.
8. Ohno T *et al.* Fatty acid composition of brown adipose tissue in genetically heat-tolerant FOK rats. *Int. J. Biometeorol.* 45: 41-44, 2001.
9. Prosser CL. Theory of adaptation. In: Biological adaptation. edited by G. Hildebrandt and H. Hensel. Stuttgart: Georg Thieme Verlag, 1982, p. 2-22.

10. Sharma HS *et al.* Pathophysiology of brain edema and cell changes following hyperthermic brain injury. In: *Progress in Brain research. Vol. 115, Brain Function in Hot Environment*, edited by Sharma HS, and Westman J. Elsevier Science B. V., Amsterdam, 1998, p. 351-412.
11. Shido O *et al.* Thermoeffector thresholds and preferred ambient temperatures of the FOK rat. Am J Physiol Regulatory Integrative Comp Physiol 274: R604 - R609, 1998.
12. Yahata T *et al.* Thermoregulatory responses of the inbred heat-tolerant. FOK rat to cold. *Am J Physiol Regulat Integrat Comp Physiol* 277: R362 - RR367, 1999.

Adaptation Biology and Medicine (Volume 4: Current Concepts)
Editors: A. Hargens, N. Takeda and P.K. Singal

3. Distinction Between Stress Resistance and Protective Effects of Adaptation in Rats of Different Genetic Strains: Role of Regulatory Systems

Maya G. Pshennikova*, Igor Yu. Malyshev, Eugenia B. Manukhina, Felix Z. Meerson

Institute of General Pathology and Pathophysiology,
Baltijskaya 8, Moscow 125315, Russia

Abstract

Review substantiates a notion, according to which the resistance to stress damage is predetermined by inherited peculiarities of regulatory stress-limiting systems restricting the stress response and its detrimental effects. Inherited or acquired higher resistance to stress damage is related to a considerable degree with the higher inherited activity of stress-limiting systems as compared to the activity of these systems in animals with lower inherited resistance to stress damage. In the process of prolonged or repeated stress impacts, the initially high efficiency of stress-limiting systems seems to become "exhausted" and cannot ensure the protective restriction of the stress response; in result the resistance to stress decreases. At the same time, the initially lower efficiency of stress-limiting systems can be increased by the process of adaptation to provide protection against stress damage; in result the resistance to stress increases.

Introduction

At present, it is above doubt that adaptation to hypoxic hypoxia, exercise, mild stress exposures and other environmental factors is an efficient means for enhancement of organism resistance to various detrimental impacts. At the same time, it is known that adaptation is not efficient always and for everybody, i.e., repeated exposures to a factor not always increase the resistance to damage. However

* Address for correspondence:
Pshennikova M.G., PhD, Sci., Prof.
Institute of General Pathology and Pathophysiology
Baltijskaya 8, Moscow 125315
Russia
Tel: +7(095)1554744; +7(095)1554748
Fax: +7(095)1511756
E-mail: manukh@orc.ru for M.G.Pshennikova

studies devoted to this phenomenon are almost absent up to the present, though urgency and prognostic value of such studies are obvious. Long-standing studies of our laboratory have demonstrated that the key role in development of adaptive defense belongs to the system responsible for stress reaction including both the stress system and systems restricting the stress reaction, i.e., stress-limiting systems (Fig.1).

The stress system includes the hypothalamo-pituitary-adrenal complex and the sympathetic nervous system with major mediators of the latter, catecholamines and corticosteroids providing the stress reaction [1, 2, 3]. Central stress-limiting systems include the GABAergic, opioidergic and dopaminergic systems, the serotonin system, nitric oxide (NO) system and other systems of brain. These systems restrict activation of the stress system and the stress response at the central level. Local stress-limiting systems include the systems of prostaglandins, adenosine, NO, antioxidants, stress proteins HSP70, etc. These systems restrict the stress response at the level of organs and cells [3 -8].

In this connection, it is natural to believe that resistance to the stress exposure and damage is directly related with the genetically or phenotypically predetermined level of stress-limiting system efficiency and with the balance of stress system and stress-limiting system activities, whereas adaptive defense depends on the effect of adaptation on the efficiency of stress-limiting systems.

This review summarizes the results obtained in studying the role of genetically predetermined, that is, inherited peculiarities of the stress system and stress-limiting systems in the mechanism of resistance to acute stress damage and ability for adaptation to environmental factors with formation of protective mechanisms.

1. Inherited Resistance to Acute Emotional Stress in August and Wistar Rats

There is abundant data, which indicate a considerable contribution of genotype to the nature of organism response to stressors. A striking example is results of studying behavior of offsprings from complete diallel crossing of inbred mouse strains in the conditions of emotional stress. It was shown that the gene pool of BALB/c and C3H/He strains contains genes of additive action responsible for the intense stress response while the gene pool of C57BL/6 and AKR/J strains contains gene of reverse action. In other words, genotype of the former two strains predetermines a higher vulnerability to stress of the strains while the genotype of the latter pair of strains predetermines relative stress resistance [9]. In studies using the open field test it was demonstrated [10] that BALB/c mice were less resistant to emotional stress and displayed the passive stress response of dying down and signs of fear, whereas C57BL/6 mice were characterized by the active stress reaction and higher resistance to emotional stressor.

Dissimilar resistance to stress impacts was demonstrated for rats of two different genetic strains, August and Wistar. In this process, August rats were more resistant than Wistar rats [13 -16] to stomach injuries induced by acute emotional stressor and to acute myocardial ischemia which is known to be associated with the arrhythmogenis stress reaction [11, 12]. In addition the open field test showed that August rats were more resistant than Wistar rats to disorders of behavior induced by acute emotional stress [15]. Furthermore the intensity of stress reaction evaluated by catecholamine and corticosterone release to blood was also lower in August than in Wistar rats [17-19]. However, in contrast, Wistar rats appeared more resistant than August rats to long-term (up to 30 hours) restraint stress [20] and severe heat stress [21] as evaluated by criteria of acute hypotension and death rate.

What are the mechanisms of these genetically predetermined differences in stress resistance? This question remains unanswered as yet. Therefore based on the above-set notions of the role of regulatory systems in stress resistance, we compared in this review the data on basal and stress-stimulated activity of stress systems and stress-limiting systems, and resistance to stress damage in rats of these two strains.

It appeared that both basal and stress-induced levels of the stress system mediators catecholamines in blood and adrenal glands [17, 22] and corticosteroids in blood [18, 19] was higher in August than in Wistar rats (Fig. 2). However the stress-induced activation of the stress system and therefore the stress response were considerably less pronounced in August than in Wistar rats. This difference was evident as a lower stress-induced increase in blood catecholamines [22] and corticosterone [18]. Another manifestation of this difference was that in Wistar rats the noradrenergic system was activated in hypothalamus, the central component of stress system, while in August rats this activation was absent [16]. Therefore it was established that the higher resistance to stress damage of August rats as compared with Wistar rats was associated with higher basal activity of the stress system but lower activation of the stress system and less intense of the stress response to emotional stressors.

Further we compared the resistance to stress-induced injuries of stomach mucose with activity of stress-limiting systems: the NO system , the brain dopaminergic system, serotoninergic system, and the cytoprotective stress proteins HSP70 in August and Wistar rats.

Nitric oxide is known as a universal regulatory factor of physiological systems. Role of NO in the stress response is determined by the presence of NOergic innervation in central and peripheral units of the stress system [23, 24], NO-ergic neurons innervate adrenal glands and NOergic neurons contact with the chromaffine cells producing catecholamines [23]. Terminals of sympathetic neurons contain not only noradrenaline (NA) but also NO, and these two transmitters are released simultaneously [25]. It was shown that NO can restrict activation of peripheral units in the stress system due to suppression of catecholamine release from adrenal glands [26] and NA from sympathetic nerve endings [27, 28]. On the contrary, suppression of NO synthesis results in sympathetico-adrenal activation [29, 30]. In addition, NO can restrict detrimental effects of the stress response due to direct inhibition of the activated free-radical oxidation, activation of antioxidant enzymes [31, 32] and expression of the enzyme encoding genes [33]. It was also shown that NO activated synthesis of stress proteins HSP70 [34], which comprise an important system of cell protection against stress and other injuries. Therefore NO can influence intensity of the stress response and stress damage by restriction of stress system activity both at the central and peripheral levels.

The baseline tissue level of NO [34] and plasma level of the stable NO metabolites nitrate and nitrite [16, 35] reflecting total NO production in the organism [36] were higher in August than in Wistar rats. We showed (Fig. 3) that 30- and 60-minute emotional stress induced increases in nitrate/nitrite in both rat strains; however this increase was significantly more pronounced in August than Wistar rats. In result, the stress-induced plasma level of nitrite/nitrate was twice higher in August rats [16]. Therefore the higher resistance of August rats to stress-induced stomach lesions might be due to the greater activation of NO system and thus higher NO production in stress. This hypothesis was confirmed by results of inhibiting NO synthesis with the NO synthase inhibitor N^{ω}-nitro-L-arginine (L-NNA). We showed (Fig. 4) stress lesions of the stomach were increased in both strains on the background of the NO deficiency created by the L-NNA treatment. In this process, the L-NNA treatment increased the area of lesions in August rats to a greater extent than in Wistar rats (Fig. 4) [37]. Similar data were obtained with L-NNA pretreatment prior to experimental myocardial infarction [14]. Inhibition of NO synthase increased the infarction-related death rate in both rat strains. However the death rate in August rats was higher than in Wistar rats in comparison to untreated rats. Therefore NO deficiency considerably decreased the interspecies difference in stress resistance of these rat strains. In other words, the higher resistance to stress damage in August than in Wistar rats was partially due to a higher level of NO production in stress exposure.

An important role in regulation of the stress response belongs also to the brain dopaminergic system, in particular the substantia nigra-striatum complex. Dopamine (DA) can restrict activation of the sympathetico-adrenal unit of stress system and, thereby, the detrimental effect of catecholamines on organ and tissues in stress [38, 39]. In addition, the striatal DA system is tightly connected with the NO systems, and the NO system activity is positively correlated with activity of the striatal DA system [40 - 42]. Therefore it can be suggested that the different resistance to stress in August and Wistar rats is due to differences in basal activity and stress reactivity of the brain DA system.

Indeed it was shown [16] that the basal striatal level of DA was significantly higher in August than in Wistar rats (Fig. 5). Furthermore the 3,4-dihydrophenylacetic acid (DOPAC) to DA ratio reflecting the intensity of DA metabolism was lower in August rats, which indicated lower basal activity of the nigro-striatal DA system. In emotional stress, the striatal DA level was also higher in August rats; the DOPAC/DA ratio and the homovanillic acid level considerably increased in August rats and remained unchanged in Wistar rats. These effects indicated a marked stress-induced activation of the nigro-striatal DA system in August rats, which was not the case in Wistar rats. This hypothesis is supported by data obtained in vivo using a well-known psychopharmacological method for evaluation of the brain DA system by dopaminergic stereotypic reactions induced by the DA mimetics apomorphine and phenamine. It was shown that responses to apomorphine and phenamine remained unchanged in Wistar rats and decreased by 40% and 21% respectively in August rats as compared to intact control [16]. This effect can signify that in August rats, the nigro-striatal DA system responds to stress with activation and increased release of endogenous DA. The DA impact on postjunctional DA-receptors attenuates the receptor response to exogenous agonists. Such stress-induced activation of DA system does not occur in Wistar rats.

Therefore the higher resistance of August rats to stress-induced stomach lesions may be due to a considerable extent to the higher activity of brain DA system, which limits activation of the stress system at the central level and, thereby, intensity of the stress response in stress exposure.

Role of the serotoninergic system in the mechanism of resistance to stress damage is yet unclear. At the same time it is known that pharmacologically induced accumulation of serotonin (5-HT) in the rat midbrain near the suture increases resistance to the heart rhythm disorders in acute myocardial ischemia, which are induced by the ischemia-concomitant stress response [11]. It appeared also that adaptation to stress of Wistar rats results in a considerable increase in 5-HT in the midbrain near the suture accompanied by the increased resistance to stress-induced and ischemic damage of the heart. Furthermore pretreatment with the 5-HT analogue 4-nitro-5-methyl-hydroxytriptamine significantly reduced the duration of arrhythmias and rate of cardiac fibrillation in acute ischemia in conscious rats, i.e., protected against the stress arrhythmogenic component of acute ischemia [43]. It is also known that chronic emotional stress induces depressive states, which are more frequent in women [44]. Analyses showed that the depression is caused by deficient functioning of the brain serotoninergic system. Animal experiments [45] have demonstrated that chronic stress results in decrease of serotonin content in the frontal cortex, hippocampus and hypothalamus of females but not males. Based on this fact authors suggested that this was just the more pronounced than in men deficiency of serotonin that underlay the predisposition of women to stress-induced depression. Therefore the resistance to stress depression can be defined by activity of this serotoninergic system.

These and other data allowed classification of the serotoninergic system as a stress-limiting system [3, 6, 7]. Therefore it was possible to suggest that the serotoninergic system participated in the pathogenesis of stress damage to the stomach. However this role is not completely elucidated. On the one hand, it was shown that central (to lateral ventricles) administration of exogenous 5-HT increased stomach lesions in stress-exposed mice while intraperitoneal injection of 5-HT antagonists diminished the lesion with different potentiating effects of 5-HT in mice of different genetic strains. [46, 47]. On the other hand, it was established that intraperitoneal injection of 5-HT and the 5-HT precursor d,1–5-hydroxytriptophan decreased stress ulceration while the elevation of 5-HT in stomach mucose induced by exogenous 5-HT accelerated healing of stress lesions [48]. It was also shown that stress ulceration was accompanied by the decreased stomach level of 5-HT [49]. Finally, it appeared that administration of 5-HT antagonists increased stress-induced stomach ulcers while the protective effect of prostaglandin E_2 against such lesions was associated with the increased content of 5-HT in the stomach [50].

In experiments on August and Wistar rats, we found that the higher resistance of August rat stomach was combined with higher basal and stress-stimulated striatal and stomach mucose levels of 5-HT and with lower stomach mucose NA/5-HT ratio as compared to Wistar rats [51]. This result is in agreement with the above-described data of literature on the protective role of endogenous 5-HT in stomach. Taken together the data suggest that the genetically-predetermined higher level of 5-HT in the stomach as a target organ as well as in the striatum is an important factor of inherited resistance to injuries in acute emotional stress.

It was also demonstrated that August and Wistar rats differed from each other by production of the cytoprotective proteins HSP70 in stress situations. The higher resistance of August rats to acute myocardial infarction and its arrhythmogenic effect [13, 14] was associated with accumulation of 2-2.5 time larger amount of HSP70 in the myocardium as compared to Wistar rats exposed to similar infarction [52]. Furthermore in August rats, the increased accumulation of HSP70 was observed not only in the ischemic left ventricle but also in non-ischemic heart divisions, which are known to be affected by stress damage in the stress reaction accompanying acute ischemia [7, 53, 54].

Therefore different resistance to stress damage is related to a considerable extent with genetically predetermined differences in the basal activity and stress-induced activation of stress-limiting systems. The higher resistance to acute stress induced stomach lesions observed in August rats as compared to Wistar rats was associated with higher inherited activity of stress-limiting systems: the NO system, the nigro-striatal DA system, the HSP70 system and also with the higher content of serotonin in stomach and striatum.

2. Dissimilar Magnitude of the Antistress Protective Effect of Adaptation in August and Wistar Rats

Studies on the role of inherited stress-limiting system activity in formation of adaptation to hypoxia and stress and adaptive protection against the damage induced by acute stress in Wistar and August rats provided paradoxical results.

Adaptation to stress exposure

Adaptation to repeated non-damaging emotional stress, both short-term (6 sessions) and more long-term (12 sessions) efficiently increased resistance to acute stress induced stomach lesions in Wistar rats, which are genetically less resistant to such damage as mentioned above, but decreased the resistance in August rats, which are genetically more resistant. Figure 6 illustrates this effect. It is seen that the number and area of acute stress induced stomach lesions was several times larger in adapted than in naive August rats, while in Wistar rats, in contrast, adaptation considerably reduced the damage. Furthermore it is important that adaptation itself induced stomach ulcers in August but not in Wistar rats; these ulcers were similar to those induced by the test stress exposure [51].

Comparison of this phenomenon with activities of stress-limiting systems showed that repeated stress exposures in the course of adaptation resulted in potentiation of stress-limiting system response to acute stress in Wistar rats and, vice versa, decreased the system responsiveness in August rats. For instance, it appeared (Fig. 7) that adapted August rats displayed a 3-fold lower level of NO production than naive ones in acute stress. Thus the decreased resistance to stress damage was associated in these rats with the absence of increased NO production in response to stress. In adapted Wistar rats, the stress-induced increase in NO production (as compared to baseline level) remained, which was associated with the enhanced resistance of stomach to stress damage (unpublished data). Therefore the decreased resistance to stress damage in adaptation to stress (August rats) was associated with the decreased responsiveness of the NO system, whereas the increased resistance (Wistar rats) was associated with the increased responsiveness of the NO system. This assumption is confirmed by that the adaptation to stress produced on the background of NO synthase inhibition with L-NNA did not provide protection against stomach damage in acute stress in Wistar rats [55].

It was also shown that responsiveness of the nigro-striatal DA system increased in the course of adaptation to stress in Wistar rats, while in August rats, the DA system responsiveness decreased rather than increased in such adaptation [8]. For instance Figure 8 shows that in pre-adapted Wistar rats the striatal level of DA increases in response to test stress as compared to the level in unadapted rats, whereas in August rats, the DA level does not increase in response to such exposure as compared to naive animals. In this process, the DOPAC/DA ratio significantly increased in stress-exposed Wistar rats and exceeded that in August rats. In adapted August rats, this ratio became lower than in stress-exposed unadapted rats and did not differ from control. This indicates that the stress response of striatal DA system increased in adapted Wistar rats, while this was not the case in adapted August rats. Therefore the increased resistance to acute stress was associated with the enhanced efficiency of brain DA system in Wistar rats, while in adapted August rats, the reduced resistance to stress damage of stomach was associated with the absence of stress activation of the DA system.

In the process of repeated stress exposures, similar changes were observed in the activity of serotoninergic system. It was shown [51] that the decreased resistance to acute stress induced stomach lesions observed in August rats after adaptation to repeated non-damaging stress was accompanied by a 35% decrease in 5-HT level and an increase in the NA/5-HT ratio in stomach mucose as compared to unadapted rats. To the contrary, in adapted Wistar rats, the protective effect of adaptation evident as the diminished stress-induced stomach ulceration was associated with the increased level of 5-HT and decreased NA/5-HT ratio in the stomach (Table). In overall, the study showed that the change in resistance to acute stress damage was specifically related with changes in activity of the endogenous 5-HT system in the stomach.

Table. Effect of acute stress exposure (30 minutes) on stomach mucose content of serotonine (5-HT) and noradrenaline (ng /mg wet tissue) in naive (unadapted) and pre-adapted to stress exposures August and Wistar rats (Ì ± m)

Rat strains	Groups of animals	5-HT	NA	NA/5-HT
	Control (unadapted) rats (10)	10.10 ± 0.50	0.86 ± 0.08	0.09 ± 0.007
AUGUST	Unadapted rats exposed to acute stress (10)	11.90 ± 0.60^{+}	0.70 ± 0.09	0.06 ± 0.002^{+}
	Pre-adapted rats exposed to acute stress (10)	7.90 ± 0.61^{++}	0.54 ± 0.07^{+}	0.07 ± 0.009
	Control (unadapted) rats (9)	6.01 ± 0.70*	0.98 ± 0.11	0.22 ± 0.02*
WISTAR	Unadapted rats exposed to acute stress (10)	6.40 ± 0.10*	0.88 ± 0.16	0.16 ± 0.01 +*
	Pre-adapted rats exposed to acute stress (10)	7.30 ± 0.40^{++}	0.50 ± 0.06	0.08 ± 0.009^{++}

+ Significant differences from control rats, p<0.05. ++ Significant differences from unadapted rats exposed to acute stress, p<0.05.

* Significant differences from August rats, p<0.05. In parentheses: a number of animals in group.

Studies of the stress protein HSP70 system [21, 56] showed that prior adaptation to repeated restraint stress increased resistance of the isolated heart from Wistar rats to thermal stress associated with myocardial accumulation of HSP70. In August rats, this adaptation did not increase the resistance to heat shock; disturbance of the heart contractile function was considerably more pronounced in hearts of August than Wistar rats. Furthermore the myocardial accumulation of HSP70 was absent in August rats during adaptation. Therefore the increased resistance to thermal stress was associated in adapted animals with accumulation of HSP70 (Wistar rats) while the absence of activation of HSP70 gene expression and HSP70 synthesis in adapted animals (August rats) was associated with the reduced resistance [21, 56].

Adaptation to hypobaric hypoxia

In August and Wistar rats adapted to high-altitude hypoxia, the antistress defense develops principally in the same way as in adaptation to stress exposure and is also associated with activation of stress-limiting systems. However the detrimental effect of repeated hypoxic sessions appears in a greater number of such sessions [16]. It was shown that a brief course of adaptation to hypoxia (6 sessions) resulted in decreased number and area of stomach lesions in Wistar rats. At the same time in August rats, the number of lesions decreased to a considerably lesser extent and the area of lesions remained unchanged. (Fig. 9). A long-term course of adaptation to hypoxia (40 sessions), as adaptation to stress, sharply potentiated stress-induced stomach lesions in August rats. In Wistar rats, this course did not potentiate the lesions but slightly decreased them in comparison with unadapted rats (Fig. 9).

Comparing the changes in stomach lesions induced by acute stress in the rats adapted to hypoxia for 6 sessions with respective changes in stress-limiting system activity showed the following. In adapted Wistar rats, the pronounced increase in stomach resistance to acute stress damage was accompanied by a 60% increase in NO production (by plasma level of nitrite/nitrate) as compared to control. In adapted August rats the absence of such increase in stress resistance was associated with the absence of increase in NO production during adaptation [16, 35]. The implication of NO in the protective antistress effect of adaptation is supported by the fact that such adaptation produced on the background of L-NNA treatment, i.e., inhibition of NO synthase did not posses the protective antistress effect [37].

It was also demonstrated [16] that adaptation to hypoxia increased striatal DA and DOPAC in rats of both strains, which indicated activation of the nigro-striatal DA system induced by hypoxia (Fig. 10). In this process, the striatal level of DA in Wistar rats increased to a considerably greater degree (47% of control) whereas the increased was twofold less in August rats (23% of control). It is important that the striatal DOPAC/DA ratio became higher in stress-exposed pre-adapted Wistar rats than in naive rats exposed to the same stress. At the same time, the ratio became lower in stress-exposed pre-adapted August rats than in stress-exposed naive rats. It means adaptation to hypoxia of Wistar rats enhanced the response of DA system to acute stress and decreased it in August rats.

Therefore adaptation to hypoxia of the same duration (6 sessions) as adaptation to stress exposure considerably enhanced the resistance to classic stress damage of stomach in Wistar rats and only slightly enhanced the resistance in August rats not reducing it however. The protective effect of adaptation to hypoxia, as that of adaptation to stress, was associated with the increased efficiency of stress-limiting systems, the NO system and brain DA system, as it was observed in Wistar rats. In contrast, the absence of pronounced antistress effect of adaptation to hypoxia was associated with the absence of activation in the brain DA system and NO system as it was observed in August rats.

On the whole it was shown that when the course of adaptation reduced efficiency of stress-limiting systems, the resistance of animals to acute stress also reduced (as in August rats); when adaptation potentiated efficiency of stress-limiting systems, the resistance of animals to stress also increased (as in Wistar rats).

In addition a definite relationship was revealed between the genetically predetermined resistance to acute stress, level of stress-limiting system efficiency and adaptability to stress and hypoxia (and perhaps to other factors). The animals with higher inherited efficiency of stress-limiting systems and resistance to acute emotional stress are less adaptable to repeated stress and hypoxia; such impacts decrease their efficiency of stress-limiting systems and resistance to acute stress. The animals possessing a lower inherited efficiency of stress-limiting systems and resistance to acute stress well adapt to repeated stresses and hypoxia; such adaptation efficiently enhance their resistance to stress damage, i.e., exerts a protective antistress effect.

The above-said allows understanding the existing in literature contradictions in evaluation of "stress-resistance" in August and Wistar rats. Initial studies using long-term (up to 30 hours) stresses [19, 20] or severe thermal stress or heat shock [21] showed that August rats died in such impacts more frequently and earlier than Wistar rats, which were more resistant. These studies have established an opinion that Wistar rats are "stress-resistant" while August rats are "non-stress-resistant". This opinion occurs in many studies [17, 19, 57, etc.].

On the other hand, August but not Wistar rats appeared more resistant to detrimental effects of less prolonged emotional stresses (30-120 min) or acute myocardial infarction [13, 15, 35] always associated with a pronounced stress response as it has been already mentioned above. The facts provided in this review allow the following explanation of these contradictions.

It can be suggested that the higher inherited efficiency of stress-limiting systems (as in August rats) does not increase or becomes even "exhausted" in the process of repeated or prolonged impacts of diverse factors and this may result in the decreased resistance of the animals to stress exposure. In other words, in this instance, adaptation and its antistress effects do not develop. In the instance of a lower inherited efficiency of stress-limiting systems (as in Wistar rats), repeated or prolonged exposures to a stressor may potentiate the efficiency of stress-limiting systems, facilitate formation of adaptation and, consistently, provide resistance to acute stress [8].

The mechanism for decreasing the efficiency of stress-limiting systems by repeated or prolonged exposure to environmental factors in animals with a higher inherited efficiency of stress-limiting systems as well as the mechanism for increasing the efficiency of stress-limiting systems by these impacts in animals with the initially lower activity of stress-limiting systems is unclear yet. As for the serotoninergic system, data of literature suggest that this system becomes "exhausted" by stress more rapidly in August rats than in Wistar rats [58]. As for the NO system, it can be suggested that the level of free NO may decrease due to more intense NO binding to NO stores in August than in Wistar rats in the process of adaptation [35, 59]; however this is only a speculation.

Mechanisms of stress resistance and its changes in adaptation to environmental factors require further investigations. However the above notions should be undoubtedly considered in developing methods of adaptive prevention and treatment because the notions indicate the necessity of evaluating the state of stress system and stress-limiting systems in patients for defining the advisability and regimens of adaptation.

References

1. Stratakis C.A., Chrousos G.P. Neuroendocrinology and pathophysiology of the stress system // Ann. N.Y. Acad. Sci. – 771: 1-18. 1995.
2. Chrousos G.P., Gold P.W. The concepts of stress system disorders: overview of behavioral and physical homeostasis. JAMA. 267: 1244-1252. 1992.
3. Meerson F.Z., Pshennikova M.G., Malyshev I.Yu. Adaptive defense of the organism: architectural trace and cross protective effects of adaptation. Ann. N.Y. Acad. Sci. 793: 371-385. 1996.
4. Manukhina E.B., Malyshev I.Yu. The stress-limiting system of nitric oxide. Ross. Fiziol. Zhurnal im. I.M. Sechenova 86: 1283-1292. 2000 (in Russian).
5. Meerson F.Z. Adaptation, stress and prophylaxis. Springer, Berlin. 294 p.1984.
6. Meerson F.Z. Essentials of adaptive medicine: protective effects of adaptation. Hypoxia Medical Ltd, Moscow, Geneva. 443 p. 1993.
7. Meerson F.Z., Pshennikova M.G. Adaptation to stress situation and physical loads. Meditsina, Moscow. 256 p. 1988. (in Russian).
8. Pshennikova M.G. Hereditary efficiency of stress-limiting systems as a factor of the resistance to stress-induced disorders. Uspekhi Fiziol. Nauk. 34 (3): 55-67. 2003. (in Russian).
9. Borodin P.M., Schuller L., Belyaev D.K. Problems of stress genetics. Information 1. Genetical analysis of mice behaviour in stress situation. Genetika. 12 (12): 62-71. 1976. (in Russian).
10. Seredinin S.B., Badyshtov B.A. Study of the hereditary differences in the cyclic nucleotide content of the blood serum in mice after exposure to stress and administration of phenazepam. Biull. Eksp. Biol. Med. 100 (11): 586-588. 1985.
11. Lown B., Desilva R., Reich P., Murawski B. Psychophysiologic factors in sudden cardiac death. Amer. J. Psychiat. 137 (11): 1325-1335. 1980.
12. Skinner J.E. Psychosocial stress and sudden cardiac death: brain mechanisms. In: Beamish R.E., Singal P.K., Dhalla N.S., eds., Stress and heart disease, Boston / Dordrecht / Lancaster. 44-59. 1985.
13. Belkina L.M., Saltykova V.A., Pshennikova M.G. Genetically determined differences in the resistance to myocardial infarction in Wistar and August rats. Bull. Exp. Biol. Med. 131 (6): 529-532. 2001.
14. Belkina L.M., Kirillina T.N., Pshennikova M.G., Arkhipenko Yu.V. August Rats are more resistant to arrhythmogenic effect of myocardial ischemia and reperfusion than Wistar rats. Bull. Exp. Biol. Med. 133 (6): 540-543. 2002.

15. Pshennikova M.G., Bondarenko N.A., Shimkovich M.V., Bondarenko O.N., Malyshev I.Yu. Differences in the behavior and resistance to stomach ulcer during stress in August and Wistar rats adapted and not adapted to hypoxia. Biull. Eksp. Biol. Med. 128 (12): 638-641. 1999.
16. Pshennikova M.G., Popkova E.V., Bondarenko N.A., Malyshev I.Yu., Shimkovich M.V., Smirin B.V., Manukhina E.B. Catecholamines, nitrogen oxide, and resistivity to stressor lesions: effect of adaptation to hypoxia. Ross. Fiziol. Zh. im I. M. Sechenova. 88 (4): 485-495. 2002. (in Russian).
17. Pertsov S.S., Koplik E.V., Krauzer V., Mikhael_N., Eme P., Sudakov K.V. Adrenal glands catecholamines of August and Wistar rats in acute emotional stress. Biull. Eksp. Biol. Med. 123 (6): 645-648. 1997.
18. Pshennikova M.G., Golubeva L.Iu., Kuznetsova B.A., Shimkovich M.V., Malysheva E.V., Malyshev I.Yu. Differences in stress reaction and development of adaptation to stress in August and Wistar rats. Biull. Eksp. Biol. Med 122 (8): 156-159. 1996.
19. Sudakov K.V., Coghlan J.P., Kotov A.V., Salieva R.M., Polyantsev Yu.V., Koplik E.V. Delta-sleep-inducing peptide sequels in the mechanisms of resistance to emotional stress. Ann. N.Y. Acad. Sci. 771: 240-251. 1995.
20. Sudakov K.V., Dushkin V.A.., Yumatov E.A. Genetical and individual differences in cardiovascular disturbances in rats during experimental emotional stress. Vestnik AMN SSSR. 12: 32-39. 1981. (in Russian).
21. Malysheva E.V., Zamotrinskii A.V., Malyshev I.Iu. The role of heat shock proteins in the formation of stress-resistance in various genetic lines of animals. Biull. Eksp. Biol. Med. 118 (7): 11-13. 1994.
22. Kvetnansky R., Belova T.N., Oprshalova Z., Ponez I., Indra A., Dushkin V.A. Plasma catecholamines in August and Wistar strains rats in emotional stress. I.M.Sechenov Fiziol. Zhurnal. 67 (4): 516-523. 1981. (in Russian).
23. Snyder S.H., Bredt D.S. Nitric oxide as a neuronal messenger. TIPS. 12: 125-128. 1991.
24. Vanhatalo S., Soinila S. Nitric oxide synthase in the hypothalamo-pituitary pathway. J. Chem. Neuroanat. 8: 165-173. 1995.
25. Toda N., Yoshida K., Okamura T. Analysis of the potentiating action of N-nitro-L-arginine on the contraction of the dog temporal artery elicited by trasmural stimulation of noradrenergic nerves. Naunyn-Schmideberg's Arch. Pharmacol. 343: 221-224. 1991.
26. Torres M., Ceballos G., Rubio R. Possible role of nitric oxide in catecholamine secretion by chromaffin cells in the presence and absence of cultured endothelial cells. J. Neurochem. 63: 988-996. 1994.
27. Addicks K., Bloch W., Feelisch M. Nitric oxide modulates sympathetic neurotransmission at prejunctional level. Microscopy Res. Tech. 29: 161-168. 1994.
28. Schwarz P., Diem R., Dun N.J., Forstermann U. Endogenous and exogenous nitric oxide inhibits norepinephrine release from rats heart sympathetic nerves. Circ. Res. 77: 841-848. 1995.
29. Goodson A.R., Leibold J.M., Gutterman D.D. Inhibition of nitric oxide synthesis augments centrally induced sympathetic coronary vasoconctriction in cats. Amer. J. Physiol. 36: H1272- H1278. 1994.
30. Zanchi A., Shaad N.C., Osterheld M.C., Grouzmann E., Nussberger J., Brunner H.R., Waeber B. Effect of chronic NO synthase inhibition in rats on renin-angiotensin system and sympathetic nervous system. Am. J. Physiol. 37: H2267-H2273. 1995.
31. Dobashi K., Pahan K., Chahal L., Singh I. Modulation of endogenous antioxidant enzymes by nitric oxide in rat C-6 glial cells. J. Neurochem. 68: 1806-1903. 1997.
32. Rotzinger S., Aragon C.M.G., Rogan F., Amir S., Amit Z. The nitric oxide synthase inhibitor N-nitro-L-arginine-methyl ester attenuates brain catalase activity in vitro. Life Sci. 56: 1321-1324. 1995.
33. Nunoshiba T., de Rojas-Walker T., Wishnok J.S., Tannenbaum S.R., Demple B. Activation by nirtic oxide of an oxidative-stress response that defends Escherichia coli against activated macrophages. Proc. Natl. Acad. Sci. USA. 90: 9993-9997. 1993.
34. Malyshev I.Yu., Manukhina E.B., Mikoyan V.D., Kubrina L.N., Vanin A.F. Nitric oxide is involved in heat-induced HSP70 accumulation. FEBS Lett. 370: 159-162. 1995.

35. Pshennikova M.G., Smirin B.V., Bondarenko O.N., Malyshev I.Iu., Manukhina E.B. Nitric oxide storage in rats of various genetic strains and its role in the antistressor effect of adaptation to hypoxia. Ross. Fiziol. Zh. Im I. M. Sechenova. 86 (2): 174-181. 2000. (in Russian).
36. Benjamin N., Vallance P. Plasma nitrate as a marker of nitric oxide production. Lancet. 344: 960. 1994.
37. Pshennikova M.G., Bondarenko N.A., Shimkovich M.V. Nitric oxide as a factor of genetically determined resistance to stress damages and adaptive protection. Bull. Exp. Biol. Med. 132 (5): 1048-50. 2001.
38. Beaulieu S., Di Paolo T., Barden N. Roles of the noradrenergic, dopaminergic and serotoninergic systems in the modulation of the ACTH response to stress by the amigdaloid central nucleus. Canad. J. Neurol. Sci. 12: 214-215. 1985.
39. Doda M., Gyorgy L. Dopaminergic inhibition of sympathetic activity in the cat. Pol. J. Pharmacol. 37: 397-401. 1985.
40. Sagach V.F., Bazilyuk O.V., Oleshko N.N., Kozuruba A.V., Appenzeller O. System of nitric oxide in the chronic deficit of cerebral dopamine and hypoxia. Fiziol. Zhunal 45 (1-2): 16-25. 1999. (in Ukrain).
41. Sagach V.F., Bazilyuk O.V., Oleshko N.N., Maiskii V.A., Costa A., Martignoni E., Qualls C., Appenzeller O. Mesostriatal lesions and endothelial function: effects of forced movements and hypoxia on levels of circulating endothelins. Neurophysiology. 30: 13-18. 1998.
42. West A.R., Galloway M.P., Grace A.A. Regulation of striatal dopamine neurotransmission by nitric oxide: effector pathways and signaling mechanisms. Synapce. 44: 227-245. 2002.
43. Shabunina E.V., Petrunin I.A., Vinograd L.Kh., Manukhina E.B., Meerson F.Z. Prevention of arrhythmia in acute ischemia in conscious animals using a serotonin analog. Biull. Eksp. Biol. Med. 106 (10): 410-412. 1988.
44. Van Praag H.M. Neurotransmitters and CNS disease: depression. Lancet. 1: 1259-1264. 1982.
45. Kennett G.A., Chaouloff F., Marcou M., Curzon G. Female rats are more vulnerable than males in an animal model of depression: the possible role of serotonin. Brain Res. 382: 416-421. 1986.
46. Koryakina L.A. Comparison of ciproheptadine and propranolol effects on development of poststress damage to stomach mucose of inbred mice. Ross. Fiziol. Zh. Im I. M. Sechenova. 79 (9): 54-60. 1993. (in Russian).
47. Koryakina L.A. Participation of serotonin $\tilde{N}_2$ -receptors in realization of stress effects on ulcerogenesis in stomach mucose of inbred mice. Ross. Fiziol. Zhurnal. Im I. M. Sechenova. 80 (11): 64-70. 1994. (in Russian).
48. Klimenko M.O., Lupaltzev V.I., Yakhnyuk A.I., Tatarko S.V. Effect of serotonin on healing of experimental gastric ulcer in vagotomy. Fiziol. Zhunal. 46 (4): 52-57.2000. (in Ukrain).
49. Orlisz-Szczesna G., Zabel M., Jaroszewski J. The effect of stress induced experimental gastric ulcers on enterochromaffin cells and on serotonin and 5-hydroxyindolacetic acid levels in stomach and duodenum of the white rat. Z. Mikrosk. Anat. Forsch. 103 (3): 504-514. 1989.
50. Ciurzynskf G., Dzierzkowska J., Maslinski S. Gastric cytoprotective activity of endogenous 5-HT. J. Physiol. Pharmacol. 45 (4): 517-532. 1994.
51. Pshennikova M.G., Popkova E.V., Shimkovich M.V. Adaptation to Stress Improves Resistance to Gastric Damage during Acute Stress in Wistar Rats and Decreases Resistance in August Rats: Role of Serotonin. Bull. Exp. Biol. Med. 134 (4): 329-332. 2002.
52. Pshennikova M.G., Belkina L.M., Bakhtina L.Iu., Bayda L.A., Popkova E.V., Malyshev I.Iu. Role of stress proteins HSP70 and the adrenergic system in different resistance to myocardial infarction in rats of the genetic strains August and Wistar. Ross. Fiziol. Zhurnal Im I. M. Sechenova. 87 (9): 1171-1177. 2001. (in Russian).
53. Meerson F.Z. Adaptive protection of the heart: protecting against stress and ischemic damage. Boca Raton: CRC Press. 340 p. 1991.
54. Samuels M.A. Neurogenic heart disease: a unifying hypothesis. Am. J. Cardiol. 60: 15J-19J. 1987.
55. Malenyuk E.B., Aimasheva N.P., Manukhina E.B., Mikoyan V.D., Kubrina L.N., Vanin A.F., Larionov N.P., Malyshev I.Yu. Is Nitric Oxide Involved in the Adaptation to the Stress-Induced Damage? Bull. Exp. Biol. Med. 126 (9): 886-889. 1998.

56. Zamotrinskii A.V., Malyshev I.Iu., Larionov N.P. A comparative analysis of the polypeptide composition of heat shock proteins 70 synthesized in Wistar and August rat myocardium. Biull. Eksp. Biol. Med. 120 (7): 30-32. 1995.

57. Davidova M.P., Tolordova I.A.,Volkov V.N., Grafov M.A., Medvedeva N.F. Altered endothelin-dependent regulation of blood pressure and vascular tone in stress-sensitive August rats. J. Cardiovascular Pharmacology. 36 (Suppl. 1): S124-S127. 2000.

58. Gorbunova A.V., Salieva R.M., Lobanova N.N., Ionochkina I.N., Petrova S.Y., Dedov V. Biogenic amine content in the brains of rats with different levels of resistance to emotional stress. Neurosci. Behav. Physiol. 27: 145-152. 1997.

59. Manukhina E.B., Malyshev I.Iu., Smirin B.V., Mashina S.Iu., Saltykova V.A., Vanin A.F. Production and storage of nitric oxide in adaptation to hypoxia. Nitric Oxide. 3 (5): 393-401. 1999.

Adaptation Biology and Medicine (Volume 4: Current Concepts)
Editors: A. Hargens, N. Takeda and P.K. Singal

4. The Mechanisms of Hypoxytherapy and the Basis of Resonant Normobaric Hypoxytherapy

A.Ya. Chizhov, A.A. Bludov

Laboratory of clinical problems of Hypoxia of Scientific Research Institute of General Pathology and Pathophysiology, Russian Academy of Medical Science, Moscow. 125315. Russia.

The concept of a possibility of protection of human organism from ionizing radiation at the moment of irradiation with the help of respiration by gas mixtures containing 10.0% ± 1.0% of Oxygen (GHA-10), for the first time was formulated in 1970 [52], and in 1980 the idea about expediency and possibility of wide replacement of hypoxic component of treatment in mountains as well as training in barocamera with dosaged controlled hypoxia framed with respiration by gas mixtures with the lowered contents of Oxygen was stated [61]. Cumulative experience of treatment of the oncologic patients with use of radial therapy and HGA-10 (hypoxyradiotherapy) allowed to verify positive medical effect of GHM-10 and at accompanying diseases (hypertention ischemic heart disease, bronchopulmonary pathology, gastroenergetic pathology and gastrointestinal path etc.) [60, 62].

It is known, that the basic intracellular frames and parts of a metabolism of a cell on the initial stages of evolution were formed in an atmosphere actually deprived of Oxygen. Therefore, initial metabolic base of intracellular processes of formation of energy were the reactions, which could proceed at a minimum of free Oxygen in medium. The himan embryo at the initial phases of the formation practically repeats evolutionary development of alive organisms and at the first stages (zygote) receives minimum Oxygen and only for the account of a simple diffusion [59]. Later, the blood from 91-92% of Oxygen goes to a placenta. This parameter is reduced up to 65 % in it. The blood, flowing to a fetus, contains 55-56 % of Oxygen, whereas the blood, flowing off from a fetus, - about 25 % of Oxygen [18].

In 1981 [69, 65] there was revealed for the first time a spontaneous cyclic reduce of Oxygen in tissues of uterus and fetus of rats, which size corresponds to a degree of hypoxia developing at respiration by gas hypoxic mixture from 10 % of Oxygen (which approximately corresponds to hypoxia developing at height 5800 m). This mechanism carries a training function and raises nonspecific resistance of a fetus to adverse influences at the moment of labors and in post-delivery period, including ionizing radiation [63, 67].

Thus, nature has created a hypoxic training as optimal physiological factor of acclimatization. Therefore at a hypoxic stimulation of the genetically determined mechanisms of acclimatization there will inevitably be rising of nonspecific resistance of an organism to the factors lying in the basis of a plenty pathological processes. Today it does not cause any more doubts that at acclimatization to hypoxia in an organism the reserve mechanisms of indemnification start at first, and later of the long-term mechanisms of acclimatization are formed. [4,9,12,39,66]. We shall stop briefly on some of them.

Pulmonary mechanisms external respiration. The system of respiration carries out the large number of functions in an organism, one of which is maintenance of ðÍ of blood. At research of the central link of regulation of respiration there was revealed an activating action on it by both lowered ðÍ, and hypoxia. At perfusion by the hypoxic the solution of the isolated oblong at a brain of rats there were revealed reactions of the central respiratory generator recorded from the ventral roots Ñ1-Ñ5 of a spinal cord [58]. Under the influence of adaptation to Interrupted normobaric Hypoxia the relative augmentation of the central inspiratory activity and that of the size of an inspiratory flow was marked and the authors connect it with the improvement of a biomechanics of respiration [34]. It is proved, that during adaptation to hypoxic conditions the efficiency of ventilating function of lungs raises at the expense of 1) decrease of resistance of various sections of a tracheobronchial tree, 2) optimization of distribution of local ventilation between various zones of a lung [12]. Hypoxic mixtures containing 12-15 % of Oxygen had their partial pressure of a carbon dioxide raised a little. The drop of ventilation reaction to a carbon dioxide [5] was subsequently marked. During the comparison of intensity of respiration with air, hyper- and hypoxic mixture [42], the hyperventilation in conditions of hypoxia has appeared the shortest and with the least total volume of ventilation. Static expiratory and inspiratory efforts straight after hyperventilation decreased. The hypercapnia raised intensity of a hyperventilation that caused faster fatigue of respiratory muscles [1].

Circulatory mechanisms are shown by augmentation of cardiac output and reorganization of a microcircular channel. There were revealed series of properties of a coronary sinus in a regulation of constrictive function of myocardium of ventricles and gas structure of a blood in an aorta and pulmonary arteria on pressure in a right auricle and coronary sinus itself [19]. The blood pressure in vessels of outflow is as higher, as higher the total pressure of gases in them [32]. Thus the concentration of gases in blood of a coronary sinus is close to those in blood of umbilical vein of a fetus and can serve criteria of a hypoxic limit for venous blood [19]. There was revealed an important role of a sinocarotid reflexogenic zone in formation of adaptive reactions of the organism - during its bilateral surgical erasing there were no adaptive reactions, at all except rising hemoglobin in blood [21]. The modern researchers pay the great attention to adaptation of cardiovascular system to hypoxia. In 1940. It was opened, that the hypoxia is potent vasodilatator for coronary vessels [94]. During drop of Oxygen in inhaled air down to 8-9 % the rate of coronary blood flow [56] considerably grows. The influence of a interrupted normobaric hypoxia on the central hemodynamics is described as well. The initial augmentation of shock and minute volumes of heart with the subsequent stabilization of these parameters [48, 66, 71] is marked. It becomes possible owing to series of bioenergetic changes of a myocardium. Not adapted animals spent the appreciable part of free energy of heart for overcoming of a power barrier of biochemical reactions. The rats trained with interrupted hypoxia [72] reveal the drop of a power barrier of biochemical processes of a myocardium in 3,3 times in rest. During acute hypoxia this parameter grew only in 1.6 times. With the help of a method of registration of currents through To K + – canals of cardiomyocytes of rats and of a man it is shown [6], that blocked in normooxic conditions the ATP-sensitive canals begin to open on 20-25th minute of a moderate hypoxia. These are only some of mechanisms of optimization of expenses of energy while intensifying function of heart in conditions of hypoxia.

The data on reorganization of a microcircular channel at acclimatization to hypoxia are received. There is a disclosing of capillaries not functioning before and induction of an angiogenesis in a direction of zones of the greatest ischemia [28]. Hypobaric hypoxic training led to the drop of a structural component of vascular resistance [30]. The hypoxia in combination with exercises accelerates a working angiogenesis in skeletal muscles of rats [44]. The adaptation results to the periodic work of a normobaric hypoxia brings to normalization of kinetics processes of oxygen metabolism determined by a of polarographic method [48,70]. There are facts about activation of fibrinolytic system of a blood under the effect of adaptation to hypoxia [91].

The most various and the least investigated are the biochemical mechanisms of adaptation to hypoxia. So, arising during respiration by hypoxic gas admixture the augmentation of concentration of a metabolic carbon dioxide is accompanied by weakening of chemical connection of Oxygen with a hemoglobin and intensification of tissue respiration [2]. During the first days of adaptation to the Alpine climate the ascending activity of hydrate carboanhydrasa of blood kept up to the end of hypoxic influence is observed [41]. An egestion of ions ÍÑÎ3 by kidneys is accompanied by loss of ions K + with urine during the first days of adaptation. With the increasing of concentration of K + in erythrocytes on a background of increasing of K + in plasma, hemoglobin insufficiency of Oxygen is enlarged, and the partial pressure of Oxygen of a blood is reduced. Further, in a process of development of long-term adaptation, the decrease of erythrocytic K + results in normalization of Ðî2 of blood (on a background of insufficiency of hemoglobin with Oxygen) [47]. Respiratory alkalosis, observed for the first days, during adaptation has leveled. Carboanhydrasa, adjusting the level of ÑÎ2 in an organism, plays the big role in a protein-lipid exchange. The resistance of an organism to low partial pressure of Î2 is caused by the step to intensification of an albuminous exchange and is connected with the restriction of fat storage in depot [41]. There are works showing the activation of glico- and glucogenesis from greasy acids during adaptation to hypoxia by rats [33]. New cell structures are produced from protein, synthesized at hypoxia, glycogen provides energetic reserve for cells.

The important meaning is given to a bioenergetic exchange, which immediately provides formation of long-term adaptation to the hypoxic factor. During hypoxic therapy realized with GHM with 10 - 12 % contents of Oxygen in a cyclic-fraction regimen, the first stage of compensative bioenergetic hypoxia develops. This stage is characterized by activation of enzymes of a substrate part of a respiratory chain and stimulation of formation of ATP. The hypoxic effect brings to the strengthening of biosynthetic processes, the increasing of mass of mitochondrions and the change of enzymes properties. All listed provides economization of a bioenergetic exchange and promotes rising of a nonspecific resistance of an organism [35,36].

Now it is known, that during the hypoxia the activation of synthesis of oxide of nitrogen (NO) is observed [37,40,50,51]. Hemalbumens of hemoglobin, myoglobin, cytochromoxidasa in mitochondrions and cytochrome Ð-450 in microsomas usually cooperating With Oxygen, in desoxiform can restore NO2 in NO and thus close the chain of transformations " L-arginine - NO - NO2/NO3 - NO " into a cycle NO [49]. Oxygen connected with them, inhibits this ability. Free-radical combinations of NO and NO2 cause formation of paramagnetic centers on albumens and lipids of membranes, and promote formation of disulfide combinations between cytoplasm and membranous albumen [50]. In the membrane-connected condition the ferment systems of synthesis of ÀÒÐ, are stimulated as well as the proliferation, transferrance of signals inside cells. Activating soluble guanilatcyclasa and ADP-ribosiltransferasa, NO adjusts intracellular concentration of ions of calcium.

NO and NO2 participate in augmentation of active zones of synaptic contacts during experimental ischemia of a brain at the cats [50,51]. The oxide of nitrogen is capable to limit the sizes of an infarct and to damage cancer cells [40]. The cellular answer to a moderate periodic hypoxia causes rising of hypoxic resistance of a cell and restriction of mechanisms of aptosis activation [37]. Hence, the rising of concentration of NO, naturally arising at adaptation to a moderate hypoxia, is a favorable factor of influence either on a sick and or a healthy organism.

Under the influence of a long acclimatization to a periodic hypoxia the activity of a key enzyme of a respiratory chain NADN cytochrome C - oxidoreductase was enlarged. It's affinity to NADN was reduced, what should raise the resistance of mitochondrions to Oxygen. It is important during blood flow restoration, when the risk of reperfussional damages is high. During the drop of intensity of oxidizing processes is marked the more effective work of a respiratory chain what can be called of "paradoxical effect" of adaptation to hypoxia [29].

In 1979 the rising activity of antioxidizing enzymes of tissues in response to periodic hypoxia effect was described. This phenomenon is named "paradoxical reaction of intracellular mechanisms of protection from Oxygen" [20]. It is shown, that the fortnight adaptation of rats to INH resulted in 20-33 % augmentation of capacity of antioxidant system while rising the content of radicals in blood plasma on 15 %. Thus the acceleration of formation of final products of a SEX, witnessing about a free-radical damage of tissues is not revealed [10,16]. Not adapted rats showed the drop, and adapted - the rise of activity of cytochrome C - oxidasa (a mitochondrial respiratory chain) and glutationreductasa (antioxidant system) in a liver, brain and heart. It reduces a possibility of acute activation of a SEX under the influence of an acute hypoxia. The rate of consumption of Oxygen at trained rats is higher, than when under control, however, the degree of coordination of respiration and oxidizing phosphorilation did not change [38].

The monooxigetic system of a liver reacts to adaptation to a hypobaric hypoxia by the drop of fermentative activity of cytochrome Ð-450, Amidopyrin-N-demethylasa and anilinhydroxylasa [73]. It is known, that it has similarity in a number of functional characteristics with immunological system and that between them exist reciprocal interactions. For example, inductors of cytochrome Ð-450 show an inhibiting effect on Immunological system and stimulators of immunity oppress monooxigetic activity. The biological sense of this relation of two systems is not clear yet. It is possible to suppose, that the drop of activity of Ð-450 is accompanied by rising of immunity, which is marked at adaptation to hypoxia [13,39,43].

It is revealed, that during adaptation to a hypobaric hypoxia a weakening of the functional activity of T-lymphocytes is observed while the number of T- and in B-cells remains constant. A level of immunoglobulins A and Ì in serum of a blood is raising [92]. Several authors mark an intensifying cytophagous ability of reticulo-endothelial system during acclimatization to height at the expense of rising the activity of its tissue without a hypertrophy [13]. On the 30-th day of adaptation to INH the intensity of the phagocytosis was lowered, while the completeness of the phagocytosis was enlarged [43].

It is fixed, that the hypoxic stimulation is capable to raise a resistance of an organism to pharmacological agents that have a toxic action (Mexaminum, Cyclophosphanum etc.) [22,56]. It allows to admit a possibility of decrease of by-effects of medicines at their simultaneous prescription with acclimatization to hypoxia. However the drop of efficiency of medical preparations during their combined use with hypoxytherapy does not occur. Actually a potentiation of effect has a place [25, 48].

The influence of hypoxia on a number of processes in the central nervous system [17] is proved. The augmentation of rate of a cerebral blood flow in hypoxic conditions is underlined [26]. After adaptation to hypoxia during a submicroscopy of a somatosensory cerebral cortex of cat there were observed the augmentation of density of barbs of dendrites pyramidal neurones, complicating of the bards device, augmentation of extent active of synaptic contacts and electron density of areas of a matrix of cytoplasma [27]. The adaptation of nervous cells to hypoxia is accompanied by rising of the contents of RNA in them [39]. It testifies to mobilization of metabolic processes and to the functional activity of a brain.

The analysis of electroencephalograms in the moment and after respiration by GHM-10 (urgent adaptation), has revealed moderate generalized changes characterized as a slow wavy inhibition [3]. The stimulation of sinocarotid and aortal chemoceptors, apparently, results in activation of a reticular formation of a trunk (trunk), which brakes a cortex [82]. It is proved by the absence of a beta rhythm during hypoxia after a denervation of chemoceptors and operative separation of a reticular formation from the large of hemispheres. During the long-term adaptation to hypoxia the stimulating action of GHM-10 on a cortex of the large hemispheres is described, that is shown by activization of the central nervous system [54]. In the experiment with electrodes implanted into a brain of the monkeys, it is shown, that a coronal cortex, hippocampus and hypothalamus are the most sensitive structures to the drop of Oxygen [62]. It is necessary to suppose, that the named formations will be the zones of the applied hypoxic influence in a brain. Taking into account, that a cortex and limbic system are the supreme parts of functional system of emotional stress [39], it is possible to prove the influence of intermittened normobaric hypoxia on psycho-emotional reactions of a person. After a long periodic adaptation to insufficiency of Oxygen in extreme conditions the leveling of differences on thresholds of aggression in groups with low and high resistance to hypoxia have been revealed. High-resistant rats show the improvement in carring out of task. Low-resistant showed the most expressive and long changes a EEG of a neocortex and ancient brain [29,31].

There are individual works about application of adaptation to hypoxia of the people with dystonias of vegetative system. Series of works are devoted to treatment by a method of hypoxytherapy of s number of psychosomatic diseases - idiopathic hypertensia, neurosolike condition [48].

In the given brief review, some basic adaptation mechanisms of an organism detoxic systems and immunity are described. Above-stated is the basis to the wide use of hypoxic factor in practical medicine [53,61,64]. Today INH is successfully applied in many countries in treatment of diseases of lungs, cardiovascular system, gastrointestinal path, neurological diseases etc.

Intermittent Normobaric Hypoxytherapy (INH) has proved its high efficiency, but as well as any method, requires the further development, which first of all should be directed to the individualization of regimens of hypoxic influence. During hypoxytherapy realization the following things are of no less importance: the estimation of duration of an individual cycle of medical hypoxic influence and the time of rest between cycles; the control of regulation of parameters of respiration according to the estimation of degree of expressiveness of hyperventilation syndrome (HVS); dynamic reactions of cardiovascular and autonomous nervous system. The monitoring of the given parameters in a real time scale and management of process of hypoxytherapy according to changes of functional parameters will allow to increase qualitatively the efficiency of hypoxytherapy and to create a new method - Resonant Normobaric Hypoxytherapy (RNH).

À.Ya. Chizhov and coauthors in the 80s of the last century [61,64]. However the choice of individual modes of hypoxytherapy should be determined by adaptive capacities of each patient. Therefore it is believed reasonable to continue the search of informative method, which would reflect the structure of individual hypoxic biorhythm incorporated in each organism of the mammals during embryo period of development. The most perspective method in this direction seems to be researches of variability of a cardiac rate (HRV).

The first domestic researches HRV were carried out under the leadership of R.M. Bayevskiy [7,8], at the end of the 50-th years. Now the definition of HRV is recognized the most informative non-invasive method of a quantitative estimation of a vegetative regulation of a heart rate [76,88]. It is considered, that the drop of HRV parameters testifies to the infringement of the vegetative control of heart activity and is adverse for the future [74,75,93].

Healthy young people and sportsmen show the best HRV parameters [89], - the patients with various organic diseases of heart, including the rhythm infringements show intermediate results [87]. The patients who have endured the episodes of a fibrillation of ventricles show the lowest HRV parameters [85].

The active HRV study by the cardiologists all over the world has resulted in the necessity of standardization of a terminology, development of optimum methods of measuring of HRV, and also description of parameters HRV and their characteristics in norm and at pathological condition. The European Society of Cardiology and the North American Society of Pacing and Electrophysiology develops the standards on measurements, physiological interpreting and clinical use of HRV in 1996 (further - Standards) [77].

The hypoxia can be surveyed as stress factor. A regulation of a heart rate, therefore, it is possible to expect remarkable of changes of HRV in response to hypoxia. Except the changes of HRV during hypoxia of a fetus, that have become classical observations, [86], there are series of researches confirming it. While the acclimatization to the Alpine climate it is shown, that at height more than 5000 m above sea level occurs a remarkable drop of capacity of HF spectrum and augmentation of the proportion of LF/HF in a position on the back, while there were no remarkable changes of these parameters in a sitting position. Thus there is revealed the authentic rising of the central frequency of HF peak from 0.25 to 0.32 Hz. The acclimatization to hypoxia (at height about 2000 m for 10 days, and then at height of about 5000 m within one month) did not result in restoration of parameters, usual for a sea level. It has allowed coming to a conclusion, that «hypoxia causes the shift in interaction of sympatic and parasympatic sections in rest to the advantage of dominance sympatic sections, similar to that that was observed on a sea level in a sitting position. The acclimatization to hypoxia does not change interaction of sections autonomic system»[90]. During the application of a special technique of HRV analysis, allowing to allocate its harmonic and "irregular" components it is shown, that hypoxic effects begin to effect HRV only on the of height more than 3500 m above a sea level. Until this height only the influence of exercise stress on HRV is shown [95]

Researches of HRV during the episodes of night dispnoe of the patients IHD, when the saturation of hemoglobin is reduced, (what is comparable to the influence of hypoxia), have revealed remarkable changes of ratio between high- and low-frequency components of HRV (spectral analysis) [83]. Moreover, the observed shifts depended on the size of the drop of a fraction of emission of a left ventricle (i.e. from an expressiveness of a heart insufficiency). It is remarkable, that practically half of the examined patients showed the spontaneous rhythmic episodes of saturation reduce for up to 20 min duration were observed, and the period of these episodes was individual.

It is well known, that during hypoxia HR increases and HRV decreases. Similar to it, but different in size, the effect of hypoxia is shown while working with the patients after a bilateral transplantation of lungs (i.e. At a total denervation of lungs), while the patients with a total denervation of heart (after the transplantation) gave a less expressed tachycardia to hypoxia. It allows to conclude, that the reflexes of lungs participate in a vegetative regulation of HR and can influence HRV [78].

Hypoxia has smaller individual fluctuations, than the influence of hypercapnia, in response to which there was observed both the increase of HR, and its decrease. In response to the hypoxic influence there was observed the augmentation of HR from 72 up to 89.5 in min (25 %) average in group. The similar results are also discovered in the search of markers of unsatisfactory acclimatization to hypoxia [1].

It is known, that the realization of sessions of INH, conjugates with remarkable reactions of cardiorespiratory and autonomous nervous systems and with the changes of a functional condition of systems of auto regulation. However until now there were no researches based on monitoring autoregulatory reactions of cardiorespiratory and independent nervous system during hypoxytherapy of sessions. In particular, it is not determined, what changes of vegetative regulation occur during the development and suppression of hyperventilate syndrome, which enough frequently accompanies hypoxytherapy. Besides it remains not found out yet, how happens the interaction between individual physiological autoregulatory hypoxic cycle and the cycle of imposed hypoxic influence. In this connection, there were the following problems of research which have been carried out for a substantiation of a method of resonant interrupted normobaric hypoxytherapy:

(A) Definition of laws of changes of a vegetative regulation at development of hyperventilate syndrome (HVS), which, as a rule, is present or can develop at realization of hypoxytherapy, and also substantiation of methods of suppression of HVS;

(B) Study of interaction between individual physiological autoregulatory hypoxic cycle and the cycle of imposed hypoxic influence;

(C) Substantiation of the methodical decisions allowing to increase the efficiency of hypoxytherapy on the basis of suppression of HVS and optimization of interaction between individual physiological autoregulatory hypoxic cycle (iah-cycle) and a cycle of external hypoxic influence.

There were performed the researches of study of 60 people (39 men, 21 women), which were divided into 2 groups: the 1st group (30 men) - practically healthy people at the age of 30- 40 years. Out of them there were 20 men, 10 women. Average age of the group - 36,3 + -2.1 years; the 2nd group (30 people) - people with neurogenic infringements of hemodynamics aged 30- 40 years. Out of them there were 19 men, 11 women. Average age in group - 35,8 + - 2,2 years. A condition of function of myocardium is determined by a method of electrocardiography and HRV. For the control of cardiac properties of a pulmonary hypertension there were estimated the dynamics of PII, III, the expressiveness of P-pulmonale, the degree of the change of tooth S5-6, and also the dynamics of the complex rSR in abduction V1 [57]. To estimate the vegetative control of a myocardium the international statistical parameters of HRV were chosen: SDNN index - standard deviation of normal RR-intervals of 5 min of recording, SDNN120 - standard deviation of normal 120 RR-intervals, RMSSD - standard deviation of differences between the next normal RR-intervals for 5 min of recording and RMSSD120 - standard deviation of differences between the next normal 120 RR-interval. The meanings of a parameter SDNN index and SDNN120 parameter, similar to it, are determined by ability of a myocardium to react to influences of all sections of vegetative nervous system. The dynamic downstroke of the given parameters specifies augmentation of a load at a myocardium. The meanings of a parameter RMSSD and RMSSD120 are determined mainly by degree of vagus control of a myocardium. The dynamic of the drop of these parameters specifies the drop of vagus control of a myocardium and augmentation of degree of influence of sympatic system on the work of a heart. For the estimation of function of cardiorespiratory system there were used HRV parameters reflecting the interaction of system heart - lung. The parameter describing the interaction of the system heart - lung was the parameter "the amount of information" (AI), necessary for organization of adequate interaction between vessel and respiratory center. AI estimates the degree of a regularity of waves of respiratory sinus arrhythmia and LF waves.

For the definition of AI the spectrum of HRV is calculated. The spectral capacity of waves of a respiratory sinus arrhythmia and LF waves is determined. The parameter (AI) is calculated, determining how much the configuration of a spectrum of waves of a respiratory sinus arrhythmia and HF waves is different from an energetically peer spectrum of "white noise" under the formula:

$$KH = \log_2 \frac{L}{L - \dfrac{\sum_{n=1}^{L} \text{abs}\left[(1/L) * \sum_{n=1}^{L} Sn - sn\right]}{2 * (1/L) * \sum_{n=1}^{L} Sn}}$$

KU - the amount of the information in bits,

L - the amount of points, which define the capacity of spectrum

Sn - spectral density in point n, taking place on the L-segment.

AI is as more, as more stable the amplitude and the period of waves of a respiratory sinus arrhythmia and HF waves, which reflect the interaction between the appropriate vegetative centers. Below is given the table of conformity of meanings of AI and of functional condition of cardiorespiratory system.

Table 1.

The quantity of the information	Functional condition
is less 1 bit	Decompensation
1,0-1,5 bit	Essentially reduced
1,6-2,0 bit	Reduced
2,1-2,5 bit	Normal more
more 2,5 bit	Optimum

The way of definition of AI on a basis of HRV parameters is offered by Bludov À.À and is described in materials of the Patent of Russian Federation on the invention [1] 2039523, 1995.

During the last 20-25 years in the world literature the increasing attention is given to neurogene hyperventilation [24]. This pathology being a consequence of stress trauma of the central nervous system (CNS) is wide-spreads and seldom is diagnosticated. In the process of accumulation of an actual material about influence of a hyperventilation (HV) on an organism it has become one of the of most serious medical problems.

According to the opinion of the psychiatrists, HVS concerns to depressions with lingering flow without psychotic exacerbations and has a rod psychosomatic structure [45].

The influence of hypocapnia is displayed in general and regional changes of circulation, the decrease of blood pressure because of some weakening of heart activity and, probably, at the expense of decrease of resistance of muscle vessels and some organs, considerate dropping of cerebral blood flow as a result of fall a general blood pressure and narrowing of brain vessels. Volume of blood per minute during hypocapnia usually does not change, but can slightly be enlarged or be decreased; coronary blood flow is lowered a little.

The hypocapnia can influence negatively the acceptability of hypoxia by an organism owing to adverse redistribution of blood flow (deterioration of a blood supply of brain and heart), and also as a result of rising of tissues needs in Oxygen. The expense of tension reduction of carbon dioxide in alveoluses the partial saturation of blood and tissues by Oxygen grows.

The influence of hyperventilation is shown by infringements of cardiorespiratory system. There are numerous facts on pathological changes of coronary blood flow, and also of the tonus of vessels in other basins of circulation [15]. At the same time the cardiac aspect of a problem in the domestic literature is covered unsufficiently. There are only individual works devoted to infringement of respiration during idiopathic hypertensia (IH) and changes of ECG at acute hyperventilation test [46]. Within the framework of known therapeutic clauses HVS is surveyed as a whole, but the pathological alterations concerning the cardiorespiratory system are not of specially discussed. In this connection a wide circle of pulmonogists and cardiologists know a little about HVS. At the same time, often when the cardiologists for the first time face the patients that suffer from neurogene hyperventilation, they frequently pay the main attention of cardio-vascular symptoms, ignoring respiratory infringements [81]. Clinical cardiologists find the greatest interest in the chronic form of neurogene hyperventilation accompanying that uninfectious cardiac pathology, in which genesis of the determining role is played by psycho-emotional trauma of the central nervous system - idiopathic hypertensia, vegetative-vascular dystonia [15].

Neurogene hyperventilation exists in paroxysmal and chronic forms. It is necessary to note the clinical form of paroxysmal neurogene hyperventilation known as an atypical asthma, when alongside with intensifying of respiration its difficulty and participation of additional muscles in the act of respiration are marked. There are so-called hyperventilation equivalents - periodic sighs, yawning, tussiculation. The special researches prove, that a pathogeny of these displays - hyperventilation [14,15].

Hyperventilational rising of tonus and the spasms of coronary arteries and arterioles reduce coronary blood flow and result in hypoxia of myocardium both at [79].

The expressiveness of hypoxic changes of myocardium at HV is aggravated by augmentation of consumption of Oxygen, which is common for hyperadrenergia. The hypoxia aggravates electrolyte infringements caused by hyperventilation; the deficiency of ATP leads to hypodynamia of myofibrils and their abasement from the contractive act, development of cardiofibrosis and the decrease of inotropism of myocardium [84]. So, hyperventilation infringements, creating those vicious circles, result in neurogene damage of cardiorespiratory system. These damages are expressed in predilection to bronchospasm and infringement of drainage function of bronchuses, electrical instability of heart, hyperdynamism and rigidity of myocardium, development of cardiosclerosis, vasopressor reactions of coronary arteries and arterioles, peripheral arteries [80].

In our researches during artificial hyperventilation the HRV of the examinees of the 2nd group which were in a relatively calm condition, was characterized by a rigidity of heart rhythm in comparison with the 1st group. The received data specify, that the average meaning of a parameter SDNN120 after a 30-minute research (reference value of a parameter SDNN120) authentically differed (p < 0,05) among each other and were the following in the groups: in the 1st group - 57,1 + - 5,2 ms, in the 2nd - 37,8 + -2,9 ms. By the end of the first minute of hyperventilation SDNN120 was authentically enlarged at the expense of augmentation of amplitude of waves of a respiratory sinus arrhythmia as in the 1st (from 57,1 + - 5,2 ms up to 87,2 + - 8,9 ms), and in the 2nd (from 37,8 + - 2,9 ms up to 58,2 + - 5,2 ms) group (ð < 0,05). During hyperventilation lasting for more than 5 minutes, all the patients of the 2nd group showed a combined change of two parameters: the decrease of HRV - SDNN120 was authentically (ð < 0,05) decreased below the reference value and the increase of the current frequency of cardiac reductions. SDNN120 of the patients of the 1st group was also decreased on the fifth minute, but only 20 men has the decrease lower than a reference value SDNN120 (66,7 % of cases). During hyperventilation lasting for more than 10 minutes the examinees of the 1st group showed the decrease of a parameter SDNN120 lower than a reference value in all cases. The augmentation of current HR was marked in all cases, both in the 1st and in the 2nd group. Thus 14 people. (46,7 %) of the 1st group and 27 people (90,0 %) of the 2nd one had the augmentation of HR on the 45th second of hyperventilation; 28 people (93,3 %) of the 1st group and 30 people (100,0 %) of the 2nd group - on the 60th second; all examinees either of the 1st or of the 2nd group - on 75th second.

The received results testify that the caused hyperventilation essentially alters vegetative regulation of cardiorespiratory system, particularly in a large measure if the parameter is initially misbalanced.

It is well known, that a HRV marker of activity of parasympatic section of autonomic system is the degree of expressiveness of waves of respiratory sinus arrhythmia [7]. The initial rising of HRV during the first minutes of hyperventilation at the expense of augmentation of respiratory sinus arrhythmia, which was observed both in a group of healthy examinees, and in a group of those with neurogene infringements of hemodynamics, specifies the presence of a phase of primary activation of parasympatic section of autonomic system. As a rule, the maximal meanings of a parameter SDNN120 were recorded on the first minute of hyperventilation. Subsequently HRV was decreased, and the decrease was faster in the 2nd group.

The given regularity allows to assume, that the hyperventilation causes an excessive stimulation of parasympatic section of autonomic system, with its subsequent attrition. As was supposed, the emaciation of parasympatic section of autonomic system, found during the study of the examinees of the 2nd group are higher, than those of the "healthy" group. Apparently, complex and various symptomatology the accompanies the hyperventilational set of symptoms [14,15], in the greater degree is connected with then attrition of a neural component of parasympatic section of autonomic system.

If the expressiveness of respiratory sinus arrhythmia is a standard HRV marker of activity of parasympatic section of autonomic system, then, concerning the marker of activity of sympatic section there is no unique opinion. In the research that we have carried out the change of current HR was chosen as the marker of change of activity of sympatic section of autonomic system.

All the examinees during hyperventilation lasting for more than 75 sec, showed the augmentation of current HR comparing to the initial meaning in a condition of relative rest. A priori it is possible to assume, that the augmentation of current HR during a proceeding hyperventilation is connected exactly with an attrition of parasympatic section of autonomic system, however the received data deny the given hypothesis. The augmentation of the current HR had always been registered before there was observed a decrease of HRV at the expense of decrease of amplitude of waves of respiratory sinus arrhythmia. The special attention should be drawn to the existence of the period, during which the beginning of a phase of activation of sympatic section is combined with properties of high activity of parasympatic section of autonomic system, i.e. the period of simultaneous high activity of the autonomous nervous system as a whole. The period of activation of autonomic system in the 1st group started later and was longer (ð < 0,05), that probably is connected with the greater resistance of parasympatic system to hyperventilation and the later beginning of a phase of activation of sympatic section of autonomic system in response to hyperventilation of the examinees of the 1st group in comparison with those of the 2nd group.

The received data have allowed to reveal a triad of HRV properties caused by hyperventilation:

(À) Initial increasing of HRV

(B) Increasing of current HR;

(C) The appearance of the tendency to decrease HRV to the meaning lower than initial.

The hyperventilation essentially changes vegetative maintenance of cardiorespiratory system. Thus the changes have a phase character: a phase of initial activation of parasympatic system; the interphase period of simultaneous high activity of parasympatic and sympatic system, the phase of activation of sympatic and the drain of parasympatic system. The people with neurogene infringements of hemodynamics the duration of the period of simultaneous activation of parasympatic and sympatic sections of autonomic system was exposed to considerable reduction.

As hyperventilation, as was shown by results of the previous research, caused essential infringements of the vegetative control of cardiorespiratory system, it was of no less importance to estimate the opportunities of effective use of respiratory training for achievement of the opposite effect, i.e. For the achievement of vegetative relaxation and restoration of the vegetative control of cardiorespiratory system. During the respiratory training the examinee was offered to synchronize the parameters of arbitrary respiration with settled optimum parameters of respiratory of cycle reflected on the screen of the monitor of the computer and allowing to suppress spontaneously developing HVS.

The patients either of the 1st, or of the 2nd groups after the realization of respiratory training for 30 minutes, had their SDNN120 authentically enlarged compared to a reference value, at the decrease of current HR compared to initial HR. The average meanings of parameters SDNN120 in the 1st group have increased in 1.44 times (ð < 0.05), in the second - in 1.52 times (ð < 0.05).

The meanings of the parameter SDNN120 in the second group at the end of the 30-th minute of respiratory training did not differ considerably from the similar parameters of the 1st group, which took place in condition of relative rest. The received results testify that the effective respiratory training allows to significantly reduce the degree of tension of autonomic system. It is important to note, that after the respiratory training, the differences between average meaning of parameter SDNN120 in condition of relative rest in the of 1st group and the meaning of parameter SDNN120 after a 30-minute respiratory training in the 2nd group stop being statistically important.

The given fact specifies that the respiratory training allows the people with neurogene infringements of regulation of hemodynamics to reach the degree of vegetative relaxation common for healthy examinees, without using pharmacological agents. The effect of vegetative relaxation is realized due to use of a biological feedback and the dynamic presence of optimum parameters of external respiration.

Our research has allowed us to reveal high physiological possibilities of use of respiratory device for achievement of effective vegetative relaxation and restoration of the control of cardiorespiratory system from the side of autonomic system.

The researched of the both groups the changes of some HRV parameters and the parameters of partial pressure of Oxygen in tissues, submitted to cyclic artificially caused by hypoxic hypoxia. Taking into account cycled character of the hypoxic influence: 5 minutes of hypoxic influence, 5 minutes of respiration by atmospheric air, - the revealed periodicity of change of some HRV parameters, multiple to 10 minutes become explained.

During the analysis of dynamics of HRV parameters, it was revealed, that the most trust-worthy parameters that reflect periodicity of artificially caused, and accordingly, the periodicity of change of partial pressure of Oxygen in tissues are the parameters RMSSD120 and LF/HF ratio. And the decrease of parameter RMSSD120 in all cases (100 %) coincided with the period of hypoxic influence and, as a consequence, with augmentation of tissue hypoxia. The ascending of parameter RMSSD120 in all cases (100 %) initial tissue Ðî2. The parameter LF/HF ratio changed twice during one hypoxic cycle. The maximums of parameter LF/HF ratio corresponded to every extremum of the diagram of change of RMSSD120 in 54 cases out of 60 (90 %), and when the standard program filters flattening casual fluctuations of parameters were applied - in 100 % of cases. The amplitude of fluctuation of parameter RMSSD120 was 28,5 + -2,8%. The parameter RMSSD120 reflects the degree of a loading on cardiorespiratory system and, in the large degree, the vagus control of myocardium. Therefore the decrease of the given parameter in the period of hypoxic stress is a physiologically natural phenomenon.

On the other hand, the change of LF/HF parameter ratio reflects short-term adaptive reactions, mainly from the side of cardiovascular system. The revealed augmentation of the given parameter in the initial period of hypoxic stress and during the termination of hypoxic influence testifies the activation of short-term adaptive reactions connected with the change of dynamics of tension of Oxygen in tissues. The received data do not contradict the data received at research of dynamics of change of HRV parameters at the occurrence of circulatory hypoxia of myocardium during the development and the subsequent cupping of stenocardia attack of the patients with ischemic heart disease. The data, received in the present research, testify that:

(A) The dynamic change of HRV parameters naturally reflects a difficult process of change of regulatory reactions when the tension of Oxygen in tissues changes.

(B) The marker of periodic change of tension of Oxygen in tissues can be a periodic change of RMSSD120 parameter;

(C) The change of LF/HF ratio parameter can serve the marker of trans-processes in the cycle "hypoxia - restoration - hypoxia"

The researched of the both groups the changes of HRV parameters - hypoxic markers (RMSSD120, LF/HF ratio), under condition of absence of imposed cyclic hypoxic influence, had the cyclic character of their own. As the process of maintenance of adequate partial pressure of Oxygen in tissues is autoregulatory, as well as any other process of maintenance of vital constants, the dynamics of HRV parameters - hypoxic markers - reflected the dynamics in the processes of autoregulation of physiological hypoxic cycle.

The LF/HF ratio parameter had the period of fluctuation twice less, than the period of fluctuation RMSSD120. The maximums of LF/HF parameter ratio corresponded to every extremum of the diagram of change RMSSD120. The given compliances were similar to the ratio of these parameters a at cyclic hypoxic stress. The amplitude of fluctuation of RMSSD120 parameter in rest were 15,1 + -2,7 %, while, the amplitude of fluctuation of this parameter at cyclic hypoxic stress GHA-10 in a mode of INH was statistically considerably bigger - 28,5 + -2,8 % (ð < 0,01). The average period of cyclic change of RMSSD120 parameter in the group of healthy people has made 612 + -42 sec., in the group of researched with neurogene infringements of regulation of hemodynamics - 543 + - 48 sec.

Oxygen in tissues, is adjusted through complex, frequently multilevel, systems of an auto regulation. Therefore the revealed regularities, in particular, periodicity and the ratio of fluctuations of HRV parameters - of hypoxic markers (HM) are physiologically reasonable. Taking into account the given reasons, and also the stability of amplitude and the period of parameters fluctuations, it is possible to make the reasonable assumption, that the fluctuations of HRV parameters - HM - reflect the process of autoregulation within the structure of functioning of individual physiological autoregular hypoxic cycle (iah-cycle). It is necessary to note, that the revealed periods of iah-cycles have the same order, as empirically chosen periods of modes of INH.

There is no doubt, the periodicity of fluctuation of RMSSD120 parameter is influenced by multilevel autoregulartory systems, with the principles of functioning are practically not studied. Therefore within the structure of the given research it is impossible to make certain conclusions about interrelation between neurogene infringements of hemodynamics and the period of an individual iah-cycle.

The revealed trust-worthy difference between the amplitude of fluctuations of RMSSD120 parameter during realization of INH and in rest specifies the large activity of regulatory systems that keep partial pressure of Oxygen in tissues constant in conditions of hypoxic hypoxia in comparison with the activity of autoregulatory systems outside without hypoxic stress.

The received results testify that:

(A) HRV parameters - are hypoxic markers (RMSSD120 and LF/HF ratio) out of artificially caused hypoxic stress possess natural autonomous cyclic character, that reflects processes of autoregulation of maintenance of adequate partial pressure of Oxygen in tissues of an organism;

(B) The amplitude of fluctuations of dynamic diagram of HRV parameters - hypoxic markers - reflects the degree of activity of processes of autoregulation providing the maintenance of adequate partial pressure of Oxygen;

(C) The numerical meanings of the periods of individual physiological autoregular hypoxic cycle have the same order as the periods hypoxic stress offered at realization of INH, but at the same time the traditional mode of INH (5 min - respiration with GHA-10, 5 min - rest) does not coincide with hypoxic own biorhythm.

The amplitude of fluctuation of RMSSD120 parameter during hypoxytherapy in a traditional mode "T" was 28,5 + -2,8 %, when during the synchronized mode "S" it was - 45,1 + -3,9 % (ð < 0,01). The augmentation of SDNN index parameter after the session of hypoxytherapy in a mode "Ò" was 16,5 + - 1,6 %, while at the use of a mode "S" it was - 23,1 + -1,8 % (ð < 0,01). The similar augmentation of RMSSD120 parameter was, accordingly, 11,8 + -1,5 % (mode "Ò") and 18,2 + -2,1 % (mode "Ñ") (ð < 0,05). During the research of cyclic structure of hypoxytherapy, carried out in modes "S" and "T", there were not any trustworthy differences revealed either in time of the total hypoxic stress, or in the duration of hypoxic influence within a hypoxic cycle. The time of hypoxic stress in a mode "S" was 29,5 + - 2,6 minutes, in a mode "T" - 30 minutes. The average period of a cycle " hypoxia - the rest " in a mode "S" was 612 + -42 seconds, in a mode "T" - 600 seconds. The period of hypoxic influence within a hypoxic a cycle in a mode "S" was 292 + -22 seconds, in a mode "T" -300 seconds.

Authentically large amplitude of fluctuations of RMSSD120 parameter and the augmentation of SDNN index parameter during the realization of hypoxytherapy in a mode "S" specifies a more expressed activation of autoregular processes in the given mode without the augmentation of total time and the period of hypoxic stress. This fact is natural and is connected with the fact that the fluctuations of HRV parameters determined by a periodic hypoxia are summarized with autoregulatory fluctuations of the given parameters. The given phenomenon - "of summarization of autoregulatory and imposed fluctuations" is specific to a mode "S" and is not observed during hypoxytherapy in a mode "T". Moreover, in certain cases during hypoxytherapy in a mode "T" it is possible autoregular fluctuations are suppressed by imposed hypoxic fluctuations. It is obvious, that for some time the given phenomenon can cause a desynchronization of autoregulatory processes and reduce a total positive effect of hypoxic stimulation. The confirmation of the assumptions stated above - is the fact of authentically smaller augmentation of RMSSD120 parameter after the session of hypoxytherapy in a mode "T". This research has allowed to reveal the following regularities:

(À) Hypoxytherapy in a mode of synchronization of autoregulatory and imposed hypoxic fluctuations causes a more expressed activation of autoregulatory systems providing an adequate regulation of partial pressure of Oxygen without increase of the total time and duration of hypoxic stimulation at the expense of the phenomena "of summarization of autoregulatory and imposed hypoxic fluctuations", specific for a mode "Ñ";

(B) The mode of synchronization autoregulatory and imposed hypoxic fluctuations provides the maximal unloading and augmentation of the level of vegetative control of cardiorespiratory system after the session of hypoxytherapy..

During the respiration with hypoxic admixture GHA-10, the time of the decrease of ÒÑÐÎ2 AND THE TIME OF THE DECREASE OF RMSSD120 PARAMETER PRACTICALLY DID NOT DIFFER (ð> 0,05). This fact specifies that the time of adaptation of regulation from the side of autonomic system of cardiorespiratory system to the hypoxic stress coincides completely with the time of the increase of Ðî2 in peripheric tissues of an organism.

During the research of time of the decrease of RMSSD120 parameter without hypoxic stress within the study of duration of the hypoxic phase of physiological autoregulatory hypoxic cycle, there was also revealed the absence of authentic differences either in the relation to the time of a tension reduction of Oxygen in tissues, measured by transcutanic method, or to the time of the decrease of RMSSD120parameter, measured also is during the respiration with GHA-10.

Nevertheless, the duration of a hypoxic phase of iah-cycle was still longer, than the time of the decrease of RMSSD120 parameter at hypoxic stress. Cardiorespiratory system, does not cause infringements of temporary characteristics of autoregulatory processes of maintenance of tension of Oxygen in tissues either while studying healthy people (group I), or - the people with neurogene infringements of hemodynamics (group II) and, consequently, is enough physiological.

The carried out researches within a clinico-physiological substantiation of the method of resonant normobaric hypoxytherapy have allowed to reveal the following most important regularities:

1. Hyperventilation causes infringements of the control of autonomic system of cardiorespiratory system.
2. Controllable use of the respiratory device in a mode of biological feedback allows to essentially increase the degree of relaxation and the level of the control of autonomic system of cardiorespiratory system, to stop the hyperventilation set of symptoms at the expense of suppression of peak, frequency and phase dispnoe, and also at the expense of synchronization of HR and the frequency of respiration in optimum ratio. The above-stated facts define the necessity of inclusion into a method of resonant normobaric hypoxytherapy (RNH) of the first element - the controllable use of the respiratory device in a mode of biological feedback.
3. The maintenance of an adequate tension of Oxygen in tissues of vital organs is an autoregulatory process, which can be authentically described during the analysis of HRV parameters - hypoxic markers.
4. The realization of hypoxytherapy with application of GHM-10 in a mode of synchronization of autoregulatory and imposed hypoxic fluctuations, causes more expressed activation of

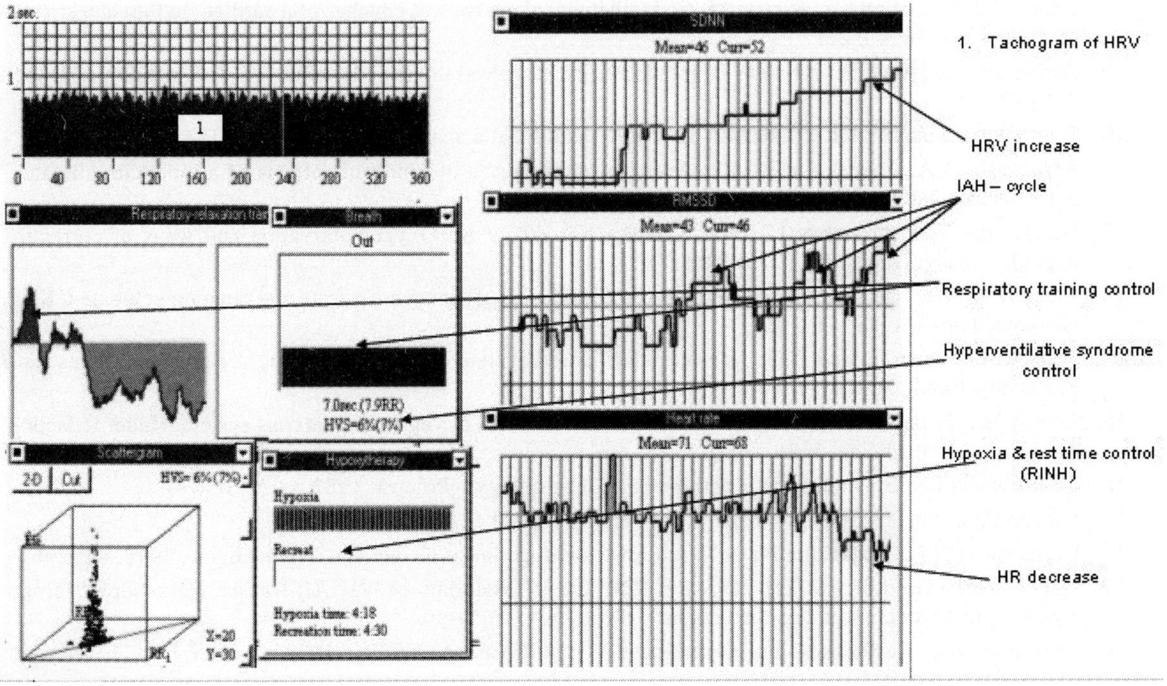

autoregulatory systems providing adequate regulation of partial pressure of Oxygen without the increase of the total time and the duration of hypoxic stimulation at the expense of a phenomena "of summarization of autoregulatory and imposed hypoxic fluctuations". The mode of synchronization of autoregulatory and imposed hypoxic fluctuations provides the maximal increase of a control level of autonomic system of cardiorespiratory system either during or after the session of hypoxytherapy.

The given regularities determine the necessity of inclusion in a method RNH the second element - the realization of hypoxytherapy in a mode of synchronization (summarization) of autoregulatory and imposed hypoxic fluctuations.

The List of the Literature

1. Agadjanyan N.À., Jelfimov À.I. - Function of an organism in conditions of a hypoxia of a hypercapnia. Ì., Medicine, 1986.-P 270.
2. Agadjanyan N.À., Krasnikov N.P., Polunin I.N. Physiological role of Carbonic dioxide and serviceability of the man. - Moscow. - 1995. – P 188.
3. Agadjanyan N.À., Old Å.Â. Bullet. exper. biol. Honey. 1991, ¹ 1, P. 11.
4. Agadjanyan N.À., Chizhov À.Yr. // Fisiologichny magazine - 1996. - Volume 42, N 3-4. - P.95-96.
5. Ànokhin M.I., Dairova Ð.À., Snegotskaya Ì.Í etc. // Materials of VII All-Russia workshops "ecologo-physiological problems of acclimatization ". - M.: 1994. - P.17.
6. Babenko À.P., Êazantseva S.Ò., Romanova J.V. Etc. // Materials of VII All-Russia workshops " ecologo-physiological problems of adaptation ". - M.: 1994. - P.24-25.
7. Baevsky R. Ì. Forecasting of condition on the verge of norm and pathology. - M.: medicine, 1979. – P 295.
8. Baevsky R. Ì., Kirilov Î. I., Kletskin S. Z. Mathematical analysis of changes of a cardiac rhythm at a stress. - M.: science, 1984. – P 221.
9. Barbashova Z.I. Acclimatization to a hypoxia and its(her) physiological mechanisms. - Ì. Ë.: edition ÀÍ USSR, 1960.-P 216.
10. White À.Ã., Gukasov V.Ì., Chukaev S.À. // a Physiological magazine. - 1992. - N 5. – P .73-76.
11. Berezovsky V.À., Deineka V.G. - Physiological mechanisms of sanogenic effects of a mountain climate. - Kiev: Íàóêîâà äóìêà, 1988.- P 224.
12. Berezovsky V.À., Levashev Ì.I., Portnichenko V.I. Etc. // An Oxygen starvation and ways of correction hypoxia. - Kiev: Íàóê.äóìêà, 1990. - P.68-75.
13. Berezovsky V.À., Deinega V.Ã. Physiological mechanisms of sanogenic effects of a mountain climate // Kiev: Naukova dumka, 1988. – P 223.
14. Vein A.M., Voznesenskaya T.G., Vorobjeva Î.V. Etc. Vegetative frustration: clinic, treatment, diagnostics // M.: honey. Èíôîðì. Agency, 1998, P. 189-209.
15. Vein A.M., Voznesenskaya T.G., Golubev V.L. Etc. Diseases of vegetative nervous system. Under redaction. À.Ì.Vein. - M.: medicine, 1991. – P 624.
16. Voskresenski Î.N. Bioantioxydants and freeradical pathology. - Poltava, 1987. - P.5-11.
17. Gaiduk Ph.Ì., Shalkevitch V.B., Koziro V.I. Patent. USSR ¹ 1223919, 1986.
18. Garmasheva N.L., Konstantinova N.N. Introduction in perinatal medicine. - M.: medicine, 1978. – P. 296.
19. Gebel G.Ya., Golostenova L.Ì., Dasaev A.N. Etc. // Materials of VII All-Russia workshops "eclogo-physiological problems of acclimatization ". - M.: 1994. - ñ.59-60.
20. Gerasimov À.Ì., Kovalenko Å.À., Kasatkina N.V. Etc. // Äîêë. ÀÍ USSR. - 1979. - 244, N 2. - ñ.492-495.

21. Jelfimov À.I., Agadjanyan N.À., Shevchenko L.V. // Fisiologichny magazine - 1996. - Volume 42, N 3-4. - ñ.102.
22. Zakoshikov K.Ph. Àâòîðåô. Äèññ. Êàíä. Honey. Sciences, Obninsk, 1986, P. 21.
23. Karash U.Ì., Strelkov R.B., Chizhov À.Yr. Normobaric hypoxia in treatment, prophylaxis and aftertreatment. - M.: medicine, 1988. - 351 with.
24. Karash U.Ì., Chizhov À.Yr., Egorova etc. - Patent. USSR. ¹ 1264949. - Ì., 1986.
25. Katukhin V.N., Ochirova A.N. // Âðà÷.äåëî. - 1979. - N 1. - P.32-35.
26. Kovalenko E.A., Chernyakov I.N. Oxygenium of tissues at the extreme factors of flight. Problems êîñìè÷. Áèîë. Ì. Medicine, 1972. Ò.21. P.-264.
27. Kositsin N.S., Reutov V.P., Ionkina E.G. // Materials of VII All-Russia workshops "ecologo-physiological problems of acclimatization ". - M.: 1994. - P.128-129.
28. Koshelev V.B., Kondashevskaya Ì.V., Rodionov I.Ì. // Materials. SA of USSR. - 1990. - Ò.311, N 3. - P.756-758.
29. Koshelev V.B., Êrushinski À.L., Ryasina Ò.V. Bull. exper. biol. 1987. Ò. 103. ¹ 3. - P. 363-376.
30. Koshelev V.B., Nemirovskaya Ò.L., Shenkman Ñ. etc. // "Interval hypoxic training (efficiency, mechanisms of action) ". - Kiev, 1992. - P.114-118.
31. Êrapivin S.V., Mazurkevich Z.B., Malitskaya E.A., Lukianova L.D. // Materials of VII All-Russia workshops " ecologî-physiological problems of acclimatization ". - M.: 1994. - P.128-129.
32. Lauer N.V., Kulikov I.À., Seredenko Ì.Ì. // Mechanisms of regulation vegetative functions. - Ì., 1970. - P.37-42.
33. Lebkova N.P., Chizhov À.Yr., Bobkov Y.I. // In: Intermittent normobaric hypoxitherapy. Mat. Àcad. Hypoxias of Russian Federation. Volume 1.- 1997. - P. 179-188.
34. Levashev Ì.I., Berezovski V.À., Nosar V.I. Etc. // Fisiologichny magazine - 1996. - Volume 42, N 3-4. - P.19-20.
35. Lukianova L.D. // Bull. of experimental biology and med. 1997. Volume 124, ¹ 9. - P. 244-254.
36. Lukianova L.D. // the Bulletin RAMS - 2000. - ¹ 9. - P. 3-12.
37. Malishev I.U., Monastirskaya Å.À., Smirin B.V. Etc. // the Bulletin of RASR - 2000. - ¹ 9. - P. 44-48.
38. Mankovskaya I.N., Nazarenko À.I., Brother L.Â. Etc. // "Interval hypoxic training (efficiency, mechanisms of action) ». - Kiev, 1992. - P.128-131.
39. Meerson Ph.Z. Adaptation medicine: mechanisms and protective effects of acclimatization. - M.: Hypoxia Medical, 1993. – P.331.
40. Meerson Ph.Z., Ìîrdvintsev P.I., Ìanukhina Å.B. Etc. // Materials of VII All-Russia workshops "ecologo-physiological problems of acclimatization ". - M.: 1994. - P.181.
41. Melnik Ò.À. // In êí. "An Oxygen starvation and ways of correction of a hypoxia ". - Kiev: sciences. Äóìêà. - 1990. - P.55-62.
42. Ìinyaev V.I., Gusev P.B., Molokov Y.G. Etc. // Materials of VII All-Russia workshops "ecologo-physiological problems of acclimatization ". - M.: 1994. - P.185.
43. Mikhalkina N.I., Zakreshev E.G. // Materials of VII All-Russia workshops "ecologo-physiological problems of acclimatization ". - M.: 1994. - P.187.
44. Nemirovskaya T.L., Tarasova T.S., Koshelev V.B. // Materials of VII All-Russia workshops "ecologo-physiological problems of acclimatization ". - M.: 1994. - P.198.
45. Îstroglazov V.G. // in: intermittent normobaric hypoxitherapy. Academy of Hypoxias Problem of Russian Federation. Volume III. - 1999. - P. 177-200.
46. Parchuf. M.L. Àâòîðåô. Äèññ. Êàíä. Honey. Sciences. - Ë.1976. – P.17.
47. Peshkova L.V., Orlova O.L., Sklyar V.E. // In êí. " An Oxygen starvation and ways of correction of a hypoxia ". - Kiev: Naukova Dumka. - 1990. - P.157-166.

48. Potievskaya V.I., Chizhov À.Yr.// a Physiological magazine. - 1992. - Ò.38, N 5. - ñ.53-57.
49. Reutov V.P., Êaushin L.P., Sorokina E.G. // Materials of VII All-Russia workshops "ecologo-physiological problems of acclimatization ". - M.: 1994. - P.229-230.
50. Reutov V.P., Kositsin E.S., Sorokina E.G. Etc. // Materials of VII All-Russia workshops «ecologo-physiological problems of acclimatization ". - M.: 1994. - P.230-231.
51. Reutov V.P., Sorokina E.G. // Fisiologichny magazine - 1996. - Volume 42, N 3-4. - P.27-28.
52. Strelkov R.B. -. Àâò. Ñâèä. On èçîáð. ¹ 389549, USSR, 1971.
53. Strelkov R.B., Êarash U.M., Chizhov À.Yr. Etc. A method of rising of a nonspecific resistance of an organism with the help of normobaric hypoxitherapy. // a Method Recommendation. ¹ 10-11/35, Ì. MINZDRAV USSR, - 1985. –P. 10.
54. Strelkov R.B., Khasabova V.À., Chizhov À.Yr. Etc. // Functional - structural bases of systemic activity and mechanisms of a plasticity of a brain, Volume. IV. Ì., Institute of a brain of AMN USSR, 1975. - P. 467-471.
55. Strelkov R.B., Chizhov À.Yr. Antiactinic protection of animals and man. - Ì., Àcad. Problems of a hypoxia, 1994. – P. 88.
56. Strelkov R.B., Chizhov À.Yr. Intermittent normobaric hypoxia in prophylaxis, treatment and ðåàáèëèòàöèè.- of Ekaterinburg. « The Ural worker ». 2001. – P. 400.
57. Sumarokov À.V., Moiseev V.S. A clinical cardiology. -M., -1995, P. 153.
58. Sushko B.S. // Ôiçiîëîãi÷íèé a magazine - 1996. - Volume 42, N 3-4. - P.109.
59. Philimonov M.V., Akinshina V.S. // an Obstetrics and gynecology, 1983. - ¹ 1. - P. 24-27.
60. Chizhov À.Yr.// Questions of an oncology .-1977. - Ò.ÕÕIII, ¹ 12. - P. 48-52.
61. Chizhov À.Yr., Karash U.M., Philimonov V.G., Strelkov R.B. // Patent ¹ 950406, USSR, 1982.
62. Chizhov À.Yr. Autoreferat of DP, Ì., 1983. - 47
63. Chizhov À.Yr., Âäîðîâà Â.Á., Karash U.M. Etc. // an Obstetrics and gynecology, 1986. - ¹ 3, - ñ.26-29.
64. Chizhov À.Yr., Karash U.M. - // Auth. Ñâèä. On èçîáð. ¹ 1628269, USSR of 1988.
65. Chizhov À.Yr., Leontievà G.V. // the Bulletin of experimental biology and medicine, 1992. Ò. 114.- ¹ 10. P. 414-416.
66. Chizhov À.Yr., Osupenko A.V. // Ïàò. Physiology and exper. therapy. - 1980. - N 1. - P.69-72.
67. Chizhov À.Yr., Strelkov R.B. // a Physiological magazine. - 1992. - Ò.38, N 5. - P.60-64.
68. Chizhov À.Yr., Strelkov R.B., Potievskaya V.I. Etc. Normobaric hypoxitherapy (method " Mountain air ") // - M.: RPFU, 1994. – P. 95.
69. Chizhov À.Yr., Philimonov V.G., Karash U.M. Etc. // Bull. of exper. biology and med., 1981. - ¹ 3.- P.392-394.
70. Chizhov À.Yr.// Àêóø. And ãèí. -1987. -11. - P. 29-32.
71. Chizhov À.Yr., Potievskaya V.I. Intermittent normobaric hypoxia in prophylaxis and treatment of an idiopathic hypertensia. - M.: RPFU 2002. – P. 187.
72. Shaov Ì.B., Shidov Z.À., Ivanov À.Ò. Etc. // Fisiologichny magazine - 1996. - Volume 42, N 3-4. - P.111.
73. Sharapov V.I., Greek Î.Ð. // Materials of VII All-Russia workshops "ecologo-physiological problems of acclimatization ". - M.: 1994. - P.323-324.
74. Adamson PB, Huang MH, Vanoli E., et al. // Circulation 1994; 90: 976-82.
75. Algra A, Tijssen JGP, Roelandt JRTC et al. // Circulation 1993; 88: 180-5.
76. Arai Y, Saul JP, Albrecht P, et al. // Am J Physiol 1989; 256: H132-41.
77. Bailey JJ, Berson AS, Garson A Jr et al. // Circulation 1990; 81: 730-9.
78. Bernardi L, Salvucci F, Suardi R et al. // Cardiovasc Res 1990; 24: 969-81.
79. Binkley PF, Haas GJ, Starling RC et al. // J Am Coll Cardiol 1993; 21: 655-61.
80. Binkley PF, Nunziata E, Haas GJ. Et al. // Am Coll Cardiol, 1991; 18: 464-72.
81. Brown HF, DiFrancesco D, Noble SJ. // Nature 1979; 280: 235-6.

82. Dell P.F. // Fam. Process. - 1989. // Vol.28, N 1. - P.1-14.
83. Ewing DJ, Neilson JMM, Shapiro JA. // Br Heart J 1991; 65: 239-44.
84. Freeman B.A., Crapo J.D. // J.Biol. Chem. - 1981. - N.10. - P.256-261.
85. Hohnloser SH, Klingenheben T, van de Loo A. Et al. // Circulation 1994; 89: 1068-1073.
86. Hon E. H., Lee S. T. // Am. J. Obstet/ Gynecol. - 1965. - Voi. 87. - P. 814 - 826
87. Huikuri HV, Valkama JO, Airaksinen KEJ et al. // Circulation 1993; 87:1220-8.
88. Kamath MV, Fallen EL. // Crit Revs Biomed Eng 1993; 21: 245-311.
89. Kleiger RE, Bigger JT, Bosner MS et. Ai. // Am J Cardiol 1991; 68: 626-30.
90. Levy MN. // Circ Res 1971; 29: 437-45.
91. Mangum M., Venable R.H., Boatwright J.D. // Aviat. Space Environ Med. - 1987. - Vol.58, N 11. - P.1093-1096.
92. Meehan R., Duncan Y., Neale L. et al. // J.Clin. Immunol. - 1988. - 8, N 5. - P.397-406.
93. Singer DH, Ori Z. // In: Malik M, Camm AJ, eds. Heart rate variability. Armonk: Futura 1995: 429-48.
94. Sugarman H., Katz L.N., Sanders A., Jochim K. // Am. J.Physiol. - 1940. - Vol.130, N 6. - P.130-143.
95. Yamamoto Y, Hughson RL. // J Appl Physiol 1991; 71: 1143-50.

Adaptation Biology and Medicine (Volume 4: Current Concepts)
Editors: A. Hargens, N. Takeda and P.K. Singal

5. Contribution of Sarcolemmal Ca^{2+}–ATPase to Free Shortening and its Energy Expenditure for Excitation-Contraction Coupling in Rat Ventricular Slices

Hisaharu Kohzuki

Department of Food and Nutrition, Okayama Gakuin University, Okayama, Japan

Abstract

Oxygen utilization for basal metabolic rate in heart has been suggested to be an important contribution to the phenomenon of cardiac hibernation. However, the origin of basal metabolism has not been fully understood. In fact, it is not known that sarcolemmal Ca^{2+}-ATPase contributes to the basal metabolism of nonbeating heart muscle as well as the energy expenditure used for total Ca^{2+}-handling in the excitation-contraction coupling in free shortening heart muscle. The aim of the present study is to clarify the effect of 5-(and-6)-carboxyeosin (CE, 20 microM), a specific blocker of sarcolemmal Ca^{2+}-ATPase, on the basal O_2 consumption (VO_2), the free shortening and its VO_2 used for total Ca^{2+} handling (total Ca^{2+} handling VO_2) of rat myocardial 300 micrometer-thick slice(s). VO_2 of quiescent slices indicates energy expenditure used for basal metabolism. Total Ca^{2+} handling VO_2 was obtained through subtracting basal VO_2 from a VO_2 during 1-Hz free shortening. Blockade of sarcolemmal Ca^{2+}-ATPase by CE did not affect basal VO_2 ($P<0.05$), although CE decreased total Ca^{2+} handling VO_2 by 8-30% of control ($P<0.05$) and the amount of the free shortening was augmented by 27% with CE ($P<0.05$). Our previous results also indicated that basal VO_2 was not decreased by a specific blocker of sarcolemmal Na^+/Ca^{2+} exchanger, KB-R7943. In the present study, free shortening was enhanced by 25% with KB-R7943 as well. All these results suggest that trans-sarcolemmal Ca^{2+} cycling due to Ca^{2+} leak via Na^+/Ca^{2+} exchanger and sarcolemmal Ca^{2+}-ATPase seems to be negligible in quiescent myocardium, and does not contributes to the basal oxygen consumption, although the energy expenditure used for trans-sarcolemmal Ca^{2+} cycling in excitation-contraction coupling to the extent less than 30% of total Ca^{2+} handling energy in free shortening myocardium of rat.

Perspectives in heart hibernation and the role of basal metabolism of heart: It will be clarified how oxygen-dependency of heart basal metabolism is related to mitochondrial energy metabolism sustained even high level to keep tissue PO_2 low under the condition of well balancing O_2 supply with O_2 demand.

Introduction

Mechanoenergetic study on whole heart has been clarifying that a linear relationship between left ventricular (LV) contractility and energy used for both total Ca^{2+} handling in excitation-contraction coupling (total Ca^{2+} handling VO_2) and basal metabolism (basal VO_2), namely oxygen costs of LV contractility, successfully characterized an O_2 saving and wasting process of heart suffered from ischemia, acidosis and inotropic agents [9, 11, 12, 13, 18, 20, 25, 27, 28]. Although the underlying mechanisms of the alteration of oxygen costs of contractility remain unclear, a change in Ca^{2+} sensitivity of contractile elements, an alteration of Ca^{2+} handling via sarcoplasmic reticulum (SR) and trans-sarcolemmal Ca^{2+} transport seem to contribute to the oxygen cost under the constant basal metabolism [17, 18, 24].

We have recently observed that the mean value of oxygen cost of LV contractility in rat hearts corresponds to that in canine hearts [29]. Ca^{2+} handling by cardiac muscle is substantially different among species [1, 4, 5]. Our previous studies supports the evidence that VO_2 of mechanically unloaded myocardial slices consists of basal VO_2 and Ca^{2+} handling VO_2 [15, 16, 26, 31]. We also reported that Ca^{2+} handling VO_2 of rat slices decreased by 70-80% with the inhibition by cyclopiazonic acid (CPA), a specific inhibitor of sarcoplasmic reticulum (SR) Ca^{2+}-ATPase [26]. It suggests that Ca^{2+} sequestration in contraction-relaxation cycles depends more on SR in rat myocardium than other species, e. g. rabbit and canine.

In mechanoenergetics and its theoretical studies [14, 17, 24], energy used for Ca^{2+} handling via SR Ca^{2+}-ATPase is more economical than that via Na^+/Ca^{2+} exchanger coupled with Na^+/K^+ ATPase. The latter is one-half economical, or twice as wasteful, although it has been proposed as the possibility that Na^+-Ca^{2+} exchange acts as an energy-saving mechanism to prevent Ca^{2+} accumulation at the junctional SR zone and thus prevents further release of Ca^{2+} in cardiac muscle [21]. Thus the similar O_2 cost of contractility between canine and rat hearts is intriguing. We hypothesized that the similar O_2 cost of rat heart resulted from higher basal metabolism and less economical process of Ca^{2+} handling, i. e. sarcolemmal Ca^{2+}-ATPase, which has a molar stoichiometry of 1 Ca^{2+}: 1ATP [10, 19, 23]. To test the hypothesis, we evaluated the effects of carboxyeosin, an inhibitor of sarcolemmal Ca^{2+}-ATPase [3, 6, 7, 8], on Ca^{2+} handling VO_2 and motility of rat myocardial slice(s).

Materials And Methods

Left ventricular myocardial slice preparation

Twenty-three adult male Wistar rats (Charles River Japan, Yokohama, Japan) weighing 375 ± 43 g were anesthetized with pentobarbital sodium (50 mg/kg, i. p.). All experimental procedures were described previously in detail [15, 16, 26, 31]. Briefly, the whole heart was excised after perfusion with Tyrode solution at 12°C gassed with 100% for 5 min. Each myocardial slice was cut into 300-μm-thick slices in parallel with the epicardium with a microslicer (DTK-3000; Dosaka EM, Kyoto, Japan). We obtained 10-15 slices from each heart. The slices were stored 30 min in 18°C Tyrode and then 30-60 min in 25°C Tyrode solution, gassed with 100% O_2. The composition of Tyrode solution (in mmol/L) was 136.0 NaCl, 5.4 KCl, 1.0 $MgCl_2$•6H2O, 0.33 NaH_2PO_4•$2H_2O$, 0.9 $CaCl_2$•$2H_2O$, 10.0 glucose, 5.0 HEPES, with pH corrected to 7.4 with NaOH at 30°C.

Image analysis of free shortening of myocardial slices

Twenty slices from 16 rats were used for image analysis of slice free-shortening. One slice was placed in the same about 2.5 ml chamber as that for oximetry. The slice was gently superfused with Tyrode solution at about 5 ml/min for 10 min, during which the magnetic stirrer was rotated. During image analysis, the transparent acrylic lid was put on the chamber and the stirrer was turned off. Slice free-shortening was evoked by 1-Hz field stimulation as described previously [26, 31].

We acquired the video image of slice free-shortening for 2 min and non-stimulated slice image for a few seconds with a photomacroscopic-image processing system (Olympus SZH-131 DA, CCD camera CS 220, Tokyo, Japan; C3163, Hamamatsu Photonics, Shizuoka, Japan). We recorded the number of pixels and individual pixel values in a selected area ($10 \times 10 <$ mm) during 2 min 1-Hz slice free shortening in a computer (PC-98, NEC, Tokyo, Japan). The free shortening was evaluated by the relative changes in slice surface area, i. e. Motility index (%) = 100 × (maximum area during diastole - minimum area during systole)/maximum area during diastole. The mean value of motility index was defined from each five pair of maximum and minimum.

Assessment of VO_2 of myocardial slices

A set of four myocardial slices on average was used to measure basal VO_2 and mechanically unloaded myocardial VO_2 during free shortening as a decreasing rate in O_2 concentration of the solution in the oximetric chamber. VO_2 of a set of slices was measured polarographically with an oxygen electrode (1T-125, Instech Labs. Plymouth Meeting, PA, USA) as described previously [15, 26, 31]. This oximetric system was calibrated at three different O_2 concentrations; 0 mg/L (5% Na_2SO_3 solution), 7.3 mg/L (Tyrode solution saturated with air), and 35.1 mg/L (Tyrode solution saturated with 100% O_2) at 30°C in each experiment. Volume (L) of Tyrode in chamber was measured at the end of the three times repeated measurements for a set of slices. The mean ± SD of volume of Tyrode was 2.65 ± 0.04 ml (number of the measurements: n=26).

We first examined the mean value of the background VO_2 without myocardial slices in the Tyrode-filled chamber at the beginning and end (0.45 ± 0.10 mg $O_2 \bullet min^{-1}$, n=26) of each measurement. We measured the wet weight of each set of slices (65.0 ± 15.1 mg; n=26 sets of slices). We calculated VO_2 of slices by subtracting background VO_2 (A mg $O_2 \bullet min^{-1}$) from the measured VO_2 (B mg $O_2 \bullet min^{-1}$) with myocardial slices. Myocardial VO_2 (ml $O_2 \bullet min^{-1} \bullet 100g\ LV^{-1}$) was calculated as [(B-A)/slice wet weight (g)] × volume of Tyrode solution in the chamber (L) × [22.4 (L)/32 (g)] × 100 (g).

Experimental procedure. Basal VO_2 without stimulation of the quiescent slices was obtained during the 1st 2 min. Total Ca^{2+} handling VO_2 is obtained by subtracting basal VO_2 from the VO_2 with 1-Hz stimulation.

Experimental protocol. After 10-min superfusion of the slice(s) with Normal Tyrode solution (NT, 0.9 mM Ca^{2+}), the 1st basal VO_2 and total Ca^{2+} handling VO_2 measurements, or video recording of free shortening were performed. Subsequently, the slice(s) were superfused with or without 20 μM 5-(and-6)-carboxyeosin (mixed isomers) (CE, Molecular Probes, Eugene, OR, USA) or 10 μM KB-R7943 (KB, Kanebo Co. LTD, Tokyo, Japan). CE and KB were dissolved in dimethyl sulfoxide (DMSO) and the solution was further diluted with NT just before use at 0.2% and 1% of final concentration of DMSO, respectively.

Statistics

All data were presented as mean ± SD. The student's paired t-test was used for the %inhibition values of CPA and KB-R7943. P values less than 0.05 were considered statistically significant.

Results

Effect of carboxyeosin on basal VO_2 and total Ca^{2+} handling VO_2 (Fig. 1)

Mean basal VO_2 values were 1.68 ± 0.24 ml O_2•min^{-1}•100g LV^{-1} in NT. Basal VO_2 of slices treated with 20 μM carboxyeosin was 1.85 ± 0.39 ml O_2•min^{-1}•100g LV^{-1}. These values were not significantly different (P>0.05). Total Ca^{2+} handling VO_2 was 0.92 ± 0.30 ml O_2•min^{-1}•100g LV^{-1} in NT. Total Ca^{2+} handling VO_2 was 0.92 ± 0.30 ml O_2•min^{-1}•100g LV^{-1} in NT. Total Ca^{2+} handling VO_2 was 0.67 ± 0.29 ml O_2•min^{-1}•100g LV^{-1} in the slices treated with 20 μM carboxyeosin. The value was significantly different from that in NT (P<0.05).

Effect of carboxyeosin and KB-R7943 on free shortening of rat myocardial slice (Figs. 2 and 3)

Motility index values were fairly constant between 10 [0.77 ± 0.33%] and 120 sec [0.76 ± 0.50 %] during the 1st measurement in NT. For the 2nd measurement in NT, motility index was fairly constant between 10 [0.80 ± 0.29%] and 120 sec [0.61 ± 0.36%]. Motility index was 0.75 ± 0.35% at 60 sec in NT. The value was significantly increased to 0.97 ± 0.41% by 26.6 ± 16.1% in the treatment with 20 μM CE (P<0.05). In KB series, motility index was 0.88 ± 0.55% at 60 sec in NT. The value was significantly increased 1.04 ± 0.59% by 25.2 ± 30.7% in the treatment with 10 μM KB (P<0.05). Motility index was 0.75 ± 0.36% for the 1st NT and 0.72 ± 0.33% for the 2nd NT. These values were not significantly different (P<0.05).

Discussion

In the present study, we reconfirmed that O_2 consumption (VO_2) used for basal metabolism in quiescent rat myocardium was higher [14, 15, 27, 31)] than that in canine KCl-arrested heart [11, 12, 18, 20, 25, 28)]. Blockade of sarcolemmal Ca^{2+}-ATPase with 20 μM carboxyeosin (CE) did not affect basal VO_2. Thus, Ca^{2+} handling VO_2 is obtained by subtracting basal metabolism from VO_2 of the stimulated slices as

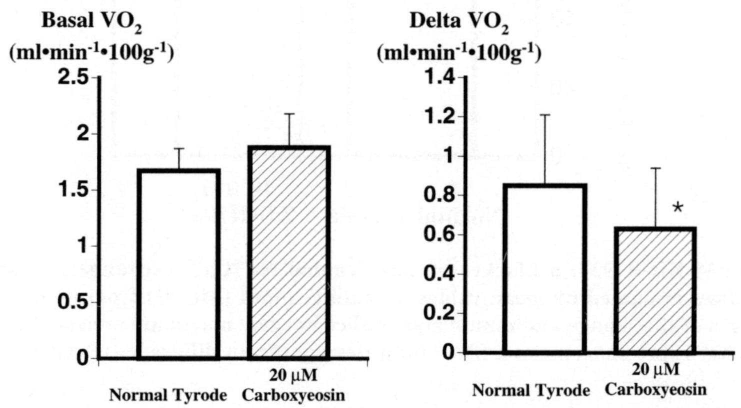

Fig. 1. Effects of 20 μM carboxyeosin, a blocker of sarcolemmal Ca^{2+}-ATPase, on basal VO_2 and total Ca^{2+} handling O_2 consumption (VO_2) of rat myocardial. Each bar expresses mean ± SD. * indicates significant difference (P<0.05).

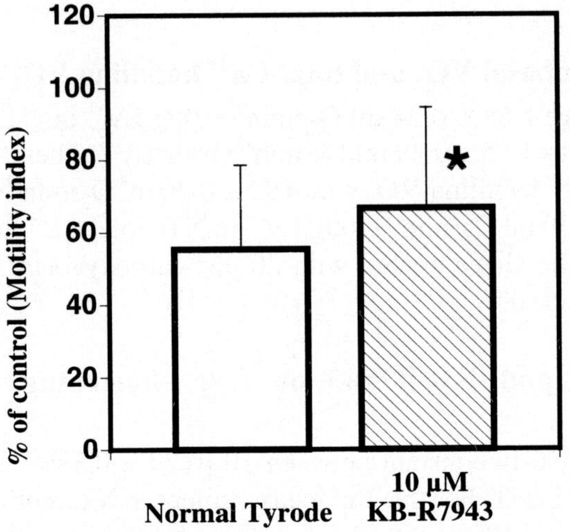

Fig. 2. Effect of 20 μM carboxyeosin, a blocker of sarcolemmal Ca^{2+}-ATPase, on free shortening of rat myocardial slices evaluated by mean values of motility index (MI, %) from each five twitch. MI = 100 × (maximum area of slice image - minimum area of slice image)/maximum area of slice image during a single twitch. Each bar expressions mean ± SD. * indicates significant difference (P<0.05).

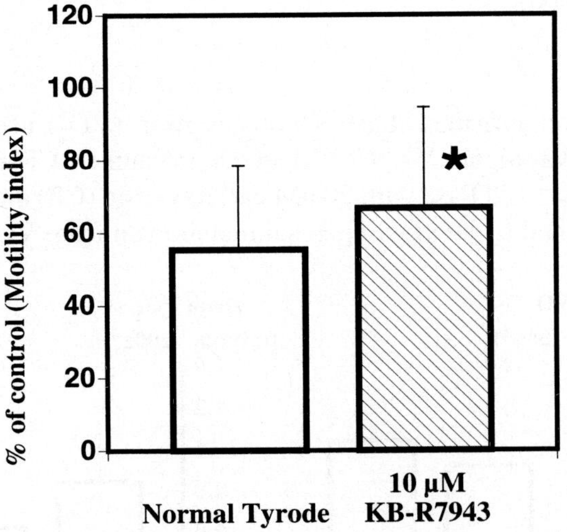

Fig. 3. Effect of 10 μM KB-R7934, a blocker of sarcolemmal Na^{+}/Ca^{2+} exchanger, on free shortening of rat myocardial slices evaluated by mean values of motility index (MI, %) from each five twitch. MI = 100 × (maximum area of slice image - minimum area of slice image) / maximum area of slice image during a single twitch. Each bar expressions mean ± SD. * indicates significant difference (P<0.05).

previously reported [25, 30]. We observed that CE induced the significant decrease in VO_2 used for total Ca^{2+} handling in excitation-contraction (E-C) coupling in rat myocardial slices. Motility of slice was not reduced by CE, but rather increased. Our present observation seems to support an evidence for the contribution of the sarcolemmal Ca^{2+}-ATPase to intracellular Ca^{2+} decay to cease free shortening [26].

Contribution of sarcolemmal Ca^{2+}-ATPase to Ca^{2+} handling VO_2 of rat heart

We have previously reported that blockade of the sarcoplasmic reticulum (SR) Ca^{2+} ATPase by 10 μM cyclopiazonic acid largely decreased free shortening and total Ca^{2+} handling VO_2 by the similar extent of 70% [26)], suggesting that handling of Ca^{2+} responsible for 70% of free shortening in E-C coupling in rat myocardium was more depend on SR Ca^{2+}-ATPase than other species [26)]. Internal Ca^{2+} recirculation fraction (RF) via SR Ca^{2+}-ATPase has been analyzed by post-extrasystolic potentiation and post-extrasystolic transient alternants [1, 2, 13, 22)]. In rat papillary muscle, RF was reported to be 0.8 [1, 2, 22)]. The figure was similar to that obtained by CPA-sensitive total Ca^{2+} handling VO_2 in rat myocardial slices [26)]. RF is essential in cardiac mechanoenergetics because total Ca^{2+} handling VO_2 is a significant fraction of LV VO_2 of whole heart, and the internal and external Ca^{2+} handling routes have Ca^{2+}: ATP molar stoichiometry with a two fold difference [17, 24)]. The Na^+/K^+ ATPase coupled with the Na^+/Ca^{2+} exchange has a net 1 Ca^{2+}: 1 ATP molar stoichiometry under Ca^{2+} and Na^+ homeostasis [20, 25, 27)]. The stoichiometry of sarcolemmal Ca^{2+}-ATPase is also 1 Ca^{2+}: 1 ATP [10, 19, 23)]. On the other hand, SR Ca^{2+}-ATPase has a 2 Ca^{2+} : 1 ATP stoichiometry.

From these considerations of the mechanoenergetic point of view, rat heart would have more economical O_2 cost of contractility than other species, e. g. canine. However our recent observation indicated that the mean value of oxygen costs of LV contractility in rat heart corresponds to that in canine heart [29)]. The present results showing a high VO_2 used for basal metabolism and the contribution of sarcolemmal Ca^{2+}-ATPase to total Ca^{2+} handling VO_2 seem to explain the similar oxygen costs between the two species.

Effect of carboxyeosin and KB-R7943 on free shortening

In the present study, we observed that blockade of sarcolemmal Ca^{2+}-ATPase did not decrease the motility but increased it. Blockade of Na^+/Ca^{2+} exchanger by KB-R7943, a specific inhibitor of Na^+/Ca^{2+} exchanger [30)], also increased the free shortening. These observation seems to be explained by the following way: 1) Because trans-sarcolemmal Ca^{2+} transport is more wasteful for handling the same amount of Ca^{2+} than SR Ca^{2+}-ATPase, blockade of trans-sarcolemmal Ca^{2+} transport increases the economy of Ca^{2+} handling thereby decreasing total Ca^{2+} handling VO_2. 2) Similar 20-30% increase in free shortening by blockade of trans-sarcolemmal Ca^{2+} transport suggest the similar fractional contribution of both sarcolemmal Ca^{2+}-ATPase and sarcolemmal Na^+/Ca^{2+} exchanger to extrude Ca^{2+} responsible for 1-Hz free shortening in rat slices. 3) As Choi and Eisner [6, 7)] discussed, blockade of sarcolemmal Ca^{2+}-ATPase were able to increase resting intracellular Ca^{2+} thereby increasing the activation of SR Ca^{2+}-ATPase and hence the SR Ca^{2+} content. They suggested that, in the intact rat myocardium, sarcolemmal Ca^{2+}-ATPase acted to decrease SR Ca^{2+} content. Present results showing the enhanced free shortening with the decreased total Ca^{2+} handling VO_2 suggest that an energetic economy significantly contributes to amount of free shortening in rat myocardial slices.

Acknowledgment

We greatly thank Mr. Yukishige Akagi, a representative of Okayama Rail Road Model Shop, for generously custom-making our oximetric chamber system.

This study was partly supported by Grants-in-Aid for Scientific Research (11470277) from the Ministry of Education, Science, Sports and Culture.

References

1. Asgrimsson, H.J., Wohlfart, B., Brandt, J., and Johannsson, M. Effect of $[Na^+]_O$, $[Ca^{2+}]_O$ and cyclopiazonic acid on decline of post-extrasystolic potentiation and twitch kinetics in guinea-pig and human myocardial preparations. Acta Physiol. Scand., 1999; 166(3): 195-201.
2. Banijamali, H.S., Gao, W-D., MacIntosh, B.R., and ter Keurs, H.E.D.J. Force-interval relations of twitches and cold contractions in rat cardiac trabeculae. Effect of ryanodine. Circ. Res. 1991; 69(4): 937-948.
3. Bassani, R.A., Bassani, J.W., and Bers, D.M. Relaxation in ferret ventricular myocytes: role of the sarcolemmal Ca ATPase. Pflugers Arch-Eur. J. Physiol. 1995; 430(4): 573-578.
4. Bers, D.M. Mechanisms contributing to the cardiac inotropic effect of Na pump inhibition and reduction of extracellular Na. J. Gen. Physiol. 1987; 90(4): 479-504.
5. Bers, D.M. Species differences and the role of sodium-calcium exchange in cardiac muscle relaxation. Ann. N. Y. Acad. Sci. 1991; 639: 375-385.
6. Choi, H.S., and Eisner, D.A. The role of sarcolemmal Ca^{2+}-ATPase in the regulation of resting calcium concentration in rat ventricular myocytes. J. Physiol. 1999; 515(1): 109-118.
7. Choi, H.S., and Eisner, D.A. The effects of inhibition of the sarcolemmal Ca-ATPase on systolic calcium fluxes and intracellular calcium concentration in rat ventricular myocytes. Pflugers Arch-Eur, J. Physiol. 1999: 437(6): 966-971.
8. Gatto, C., Hale, C.C., Xu, W., and Milanick, M.A. Eosin, a potent inhibitor of the plasma membrane Ca pump, does not inhibit the cardiac Na-Ca exchanger. Biochemistry 1995; 34(3): 965-972.
9. Goto, Y., Slinker, B.K., and LeWinter, M.M. Effects of amrinone and isoproterenol on mechanoenergetics of blood-perfused rabbit heart. Am. J. Physiol. Heart Circ. Physiol. 1992; 262(2): H719-H727.
10. Hao, L., Rigaud, J.L., and Inesi, G. Ca^{2+}/H^+ countertransport and electrogenicity in proteoliposomes containing erythrocyte plasma membrane Ca-ATPase and exogenous lipids. J. Biol. Chem. 1994; 269(19): 14268-14275.
11. Hata, K., Goto, Y., Kawaguchi, O., Takasago, T., Saeki, A., Nishioka, T., and Suga, H. Hypercapnic acidosis increases oxygen cost of contractility in the dog left ventricule. Am. J. Physiol. Heart Circ. Physiol. 1994; 266(2): H730-H740.
12. Hata, K., Takasago, T., Saeki, A., Nishioka, T., and Goto, Y. Stunned myocardium after rapid correction of acidosis. Increased oxygen cost of contractility and the role of the Na^+-H^+ exchange system. Circ. Res. 1994; 74(5): 794-805.
13. Hata, Y., Shimizu, J., Hosogi, S., Matsubara, H., Araki, J., Ohe, T., Takaki, M., Takasago, T., Taylor, T.W., and Suga, H. Ryanodine decreases internal Ca^{2+} recirculation fraction of the canine heart as studied by postextrasystolic transient alternans. Jpn. J. Physiol. 47(6): 521-530, 1997.
14. Hata, Y., Sakamoto, T., Hosogi, S., Ohe, T., Suga, H., and Takaki, M. Effects of thapsigargin and KCl on the O_2 use of the excised blood-perfused rat heart. J. Mol. Cell Cardiol. 1998; 30(10): 2137-2144.
15. Kohzuki, H., Misawa, H., Sakata, S., Ohga, Y., Suga, H., and Takaki, M. Energy expenditure by Ba^{2+} contracture in rat ventricular slices derives from cross-bridge cycling. Am. J. Physiol. Heart Circ. Physiol. 1999; 277(1): H74-H79.
16. Kohzuki, H., Misawa, H., Sakata, S., Takaki, M. Barium contracture in rat ventricular slices and its energy expenditure: Inhibitory effect of pretreatment with cyclopiazonic acid. In: *The First International Conference on Control and Diseases of Sodium Dependent Transportation Proteins and Ion Channels.* Edited by Suketa Y. Amsterdam: Elsevier Science, 1999; pp439-440.
17. Lee, S., Araki, J., Imaoka, T., Maesako, M., Iribe, G., Miyaji, K., Mohri, S., Shimizu, J., Harada, M., Ohe, T., Hirakawa, M., and Suga, H. Energy-wasteful total Ca^{2+} handling underlies increased O_2 cost of contractility in canine stunned heart. Am. J. Physiol. Heart Circ. Physiol. 2000; 278(5): H1464-H1472.
18. Mikane, T., Araki, J., Suzuki, S., Mizuno, J., Shimizu, J., Mohri, S., Matsubara, H., Hirakawa, M., Ohe, T., and Suga, H. O_2 cost of contractility but not of mechanical energy increases with temperature in canine left ventricle. Am. J. Physiol. Heart Circ. Physiol. 1999; 277(1): H65-H73.

19. Niggli, V., Sigel, E., and Carafoli, E. The purified Ca^{2+} pump of human erythrocyte membranes catalyzes an electroneutral Ca^{2+}-H^+ exchange in reconstituted liposomal systems. J. Biol. Chem. 1982; 257(5): 2350-2356.
20. Ohgoshi, Y., Goto, Y., Futaki, S., Yaku, H., Kawaguchi, O., and Suga, H. Increased oxygen cost of contractility in stunned myocardium of dog. Circ. Res. 1991; 69(4): 975-988.
21. Ponce-Hornos, J.E., Philipson, K.D., Bonazzola, P., and Langer, G.A. Energetics of Na^+-Ca^{2+} exchange in resting cardiac muscle. Biophys. J. 1999: 77: 3319-3327.
22. Ragnarsdottir, K., Wohlfart, B., and Johannsson, M. Mechanical restitution of the rat papillary muscle. Acta Physiol. Scand. 1982: 115(2): 183-191.
23. Salvador, J.M., Inesi, G., Rigaud, J.L., and Mata, A.M. Ca^{2+} transport by reconstituted synaptosomal ATPase is associated with H^+ countertransport and net change displacement. J. Biol. Chem. 1998; 273(29): 18230-18234.
24. Shimizu, J., Araki, J., Mizuno, J., Lee, S., Syuu, Y., Hosogi, S., Mohri, S., Mikane, T., Takaki, M., Taylor, T.W., and Suga, H. A new integrative method to quantify total Ca^{2+} handling and futile Ca^{2+} cycling in failing hearts. Am. J. Physiol. Heart Circ. Physiol. 1998; 275(2): H2325-H2333.
25. Suga, H. Ventricular energetics. Physiol. Rev. 1990; 70(2): 247-277.
26. Takaki, M., Kohzuki, H., Kawatani, Y., Yoshida, A., Ishidate, H., and Suga, H. Sarcoplasmic reticulum Ca^{2+} pump blockade decreases O_2 use of unloaded contracting rat heart slices: Thapsigargin and cyclopiazonic acid. J. Mol. Cell Cardiol. 1998; 30: 649-659.
27. Takaki, M., Matsubara, H., Araki, J., Zhao, L.Y., Ito, H., Yasuhara, S., Fujii, W., and Suga, H. Mechanoenergetics of acute failing hearts characterized by oxygen costs of mechanical energy and contractility. In: *New Horizons for Failing Heart Syndrome.* Edited by Sasayama S. Tokyo: Springer-Verlag Tokyo, 1996; pp 133-164.
28. Takasago, T., Goto, Y., Kawaguchi, O., Hata, K., Saeki, A., Nishioka, T., and Suga, H. Ryanodine wastes oxygen consumption for Ca^{2+} handling in the dog heart. A new pathological heart model. J. Clin. Invest. 1993; 92(2): 823-830.
29. Tsuji, T., Ohga, Y., Yoshikawa, S., Sakata, S., Kohzuki, H., Misawa, H., Abe, T., Tabayashi, N., Kobayashi, S., Kitamura, S., Taniguchi, S., Suga, H., and Takaki, M. New index for oxygen cost of contractility from curved end-systolic pressure-volume relations in cross-circulated rat hearts. Jpn. J. Physiol. 1999; 49(6): 513-520.
30. Watano, T., Kimura, J., Morita, T., and Nakanishi, H. A novel antagonist, No. 7943, of the Na^+/Ca^{2+} exchanger current in guinea-pig cardiac ventricular cells. Brit. J. Pharmacol. 1996; 119(3): 555-563.
31. Yasuhara, S., Takaki, M., Kikuta, A., Ito, H., and Suga, H. Myocardial VO_2 of mechanically unloaded contraction of rat ventricular slices measured by a new approach. Am. J. Physiol. Heart Circ. Physiol. 1996; 270(2): H1063-H1070.

Adaptation Biology and Medicine (Volume 4: Current Concepts)
Editors: A. Hargens, N. Takeda and P.K. Singal

6. Cardiovascular Adaptation to Gravity: Lessons from Comparative Studies of Snakes

Harvey B. Lillywhite

Department of Zoology
The University of Florida
Gainesville, Florida 32611-8525 USA

Introduction

Gravity is a pervasive feature of the environment and one to which virtually every organism has adapted in various ways over eons of evolutionary history. From a human perspective, we are impressed with larger terrestrial organisms and recognize that gravity's effects on blood circulation are more pronounced in terrestrial species with upright posture and greater height. In comparison with the majority of vertebrates, humans are relatively large and tall. As a consequence, the human cardiovascular system has evolved extensive and sophisticated regulatory mechanisms to counteract gravitational disturbance during upright posture (Rowell, 1993). Taller animals such as giraffes, some flightless birds, climbing snakes, and extinct dinosaurs require(d) more intense responses to cope with problems associated with upright posture. Various sophisticated mechanisms have evolved to provide adequate blood flow to the brain while restricting blood flow and swelling of tissues in the lower body where large gravitational pressures can prevail.

What we consider to be "normal" cardiovascular behavior or performance is the result of adaptation to Earth gravity, and we do not know how different these parameters might be if humans had experienced long evolutionary history in a different gravitational field. We are aware of responses to loss of gravity in space flight and the difficulties of re-acclimation to gravity following return to Earth (Watenpaugh and Hargens, 1996). These responses range from moderate to severe. They reflect comparatively short-term adjustments of phenotypic expression, but they cannot predict the genetic-based changes that might occur if humans were subjected to microgravity over evolutionary periods.

The objective of this paper is to examine a suite of characters related to cardiovascular performance in a group of gravity-sensitive vertebrates having variable evolutionary histories with respect to gravity stress. The evolutionary radiation of snakes provides living material from a natural experiment in long-term responses to the gravity environment. Clearly, the results of this experiment provide insights into the probable biological adjustments that are required for successful life in variable gravity environments, including space.

Why Snakes?

Snakes are elongate in body form and therefore potentially highly susceptible to shifts of blood volume and disturbance to integrated cardiovascular functions when they assume upright or vertical postures. Upright snakes in terrestrial environments experience significant gradients of intravascular pressures, which must be counteracted to prevent blood pooling and excess plasma filtration in dependent tissues. In aquatic environments, however, gravitational pressures in blood vessels are counterbalanced by parallel gradients in the surrounding water column, and the distribution of blood volume is not strongly affected by changes of body position or posture (Lillywhite, 1996).

More than 2500 species of snakes are recognized, and the earliest fossil species dates from the mid-Cretaceous approximately 100 million years ago. These vertebrates have radiated extensively and are cosmopolitan with representatives above the Arctic Circle in Europe, and above timberline in the Himalayas and Andes. Snakes occupy a diversity of habitats, and several lineages have evolved aquatic or semi-aquatic forms. Some groups, such as sea snakes (Elapidae: Hydrophiinae) and file snakes (Acrochordidae), have evolved aquatic specializations, with member species having long evolutionary histories entirely in water where conditions simulate microgravity. Thus, from a comparative and phylogenetic perspective, snakes include forms that routinely experience gravity stress (arboreal/scansorial species) as well as others that might be regarded as evolutionarily "deconditioned" to gravity (aquatic species). Thus, within a single taxon having a body form that is sensitive to gravity stress, it is possible to sample a range of gravitational adaptation attributable to diversification of habitat demands and behaviors.

Gross Anatomy

The Heart

Various traits related to the cardiovascular system must co-evolve to meet cardiovascular performance in response to selection forces that are induced by gravitational stress. Thus, ventricle mass scales to the 0.95 power in snakes, whereas the scaling exponent is only 0.77 to 0.91 in other reptiles that are less subject to gravitational stress (Seymour, 1987). The data from other reptiles were taken from species that are small or compact (lizards, turtles) or do not raise the head much above the heart (crocodilians). Therefore, these animals do not develop large gravitational pressures between the heart and head. Elongated snakes, however, become increasingly subject to gravitational pressure loads on the heart, especially if behaviors elevate the head above the heart, as in climbing. There is a tendency for aquatic and strictly ground-dwelling species of snakes to have smaller hearts than do other species of snakes, however there are no significant correlations within habitat groups (Seymour, 1987). Larger sample sizes from fresh material are needed before firm conclusions might be made regarding correlation between heart size and gravity stress.

A relation between gravity and the anatomic position of the heart in snakes is more clear. The hearts of aquatic species are significantly closer to the body center than are those of arboreal and scansorial species, while semi-aquatic and relatively non-climbing terrestrial species are intermediate (Seymour and Lillywhite, 1976; Lillywhite, 1987; Seymour, 1987). At extremes, the heart occupies positions as little as 15% of the body length from the head in some arboreal species, whereas the heart position of aquatic species is at nearly 45% of body length from the head. The relative heart position is independent of body mass and length, and there is no tendency for a reduction of head-heart distance in longer snakes within a habitat category (Seymour, 1987). Indeed, head-heart distance increases linearly in longer snakes within a given group. Thus, the anatomic differences in heart position observed among snakes appear strongly related to habitat and behavior.

A heart position near body center is relatively more efficient energetically, and offers likely explanation for the anatomy seen in aquatic species living in zero gravity environments. Counteracting selection pressures must account for the anterior heart position seen among species that are subject to gravity stress on the heart while climbing or in upright positions out of water. These may be stated as advantages and include the following. 1) The anterior position favors perfusion of the brain at all body angles and (2) minimizes pressure against which the heart must work when the head is up (proportional to the effective vertical distance between heart and head). Thus, proximity of the heart to the head maximizes cerebral perfusion pressures during head-up postures. (3) An anterior heart position may strategically locate baroreceptors (see below) anterior to the hydrostatic indifferent point to detect and neurogenically correct shifts of gravitational pressures whenever postures depart from horizontal. Of course, the anterior heart position increases the relative length of the venous blood column below the heart and thereby renders the inferior venous return more difficult in vertical, head-up postures outside of water.

Lung Morphology and Gravity

As in other reptiles and probably all tetrapod vertebrates, the ophidian lung is a low resistance, low-pressure vascular circuit. Pulmonary arterial pressures may exceed mammalian values, however, while the converse is true of plasma oncotic pressure. Consequently, the reptilian lung is prone to filter relatively large amounts of fluid across highly permeable capillaries and is sensitive to edema (Burggren, 1982; Smits, 1989).

The lungs of snakes are elongated structures, in conformance with the ophidian body plan, and consist of a single, large axial chamber in most species. They are, however divisible into anatomically and functionally discrete segments. Gas exchange takes place through membranous walls of radial chambers, termed faveoli, which surround the central lumen of the respiratory organ and give a spongy appearance to the wall of the lung. This respiratory region is highly vascular and will be termed the *vascular lung* for purposes of the present discussion. The remainder of the lung, having lumen continuity with the vascular lung, lacks respiratory parenchyma and continues for variable distances as a *saccular lung*, terminating posteriorly in a blind-ending sac. Blood flow through the pulmonary artery and pulmonary veins services only the vascular lung. The saccular lung is relatively non-vascular and is usually a thin, membranous sheet or may be thick and muscular (in sea snakes).

While the entire lung structure extends for much of the length of the body cavity, the relative lengths of the vascular and saccular segments vary considerably among different species. In arboreal and scansorial species, the vascular segment is always very short, beginning usually near the heart and extending less than 20% of the body length. In some species, the vascular segment is less than 9% of the body length (Wallach, 1998). On the other hand, vascularized parenchyma in lungs of totally aquatic species extend virtually the entire length of the body cavity, except in some species in which there is a short saccular segment. The lungs of some ground-dwelling viperid species of snakes are intermediate to those of scansorial and aquatic species.

The differences in vascular segments appear to represent an absolute constraint on the length of pulmonary vasculature in the scansorial species, for gravitational pressures develop in the pulmonary vasculature in proportion to the height of the blood column (Lillywhite, 1987). These pressures exceed the threshold for inducing serious pulmonary edema. Indeed, when sea snakes having elongate vascular lungs are tilted to vertical postures in air outside of water, histological studies confirm the occurrence of severe pulmonary edema and the actual rupture of pulmonary capillaries (Fig. 1). Thus, pulmonary vessels comprise fluid columns that vary in length according to habitat and risk of hydrostatic disturbance. Elongate pulmonary vessels, characteristic of aquatic snakes, develop significant gravitational pressures if they are positioned vertically in air. Because these pressures develop in both arterial and venous blood columns, they are transmitted to capillaries and the lung is at risk of severe edema and capillary rupture. These problems are avoided entirely by the short lung morphology that is seen in all scansorial species examined to date. In the aquatic environment, gradients of transmural pressures do not develop in the pulmonary vasculature because lung gases are pressurized as snakes dive to depth, and external water pressures approximate the gravitational pressures within the blood columns regardless of a snake's position or posture. Without the risk of gravity-induced edema, aquatic snakes evolved elongated vascular lung segments presumably because selection for short segments was relaxed and the elongate parenchyma permitted more effective, or efficient, uptake of oxygen from the lung air.

General Body Form

With few exceptions, arboreal and scansorial species of snakes tend to be relatively short and slender in comparison with more terrestrial, or aquatic, relatives within the same family (Lillywhite and Henderson, 1993). In relative terms, this morphology has the hemodynamic advantages of limiting the absolute length of vertical blood columns and, according to principles in the Law of Laplace, providing resistance to distending forces that might be caused by gravity-induced pooling of fluids within the body. Of course, the slender shape can also be related to selection forces other than gravity, e.g. camouflage, locomotion, etc., but hemodynamics might well contribute to the overall selective advantage involved in the evolution of a gracile body.

Many snakes of varying length are capable of climbing in vegetation or other objects by moving at low angles and using "switchback" tactics, as roads on a mountainside. However, we are concerned here with climbing behaviors that result in significant vertical posture and gravity stress on the body fluids. The majority of species with such arboreal/scansorial behaviors have evolved within three families of snakes: Boidae, Colubridae and Viperidae. The slenderness of body form is accomplished in various species by the evolution of narrow vertebrae and ribs that are directed downward rather than outward (Lillywhite and Henderson, 1993).

Another feature of arboreal snakes is a tendency for species to have proportionately long tails, which may comprise up to 40% of the total body length in some species (Lillywhite and Henderson, 1993). The tail provides a relatively "tighter" (low compliance) compartment surrounding blood vessels than does the precaudal segment, which accommodates the body cavity. Thus, for a given body length, the elongate tail provides additional hemodynamic advantage in counteracting tendencies for blood pooling in dependent tissues when the animal is upright. A possible parallel among humans is the relative elongation of the lower limbs in comparison with the torso during the evolution of stature.

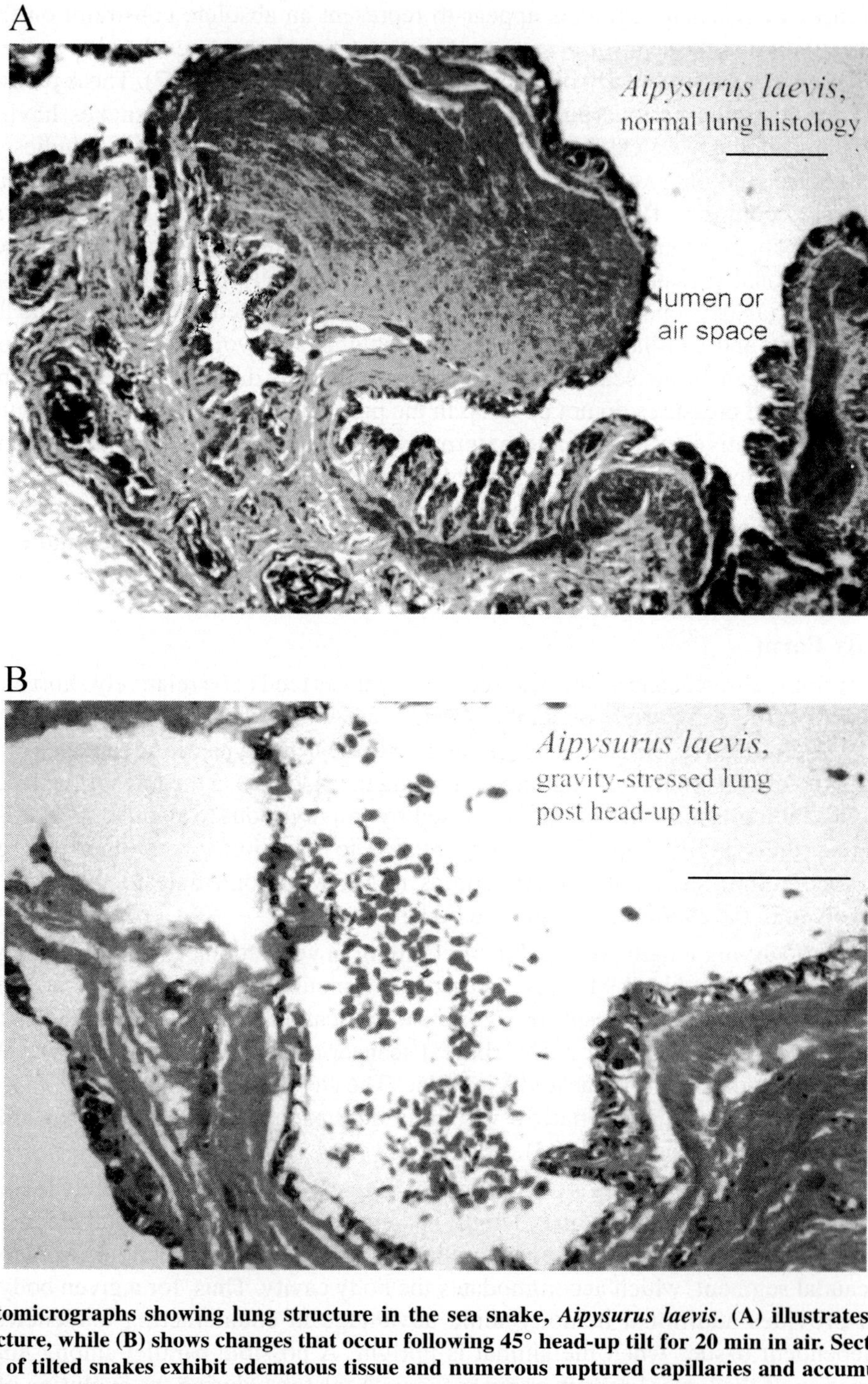

Fig. 1. Photomicrographs showing lung structure in the sea snake, *Aipysurus laevis*. (A) illustrates normal lung structure, while (B) shows changes that occur following 45° head-up tilt for 20 min in air. Sections from the lung of tilted snakes exhibit edematous tissue and numerous ruptured capillaries and accumulation of red blood cells within the faveoli. Sections were taken approximately 42 cm posterior to the lung apex. Scale bars = 100 mm. (Lillywhite, unpublished)

Morphology and the "Antigravity Suit"

Arboreal and scansorial species of snakes are characterized by comparatively "tight" external anatomy and by having perivascular tissues of comparatively low compliance in relation to non-scansorial species. In addition to features already mentioned, the integument of scansorial species appears to have tighter and more extensive attachment to underlying tissues than does that of non-scansorial species (Lillywhite and Smits, 1992; Lillywhite and Henderson, 1993). Such differences presumably reflect adaptive structural modifications related to requirements for counteracting gravity stresses in the various forms. Studies of snakes incorporating use of a tail plethysmograph found that the magnitude of change in tail volume attributable to combined blood pooling and plasma filtration varied from about 1% in arboreal species to as much as 9% in aquatic species during head-up tilt in air (Lillywhite, 1985a). Such differences might be attributed to combined morphological attributes and the vasomotor status of resistance and capacitance vessels in the dependent tissues of the various species. However, further investigations found that compliance of the subcutaneous tissue space was nearly tenfold greater in aquatic and non-scansorial species than in scansorial species of snakes that were investigated (Lillywhite, 1993a).

It is of interest to mention here experiments in which the tolerance of snakes to graded acceleration force were studied by use of a centrifuge (Lillywhite et al., 1996). It was found that mechanical enhancement of the antigravity suit, accomplished by having snakes within a tight-fitting tube, increases the level of acceleration which a snake can withstand without cessation of carotid arterial blood flow. The tight tube prevents expansion of the snake's body, and the acceleration tolerance increases from roughly +2 to +3 G_z. The impressive finding is the improvement of acceleration tolerance was accomplished solely by the mechanical countermeasure rather than to changes in physiology.

The combined morphological characters that limit tissue and vascular expansion have been referred to as an anatomical "antigravity suit" that evolves tighter properties under natural selection related to gravitational stress (Lillywhite, 1996). Convergent examples can be found among taller upright mammals, such as giraffes, in which very tight skin invests the feet and legs (Hargens et al., 1987, 1988).

Arterial Blood Pressure and Hemodynamic Regulation

There are distinct trends in the level of arterial blood pressure among snakes in relation to habitat and potential gravitational stress on the circulation. Among vertebrates generally, there is a phylogenetic trend for increase in systemic arterial pressure as one progresses from smaller ectothermic taxa to larger endothermic taxa (Johansen, 1972; Burggren et al., 1997). The higher levels of arterial pressure appear to have evolved in relation to endothermy (birds, mammals), metabolic demands of activity (endotherms, some fishes and varanid lizards), separation of systemic and pulmonary circulation (crocodilians and varanids), and the gravitational demands of the habitat (snakes, possibly varanids).

Among snakes, mean resting arterial pressure correlates significantly with body mass, but also tends to be significantly higher in scansorial species and lowest in fully aquatic species, irrespective of size (Seymour and Lillywhite, 1976; Seymour, 1987). Systemic pressures in scansorial species range generally between 40 and 90 mm Hg, whereas those in aquatic and amphibious species are generally between 18 and 30 mm Hg and may approach values (10-20 mm Hg) approximating critical closing pressures of mammals (Lillywhite and Pough, 1983). The higher relative pressures observed in scansorial species of snakes appear to reflect generally greater levels of vascular tone and peripheral resistance (Fig. 2) that are important for regulation of hemodynamics during postural disturbance (Lillywhite and Donald, 1994).

The higher pressures of scansorial species are advantageous insofar as they help to ensure adequate perfusion of the head and cerebral vasculature at all attitudes of posture (Seymour and Lillywhite, 1976; Lillywhite, 1987). Both theoretic considerations and empirical evidence indicate that the ventricle must produce a pressure in excess of the hydrostatic column above it in order to produce flow in the cephalad direction (Lillywhite and Donald, 1994). Turning to mammalian comparisons, the well-known "hypertension" of giraffes (arterial pressures roughly twice that of humans) seems related to the elongate neck and long blood column between the head and heart of upright animals (Seymour et al., 1993). Indeed, there is a crude correlation between the characteristic arterial blood pressure and height of larger terrestrial mammals (Patterson et al., 1975). It thus appears that levels of systemic arterial pressure have evolved to exceed those of the hydrostatic column above the heart when animals are in an upright position and, thus, are related to the degree of gravitational stress which a species experiences as a result of its height and postural behavior. Aquatic species must have experienced relaxed selection for high levels of arterial pressure following their secondary invasion of liquid

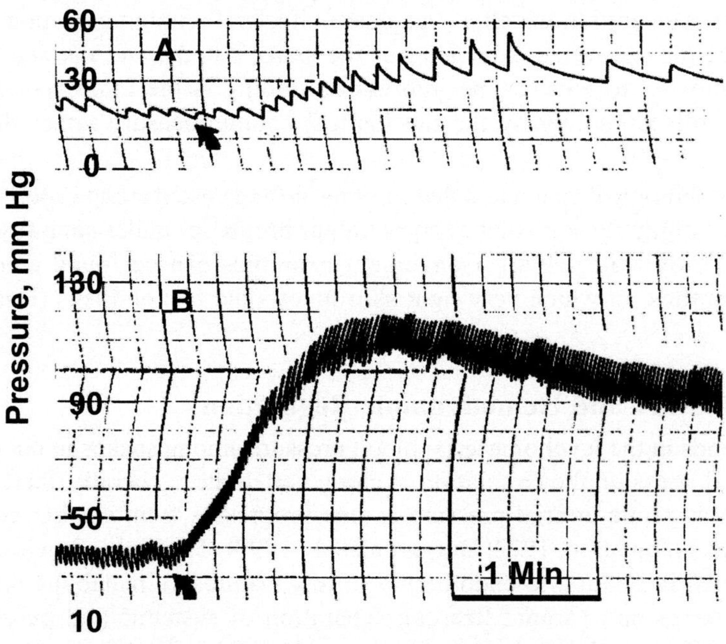

Fig. 2. Pressor responses to 100 μg/kg (A) or 10 μg/kg (B) of norepinephrine, injected intravenously at points in time indicated by the arrows. The level of hypertension induced by the exogenous catecholamine in the aquatic snake *Acrochordus granulatus* (A) is about maximal for this species. Similarly induced hypertension in the semi-arboreal snake *Elaphe obsoleta* (B) exceeds that of the aquatic species considerably, even at lower doses. Pressures were recorded from indwelling, non-occluding intraaortic catheters in conscious snakes, and norepinephrine was injected in small carrier volumes of 50 ml saline. Illustration adapted from Lillywhite (1987).

habitats. Low arterial pressure and poor compensation for gravitational disturbance to pressure, prevalent among aquatic species, also characterize non-climbing terrestrial snakes such as heavy-bodied vipers that spend much time inactive in horizontal postures (Lillywhite and Smits, 1992; Lillywhite, 1993b).

Scansorial snake species are characterized by robust control of arterial pressure and exhibit superior regulation of pressure in the face of gravitational disturbance to hemodynamics, relative to aquatic or terrestrial viperid species (Lillywhite and Gallagher, 1985; Lillywhite and Donald, 1994; Lillywhite et al., 1996). Regulation of arterial pressure in snakes is fundmentally similar to that in mammals and involves neural activation of baroreflexes involving cardiovascular mechanoreceptors, in addition to chronic adjustments that preserve the blood volume (Smits and Lillywhite, 1985). Endocrine, autocrine, and paracrine mechanisms are also undoubtedly important to stability of arterial pressure, but these are relatively not well studied (Chiu et al., 1986; Mifune et al., 1996; Wang et al., 2000).

Head-up posture tends to displace a large fraction of the blood volume posteriorad and immediately reduces the ventricular output and central arterial pressure. Partial or full recovery of the pressure is achieved by reflexogenic increases in both heart rate and peripheral vascular resistance during a compensatory period in which events are basically similar to those seen in mammals (Lillywhite and Donald, 1994). In scansorial species of snakes, the regulated arterial pressure during head-up tilt exceeds the pre-tilt baseline at the body center, and tends to compensate for the passive fall of pressure at the level of the elevated head. As a consequence, carotid artery and cerebral blood flow are maintained during postural gravity stress. On the other hand, in the aquatic species there is tendency for blood pooling in the lower body during similar circumstances to overwhelm comparatively weaker reflexogenic mechanisms, and both central arterial pressure and cephalic blood flow fall to zero during head-up postures exceeding 30-45°. Similar loss of cardiovascular homeostasis during gravity stress is observed also in strictly ground-dwelling species of viperid snakes (Fig. 3). In these non-scansorial species, the degree of effector stimulation is relatively feeble (Fig. 2) in addition to pronounced tendencies to blood pooling (Lillywhite and Pough, 1983; Lillywhite, 1985a; Lillywhite, 1987; Lillywhite 1993b).

Studies of the scansorial rat snake (*Elaphe obsoleta*) demonstrate that ventricular output is reduced about 50% during head-up tilt, in spite of increases of heart rate (Lillywhite and Gallagher, 1985). In these same investigations, measurements of regional blood flows using radioactively labeled microspheres demonstrate that blood flow is reduced primarily in visceral organs, posterior skin and posterior skeletal muscle, concomitant with 2-3-fold increases in peripheral resistance, while blood flow is maintained to the heart, brain and lung. These responses are blocked by the adrenoceptor antagonists phentolamine and nitroglycerin. In aquatic or non-climbing species that fail to regulate arterial pressure during head-up tilt, carotid blood flow falls to zero, coincident with reduction of arterial pressure below levels equivalent to the hydrostatic column above the heart (Lillywhite and Donald, 1994).

There are two novel aspects of blood pressure regulation that are seen in *Elaphe obsoleta* and probably other arboreal species. First, small-diameter and richly innervated vessel segments connecting the right aortic arch and dorsal aorta create a posterior-to-anterior shunt of blood flow during head-up posture (Lillywhite and Donald, 1988) (Fig. 4). The vessels in question are of larger diameter in a number of non-climbing species of snakes that have been examined, and the mechanism is probably lacking in these species (unpublished data). Second, arboreal species of snakes are noted to

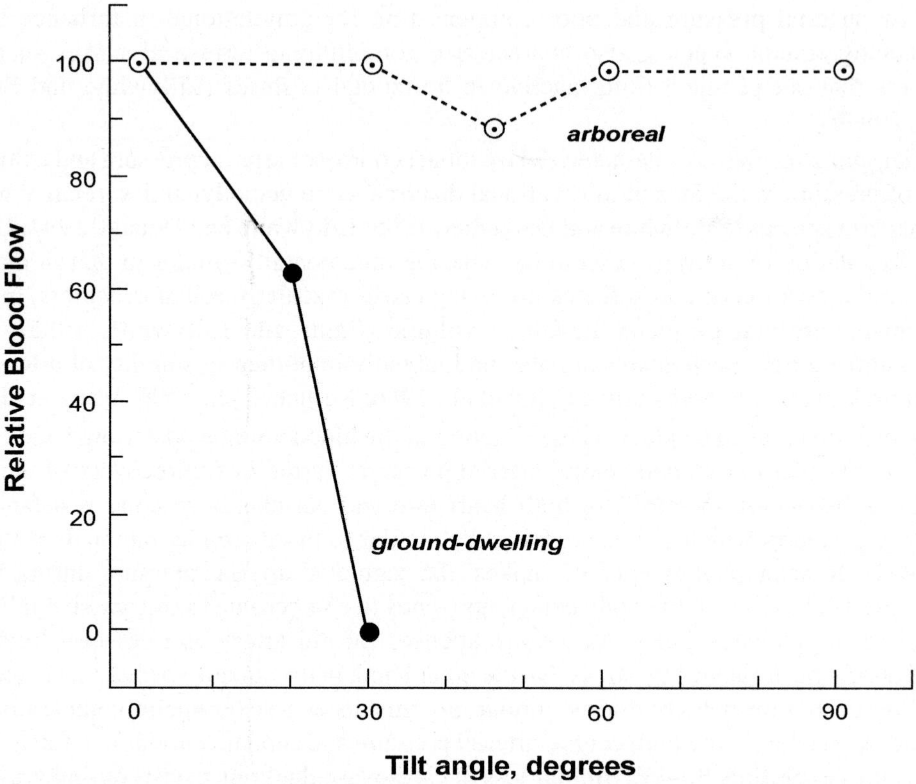

Fig. 3. Changes of carotid arterial blood flow in the ground-dwelling snake *Bitis gabonica* (lower left trace) and the arboreal species *Philodryas baroni* (upper trace), both subjected to progressive, graded, head-up tilt in air. Blood flows are expressed relative to those measured at horizontal position (100%) and reflect steady state flows attained during 3 min of tilt. Blood flows were measured by means of miniaturized Doppler blood flow cuffs positioned near the base of the carotid artery in conscious snakes. Data from Lillywhite (1993b).

engage in stereotyped wiggling behaviors during postural hypotension. These consist of lateral undulations that pass craniad along the body and have the effect of increasing venous return, hence the ventricular output and arterial pressure (Lillywhite, 1985b). Insofar as anatomical valves appear to be lacking from the major veins of snakes (Lillywhite, 1987), body movements are potentially very important to maintenance of blood circulation. For reasons not entirely understood, body movements have relatively less effect in correcting circulatory deficiency in aquatic and viperid species that are subjected to head-up tilt.

Efferent autonomic mechanisms play an important role in the regulation of hemodynamics in snakes. Baroreceptors have been identified in the truncus arteriosus, and mechanoreceptive sites have been implicated in distal as well as proximal sites in the pulmonary artery, aorta, and carotid arteries (Berger, 1987; Backhouse et al., 1989; Lillywhite and Donald, 1994; Van Vliet and West, 1994). The heart is richly innervated by cholinergic inhibitory nerves as well as dense but variable adrenergic and peptidergic cardiac nerves. Similarly, neuropeptides as well as catecholamines are extensively distributed and colocalized in perivascular nerves innervating arteries and veins of snakes (Davies and

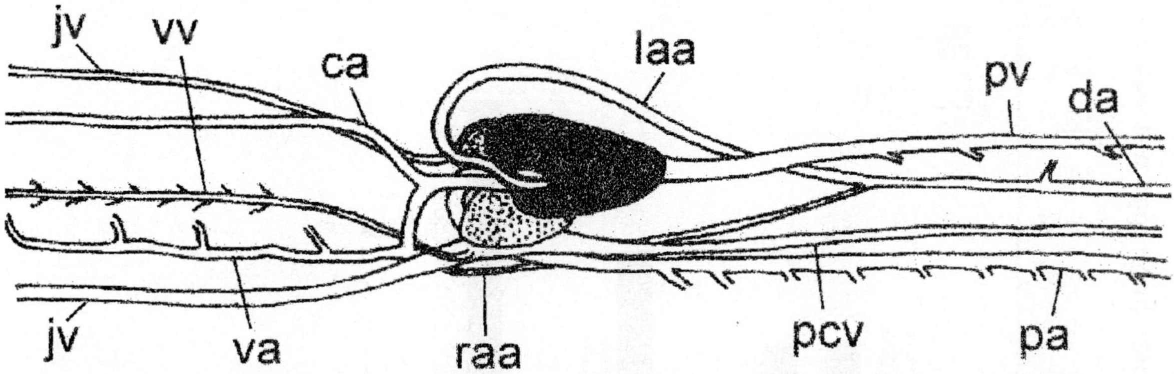

Fig. 4. **Schematic illustration of the central blood vessels in an arboreal snake. Cephalic arterial blood flow is derived from the carotid artery (ca) and vertebral artery (va) (arrows), both being derived from the right aortic arch (raa). The distal terminal segment of the right aortic arch is comparatively small diameter in comparison with the left arch (laa), prior to its juncture with the dorsal aorta (da). During head-up posture, blood flow in the distal segment of the right arch is reduced to near zero, presumably by means of vasoconstriction, and the total right aortic blood flow is directed toward the head via the carotid and vertebral arteries. Additionally, increased peripheral resistance in the left aortic arch, attributable largely to vasoconstriction in the posterior and visceral vessels, elevates its resistance and potentially creates a shunting of blood from left to right arch by means of an interaortic foramen at the base of the outflow tracts (Young et al., 1993). Other vessel abbreviations: jv = jugular vein; pa = pulmonary artery; pcv = posterior vena cava; vv = vertebral vein. Figure adapted from Donald and Lillywhite (1988).**

Donald, 1992; Lillywhite and Donald, 1994). Neurogenic peripheral vasoconstriction is mediated by baroreflexes involving alpha adrenoceptors in the peripheral vessels (Lillywhite and Seymour, 1978; Lillywhite and Gallagher, 1985), and catecholamines are strongly implicated in the regulation of venomotor tone to promote venous return and cardiac filling (Lillywhite and Smith, 1981; Lillywhite, 1987). The combined data indicate there is functional specialization within components of the peripheral autonomic system controlling the circulation, especially with regard to regulation of venous capacity.

Comparative investigations indicate clear interspecific variation in the density of adrenergic innervation of the larger arteries and veins of snakes and suggest the patterns of innervation differences are adaptive with respect to the gravitational environment (Lillywhite and Donald, 1994). Scansorial species demonstrate a substantially denser innervation of posterior arteries and veins than do species that are primarily terrestrial or aquatic. The evolution of densely innervated posterior vessels may be a key regulatory feature that facilitates regulation of central arterial pressure and flow of blood to vital anterior organs such as heart and brain during upright posture. Indeed, catecholamines stimulate several-fold greater tension in posterior than in anterior vessels, which were shown to have lesser inherent contractility *in vitro* (Conklin et al., 1996). Such data correlate nicely with innervation patterns that most likely evolved in response to the gravitational influence on postural hemodynamics (Fig. 5). Peptidergic innervation of capacity vessels is exceptional and can exceed that of the arteries, which further emphasizes the importance of venous tone in the regulation of cardiovascular hemodynamics.

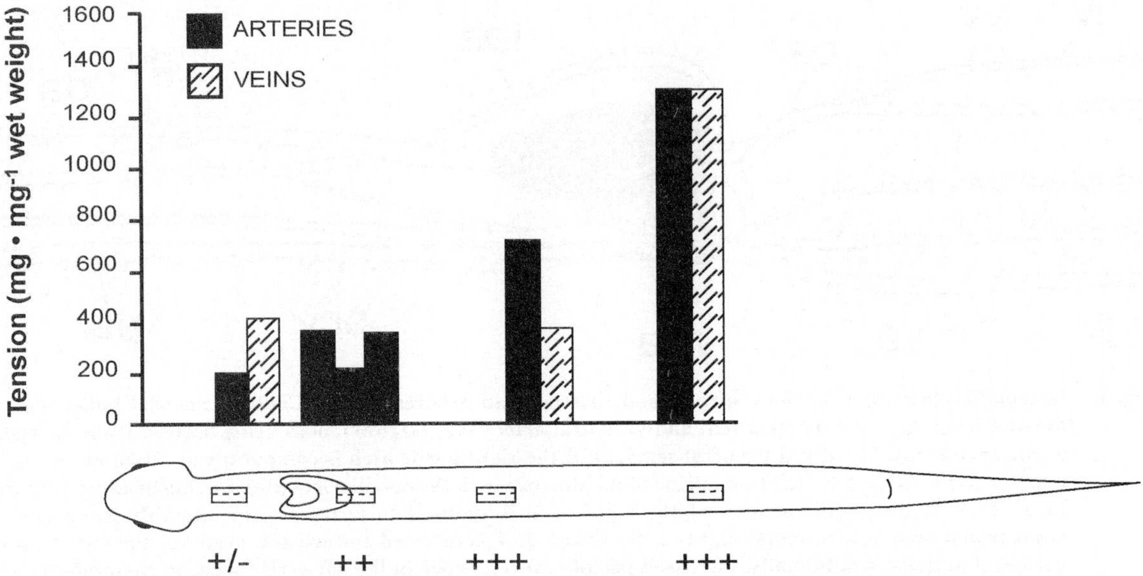

Fig. 5. Anatomic distribution of maximal tension development in isolated vascular rings exposed to 80 mM potassium bath *in vitro*. Measurements were from 4-8 individuals of the semi-arboreal snake *Elaphe obsoleta* for each vessel segment tested (differences between anterior and posterior vessels were statistically significant). Corresponding levels of adrenergic innervation density are shown at the bottom of the figure. Data are from Conklin et al. (1996) and J. Donald (unpublished).

Responses of Snakes to Hypergravic Acceleration on a Centrifuge

The cardiovascular responses of snakes to increasing acceleration force measured during G_z acceleration parallel those which are observed during graded, head-up tilt, with scansorial species being more tolerant of hypergravic force (Lillywhite et al., 1996, 1997). Maximal heart rates measured during acceleration are similar in scansorial and non-scansorial species, suggesting that differences in tolerance are strongly dependent on factors related to vascular compliance and peripheral vascular tone (Lillywhite and Seymour, 1978; Lillywhite and Pough, 1983; Lillywhite and Gallagher, 1985). Scansorial species of snakes can withstand acceleration forces 2-3 times that of Earth g for periods up to 1 h without cessation of carotid blood flow or loss of normal behaviors such as body or head movements and tongue flicking. Aquatic species, on the other hand, cannot withstand an acceleration force equivalent to +1 G_z without debilitating loss of carotid blood flow. Intraspecific regression analyses indicate that G_z tolerance of scansorial rat snakes correlates with shorter body length, higher arterial pressures, comparatively higher blood volume, comparatively lower maximal heart rate, and chronic acclimation to G_z force. These characters tend to be associated with G tolerance in vertebrates generally (Burton and Smith, 1996).

From Snakes to Humans

Fundamentally, many of the adaptive traits of snakes that are discussed in the preceding pages appear to represent general features of gravity adaptation that are applicable to vertebrates as a whole

(Lillywhite, 1996). In view of the short-term stresses on the cardiovascular system that are known in astronauts (Watenpaugh and Hargens, 1996), and the divergent features seen in related taxa having long evolutionary histories in aquatic and arboreal environments, a number of adaptive changes seem likely to occur in humans if they were exposed to microgravity of space or other environments for evolutionary time. Such likely changes include: 1) lower levels of arterial blood pressure; 2) decreased vascular tone; 3) "looser" tissue spaces; 4) possibly larger body size with relatively elongated torso; 5) some reorganization of gross anatomy; 6) loss of gradients of vascular characters; and 7) alterations of vascular structure and function. Of course, long-term evolutionary exposure to microgravity seems unlikely without technological countermeasures to deconditioning, but changes of structure and function in the suggested directions might occur on a lesser and perhaps more subtle scale if humans were to live permanently in a circumstance of reduced, but not virtual zero, g force.

One important overall conclusion emerges from the comparative investigations of snakes that are reviewed here. Adaptive changes in response to evolutionary histories in different gravitational environments involve substantial alterations of features related to the cardiovascular system. These reflect not merely minor shifts in anatomy or physiological mechanisms, but, rather, profound changes in both structure and function. Underlying causation of these changes can be inferred from the demonstrations of altered molecular structure and gene expression in cells that are cultured in microgravity (Morey-Holton, 2003).

Acknowledgements

The author wishes to thank numerous persons and collaborators who were involved in the many studies of snake physiology that form the basis of this synthesis. Special thanks are due to Roger Seymour, with whom these investigations began, and to Alan Hargens who nurtured an interest in space biology and its relations to comparative investigations. Support for the various studies was provided by the National Science Foundation, National Institutes of Health, NASA, and the National Research Council.

References

Backhouse SS, Harper AA, VanVliet BN, West NH. Localization and conduction velocities of arterial baroreceptors in the anesthetized snake. *J. Physiol. Lond.* 1989; 418:135P.

Berger, PJ. The reptilian baroreceptor and its role in cardiovascular control. *Am. Zool.* 1987;27:111-120.

Burggren W. Pulmonary blood plasma filtration in reptiles: a "wet" vertebrate lung? *Science* 1982;215:77-78.

Burggren W, Farrell A, Lillywhite H. Vertebrate cardiovascular systems. In: Dantzler WH, ed., *Handbook of Physiology: Comparative Physiology, Sec. 13*, Oxford University Press, new York, 1997:215-308.

Burton RR, Smith AH. Adaptation to acceleration environments. In: Fregly MJ, Blatteis, CM, eds., *Handbook of Physiology: Environmental Physiology, Sec 3*, Oxford University Press, New York, 1996:943-970.

Chiu KW, Wong VCK, Chan MY, Pang PKT. Blood pressure homeostasis in the snake, *Ptyas korros. Gen. Comp. Endocrinol.* 1986; 64:300-304.

Conklin DJ, Lillywhite HB, Olson KR, Ballard RE, Hargens AR. Blood vessel adaptation to gravity in a semi-arboreal snake. *J. Comp. Physiol.* 1996; B165:518-526.

Davies PJ, Donald JA. Distribution and colocalisation of neuropeptides in the large systemic arteries and veins of the ratsnake, *Elaphe obsoleta. Cell Tissue Res.* 1992; 269:495-504.

Donald JA, Lillywhite HB. Adrenergic innervation of the large arteries and veins of the semiarboreal rat snake *Elaphe obsoleta. J. Morphol.* 1988; 198:25-31.

Hargens AR, Millard RW, Pettersson K, Johansen K. Gravitational haemodynamics and oedema prevention in the giraffe. *Nature* 1987;329:59-60.

Hargens AR, Gershuni DH, Danzig LA, Millard RW, Pettersson K. Tissue adaptations to gravitational stress: Newborn versus adult giraffes. *Physiologist* 1988;31:S110-S113.

Johansen K. Heart and circulation in gill, skin and lung breathing. *Respir. Physiol.* 1972;14:193-210.

Lillywhite HB. Postural edema and blood pooling in snakes. *Physiol. Zool.* 1985a;58:759-766.

Lillywhite HB. Behavioral control of arterial pressure in snakes. *Physiol. Zool.* 1985b;58:159-165.

Lillywhite HB. Circulatory adaptations of snakes to gravity. *Amer Zool* 1987;27:81-95.

Lillywhite HB. Subcutaneous compliance and gravitational adaptation in snakes. *J. Exp. Zool.* 1993a;267:557-562.

Lillywhite HB. Orthostatic intolerance of viperid snakes. *Physiol. Zool.* 1993b;66:1000-10014.

Lillywhite HB. Gravity, blood circulation, and the adaptation of form and function in lower vertebrates. *J. Exp. Zool.* 1996;275:217-225.

Lillywhite HB, Donald JA. Anterograde bias of blood flow in arboreal snakes. *Am Zool.* 1988;28:8A.

Lillywhite HB, Donald JA. Neural regulation of arterial blood pressure in snakes. *Physiol. Zool.* 1994;67:1260-1283.

Lillywhite HB, Gallagher KP. Hemodynamic adjustments to head-up posture in the partly arboreal snake, *Elaphe obsoleta. J. Exp. Zool.* 1985;235:325-334.

Lillywhite HB, Henderson RW. Behavioral and functional ecology of arboreal snakes. In: Seigel, R, Collins J, eds., *Snakes: Ecology and Behavior*, MacMillan, New York, 1993:1-48.

Lillywhite HB, Pough FH. Control of arterial pressure in aquatic sea snakes. *Am. J. Physiol.* 1983;244:R66-R73.

Lillywhite HB, Seymour RS. Regulation of arterial blood pressure in Australian tiger snakes. *J. Exp. Biol.* 1978;75:65-79.

Lillywhite, HB, Smith LH. Haemodynamic responses to haemorrhage in the snake *Elaphe obsoleta obsoleta. J. Exp. Biol.* 1981;94:275-283.

Lillywhite HB, Smits AW. Cardiovascular adaptations of viperid snakes. In: Campbell JA, Brodie ED Jr, eds., *Biology of Pitvipers*, Selva, Tyler, Texas, 1992:143-153.

Lillywhite HB, Ballard RE, Hargens AR. Tolerance of snakes to hypergravity. *Physiol. Zool.* 1996;69:293-303.

Lillywhite HB, Ballard RE, Hargens AR, Rosenberg HI. Cardiovascular responses of snakes to hypergravity. *Grav. Space Biol. Bull.* 1997;10:145-152.

Mifune H, Suzuki S, Nokihara K, Noda Y. Distribution of immunoreactive atrial and brain natriuretic peptides in the heart of the chicken, quail, snake and frog. *Exper. Anim. Tokyo* 1996; 45:125-133.

Morey-Holton ER. The impact of gravity on life. In: Rothschild L, Lister A, eds., Evolution on Planet Earth: The Impact of the Physical Environment, Elsevier, Oxford, 2003:142-159.

Patterson JL Jr., Goetz RH, Doyle JT, Warren JV, Gauer OH, Detweiler DK, Said SI, Hoernicke H, McGregor M, Keen EN, Smith MH Jr., Hardie EL, Reynolds M, Flatt WP, Waldo DR. Cardiorespiratory dynamics in the ox and giraffe, with comparative observations on man and other mammals. *Ann. N.Y. Acad. Sci.* 1975;127:393-413.

Rowell LB. *Human Cardiovascular Control.* Oxford University Press, New York, 1993.

Seymour, RS. Scaling of cardiovascular physiology in snakes. *Amer. Zool.* 1987;27:97-109.

Seymour, RS, Lillywhite, HB. Blood pressure in snakes from different habitats. *Nature* 1976;264:664-666.

Seymour RS, Hargens AR, Pedley TJ. The heart works against gravity. *Am. J. Physiol.* 1993;265:R715-R720.

Smits, AW. Fluid balance in vertebrate lungs. In: Wood, S.C., ed., *Comparative Pulmonary Physiology.* Current Concepts, Marcel Dekker, New York, 1989:503-537.

Smits AW, Lillywhite HB. Maintenance of blood volume in snakes: transcapillary shifts of extravascular fluids during acute hemorrhage. *J. Comp. Physiol.* 1985;155B:305-310.

Van Vliet BN, West NH. Phylogenetic trends in the baroreceptor control of arterial blood pressure. *Physiol. Zool.* 1994; 67:1284-1304.

Wallach V. The lungs of snakes. In: Gans C, Gaunt AS, eds., *Biology of the Reptilia. Vol. 19, Morphology G, Visceral Organs*, Soc. Study Amphibians Reptiles, Ithaca, New York, 1998:93-295.

Wang T, Axelsson M, Jensen J, Conlon JM. Cardiovascular actions of python bradykinin and substance P in the anesthetized python, *Python regius. Am. J. Physiol.* 2000; 279:R531-R538.

Watenpaugh DE, Hargens AR. The cardiovascular system in microgravity. In: Fregly MJ, Blatteis CM, eds., *Handbook of Physiology: Environmental Physiology, Sec. 3*, Oxford University Press, New York, 1996:631-674.

Young BA, Lillywhite HB, Wassersug RJ. On the structure of the aortic valves in snakes (Reptilia: Serpentes). *J. Morphol.* 1993; 216:141-159.

Adaptation Biology and Medicine (Volume 4: Current Concepts)
Editors: A. Hargens, N. Takeda and P.K. Singal

7. Role of Free NO and NO Stores in Protective Effects of Adaptation to Hypoxia

E.B. Manukhina and I.Yu. Malyshev

Institute of General Pathology and Pathophysiology, Moscow

Abstract

Hypoxia can exert both detrimental and protective effect on the organism. Acute hypoxia induces diverse responses of intracellular signaling pathway and, accordingly, different physiological responses. This fact has called attention to the most universal physiological processes, such as metabolism of nitric oxide (NO), which is extensively regulated by oxygen level in the environment. Direction of the changes in NO synthesis induced by hypoxia depends on the severity and duration of hypoxia. Chronic hypoxia can suppress not only NO synthase activity but also expression of eNOS gene in blood vessels of systemic circulation. At the same time, chronic hypoxia stimulates NO synthesis in pulmonary blood vessels. Opposite to chronic hypoxia, intermittent hypoxia is an efficient stimulator of NO synthesis. Therefore an adapting organism, which progressively increases its NO production has a possibility to "detoxicate" excessive NO by binding it to complexes, which form physiologically active NO stores in the vascular wall. Experiments on rats of different strains possessing different inherited intensity of NO production and storage showed that 1) NO stores can serve as an additional non-enzymic source of free NO in the conditions of NO deficiency; 2) NO binding to NO stores prevents detrimental effects of NO overproduction; and 3) excessive NO storage is possible in certain conditions, which may be unfavorable for stress-resistance of the organism. Therefore NO plays an important role in development of adaptation to hypoxia. Both intensity of NO production and extent of NO storage should be taken into account in developing regimens of adaptation to hypoxia for clinical and experimental applications.

Periodic hypoxic episodes can exert both detrimental and protective effects on the organism, which are defined to a considerable extent by the regimen, that is, ratio of duration and intensity of hypoxic exposures. It was shown that acute, chronic and intermittent hypoxia induce different responses of intracellular signaling pathways for transcription of different genes; physiological responses to hypoxic exposures differ correspondingly [24]. It is well known that chronic periodic hypoxia, which is observed, for example, in sleep apnea syndrome, can result in development of pulmonary and systemic hypertension, myocardial infarction and cognitive disorders [22]. At the same time, dosed adaptation to intermittent hypobaric or normobaric hypoxia possesses a spectrum of direct and cross protective effects, which have been widely used for treatment and prevention of many diseases and to increase efficiency of exercise training [18]. This is why studying the effect of hypoxia on key physiological processes is so important. One of such universal processes is metabolism of nitric oxide (NO) tightly regulated by environmental oxygen [12].

Synthesis of NO is a five-electron nitrogen oxidation at the terminal guanidine group of L-arginine. This oxygen-dependent reaction occurs in the presence of NADPH, BH_4, FAD and FMN as cofactors and is catalyzed by the heme-containing enzyme NO synthase (NOS), which exists as three isoforms. The isoenzyme NOS I (neuronal NOS, nNOS) is constitutively expressed in primarily central and peripheral neurons, though it was later shown to be present also in some epithelial and vascular smooth muscle cells (including pulmonary vessels) [28]. Activity of nNOS is regulated by Ca^{2+}-dependent calmodulin binding. The isoenzyme NOS II (inducible NOS, iNOS) is normally absent in cells; NOS II is induced by various factors related to inflammatory and free radical oxidation processes. This isoenzyme is only regulated at the expression level, and its activity does not depend on Ca^{2+} and calmodulin. NOS II produces NO in the amounts three orders of magnitude exceeding those produced by constitutive NOS isoforms. The third isoform, NOS III (endothelial NOS, eNOS) is present in endothelial and some other types of cells and is regulated at both transcriptional and translational level and at the level of enzyme activity. Activity of eNOS is regulated by intracellular Ca^{2+}/calmodulin. Synthesis of NO takes a start within a few seconds of any stimulation increasing intracellular Ca^{2+}, such as acetylcholine, bradykinin, ATP, serotonin, thrombin, etc. The major physical factors regulating both eNOS gene expression and eNOS activity are shear stress and concentration of molecular oxygen [7, 30].

Effect of NO depends on NO level. High concentrations of NO are toxic and provide cytostatic and cytotoxic effects on tumor and bacterial cells. In addition, excessive NO readily reacts with superoxide and forms even more toxic peroxynitrite. Comparatively low concentrations of NO provide regulatory function through activation of cyclic guanylate cyclase and cGMP production in target cells. For example, in blood vessels, the NO synthesized in the endothelium diffuses to neighboring smooth muscle cells and activates cGMP-dependent protein kinase (G kinase) therein with subsequent decrease in intracellular Ca^{2+}, vascular smooth muscle relaxation and vasodilation [3].

Molecular oxygen is a key substrate for NOS. However a direct dependence of NO synthesis on O_2 level in the environment is absent. Studies performed on a whole organism, isolated organs and cultured cells have shown that the direction of changes in NO synthesis is related with the extent and duration of hypoxia with different mechanisms of these changes.

It was demonstrated on cell culture that after the first 10 minutes of moderate hypoxia, Ca^{2+} begins to enter the cell to activate eNOS. More prolonged hypoxia terminates the Ca^{2+} entry and decreases the NO synthesis [10]. Luckhoff and Busse [13] showed a close positive correlation between increases in intracellular Ca^{2+} and release of NO in endothelial cells exposed to hypoxia.

Hypoxic inhibition of eNOS is evident as attenuation of endothelium-dependent vascular relaxation. After 48 hours of exposing rats to hypoxia, endothelium-dependent relaxation of the isolated aorta was twofold reduced [33].

The level of NO remained virtually unchanged in acute 3-min hypoxia until the oxygen concentration decreased below 10%; NO level was only significantly decreased when oxygen concentration was reduced to 5% [4, 34]. This oxygen level corresponds to the composition of hypoxic mixtures used for adaptation to hypoxia [32].

The decrease in NO production in acute hypoxia is reversible. For example, after 90-min hypoxia, plasma levels of the NO metabolites nitrite and nitrate in the blood from aorta and renal artery were decreased to 48% and 73% of the initial level, respectively. After 1 hour of reoxygenation, the parameters returned to baseline [23].

Activity of NOS directly depends on the level of synthesized NO since NO regulates the NOS activity by the negative feedback mechanism. The synthesized NO binds to iron of NOS heme thereby inhibiting NOS; simultaneously apparent KM for O_2 increases [1]. Since O_2 and NO compete for NOS heme iron, the extent of NOS dependence on O_2 is related with decomposition rate of the NO/heme iron complex, which depends, in its turn, on O_2 concentration [2]. The level of O_2 as a substrate can limit NO production in hypoxia because the apparent sensitivity of NOS isoforms to O_2 is within the range of normal tissue O_2 concentrations [26].

Another possible mechanism for hypoxic inhibition of NO production is the decrease in heat shock proteins HSP90 characteristic of hypoxia [31]. These proteins bind to eNOS and provide its activation in response to NO-stimulating agonists [8].

Sensitivity of eNOS to O_2 shortage increases on the background of iNOS induction. Indeed, a moderate decrease in O_2 tension in a cell culture, which generally does not induce any attenuation of NO synthesis, suppresses eNOS activity following the iNOS gene expression stimulated by bacterial lipopolysaccharide [11].

Importantly, the decreased NO production in acute hypoxia is due to inhibition of eNOS activity but not downregulation of the enzyme protein synthesis [31]. However chronic hypoxia can suppress both eNOS activity and eNOS gene expression in vessels of systemic circulation simultaneously stimulating the latter in pulmonary circulation. The amount of eNOS protein sharply falls in rat aorta while it increases in lungs as early as after 12 hours of hypoxia [33]. Percentage of pulmonary arterioles expressing eNOS begins to increase after 1 day of hypoxia. After that this parameter increases for several days and then remains unchanged for 4 weeks. The NO overproduction in pulmonary arterioles is not always beneficial and may even contribute to development of pulmonary hypertension depending on the relationship between NO and free oxygen species [10].

In contrast to chronic hypoxia, dosed periodic hypoxia is an efficient stimulator of NO synthesis and eNOS expression. However when developing regimens for practical application of adaptation to hypoxia one should take into account the following important issue. Intermittent hypoxia stimulates both activity and expression of all three NOS isoforms. Potentiation of constitutive NO production is generally beneficial for the organism because it protects the organism against hypertension, thromboses, vasospasm, oxidative stress, etc. At the same time, expression of iNOS results in NO overproduction and toxic effects of excessive NO. During a hypoxic exposure, expression of iNOS takes a start only after 6 hours of continuous hypoxia while the constitutive isoforms eNOS and nNOS become activated almost immediately [9]. Therefore duration of an adapting session of hypoxia should not exceed 6 hours.

In our experiments, adaptation to intermittent hypobaric hypoxia was used for stimulation of endogenous NO production [15]. Adaptation was performed in the altitude chamber at the simulated altitude corresponding to 4000 m above sea level. The duration of hypoxic exposure was gradually increased from 10 minutes to 5 hours. The complete course of adaptation consisted of 40 daily sessions. The NO production was evaluated spectrophotometrically by total plasma concentration of nitrite and nitrate. Figure 1 shows that adaptation induced a gradual increase in plasma nitrite plus nitrate, and by the end of adaptation course this parameter twice exceeded the control level.

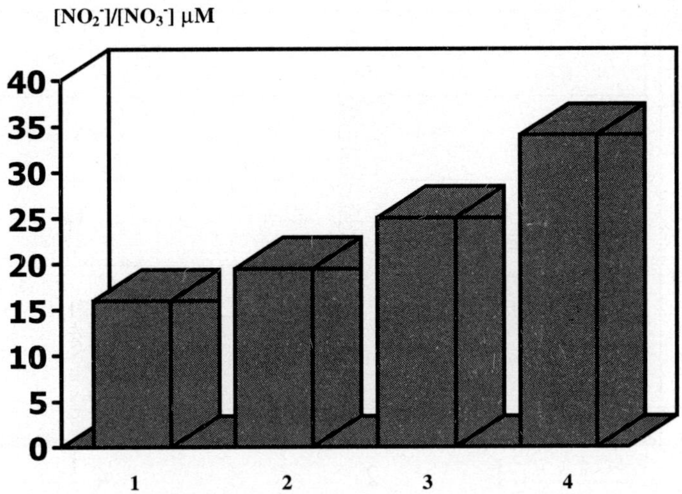

Fig. 1. Effect of adaptation to hypoxia on plasma level of nitrite+nitrate in rats. Bars reflect the total concentration of plasma nitrite and nitrate in μM. 1, control; 2, 3 sessions of adaptation; 3, 6 sessions of adaptation; 4, 40 sessions of adaptation. *Significant differences from control, $p<0.05$.

Protective effect of 8-day adaptation to hypoxia was evident as a significant increase in survival of rats exposed to acute, severe hypoxia at a simulated altitude of 11,000 m above sea level (Fig. 2) [14]. The NOS inhibitor N^{ω}-nitro-L-arginine itself reduced the resistance of rats to acute hypoxia and abolished the protective effect of adaptation. Results of this experiment support the role of the adaptive potentiation of NO production in protective effects of adaptation to hypoxia.

Obviously, an adapting organism, which increases the NO production, should possess some additional mechanisms of protection against NO overproduction. Indeed NO can be stabilized by binding to the complexes which form physiologically active NO stores. NO stores can gradually release NO and therefore serve as an additional non-enzymic source of free NO. Formation of NO stores can be induced by any increase in NO level no matter what was the reason for this increase. For instance, the increase in NO level can result from both stimulation of endogenous NO synthesis and injection of exogenous NO donor. In basal conditions, NO stores are undetectable [16].

S-nitrosothiols and dinitrosyl iron complexes (DNIC) are two major forms of NO storage and transportation in the organism (Fig. 3). These two types of compounds can transform into each other depending on the intracellular level of iron, low molecular weight thiols and NO. S-nitrosothiols are apparently the major carriers of NO. When S-nitrosothiols enter a region with high levels of non-heme iron and thiols, S-nitrosothiols initiate formation of DNICs, which degrade and release NO. S-nitrosothiols and DNICs exist in two forms, a high molecular weight, that is, protein-bound form and a low molecular weight form containing low molecular weight thiol ligands such as cysteine or reduced glutathione. Protein-bound complexes are much more stable than low molecular weight ones and they are regarded as intracellular NO stores. Biological activity of DNICs is due to release of NO, transfer of NO to protein SH-groups or transfer of dinitrosyl iron to protein dithiols with formation of high molecular weight DNICs [35].

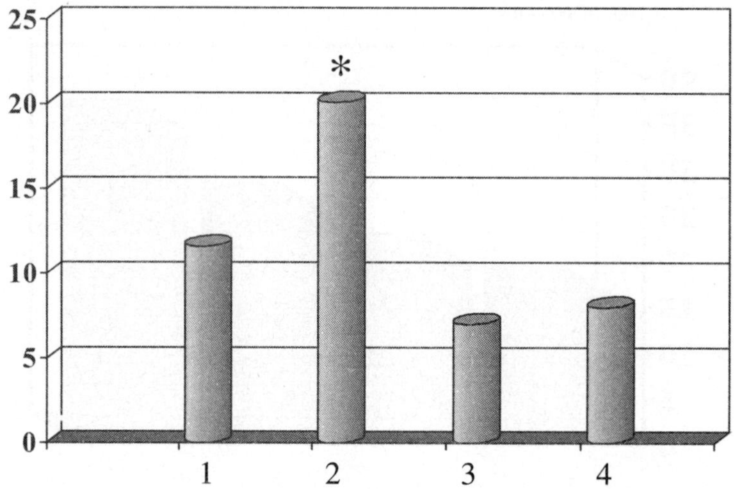

Fig. 2. **Role of NO in the increased resistance of hypoxia-adapted rats to acute hypoxia. Bars show survival time of rats (min) at a simulated altitude of 11,000 m. 1, control; 2, adaptation to hypoxia; 3, L-NNA; 4, adaptation + L-NNA. *Significant differences from control, $p<0.05$.**

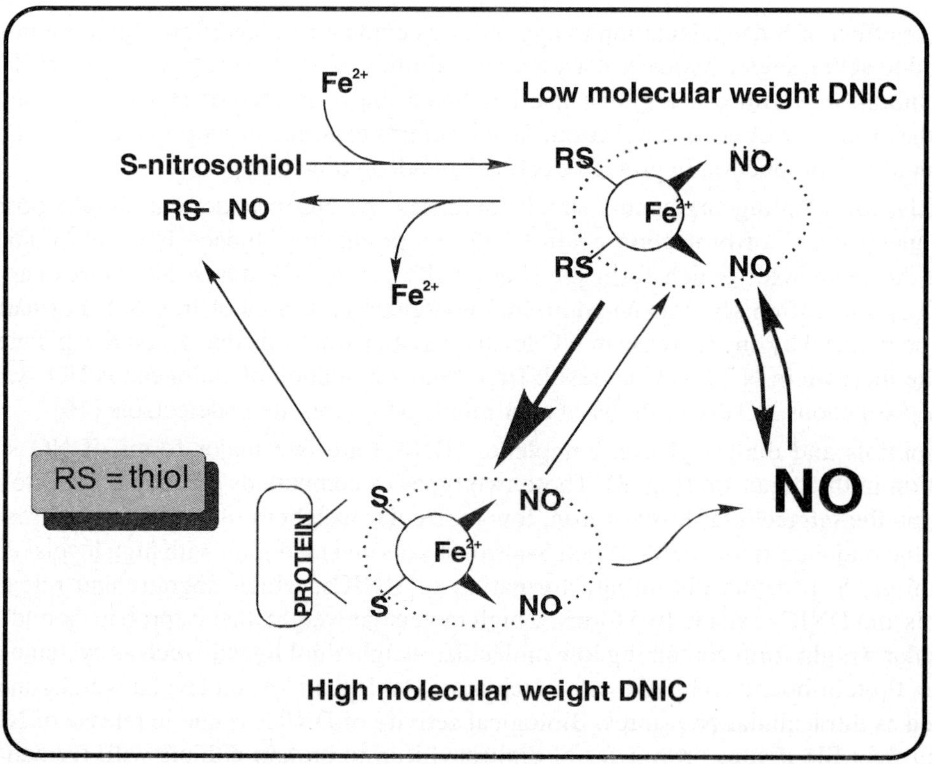

Fig. 3. **NO stores in the form of S-nitrosothiols (RS-NO), high molecular weight dinitrosyl iron complexes (DNIC) with protein ligands and low molecular weight DNIC.**

The NO stores in blood vessels have been detected using the electron paramagnetic resonance (EPR) method [36], histochemical staining for bivalent iron [6], or photorelaxation response of isolated blood vessels [19]. In our experiments we used the reaction of diethyldithiocarbamate (DETC) with DNIC and S-nitrosothiols, which results in the release of vasorelaxing products [21, 29].

Figure 4 shows a schematic record of experiment for detection of NO stores in the isolated rat aorta. NO stores were revealed in the blood vessels precontracted with noradrenaline against the background of the NO synthase inhibitor L-NNA. Control preparations have never relaxed to DETC. Apparently, in the basal conditions, the DETC-sensitive NO stores are absent or their volume is below the level of detection. The aorta isolated from rats after stimulation of NO synthesis or injection of exogenous DNIC with glutathione as a ligand as well as the preparations preincubated with a NO donor responded to DETC with relaxation. The magnitude of relaxation reflected the volume of NO stores. Adaptation to hypoxia resulted in formation of NO stores and progressive increase in their size. The size of NO stores significantly positively correlated with plasma levels of nitrite and nitrate [15].

A possible mechanism of increased NO synthesis in adaptation to intermittent hypoxia involves alternations of hypoxia and reoxygenation (Fig. 5). Hypoxia activates so-called hypoxia-inducible factor-1 (HIF-1), a transcriptional regulator of certain genes including the NOS gene. HIF-1 is a heterodimer consisting of two components, HIF-1α and HIF-1β [27]. Expression of HIF-1α dose-dependently increases at O_2 tension below 20% whereas HIF-1β is expressed constitutively. HIF-1 decomposes after less than one minute of reoxygenation [38]. Such rapid dynamics of HIF-1 may provide adaptation to periodic hypoxia at the transcriptional level, with hypoxic stimulation not only of NO synthesis but also erythropoiesis, angiogenesis and glycolysis [22]. Due to activation of HIF-1, expression of the NOS gene progresses during adaptation to make adaptation more reliable and long-term.

The intensity of NO production is predetermined at the genetic level. For example, in spontaneously hypertensive rats of SHR and SHRSP strains, endothelial NO synthesis is decreased [37], while in rats of the August strain, NO synthesis is increased [20]. We studied the relationship between NO production and storage in rats of different genetic strains in the conditions of increased NO synthesis. Adaptation to intermittent hypobaric hypoxia was used for stimulation of endogenous NO production. Adaptation was started in WKY and SHRSP aged 5-6 weeks, which corresponded to the early hypertensive stage in SHRSP, and was completed in 13 week old rats, that is at the stage of advanced hypertension.

Adaptation to hypoxia significantly increased urinary nitrate and nitrite in both SHRSP and their genetic normotensive control Wistar-Kyoto (WKY). At the same time, adaptation decreased blood pressure (BP) in SHRSP and left BP unchanged in WKY. [17].

Figure 6 demonstrates the volume of NO stores in the aortic wall, which has been formed during adaptation to hypoxia. The NO stores were formed in aortas from rats of both strains but the size of NO store was twice greater in WKY than in SHRSP (19.6% and 9.4% respectively). Bottom diagrams on Figure 6 demonstrate another important parameter, so-called "potential capacity" of NO stores. The potential capacity of NO stores was measured as maximum size of NO stores formed during incubation of an isolated blood vessel with abundant NO donor. This parameter, which characterizes the ability of blood vessels to accumulate NO stores, was significantly lower in SHRSP than in WKY.

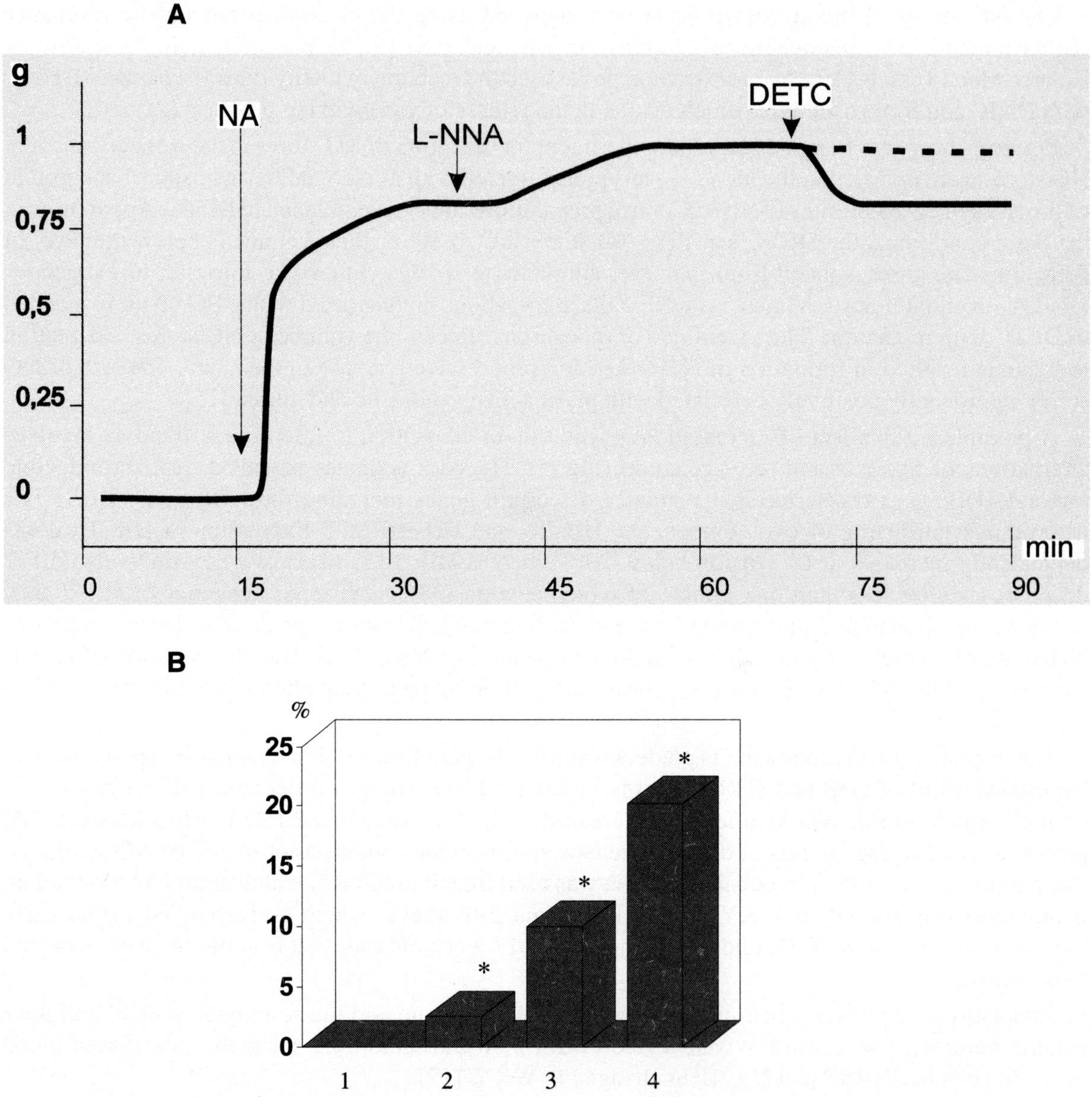

Fig. 4. Effect of adaptation to hypoxia on formation of NO stores in the wall of rat aorta.
À: Schematic record of an experiment on detection of NO stores in the isolated rat aorta. Abscissa, time in minutes; ordinate, contraction of aorta in g. NA, noradrenaline; L-NNA, Nw-nitro-L-arginine; DETC, diethyldithiocarbamate. Arrows indicate addition of reagents to the incubation chamber. Solid line: relaxation response to DETC in the aorta from adapted rat; dotted line: absence of relaxation response to DETC in the aorta from control rat.
B: Formation of NO stores in the course of adaptation to hypoxia. Bars reflect the magnitude of rat aorta relaxation in response to DETC (estimated size of NO stores) in % of the contractile response to noradrenaline. 1, control; 2, 3 sessions of adaptation; 3, 6 sessions of adaptation; 4, 40 sessions of adaptation. *Significant differences from control, $p<0.05$.

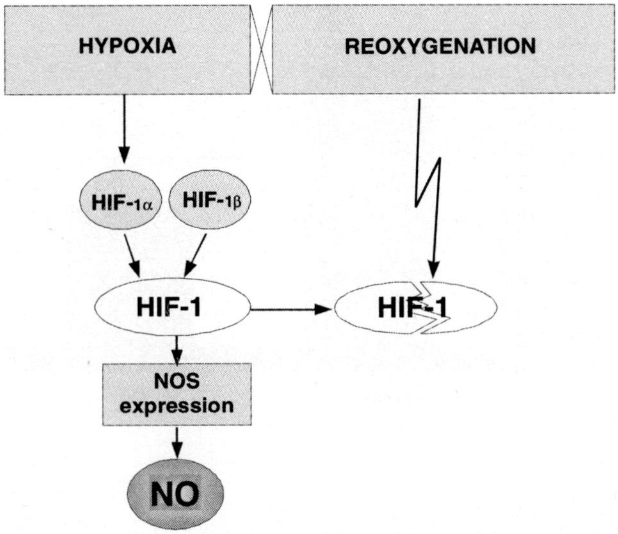

Fig. 5. Tentative mechanisms of the increased NO synthesis in adaptation to hypoxia. NOS, NO synthase; HIF, hypoxia inducible factor.

A tentative relationship between the NO level, NO stores and BP in normotensive and spontaneously hypertensive rats can be represented as follows. When adaptation to hypoxia stimulates NO synthesis, a part of excessive NO binds to the NO store whereas the unbound part of NO exerts its biological effect, that is, induces vasodilation and decrease in BP. When the efficiency of NO storage is high, the volume of NO stores is large while the hypotensive effect is slight. This situation apparently takes place in normotensive rats. On the contrary, when the efficiency of NO storage is low, much NO remains unbound and exerts a more pronounced hypotensive effect. This is the case in spontaneously hypertensive rats.

Thus blood vessels of spontaneously hypertensive rats have a lower capacity for NO storage than blood vessels of normotensive animals. This fact apparently explains the absence of hypotensive effect of adaptation to hypoxia in normotensive rats as distinct from spontaneously hypertensive rats despite a similar increase in NO production in both strains.

Further it was interesting to study the protective effect of adaptation to hypoxia in August rats displaying higher basal and stimulated production of NO than Wistar rats. [20]. We suggested that August rats possessed more potent system of NO biding to stores for protection of the organism against the detrimental effect of excessive NO.

Indeed, adaptation to hypoxia consistently increased the plasma level of nitrite and nitrate in rats of both strains (Fig. 7). However this increase proceeded slower in August rats. In result by the end of adaptation, the level of nitrite and nitrate was lower in August rats though it had been higher than in Wistar rats at baseline. NO stores appeared after the first three sessions of adaptation. Then their volume consistently increased. The formation of NO stores proceeded more rapidly in August than in Wistar rats and by the end of adaptation, the volume of NO stores in August rats was almost twice as large as in Wistar rats [25].

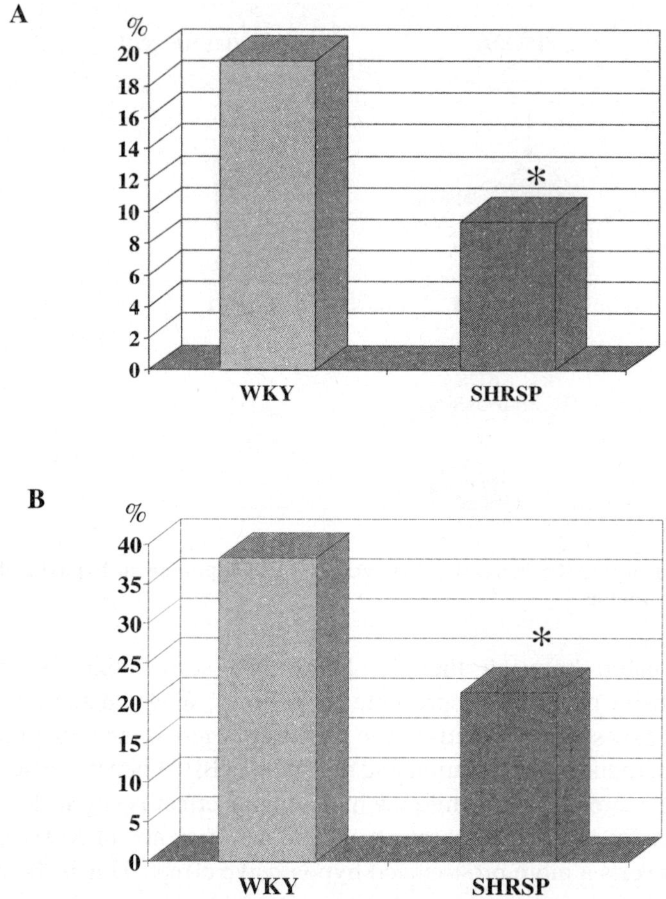

Fig. 6. Formation of NO stores in stroke-prone spontaneously hypertensive rats (SHRSP) and normotensive Wistar-Kyoto (WKY) rats. À: estimated size of NO stores formed in the aortic wall of rats adapted to hypoxia. B: Potential capacity of NO stores. Estimated size of NO stores is expressed as relaxation response to DETC in % of the contractile response to noradrenaline. *Significant differences from WKY, $p<0.05$.

Therefore August rats possess not only a higher level of basal NO production but they also are able to accumulate NO more efficiently during stimulation of NO synthesis induced by adaptation to hypoxia. In order to evaluate the physiological significance of higher NO production and storage efficiency we compared the extent of stress-induced stomach ulcers in Wistar and August rats. It is known that stress-induced stomach ulcers result from the adrenergic vasoconstriction in stomach mucose whereas NO provides an efficient protection against this injury [5].

Indeed, naive August rats displaying a higher intensity of NO production were considerably more resistant to stress-induced stomach ulceration than naive Wistar rats. Stomach ulcers developed 3 times more frequently and their total area was significantly larger in Wistar rats. After 6 days of adaptation to hypoxia, a protective "anti-ulcerogenic" effect was observed in rats of both strains; however the difference between the strains remained. The most interesting fact was that the 40-day adaptation to

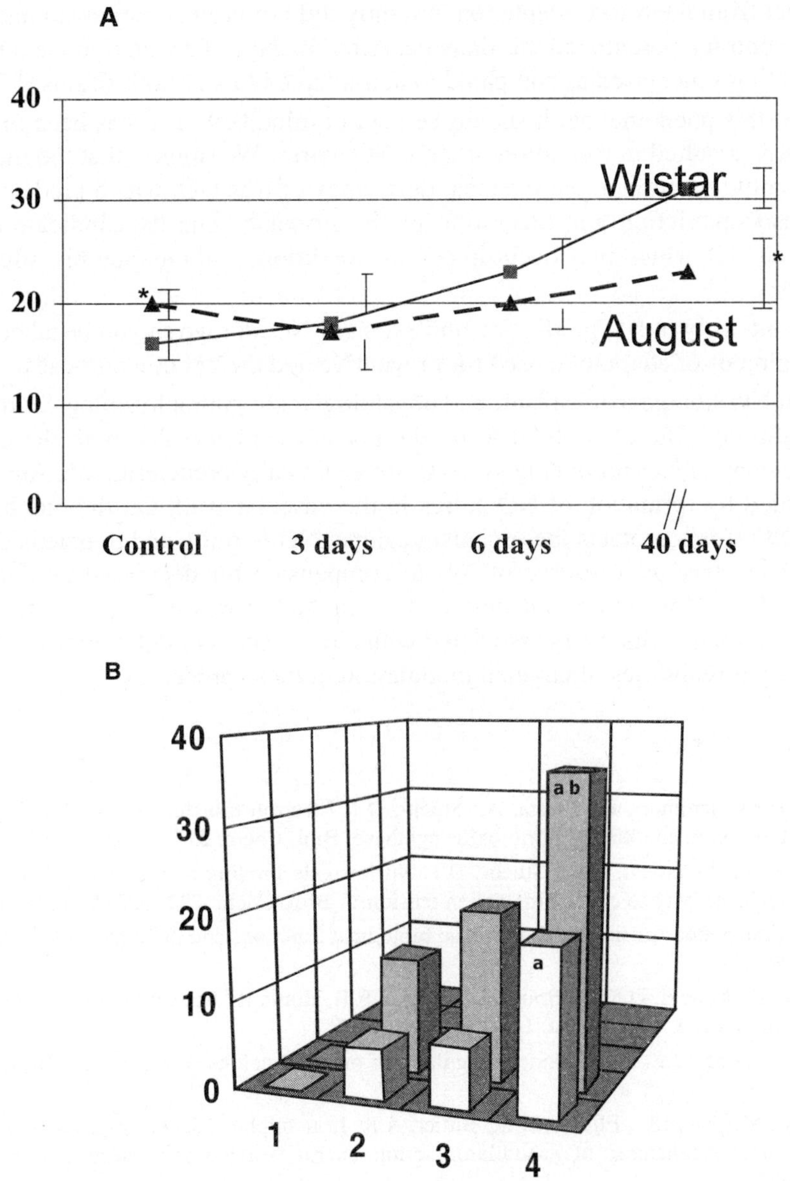

Fig. 7. Effect of adaptation to hypoxia on plasma level of nitrite+nitrate (A) and formation of NO stores in the aortic wall of Wistar and August rats (B).

À: abscissa, duration of adaptation (days); ordinate, total plasma level of nitrite and nitrate, mM. *Significant differences from baseline, p<0.05. [+]Significant differences between Wistar and August, p<0.05.

B: magnitude of aorta relaxation response to DETC reflecting the estimated size of NO stores (% of contractile response to noradrenaline).

Light bars: Wistar; dark bars: August. 1, control; 2, 3 sessions of adaptation; 3, 6 sessions of adaptation; 4, 40 sessions of adaptation.

a: significant differences from 3 sessions of adaptation, p<0.05; b: significant differences between Wistar and August, p<0.05.

hypoxia, as distinct from the 6-day adaptation, not only did not protect the rat stomach against stress ulcers but, on the contrary, potentiated this damage. After 40 days of adaptation the total area of stress ulcers was 3 to 10 times increased as compared to non-adapted rats of both strains [25].

In evaluation of this phenomenon, it should be kept in mind that, as it has been mentioned above, long-term adaptation resulted in formation of large NO stores. We suggest that the intense binding of NO to NO stores could result in a relative local deficiency of free NO, which predisposed animals to stress-induced vasoconstriction and ulceration of the stomach. The data indicate a possibility of excessive storage of NO, which may occur in certain conditions and unfavorably affect the organism resistance to stress.

Therefore both intensity of NO production and extent of NO storage should be taken into account in developing the regimens of adaptation used for preventive and therapeutic purposes.

Investigation of NO storage mechanisms and physiological or pathophysiological role of NO stores is at the very beginning. The data obtained by the present evidence that both the capacity for NO storage and the potency of NO-producing systems are genetically predetermined. Any increase in NO level is accompanied by formation of NO stores in the vascular wall. On the one hand, binding of excessive NO to NO stores protects the organism against NO toxicity and hypotension. On the other hand, NO stores can serve as a reserve of NO to compensate for decreased production of NO by endothelial cells. Thus, formation and degradation of NO stores can apparently play a role in prevention of cardiovascular disorders associated with either excess or deficiency of NO. Therefore it is important to study possibilities of targeted modulation of these processes.

References

1. Abu-Soud, H.M., Ichimori, K., Presta, A., Stuehr, D.J. Electron transfer, oxygen binding and nitric oxide feedback inhibition in endothelial nitric-oxide synthase. Biol. Chem. **275**: 17349-17357, 2000.
2. Abu-Soud, H.M., Rousseau, D.L., Stuehr, D.J. Nitric oxide binding to the heme of neuronal nitric-oxide synthase links its activity to change in oxygen tension. J. Biol. Chem. **271**: 32515-32518, 1996.
3. Bredt, D.S. Endogenous nitric oxide synthesis: biological functions and pathophysiology. Free Rad. Res. **31**: 577-596, 1999.
4. Dweik, R.A., Laskowski, D., Abu-Soud, H., Kaneko, F.T., Hutte, R., Stuehr, D.J., Erzurum, S.C. Nitric oxide synthesis in the lung. J. Clin. Invest. **101**: 660-666, 1998.
5. Elliott, S.N., Wallace, J.L. Nitric oxide: a regulator of mucosal defense and injury. J. Gastroenterol. **33**: 792-803, 1998.
6. Flitney, F.W., Megson, I.L., Flitney, D.E., Butler, A.R. Iron-sulphur cluster nitrosyls, a novel class of nitric oxide generator: mechanism of vasodilator action on rat isolated tail artery. Br. .J. Pharmacol. **107**: 842-848, 1992.
7. Förstermann, U., Biossel, J.-P., Kleinert, H. Expressional control of the "constitutive isofiorms of nitric oxide synthase (NOS I and NOS III). FASEB J. **12**: 773-790, 1998.
8. Garcia-Carderia, G., Fan, R., Shah, V., Sorrentino, R., Cirino, G., Papapetropoulos A., Sessa W.C. Dynamic activation of endothelial nitric oxide synthase by Hsp90. Nature **392**: 821-824, 1998.
9. Gess, B., Schricker, K., Pfeifer, M., Kurtz, A. Acute hypoxia upregulates NOS gene expression in rats. Am. J. Physiol. **273**: R905-R910, 1997.
10. Hampl, V., Herget, J. Role of nitric oxide in the pathogenesis of chronic pulmonary hypertension. Physiol. Rev. **80**: 1337-1372, 2000.

11. Hong, Y., Suzuki, S., Yatoh, S., Mitzutani, M., Nakajima, T., Bannai, S., Sato, H., Soma, M., Okuda, Y., Yamada, N. Effect of hypoxia on nitric oxide production and its synthase gene expression in rat smooth muscle cells. Biochem. Biophys. Res. Commun. **268**: 329-332, 2000.
12. Le Cras, T., McMurtry, I.F. Nitric oxide production in hypoxia. Amer. J. Physiol. **280**: L575-L582, 2001.
13. Luckhoff, A, Busse, R. Refilling of endothelial calcium stores without bypassing the cytosol.FEBS Lett. **271**:108-110, 1990.
14. Malyshev, I.Yu., Zenina, T.A., Golubeva, L.Yu., Saltykova, V.A., Manukhina, E.B., Mikoyan, V.D., Kubrina, L.N., Vanin, A.F. NO-dependent mechanisms of adaptation to hypoxia. Nitric Oxide **3**: 105-113, 1999.
15. Manukhina, E.B., Malyshev, I.Yu., Smirin, B.V., Mashina, S.Yu., Saltykova, V.A., Vanin, A.F. Production and storage of nitric oxide in adaptation to hypoxia. Nitric Oxide **3**: 393-401, 1999.
16. Manukhina, E.B., Smirin, B.V., Malyshev, I.Yu., Stoclet, J.-C., Muller, B., Solodkov, A.P., Shebeko, V.I., Vanin, A.F. Nitric oxide storage in the cardiovascular system. Biology Bulletin, **5**: 595-606, 2002.
17. Mashina, S.Yu., Smirin, B.V., Malyshev, I.Yu., Lyamina, N.P., Senchikhin, V.N., Pokidyshev, D.A., Manukhina, E.B. Correction of NO-dependent cardiovascular disorders by adaptation to hypoxia. Rossijsky fiziologichesky zhurnal. **87**: 110-117, 2001 (in Russian).
18. Meerson, F.Z. Essentials of Adaptive Medicine: Protective Effects of Adaptation. Hypoxia Medical LTD. Moscow, 1994.
19. Megson, I.L., Holme, S.A., Magid, K.S. Selective modifiers of glutathione biosynthesis and 'repriming' of vascular smooth muscle photorelaxation. Br. J. Pharmacol. **130**: 1575-1580, 2000.
20. Mikoyan, V.D., Kubrina, L.N., Manukhina, E.B., Malysheva, E.V., Malyshev, I.Yu., Vanin, A.F. Differences in stimulation of NO synthesis by heat shock in rats of genetically different populations. Bull. Exper. Biol. Med. **121**: 634-637, 1996.
21. Muller, B., Kleschyov, A.L., Stoclet, J.-C. Evidence for N-acetylcysteine-sensitive nitric oxide storage as dinitrosyl iron complexes in lipopolysaccharide-treated rat aorta. Brit. J. Pharmacol. **119**: 1281-1285, 1996.
22. Neubauer, J.A. Physiological and pathophysiological responses to intermittent hypoxia. J. Appl. Physiol. **90**: 1593-1599, 2001.
23. Pearl, J.M., Nelson, D.P., Wellmann, S.A., Raake, J.L., Wagner, C.J., McNamara, J.L., Duffy, J.Y. Acute hypoxia and reoxygenation impairs exhaled nitric oxide release and pulmonary mechanics. J. Cardiovasc. Surg. **119**: 931-938, 2000.
24. Prabhakar, N.R., Fields, R.D., Baker, T., Fletcher, E.C. Intermittent hypoxia: cell to system. Amer. J. Physiol. **281**: L524-L528, 2001.
25. Pshennikova, M.G., Smirin, B.V., Bondarenko, O.N., Malyshev, I.Yu., Manukhina, E.B. Nitric oxide storage in rats of different strains and its role in the antistress effect of adaptation to hypoxia. Rossijsky fiziologichesky zhurnal. **86**: 174-181, 2000 (in Russian).
26. Rengasamy, A., Johns, R.A. Determination of Km for oxygen of nitric oxide synthase isoforms. J. Pharmacol. Exp. Ther. **276**: 30-33, 1996.
27. Semenza, G.L. HIF-1 and mechanisms of hypoxia sensing. Curr. Opin. Cell Biol. **13**: 167-171, 2001.
28. Sherman, T.S., Chen, Z., Yuhanna, I.S., Lau, K.S., Margaf, L.R., Shaul, P.W. Nitric oxide synthase isoform expression in the developing lung epithelium. Amer. J. Physiol. **276**: L383-L390, 1999.
29. Smirin B.V., Vanin A.F., Malyshev, I.Yu., Pokidyshev, D.A., Manukhina, E.B. Nitric oxide storage in blood vessels in vivo. Bull. Exper. Biol. Med. **127**: 629-632, 1999.
30. Stuehr, D.J. Structure-functional aspects in the nitric oxide synthesases. Annu. Rev. Pharmacol. Toxicol. **37**: 339-359, 1997.
31. Su, Y., Block, E.R. Role of calpain in hypoxic inhibitio of nitric oxide synthase activity in pulmonary endothelial cells. Am. J. Physiol. **278**: L1204-1212, 2000.

32. Tkatchouk, E.N., Gorbachenkov, A.A., Kolchinskaya, A.Z., Kondrykinskaya, I.I., Ehrenbourg, I.V. Adaptation to interval hypoxia for prophylaxis and treatment. Essentials of Adaptive Medicine: Protective Effects of Adaptation. (F.Z. Meerson, Ed.) Hypoxia Medical LTD. Moscow, 303-331, 1994.

33. Toporsian, M., Govindaraju, K., Nagi, M., Eidelman, D., Thibault, G., Ward, M.E. Downregulation of endothelial nitric oxide synthase in rat aorta after prolonged hypoxia in vivo. Circ. Res. **86**: 671-675, 2000.

34. Tsujino, I., Miyamoto, K., Nishimura, M., Shinano, H., Makita, H., Saito, S., Nakano, T, Kawakami, Y. Production of nitric oxide (NO) in intrathoracic airways of normal humans. Am. J. Respir. Crit. Care Med. **154**: 1370-1374, 1996.

35. Vanin, A.F. Dinitrosyl iron complexes and S-nitrosothiols: two possible forms of nitric oxide stabilization and transport in biological systems. Biochemistry (Moscow); **7**: 924-238, 1998.

36. Vanin, A.F., Kleschyov, A.L. EPR detection and biological implication of nitrosyl non-heme iron complexes. Nitric Oxide in Transplant Rejection and Anti-Tumor Defense. Eds. Lukiewicz S.J., Zweier J.L. Kluwer Academic Publ., Norwell, MA, 1998, 49-82.

37. Wu, C.-C., Yen, M.-H. Nitric oxide synthase in spontaneously hypertensive rats. Biomed. Sci. **4**: 249-255, 1997.

38. Yu, A.Y., Frid, M.G., Shimoda, L.A., Wiener, C.M., Stenmark, K., Semenza, G.L. Temporal, spatial, and oxygen-regulated expression of hypoxia-inducible factor-1 in the lung. Am. J. Physiol. **275**: L818-L826, 1998.

Adaptation Biology and Medicine (Volume 4: Current Concepts)
Editors: A. Hargens, N. Takeda and P.K. Singal

8. The Thioredoxin-Thioredoxin Reductase System Adapts to Human Cancer Growth by Overexpression

D. T. Lincoln[1], P. K. Singal[2], E. M. Ali Emadi[3], M. M. Al-Khaledi[4], F. M. A. Mohammed[5], F. Al-Yatama[5], K. F. Tonissen[6] and F. M. Clarke[6].

[1]Independent Research Foundation, Chapel Hill, Qld. 4069, Australia.

[2]Division of Cardiovascular Sciences, St. Boniface General Hospital Research Centre, Faculty of Medicine, The University of Manitoba, Canada.

[3] Department of Histology, Maternity Hospital, Sulaibikhat, Kuwait.

[4]School of Health and Rehabilitation Sciences, University of Queensland, Brisbane, Australia.

[5]Department of Medical Laboratory Sciences, Faculty of Allied Health Sciences, Kuwait University, Kuwait.

[6]School of Biomolecular and Biomedical Science, Faculty of Science and Technology, Griffith University, Australia.

Abstract

Redox control has emerged as a fundamental biological control mechanism. One of the major redox control systems is the thioredoxin system comprised of thioredoxin (TRX) and thioredoxin reductase (TR). Together they form a powerful system involved in many central intracellular and extracellular processes including cell proliferation, the redox regulation of gene expression and signal transduction, protection against oxidative stress, anti-apoptotic functions, growth factor and co-cytokine effects, and regulation of the redox state of the extracellular environment. Over recent years this system has increasingly been linked to the development and expression of cancer phenotypes. In this report, immunocytochemical approaches have been used to simultaneously determine the expression and localisation of both TRX and TR in primary human cancers, including breast cancer, thyroid, prostate and colorectal carcinoma, and malignant melanoma. In aggressive invasive mammary carcinomas and advanced malignant melanomas, thioredoxin was highly over-expressed compared to tumours of lesser, aggressive nature. TRX expression was found in both nuclear and cytoplasmic location in the neoplastic cells. Furthermore, increased levels of TRX positively correlate with thioredoxin reductase (TR) expression and localisation. These results, which are the first immunocytochemical studies on the in vivo expression and localisation of TRX and TR in melanomas, thyroid, prostate and colorectal carcinomas and the first reports of TR expression in breast carcinomas, significantly extend the range of human cancers for which such data is available. Overall, the results support the conclusion that aggressive tumours greatly over-express both TRX and TR. Such tumours have a high proliferation capacity, a low apoptosis rate and an elevated metastatic potential, strongly implicating the involvement of the TRX system in the processes of oncogenesis and tumourogenesis and confirming its potential as a target for anti-cancer therapy for a wide range of human tumours.

Introduction

The thioredoxin system is a major redox control system in mammalian cells and tissues which has been increasingly implicated in the development and expression of the cancer phenotype of several human cancers. Thioredoxins (TRXs) are small (12 KDa) redox active proteins with highly conserved active sites of -C-G-P-C- which participate in redox reactions through the reversible oxidation of this active site dithiol (Holmgren, 1985). The oxidised thioredoxin is reduced by an NADPH dependent thioredoxin reductase (TR) and the reduced thioredoxin is a very effective protein disulphide reductase. Through this action, it is able to effect the disulphide-dependent structural changes in other molecules, causing the activation or inhibition of target proteins (Holmgren, 1985). Thioredoxin reductases are the only enzymes known to be able to reduce the active site of TRX (Arner and Holmgren, 2000). Mammalian thioredoxin reductases are homodimeric, flavin adenine dinucleotide-containing proteins with a C-terminal selenocysteine residue (Gladyshev et al., 1996; Powis et al., 1997) that is essential for the activity of the mammalian thioredoxin reductases (Gasdaska et al., 1999). In addition to catalysing TRX reduction, mammalian TRs are notable in having a wide substrate specificity encompassing many low molecular weight disulphide compounds and nondisulphide compounds such as lipid hydroperoxides, dehydroascorbate and lipoic acid (Nordberg and Arner, 2001).

Human thioredoxin-1 forms covalently-linked dimers in solution (Tan et al., 1998), especially in the presence of an oxidant or when stored at high concentrations (Stuehr and Nathan, 1989). This is due to an 1100 $Å^2$ hydrophobic patch, five hydrogen bonds, and a Cys^{73}-Cys^{73} disulphide bond. The hydrophobic patch is composed of 12 hydrophobic amino acids, 10 of which are invariant in vertebrate species but not found in lower species, which suggests that dimer formation may be a recent occurrence in evolution (Tan et al., 1998). The apparent dissociation constant for noncovalent thioredoxin dimer formation is between 6 and 166 μM at pH levels of 3.8 to 8.0 respectively (Albina et al., 1993). When formed, the hydrophobic dimer interface excludes all water molecules and is held together by Cys^{73}-Cys^{73} disulphide bond formation, which can occur even under strong reducing conditions (Tan et al., 1998). Covalently linked dimer formation is not seen with mutant Cys^{73}→Ser thioredoxin [Tan et al., 1998; Stuehr and Nathan, 1989). The dimer forming the Cys^{73} residue is found in all mammalian thioredoxins so far examined, but not in thioredoxins from bacteria, plants and invertebrates that do not form dimers (Knowles and Moncada, 1992). A study using analytical ultracentrifugation and nuclear magnetic resonance spectroscopy failed to find evidence of dimer formation in solution, but whether these experiments were conducted under oxidising conditions necessary for dimer formation is not clear (Sari et al., 1993). The concentration of human thioredoxin in tissues has not yet been accurately determined but is about 0.5-5.0 μM in bovine tissues (Ankacrona et al., 1994) and possibly higher in tumour tissues that overexpress thioredoxin. Whether thioredoxin dimer formation occurs under physiological conditions and the function of dimerisation are not known. However, it is known that the dimerised thioredoxin is no longer a substrate for reduction by thioredoxin reductase and does not stimulate cell growth (Stuehr and Nathan, 1989).

Together TRX and TR constitute the TRX system, a key cellular redox control system. Multiple protein substrates have been identified for thioredoxin, including ribonucleotide reductase (Holmgren, 1985) and various transcription factors (Arrigo, 1999), and so TRX is an essential part of the cell proliferation machinery and a key component in the redox regulation of gene expression. TRX is also involved in the redox regulation of apoptosis. Reduced TRX (but not oxidised TRX) inhibits apoptosis by an inhibitory binding to ASK-1 (Ueda et al., 2002). Furthermore, TRX possesses reactive oxygen reducing activity and so acts as a scavenger for reactive oxygen species (ROS) (Das and Das, 2000). TRX is also the electron donor to thioredoxin peroxidases (peroxiredoxins) important in the reduction peroxides and protecting cells from oxidative stress (Das and Das, 2000). Thioredoxin also has extracellular functions. TRX can be secreted by cells by a non classical pathway and can act as an autocrine growth factor as well as displaying co-cytokine activity augmenting the effects of other cytokines (Schenk, 1996). Extracellular TRX may be bound to the external cell membrane where it may participate in and regulate cell to cell contact and contribute to redox regulation in the extracellular space (Sahaf, 1997).

TRX and TR are over-expressed in several tumour cells and both are secreted (Rubartelli et al., 1992; Soderberg et al., 2000) and recent work indicates the TRX system may have important roles to play in tumour development and malignancy. TRX and TR have been reported to be expressed at a high level in a number of cancers and transformed cell lines. For example, TRX mRNA is present in 3 to 100 fold elevated levels in almost half of the human primary lung and colon tumours examined, compared to adjacent normal tissues from the same patients (Berggren et al., 1996). A number of human transformed cell lines have also been analysed and found to have 10 fold higher levels of TRX mRNA and 23 fold higher levels of TR mRNA (Berggren et al., 1996). Thioredoxin stimulates the proliferation of both normal fibroblasts and a variety of human solid and leukaemic cancer cell lines (Gasdaska et al., 1995). It is secreted by these cells and so may act as an autocrine growth factor. Redox activity is essential for these growth stimulatory effects of TRX since redox-inactive mutant forms lacking the active site cysteine residues are devoid of these functions (Gasdaska et al., 1995). Transfection of cells with TRX constructs increases cellular TRX expression and the density to which NIH3T3 cells will grow in culture, and stimulates many fold the anchorage-independent colony formation by MCF-7 breast cancer cells (Gallegos et al., 1996). Transfection of WEHI 7.2 mouse thymoma derived cells with TRX constructs stimulates tumour growth and inhibits apoptosis in vivo (Baker et al., 1997). Transfection of breast cancer cells with the gene encoding a redox inactive TRX mutant reversed the transformed phenotype of the cancer cells with the expressed protein acting as a dominant negative. Tumour formation by the redox mutant transfected MCF-7 cells on inoculation into scid mice was almost completely suppressed, with only microscopic tumour cell deposits being observed and there was no evidence of metastasis to other organs (Gallegos et al., 1996).

While such studies implicate the TR system in the process of tumour development, there have been relatively few studies on the expression and localisation of TRX and TR in solid tumours. There have been reports of TRX expression and localisation in breast (Ueno et al., 2000; Matsutani et al., 2001), lung (Kakolyris et al., 2001), gastric (Grogan et al., 2000), pancreatic (Nakamura et al., 2000), hepatocellular (Nakamura et al., 1992) and cervical carcinomas (Fujii et al., 1991) as well as in some leukaemias (Shao et al., 2001). There have however, been only two reports of the expression and localisation of TR in tumours namely in small cell carcinoma (Soini et al., 2001) and mesothelioma (Kahlos et al., 2001), and these are the only two studies in which the expression of both TRX and TR in the same samples has been investigated. In this report we extend these studies by examining the expression and cellular localisation of both TRX and TR in a range of human tumours including breast, thyroid, prostrate, colorectal and melanoma. The results show that aggressive tumours greatly over-express TRX and TR. The relevance of these observations to the high proliferation rate, low apoptosis rate and elevated metastatic potential of the tumours is discussed in terms of the involvement of the TRX system in the processes of oncogenesis and tumourogenesis, and the potential of the TRX system as a target in anti-cancer therapies.

Materials and Methods

Tumour and normal tissues

Tumours were obtained from the Kuwait Cancer Control Centre. The following tumours were investigated: (1) mammary neoplasms (n=49), consisting of infiltrating ductal carcinoma (n=10), ductal carcinoma (n=10), lobular carcinoma (n=10), signet ring carcinoma (n=2), mucin producing adenocarcinoma (n=2), fibrocystic disease (n=5), the tumours are lymph node positive and have a high nuclear proliferative index; (2) malignant melanomas (n=26), consisting of superficial spreading melanoma (n=10), nodular melanoma (n=10), metastatic melanoma (n=6); (3) thyroid neoplasms (n=30), consisting of papillary carcinoma (n=10), papillary oncocytic neoplasm (n=2), invasive follicular carcinoma (n=8), follicular carcinoma (n=10); (3) prostate neoplasms (n=20), consisting of benign hyperplasia neoplasm (n=10), carcinoma (n=10); (4) colorectal carcinomas (n=10). Tissue was fixed in phosphate buffered 4% paraformaldehyde (pH 7.4) overnight at 4°C, washed in several changes of Tris buffer at pH 7.4, routine processed and embedded in paraffin wax. Sections were cut at 5 μm thickness and mounted on 2% aminopyroethylsaline (APS) coated microscope slides. Sections of 5 μm formalin-fixed, paraffin wax embedded tissues, obtained from locations adjacent to the tumours, were used as normal control tissue.

TRX and TR antibodies

Immunohistochemical localisation of TRX in tissue sections was performed using purified mouse anti-human TRX monoclonal antibody which had previously been characterised and used for TRX localisation in human (Perkins et al., 1995) and marmoset (Lopota et al., 2001) tissues. Immunohistochemical expression of TR was demonstrated using an anti-human TR antiserum prepared by immunisation of rabbits against purified human placental TR. The antiserum was assessed for specificity by Western Blot analysis against purified human TR and human cell and tissue extracts and detected a single 56K band of human TR.

Immunohistochemistry

Paraffin embedded tissue sections were cut at 5 μm thickness and mounted on 2% aminopyroethylsaline (APS) coated microscope slides. Sections were deparaffinised with xylene and brought to distilled water via descending series of alcohols. Endogenous peroxidase was blocked by application of 3% hydrogen peroxide in Tris buffer for 5 min at room temperature. Sections were rinsed in Tris buffer and placed in blocking solution of 20% normal goat serum in Tris buffer for 20 minutes at room temperature. Excess serum was tapped off and sections were incubated with diluted (1:100) purified mouse anti-human TRX monoclonal or rabbit anti-human TR antiserum, in a humidified chamber overnight at 4°C. Sections were then rinsed in Tris buffer and incubated with biotinylated goat anti-mouse or anti-rabbit gammaglobulin secondary antibody (Dako, Glastrup, Denmark), diluted 1:200, for 1 hour at room temperature. Sections were then rinsed in Tris buffer and incubated in avidin horseradish peroxidase link complex (Dako, Glastrup, Denmark) solution for 1 hour at room temperature. Following washing in three changes of Tris buffer, visualisation of the peroxidase was by application of 3- acetyl 9-ethylcarbazole (AEC) as chromogen (Dako, Glostrup, Denmark) and 0.09% hydrogen peroxide in Tris buffer. The sections were rinsed in Tris buffer, nuclei counterstained in Mayer's haematoxylin, and finally dehydrated in ascending series of alcohols, cleared in three changes of xylene and mounted with DePex. Controls for thioredoxin and thioredoxin reductase specificity were performed by omission of the anti-human TRX monoclonal antibody and anti-human TR rabbit antiserum respectively.

Results

Thioredoxin

The results of these immunocytochemical analyses, using anti-human TRX and TR antibodies (Table 1), show that TRX and TR are both overexpressed in the cytoplasm and nuclei in the majority of mammary carcinomas (Table 1, Fig. 1), thyroid carcinoma (Table 1, Fig. 2), malignant melanomas (Table 1, Fig. 3), prostate carcinomas (Table 1) and colorectal carcinomas (Table 1), compared to their normal tissues counterparts. In the case of the mammary carcinomas investigated, TRX overexpression was found in 40% of the lobular carcinomas, 100% of the signet ring carcinomas, 80% of the infiltrating ductal carcinomas (Fig. 1), 70% of the ductal carcinomas, 60% of the intraductal carcinomas, and 100% of the mucin producing carcinomas (Table 1). In contrast, only 20% of the fibrocystic diseases investigated showed TRX over-expression (Table 1). In the case of the thyroid carcinomas investigated, TRX overexpression (Fig. 2) was found in 70% of the papillary carcinomas, 50% oncocytic papillary carcinomas, 60% of the follicular carcinomas and 70% of the invasive follicular carcinomas (Table 1). In the case of the malignant melanomas investigated, TRX was over-expressed in 40% superficial spreading malignant melanomas, 80% of the nodular malignant melanomas (Fig. 3) and 40% of the metastatic melanomas were over-expressed (Table 1). Of the prostate neoplasms investigated, 10% of the benign prostatic hyperplasia diseases and 30% of the prostate carcinomas were TRX over expressed (Table 1). In the case of the colorectal carcinomas investigated, TRX was over expressed in 40% of the cases (Table 1).

Thioredoxin reductase

TR, the enzyme involved in the reduction of TRX, was also present in large amounts in the cancer tissues, probably reflecting that a large amount of its substrate(TRX) was also present. In the case of the mammary carcinomas investigated, overexpression of TR was found in 30% of the lobular carcinomas, 60% of the ductal carcinomas, 60% of the intraductal carcinomas, 100% of the signet ring carcinomas, 80% of the infiltrating ductal carcinomas and 100% of the mucin producing carcinomas (Table 1). In the case of the malignant melanomas investigated, 30% of the superficial spreading melanomas, 70% of the nodular melanomas (Fig. 4) and 30% of the metastatic melanomas were TR over-expressed (Table 1). In the case of the thyroid carcinomas investigated, over-expression was found in 70% of the papillary carcinomas, 50% oncocyticpapillary carcinomas, 70% of the follicular carcinomas and 80% of the invasive follicular carcinomas (Table 1). Of the prostate neoplasms investigated, 30% of the carcinomas were TR over-expressed, while no increase was observed in the benign prostatic hyperplasia diseases (Table 1). In the case of the colorectal carcinomas investigated, TR was over expressed in 40% of the cases investigated (Table 1).

Table 1. Thioredoxin (TRX) and thioredoxin-reductase (TRX-R) over-expression in human mammary carcinomas, malignant melanomas, thyroid neoplasms, prostate neoplasm and colorectal carcinomas

Tumour	Type	Number of subjects	% Overexpressed	
			TRX*	TRX-R*
Mammary-carcinoma	Lobular	10	40.0	30.0
	Ductal	10	70.0	60.0
	Intraductal	10	60.0	60.0
	Signet ring	2	100.0	100.0
	Infiltrating ductal	10	80.0	80.0
	Mucin producing	2	100.0	100.0
	Fibrocystic	5	20.0	10.0
Melanoma	Superficial spreading	10	40.0	30.0
	Nodular	10	80.0	70.0
	Metastatic	6	40.0	30.0
Thyroid neoplasm	Papillary carcinoma	10	70.0	70.0
	Papillary oncocytic	2	50.0	50.0
	Follicular carcinoma	10	60.0	70.0
	Invasive follicular carc.	8	70.0	80.0
Prostate neoplasm	Hyperplasia	10	10.0	0
	Carcinoma	10	30.0	30.0
Colorectal	Carcinoma	10	40.0	40.0

*Compared to corresponding normal tissue from the same subject.

Discussion

The results reported here are the first immunocytochemical studies on the in vivo expression of TRX and TR in melanomas, thyroid, prostate and colorectal carcinomas, and the first reports of TR expression in breast carcinomas. TRX and TR were found in both nuclear and cytoplasmic locations in the neoplastic cells. Furthermore, increased levels of TR positively correlated with TRX expression in all tumours examined. There have been two previous reports of TRX over-expression in breast carcinoma (Ueno et al., 2000; Matsutani et al., 2001). Also, Bini et al (1997), by determining protein expression profiles detected the consistent high expression of TRX in breast ductal carcinoma compared to normal tissue. The present results confirm and extend these observations by also demonstrating the over-expression of TR. Furthermore, the association of TRX and TR staining with advanced tumour grades suggest a positive association of enhanced expression of these two proteins with the more aggressive phenotypes.

To our knowledge, there have been no previous reports of TRX or TR expression in melanomas in vivo. However, Barral et al. (2000) have reported that TRX and TR are highly expressed in cultured

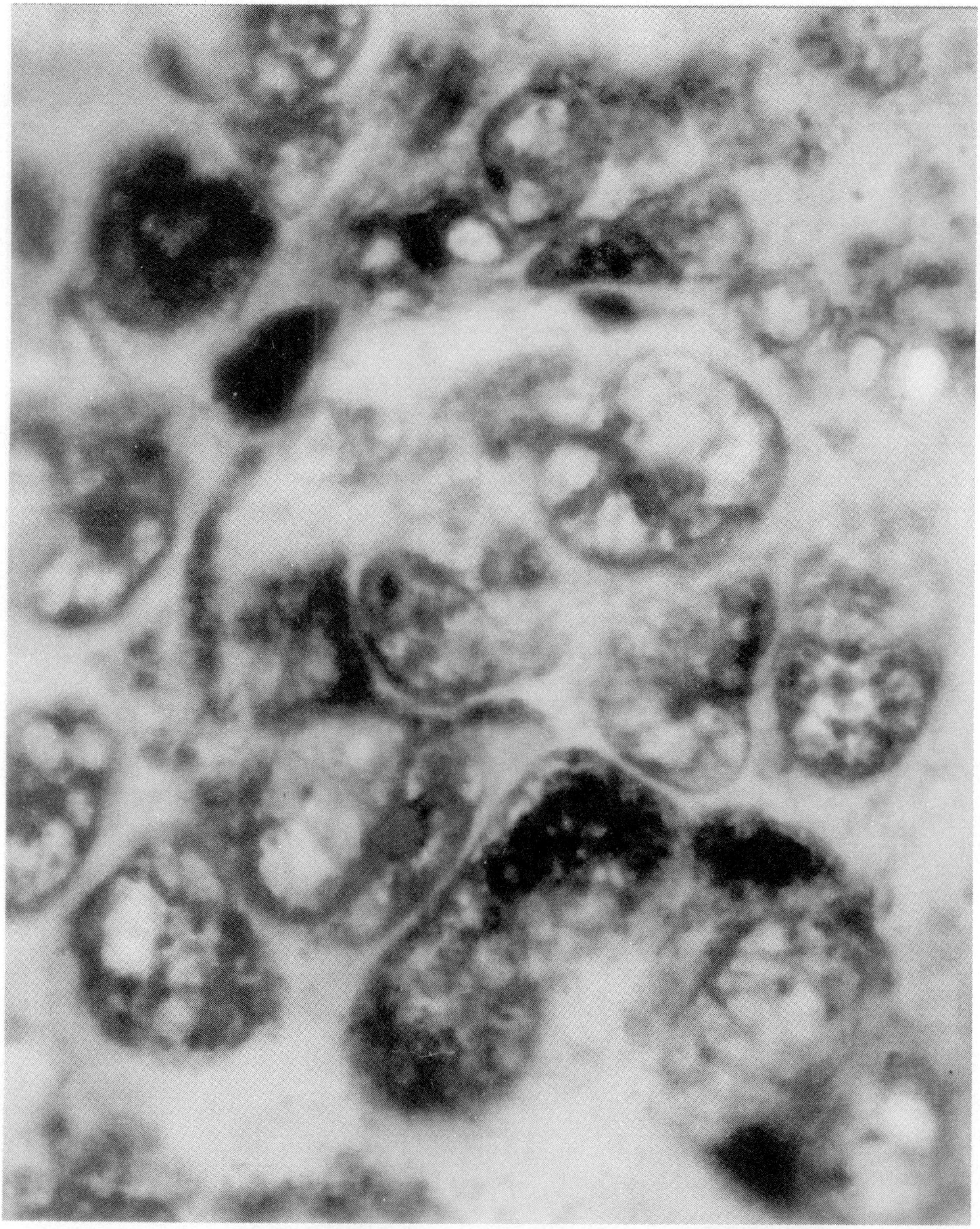

Fig. 1. **Nuclear and cytoplasmic thioredoxin immunoreactivity (red) in a Grade 5b infiltrating ductal mammary gland carcinoma of a 26 year old patient. Note intense cytoplasmic thioredoxin immunoreactivity. Majority of lymph nodes are tumour positive. Thioredoxin is over-expressed 80% of all infiltrating ductal carcinomas investigated. Magnification x 1000.**

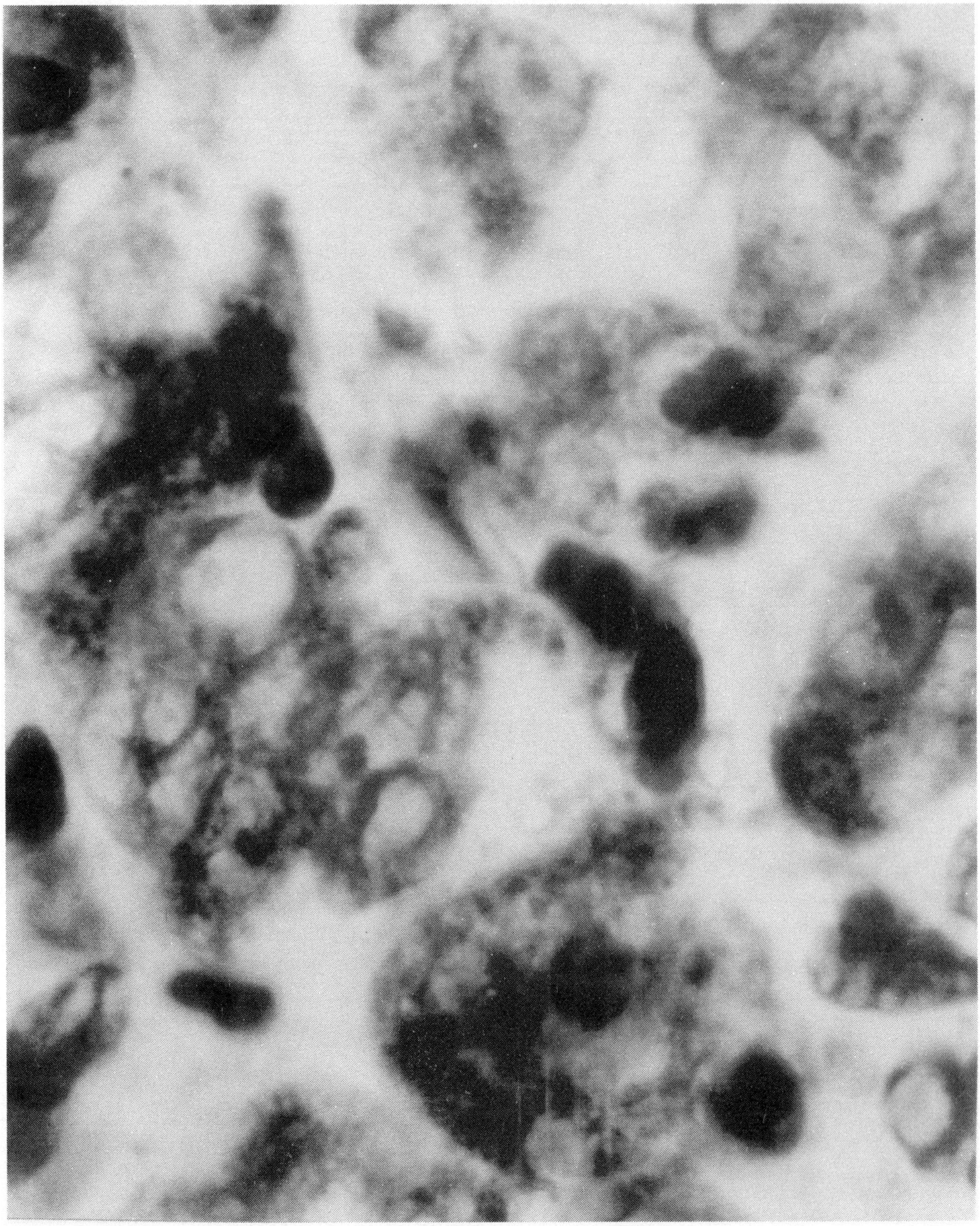

Fig. 2. **Thioredoxin (TRX) overexpression in a papillary carcinoma of the thyroid gland. Note intense cytoplasmic immunoreactivity (red). Majority of nuclei are negative. TRX is overexpressed 70% of all papillary carcinomas investigated. Magnification x 1000.**

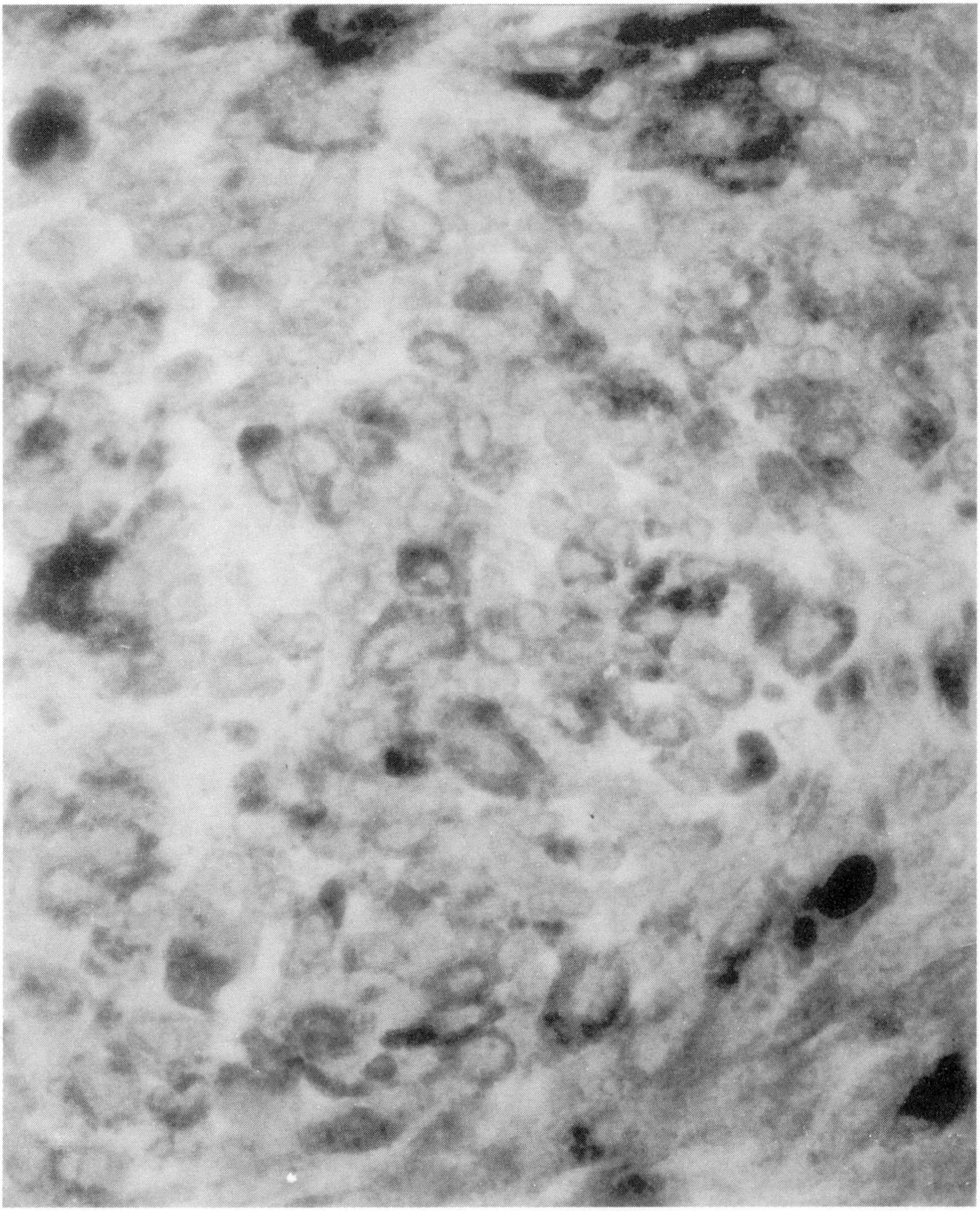

Fig. 3. Thioredoxin (TRX) immunoreactivity (red) in a nodular melanoma of Clark IV level. Thioredoxin is over-expressed 80% of all nodular melanomas investigated. Majority of lymph nodes are tumour positive. Magnification x 400.

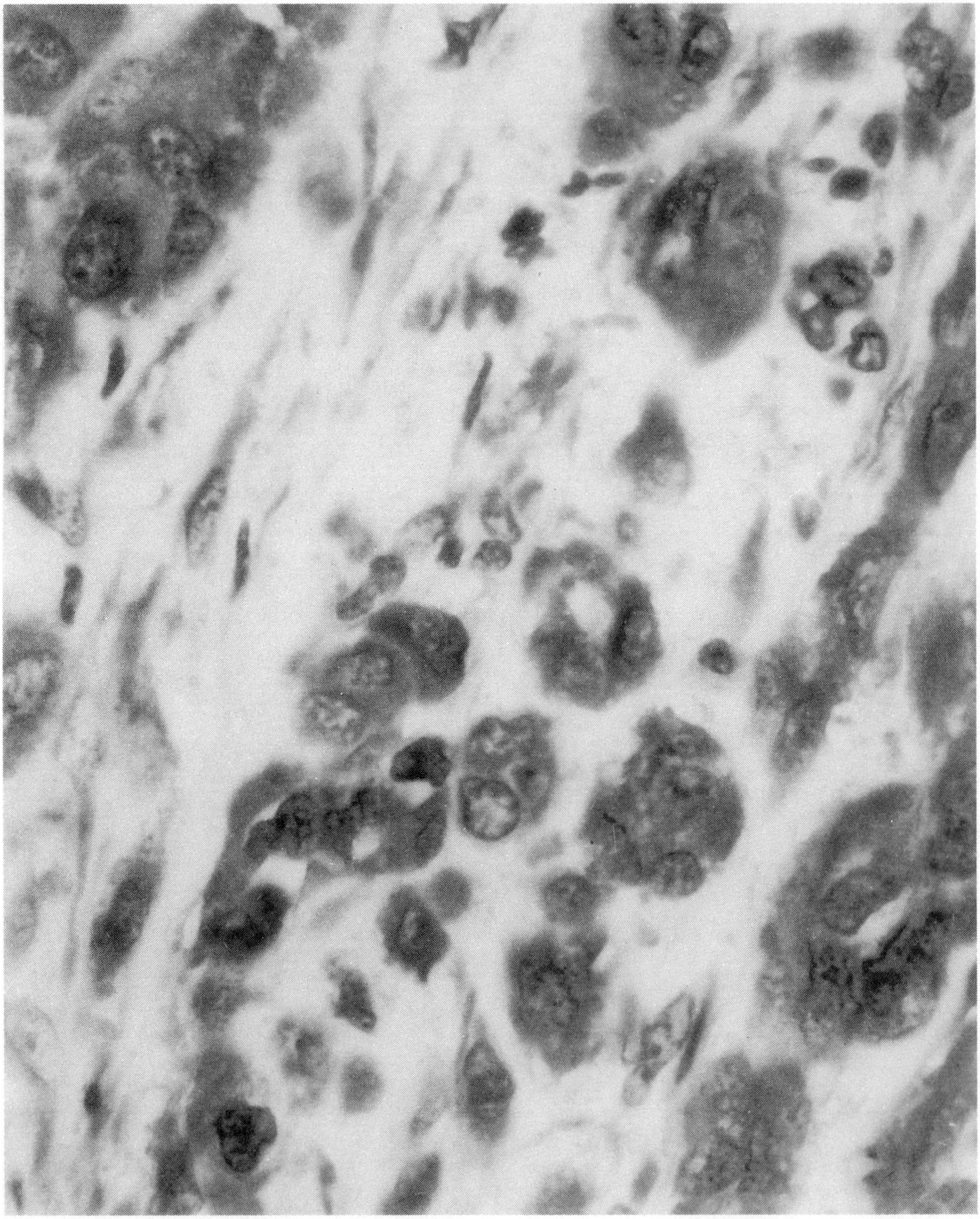

Fig. 4. Nuclear and intense cytoplasmic thioredoxin reductase (TRX-R) immunoreactivity in a nodular melanoma of Clark IV level. TRX-R is over-expressed in 70% of all nodular melanomas investigated. Majority of lymph nodes are tumour positive. Magnification x 400.

malignant melanoma cell lines. With prostate cancer, Suzuki et al (2000) have noted elevated expression of TRX in hormone–independent prostate cell lines derived from bone metastases and suggest that this, and elevated levels of other antioxidant systems observed, may contribute to the resistance of metastatic prostate cancer to chemotherapy. The present immunocytochemical results on the expression of TRX and TR in colorectal carcinomas are also in keeping with previous observations. Berggren et al (1996) reported that TRX mRNA levels were increased 3 to 100-fold in 50% of human primary colorectal carcinomas compared to adjacent normal colonic mucosa form the same subject. Also, in the same carcinomas TR activity and protein levels were increased at least 2-fold compared to normal mucosa.

From our present studies and the previous reports of TRX expression of tumours in vivo and by tumour cell lines in vitro, a general picture emerges of increased TRX/TR expression associated with tumourigenesis. While there are, no doubt, very significant differences between individual cancer types the overall results suggest that over-expression of the TRX system contributes significantly to various aspects of the different cancer phenotypes. Indeed there is significant evidence which correlates the expression of these proteins with the proliferative capacity, apoptotic resistance and metastatic potential of different cancers.

Thioredoxin has been reported to selectively activate the DNA binding of certain transcription factors. This includes the dimeric transcription factor NF-κB, which is involved in cellular response to oxidative stress, apoptosis and tumourigenesis (Venturini et al., 1998; Michetti et al., 1995). The binding of NF-κB to DNA measured by gel shift assays is inhibited by oxidising conditions (Lipton, 1997; Smeyne et al., 1993). Thioredoxin increases the DNA binding of NF-κB to DNA and is more active than L-cysteine, reduced glutathione and nonphysiological reducing agents such as N-acetyl cysteine, 2-mercaptoethanol and dithiothreitol (Smeyne et al., 1993; Mannick et al., 1999; Dimmeler et al., 1997). Oxidised thioredoxin inhibits the binding of NF-κB to DNA(Hebestreit et al., 1998). Activation of the DNA binding of NF-κB requires that the Cys^{62} of one subunit is linked by a disulphide bridge with the Cys^{62} of the other in uncomplexed NF-κB, the DNA can no longer gain access to the binding surface of the p50 homodimer; also, if the p50 Cys^{62} is disulphide-linked to DNA, it can no longer be released from the complex (Estevez et al., 1998; Kim et al., 1997). Nuclear magnetic resonance has been used to show a disulphide-bonded complex between a catalytically inactive mutant human thioredoxin (Cys^{35}→Ala.Cys^{62}→Ala.Cys^{69}→Ala.Cys^{73}→Ala) and a 13 residue peptide comprising residues 56-68 of the p50 subunit of NF-κB encompassing the critical Cys^{62} residue (Tenneti et al., 1997). Both stable and transient transfection of cells with human thioredoxin has been found to increase NF-κB transactivation measured with a reporter construct (Mannick et al., 1997; Kim et al., 1998). However, other studies have reported that transient transfection with thioredoxin or addition of thioredoxin to the medium results in a dose-dependent inhibition of constitutive as well as phorbol ester-stimulated NF-κB DNA binding and transactivation (Tzeng et al., 1998). This difference may be due to the use of reporter constructs containing different NF-κB promoter elements. Recent studies have found that NF-κB transactivation is increased in both human MCF-7 breast cancer and mouse WEHI7.2 lymphoid cells stably transfected with human thioredoxin and with the catalytic site mutant Cys^{32} Ser/Cys^{35}→Ser thioredoxin, suggesting that catalytic site redox activity may not be necessary for NF-κB activation by thioredoxin (Ernster and Dallner, 1995).

A second transcription factor whose activity is regulated by thioredoxin is the glucocorticoid receptor, which is known to be subject to redox modulation through critical cysteine residues in which oxidation leads to decreased ligand binding activity (Haendeler et al., 1997) and decreased DNA binding (Li et al., 1997). Transfection of cells with thioredoxin has been shown to increase the expression of glucocorticoid receptor-mediated genes and to increase glucocorticoid receptor reporter activity in oxidant-treated cells, while transfection with antisense thioredoxin leads to decreases (Rossig et al., 1999; Thor et al., 1982). Thioredoxin associates with the DNA binding domain of the glucocorticoid receptor in the nucleus, which may account for the increased glucocorticoid receptor activity (Nguyen et al., 1992).

The transcription factor AP-1 (Fos and Jun homo- and heterodimers), in which activation is closely correlated with increased cell growth, is also redox-regulated (Tzeng et al., 1998; Sata et al., 1997). DNA binding of AP-1 is increased by the reduction of a single conserved Cys residue in the DNA binding domain of each of the homodimers (Nicholson et al., 1995). Mutant Fos and Jun proteins in which this Cys residue is replaced by Ser show constitutive DNA binding (Nicholson et al., 1995). Cells transfected with human thioredoxin show an increase in AP-1 activity measured with a reporter construct (Kim et al., 1998). Thioredoxin does not reduce AP-1 directly but does so through another nuclear redox protein Ref-1 (Di Monte et al., 1997). Ref-1 is a 37 kDa protein that also has an apurine/apyrimidine endonuclease repair activity and a core domain that is highly conserved in a family of prokaryotic and eukaryotic DNA repair enzymes (Leist et al., 1997). Sequences in the N-terminal domain of Ref-1 are required for redox activity, whereas C-terminal sequences are necessary for DNA repair activity (Leist et al., 1997). DNA binding by the transcription factor AP-2 is also increased by thioredoxin (Chesis et al., 1984).

In addition to its roles in cell proliferation and control of gene expression, secreted TRX can also act as an extracellular growth factor for both normal and tumour cells and can enhance the sensitivity of the cells to other growth factors (Schenk, 1996). Breast cancer cells transfected with TRX show increased anchorage-independent growth, while a redox inactive TRX mutant acts in a dominant negative fashion to inhibit proliferation and tumour formation in scid mice (Gallegos et al., 1996). Consistent with this Grogan et al (2000) have observed in vivo a positive correlation between TRX over-expression and cancer cell proliferation in primary gastric carcinomas. In addition to its proliferative effects TRX is also known to express anti-apoptotic effects. TRX inhibits apoptotic signalling by scavenging ROS and also by inhibiting the activity of ASK-1 (Ueda et al., 2002). In studies of TRX expression in gastric cell carcinoma, Grogan et al (Grogan et al., 2000) also noted a significant negative correlation between TRC over-expression and apoptosis suggesting a role for TRX in decreased apoptosis and increased carcinoma cell survival. In a study of non small cell lung carcinomas Soini and co-workers (2001) also observed that apoptosis was inversely associated with TRX and TR expression, again indicating that an anti-apoptotic effect of the TRX system may contribute to tumour cell survival.

Both TRX and TR are known to be secreted by normal and cancer cells. Indeed elevated TRX levels have been observed in the plasma of patients with hepatocarcinomas (Miyazaki et al., 1998) and pancreatic cancer (Nakamura et al., 2000). Recently, it has been shown that secreted TRX can regulate the redox state of specific cell surface receptors (Matthias et al., 2002) and of the extracellular environment (Angelini et al., 2002). Consequently, TRX may exert a redox control over cellular mechanisms that are involved with cell attachment, invasion and metastasis. In keeping with this, Farina et al. (2001) have also provided direct evidence that the extracellular TRX system contributes to the invasive capacity of SK-N-SH neuroblastoma cells in vitro and this is due in part to redox regulation of the functional MMP/TIMP balance governing MMP activity expression. In this pivotal study, Farina et al., (2001) demonstrated that TRX stimulated the invasive capacity of SK-N-SH neuroblastoma cells in a Matrigel invasion assay, and that the TR inhibitor aurothioglucose inhibited the capacity of TRX to stimulate invasion, indicating that the redox activity of the TRX system was required for this function. Moreover, it was shown that TRX inhibited the activities of both TIMP-1 and TIMP-2. It also inhibited MMP-2 at higher doses but did not inhibit MMP-9. It was further shown that TRX not only stimulated basal neuroblastoma cell invasion, but also reversed the capacity of exogenous TIMP-1 to inhibit both basal and MMP-9 stimulated invasion. In the present studies we noted in aggressive invasive breast carcinomas and advanced melanomas for example, TRX and TR were over expressed compared to tumours of a less aggressive nature. Similar observations have been made for a number of other tumours in vivo, for example Kakolyris and co-workers (2001) noted that the over expression of TRX in small cell carcinomas was correlated with the more aggressive phenotype and was associated with poor prognostic features. Similarly, Nakamura et al (2000) have reported on a possible association of TRX over expression with the malignant potential in pancreatic ductal carcinoma.

Given the association of the over-expression of the thioredoxin system with the processes of tumourigenesis and malignancy reported here and elsewhere, the targeted inhibition of the TRX system has been suggested as a novel approach for the treatment of some cancers. Indeed, specific chemical inhibitors of TRX and TR are known to inhibit cancer cell growth and exhibit anti-tumour activity in vivo. For example, some alkyl 2-imidazolyl disulfide inhibitors of TRX have been shown to have anti-tumour activity against human tumour xenografts growing in scid mice (Kirkpatrick et al., 1998). Also, Kunkel et al (1997) utilised an algorithm to search the NCI investigational drug database of known cytotoxic agents for similar compounds to known TRX/TR inhibitors. Of the 46 compounds identified, 37 exhibited anti TR activity, 3 were TRX inhibitors and several were already known to be potent anti-tumour drugs. Moreover, other studies indicate that other potential therapeutics may achieve their anti-tumour effects through down-regulation of the TRX system. The recent work of Butler et al (2002) demonstrates that such downregulation accounts at least in part for the action of histone deacetylase inhibitors such as SAHA which induce growth arrest, differentiation and /or apoptosis of transformed cells in vitro and inhibit tumour growth in vivo. SAHA induces the expression of thioredoxin-binding protein-2 (TBP-2), also known as vitamin D upregulated protein (VDUP), which binds to and inhibits TRX activity and also results in a decreased expression of TRX. TRX/TR over expression was also associated with the development of drug resistance in several tumour cells and cell lines. For example, Yokomizo et al. (1995) demonstrated that increased levels of TRX in prostatic and bladder cancer cell lines are associated with drug sensitivity to cisplatin, mitomycin C, doxorubicin and etoproside. Further studies show that inhibition/downregulation of TRX/TR expression sensitises drug resistant tumour cells to drug action, clearly establishing the link between the TRX system and drug sensitivity (Sinha et al., 1998; Sasada et at., 2000). Clearly, drugs that target the TRX system either directly or indirectly have potential as therapeutic drugs either singularly or in combination with other therapeutic agents.

In conclusion these studies have demonstrated the over-expression of the TRX system in a range of human tumours including breast, thyroid, prostate and colorectal carcinomas, as well as melanomas, and an association with the more aggressive tumour phenotypes. Such tumours have a high proliferation rate, a low apoptosis rate and an elevated metastatic potential, all of which can be influenced by the actions of the TRX system. As such, these studies further emphasis the potential of anti-TRX system agents as anti-cancer therapeutics in the treatment of a wide range of human tumours.

References

Albina J.C., Cui S., Mateo R.B., Reichner J.S. (1993). Nitric oxide-mediated apoptosis in murine peritoneal macrophages. J. Immunol. 150: 5080-5085.

Angelini G., Gardella S., Ardy M., Ciriolo M.R., Filomeni G., Di Trapani G., Clarke F.M., Sitia R., Rubartelli A. (2002). Antigen-presenting dendritic cells provide the reducing extracellular microenvironment required for T lymphocyte activation. Proc. Acad. Natl. Sci. USA. 99: 1491-1496.

Ankarcrona M., Dypbukt J.M., Brune B., Nicotera P. (1995). Interleukin-1 beta-induced nitric oxide production activates apoptosis in pancreatic RINm5F cells. Exp. Cell. Res. 213: 172-177.

Arner E.S. and Holmgren A. (2000). Physiological functions of thioredoxin and thioredoxin reductase. Eur. J. Biochem. 267: 6102-6109.

Arrigo A. (1999). Gene expression and the thiol redox state. Free Radic. Biol. Med. 27: 936-944.

Baker A., Payne C., Briehl M., Powis G. (1997). Thioredoxin, a gene found over-expressed in human cancer, inhibits apoptosis in vitro and in vivo. Cancer Res. 57: 5162-5167.

Barral A.M., Kallstrom R., Sander B., Rosen,A (2000). Thioredoxin, thioredoxin reductase and tumour necrosis factor-alpha expression in melanoma cells: correlation to resistance against cytotoxic attack. Melanoma Res. 10: 331-443.

Berggren M., Gallegos A., Gasdaska J., Gasdaska P., Warneke J., Powis G. (1996). Thioredoxin and thioredoxin reductase gene expression in human tumors and cell lines, and the effects of serum stimulation and hypoxia. Anticancer Res. 16: 3459-3466.

Bini L., Magi B., Marzocchi B., Arcuri F., Tripodi S., Cintorino M., Sanchez J.C., Frutiger S., Hughes G., Pallini V., Hochstrasser D.F., Tosi P. (1997). Protein expression profiles in human breast ductal carcinoma and histologically normal tissue. Electrophoresis. 18: 2832-2841.

Butler L.M., Zhou X., Xu W.S., Scher H.I., Rifkind R.A., Marks P.A., Richon V.M. (2002). The histone deacetylase inhibitor SAHA arrests cancer cell growth, up-regulates thioredoxin-binding protein-2, and down-regulates thioredoxin. Proc. Acad. Natl. Sci. USA 99: 11700-11705.

Chesis P.L., Levin D.E., Smith M.T., Ernster L., Ames B.N. (1984). Mutagenicity of quinones: pathways of metabolic activation and detoxification. Proc. Natl. Acad. Sci. USA. 81: 1696-1700.

Das K.C. and Das,C.K:. (2000). Thioredoxin, a singlet oxygen quencher and hydroxyl radical scavenger: redox independent functions. Biochem. Biophys. Res. Commun. 277: 443-447.

Dimmeler S., Haendeler J., Nehls M., Zeiher A.M. (1997). Suppression of apoptosis by nitric oxide via inhibition of interleukin-1 beta-converting enzyme (ICE)-like and cysteine protease protein (CPP)-32-like proteases. 1997. J. Exp. Med. 185: 601-607.

Di Monte D., Bellomo G., Thor H., Nicotera P., Orrenius S. (1984). Medadione-induced cytoxicity is associated with protein thiol oxidation and alteration in intracellular Ca2+ homeostasis. 1984. Arch. Biochem. Biophys. 235: 343-360.

Ernster L., Dallner G. Biochemical, physiological and medical aspects of ubiquinone function. (1995). Biochem. Biophys. Acta. 1271: 195-204.

Estevez A.G., Spear N., Thompson J.A., Cornwell T.L., Radi R., Barbeito L., Beckman J.S. (1998). Nitric oxide-dependent production of cGMP supports the survival of rat embryonic motor neurons cultured with brain-derived nitrotrophic factor. J. Neurosci. 18: 3708-3714.

Farina A.R., Tacconelli A., Cappabianca L., Masciulli M.P., Holmgren A., Beckett G.J., Gulino A., MacKay A. (2001). Thioredoxin alters the matrix metalloproteinase/tissue inhibitors of metalloproteinase balance and stimulates human SK-N-SH neuroblastoma cell invasion. Eur. J. Biochem. 268: 405-413.

Fujii S., Nanbu Y., Nonogaki H., Konishi I., Mori T., Masutani H., Yodoi J. (1991). Coexpression of adult T-cell leukemia-derived factor, a human thioredoxin homologue, and human papillomavirus DNA in neoplastic cervical squamous epithelium. Cancer. 68: 1583-1591.

Gallegos A., Gasdaska J., Taylor C., Paine-Murrieta G., Goodman D., Gasdaska P., Berggren M., Briehl M., Powis G. (1996). Transfection with human thioredoxin increases cell proliferation and a dominant-negative mutant thioredoxin reverses the transformed phenotype of human breast cancer cells. Cancer Res. 56: 5765-5770.

Gasdaska J.R., Berggren M., Powis G. (1995). Cell growth stimulation by the redox protein thioredoxin occurs by a novel helper mechanism. Cell Growth Differ. 6: 1643-1650.

Gasdaska J.R., Harney J.W., Gasdaska P.Y., Powis G., Berry M.J. (1999). Regulation of human thioredoxin reductase expression and activity by 3'-untranslated region selenocysteine insertion sequence and mRNA instability. J. Biol. Chem. 274: 25379-25385.

Gladyshev V.N., Jeang K.T., Stadtman T.C. (1996). Selenocysteine, identified as the penultimate C-terminal residue in human T-cell thioredoxin reductase, corresponds to TGA in the human placental gene Proc. Acad. Natl. Sci. USA 93: 6146-6151.

Grogan T.M., Fenoglio-Prieser C., Zeheb R., Bellamy W., Frutiger Y., Vela E., Stemmerman G., Macdonald J., Richter L., Gallegos A., Powis G. (2000). Thioredoxin, a putative oncogene product, is over expressed in gastric carcinoma and associated with increased proliferation and increased cell survival. Hum. Pathol. 31: 475-481.

Haendeler J., Weiland U., Zeiher A.M., Dimmeler S. (1997). Effects of redox-related congeners of NO on apoptosis and caspase-3 activity. Nitric Oxide. 1: 282-293.

Hebestreit H., Dibbert B., Balatti I., Braun D., Schapowal A., Blaser K., Simon H.U. (1998). Disruption of fas receptor signaling by nitric oxide in eosinophils. J. Exp. Med. 187: 415-425.

Holmgren A. (1985). Thioredoxin. Ann. Rev.. Biochem. 54: 237-271.

Kahlos K., Soini Y., Saily M., Koistinen P., Kakko,S., Paakko P., Holmgren A., Kinnula V.L. (2001). Up-regulation of thioredoxin and thioredoxin reductase in human malignant pleural mesothelioma. Int. J. Cancer. 95: 198-204.

Kakolyris S., Giatromanolaki A., Koukourakis M., Powis G., Souglakos J., Sivridis E., Georgoulias V., Gatter K.C., Harris A.L. (2001). Thioredoxin expression is associated with lymph node status and prognosis in early operable non-small cell lung cancer. Clin. Cancer Res. 7: 3087-3091.

Kim Y.M., Talanian R.V., Li J., Billiar T.R. (1997). Nitric oxide inhibits apoptosis by preventing increases in caspase-3-like activity via two distinct mechanisms. J. Biol. Chem.: 272: 31138-31148.

Kim Y.M., Talanian R.V., Li J., Billiar T.R. (1998). Nitric oxide prevents IL-1 beta and IFN-gamma-inducing factor (IL-18) release from macrophages by inhibiting caspase-1 (IL-1 beta-converting enzyme). J. Immunol. 161: 4122-4128.

Kirkpatrick D.L., Kuperus M., Dowdeswell M., Potier N., Donald L.J., Kunkel M., Berggren M., Angulo M., Powis G. (1998). Mechanisms of inhibition of the thioredoxin growth factor system by antitumor 2-imidazolyl disulfides. Biochem. Pharm. 55: 987-994.

Knowles R.G., Moncada S. (1992). Nitric oxide is a signal blood vessels. Trends Biochem. Sci. 17: 399-402.

Kunkel M.W., Kirkpatrick D.L., Johnson J.I., Powis G. (1997). Cell line-directed screening assay for inhibitors of thioredoxin reductase signaling as potential anti-cancer drugs. Anticancer Drug Des. 12: 659-670.

Leist M., Volbracht C., Kuhnle S., Fava E., Ferrando-May E., Nicotera P. (1997). Caspase-mediated apoptosis in neuronal excitotoxicity triggered by nitric oxide. Mol. Med. 3: 750-764.

Li J., Billiar TR., Talanian R.V., Kim Y.M. (1997). Nitric oxide reversibly inhibits seven members of the caspase family via S-nitrosylation. Biochem. Biophys. Res. Commun. 240: 419-424.

Lipton S.A. Janus faces of NF-κN: neurodestruction versus neuroprotection. (1997). Nat. Med. 3: 20-22.

Lopata A., Sibson M.C., Enders A.C., Bloomfield K.L, Gregory M.S., Trapani G.D., Perkins A.V., Tonissen K.F., Clarke F.M. (2001). Expression and localization of thioredoxin during early implantation in the marmoset monkey. Mol. Hum. Reprod. 7: 1159-1165.

Mannick J. B., Hausladen A., Liu L., Hess D.T., Zeng M., Miao Q.X., Kane L.S., Gow A.J., Stamler J.S. (1999). Fas-induced caspase denitrosylation. Science. 284: 651-654.

Mannick J.B., Miao X.Q., Stamler J.S. (1997). Nitric oxide inhibits Fas-induced apoptosis. J Biol. Chem. 272: 24125-24128.

Matsutani Y., Yamauchi A., Takahashi R., Ueno M., Yoshikawa K., Honda K., Nakamura H., Kato H., Kodama H., Inamoto T., Yodoi J., Yamaoka Y. (2001). Inverse correlation of thioredoxin expression with estrogen receptor- and p53-dependent tumor growth in breast cancer tissues. Clin. Cancer Res. 7: 3430-3436.

Matthias L.J., Yam P.T., Jiang X.M., Vandegraaff N., Li P., Poumbourios P., Donoghue N., Hogg P.J. (2002). Disulfide exchange in domain 2 of CD4 is required for entry of HIV-1. Nat Immunol. 3: 727-732.

Michetti M., Salamino F., Melloni E., Pontremoli S. (1995). Reversible inactivation of calpain isoforms by nitric oxide. Biochem. Biophys. Res. Commun. 207: 1009-1014.

Miyazaki K., Noda N., Okada S., Hagiwara Y., Miyata M., Sakurabayashi I., Yamaguchi N., Sugimura T., Terada M., Wakasugi H. (1998). Elevated serum level of thioredoxin in patients with hepatocellular carcinoma. Biotherapy. 11: 277-288.

Nakamura H., Masutani H., Tagaya Y., Yamauchi A., Inamoto T., Nanbu Y., Fujii S., Ozawa K., Yodoi J. (1992). Expression and growth-promoting effect of adult T-cell leukemia-derived factor. A human thioredoxin homologue in hepatocellular carcinoma. Cancer. 69: 2091-2097.

Nakamura H., Bai J., Nishinaka Y., Ueda S., Sasada T., Ohshio G., Imamura M., Takabayashi A., Yamaoka Y., Yodoi J. (2000). Expression of thioredoxin and glutaredoxin, redox-regulating proteins, in pancreatic cancer. Cancer Detect. Prev. 24: 53-60.

Nicholson D.W., Ali A, Thornberry N.A., Vaillancourt J.P., Ding D.K, Gallant M., Gareau Y., Griffin P.R., Labelle M., Yamin T.-T., Yu V.L., Miller D. (1995).Identification and inhibition of the ICE/CED-3 protease necessary for mammalian apoptosis. Nature 376: 37-43.

Nordberg J. and Arner E.S. (2001). Reactive oxygen species, antioxidants, and the mammalian thioredoxin system(1). Free Radic. Biol. Med. 31: 1287-1312.

Nguyen T., Brunson D., Crespi C.L., Penman B.W., Wishnok J.S., Tannenbaum S.R. (1992). DNA damage and mutation in human cells exposed to nitric oxide in vitro. Proc. Natl. Acad. Sci. USA 89: 3030-3034.

Perkins A., Di Trapani G., McKay M., Clarke F.M. (1995). Immunocytochemical localisation of thioredoxin in human trophoblasts and decidua. Placenta. 16: 635-642.

Powis G., Gasdaska J., Gasdaska P., Berggren M., Kirkpatrick D., Engman L., Cotgreave I.., Angulo M., Baker A. (1997). Selenium and the thioredoxin redox system: effects on cell growth and death. Oncol. Res. 9: 303-312.

Rossig L., Fichtischerer B., Breitschopf K., Haendeler J., Zeiher A.M., Mulsch A., Dimmeler S. (1999). Nitric oxide inhibits caspase-3 by S-nitrosation in vivo. J. Biol. Chem. 274: 6823-6826.

Rubartelli A., Bajetto A., Allavena G., Wollman E., Sitia R. (1992). Secretion of thioredoxin by normal and neoplastic cells through a leaderless secretory pathway. J. Biol. Chem. 267: 24161-24164.

Sahaf B., Soderberg A., Spyrou G., Barral A., Pekkari K., Holmgren A., Rosen A. (1997). Thioredoxin expression and localization in human cell lines: detection of full-length and truncated species. Exp. Cell Res. 236: 181-192.

Sarih M., Souvannavong V., Adam A. (1993). Nitric oxide synthase induces macrophage death by apoptosis. Biochem. Biophys. Res. Commun. 191: 503-508.

Sasada T., Nakamura H., Ueda S., Iwata S., Ueno M., Takabayashi A., Yodoi J. (2000). Secretion of thioredoxin enhances cellular resistance to cis-diamminedichloroplatinum (II). Antioxid Redox Signal. 2: 695-705.

Sata N., Klonowski-Stumpe H., Han B., Haussinger D., Niederau C. (1997). Medanione induces both necrosis and apoptosis in rat pancreatic acinar AR4-2J cells. Free Radic. Biol. Med. 23: 844-850.

Schenk H., Vogt M., Droge W., Schulze-Osthoff K. (1996). Thioredoxin as a potent costimulus of cytokine expression. J. Immunol. 156: 765-771.

Shao L., Diccianni M.B., Tanaka, T., Gribi R., Yu A.L., Pullen J.D., Camitta B.M., Yu J. (2001).Thioredoxin expression in primay T-cell acute lymphoblastic leukemia and its therapeutic implication. Cancer Res. 61: 7333-7338.

Sinha P., Hutter G., Kottgen E., Dietel M., Schadendorf D., Lage H. (1998). Increased expression of annexin I and thioredoxin detected by two-dimensional gel electrophoresis of drug resistant human stomach cancer cells. J Biochem Biophys Methods. 37: 105-116.

Smeyne R.J., Vendrell M., Hayward M., Baker S.J., Miao G.G., Schilling K., Robertson L.M., Curran T., Morgan J.I. (1993). Continuous c-fos expression precedes programmed cell death in vivo. Nature 363: 166-169.

Soderberg A., Sahaf B., Rosen A. (2000). Thioredoxin reductase, a redox-active selenoprotein, is secreted by normal and neoplastic cells: presence in human plasma. Cancer Res. 60: 2281-2289.

Soini Y., Kahlos K., Napankangas U., Kaarteenaho-Wiik R., Saily M., Koistinen P., Paaakko P., Holmgren A., Kinnula V.L. (2001). Widespread expression of thioredoxin and thioredoxin reductase in non-small cell lung carcinoma. Clin. Cancer Res. 7: 1750-1757.

Stuehr D. J. and Nathan C.F. (1989). Nitric oxide. A macrophage product responsible for cystostasis and respiratory inhibition in tumour target cells. J. Exp. Med. 169: 1543-1555.

Suzuki Y., Kondo Y., Himeno S., Nemoto K., Akimoto M., Imura N. (2000). Role of antioxidant systems in human androgen-independent prostate cancer cells. Prostate. 43: 144-149.

Tan S., Sagara Y., Liu Y., Maher P., Schubert D. (1998). The regulation of reactive oxygen species production during programmed cell death. J. Cell. Biol. 141: 1423-1432.

Tenneti L., D' Emilia D.M., Lipton S.A. (1997). Suppression of neuronal apoptosis by S-nitrosylation of caspases. Neurosci. Lett. 236: 139-142.

Thor H., Smith M.T., Hartzell P., Bellomo G., Jewell S.A., Orrenius S. (1982). The metabolism of menadione (2-methyl-1.4-napthoquinone) by isolated hepatocytes. A study of the implications of oxidative stress in intact cells. 1982. J. Biol. Chem. 257: 12419-12425.

Tzeng E., Billiar T.R., Williams D.L., Li J., Lizonova A., Kovesdi I., Kim Y.M. (1998). Adenovirus-mediated inducible nitric oxide synthase gene transfer inhibits hepatocyte apoptosis. Surgery. 124: 278-283.

Ueda S., Masutani H., Nakamura H., Tanaka T. Ueno M., Yodoi J. (2002). Redox control of cell death. Antioxid. Redox. Signal 4: 405-414.

Ueno M., Matsutani Y., Nakamura H., Masutani H., Yagi M., Yamashiro H., Kato H., Inamoto T., Yamauchi A., Takahashi R., Yamaoka Y., Yodoi J. (2000). Possible association of thioredoxin and p53 in breast cancer. Immunol. Lett. 75: 15-20.

Venturini G., Fioravanti E., Colasanti M., Persichini T., Ascenzi P. (1998). Cys25-nitrosylation inactivates papain. Biochem. Mol. Biol. Int. 46: 425-428.

Yokomizo A., Ono M., Nanri H., Makino Y., Ohga T., Wada M., Okamoto T., Yodoi J., Kuwano M., Kohno K. (1995). Cellular levels of thioredoxin associated with drug sensitivity to cisplatin, mitomycin C, doxorubicin, and etoposide. Cancer Res. 55: 4293-4296.

Adaptation Biology and Medicine (Volume 4: Current Concepts)
Editors: A. Hargens, N. Takeda and P.K. Singal

9. Membranoprotective Effects of Adaptation in the Heart and Skeletal Muscle

Sazontova T.G., *Arkhipenko Yu.V.

Institute of General Pathology and Pathophysiology, Russian Academy of Medical Sciences; *M.V.Lomonosov Moscow State University, Moscow, Russia

Abstract

The effect of adaptation on various membrane structures is strongly tissue-specific, *i.e.,* the same factor or influence elicits different responses in various tissues which vary from protective to damaging. Membrane responses during adaptation to physical load by swimming (32°C; 1 h daily for 4, 15 and 30 days) were studied in two types of muscle (myocardium and skeletal muscle) tissues, which differ essentially in sensitivity to reactive oxygen species (ROS). In the heart, adaptation to physical load was accompanied by increasing resistance of the SR membrane to ROS without significant increase in the activity of the SR Ca-pump at initial stages. However, the enzyme activity increased 1.3-2.3-fold on days 15 and 30. Contrariwise, in skeletal muscle adaptation caused a 3.5-fold increase in SR Ca-pump activity, but the resistance of the enzyme to ROS and high level of Ca^{2+} decreased dramatically. The resistance of the enzyme increased to the control level only after a drop in Ca-pump activity on day 15. On day 30, the activity and resistance of the skeletal muscle enzyme remained at a high level.

As early as 1986, Professor Felix Meerson published an article entitled "On the price of adaptation". The ideas stated therein were developed and further enriched in our studies. This subject is virtually boundless, but nevertheless extremely important for the modern adaptation science, since specialists in this field who endeavor to solve concrete practical tasks begin to focus their attention on the functional states of different body organs and their improvement using adaptational training.

However, the problem of tissue specificity is directly related to the effect of adaptation on the whole organism as it takes place in the living Nature, whereas the responses of different organs vary widely from protective to damaging under the influence of the same factor. We are often faced with this problem during a comparison of functional states of membrane structures in various tissues, such as liver and brain, heart and liver, heart and skeletal muscles, etc. [Sazontova T.G., 1998]. Thus, it was shown that tissue specificity varies within very broad limits depending on the type of training, and the sensitivity of body organs to the active factor must be taken into consideration in each concrete case, especially where specific protection is required. Our previous studies established pronounced tissue specificity of adaptation to stress and intermittent hypoxia. It was found, in particular, that factors of similar origin and intensity may produce quite different effects on tissues, which vary from protective to damaging. This can be attributed to the difference in the sensitivities of concrete tissues, cells or intracellular structures to reactive oxygen species (ROS), different ratios of prooxidant and antioxidant systems of the cell at the moment of cell exposure to exogenous factors, etc. The involvement of one or another tissue in the formation of an adaptive response to a specific factor, i.e., its relatedness to a "working" organ, also plays a role. In this context, the detection of the most sensitive organs and development of methods protecting against possible side effects become the main challenge for modern-day adaptation medicine.

This study is devoted to the analysis of the functional state of the sarcoplasmic reticulum (SR) Ca-pump, an intracellular membrane-bound system responsible for the transport of excess Ca to the intracellular depots in the heart and skeletal muscle during adaptation of the organism to physical training by swimming.

Adaptation to physical training has a broad spectrum of protective effects on the heart. Significant reduction of the risk of cardiovascular diseases and increased resistance to stress and ischemia makes such adaptation a currently central task [Meerson F.Z., Pshennikova M.G., 1988]. However, no such unambiguous protective effect was established for other organs. Thus, the structural resources of liver, kidney and adrenals in contrast with heart [Guski H et al., 1981] decrease considerably after adaptation to physical training [Bloor C. et al., 1968]. The development of conditioned reflexes is impaired with an increase in the training intensity [Meerson F.Z., Pshennikova M.G., 1988]. The data on skeletal muscles are often controversial. The increase in the muscle mass is paralleled either with an increase or a decrease in the number of mitochondria and mitochondrial enzymes, the rate of oxidative phosphorylation and the activities of antioxidant protection systems [Bloor C. et al., 1968; Yakovlev N. et al., 1981; Leeuwenburgh C. et al., 1994; Powers S.K. et al., 1994; Schluter J.M., Fitts R.N., 1994]. The experiments with chronic stimulation of fast muscles [Leberer E. et al., 1990; Hicks A. et al., 1997] or with long term physical training [Belcastro A. et al., 1993] have shown that the rate of Ca^{2+} transport into SR decreases under the influence of this factor due to the changes in the kinetic parameters of Ca^{2+} -ATPase. The data obtained are strongly suggestive of metabolic changes induced by adaptation to physical load. After periodic training, the initial type of skeletal muscle fibers is preserved in the overwhelming majority of tested individuals (95%), whereas their metabolic characteristics, e.g., energy profile, change dramatically in 56% of cases. [Piskova D.Ì., Son'kin V.D., 1996]. It was detected different kind of isozymes of the Ca^{2+} -ATPase of SR with high and low resistance to endogenous damaging factors [Belcastro A. et al., 1993; Kandarian S. et al., 1994; Favero T. et al., 1995]

These data altogether demonstrate the ambiguity of processes associated with the functional activities of various cellular structures of the heart and, particularly, of skeletal muscles in the course of adaptation to physical training.

This study was an attempt to answer the question "What is the price of adaptation in the heart and skeletal muscles under physical load?"

Methods

The experiments were performed on male Wistar rats weighing 250 g (n=54).

Acute physical training was carried out by 1-hr swimming of rats in water (32°C). The animals were sacrificed 1 hr after cessation of the training course.

Adaptation of rats to physical training was studied during 1-hr swimming of animals in water (32°C, 1 h daily for 30 days). The heart and skeletal muscles were extracted on the next day after termination of 4, 11, 15 and 30 swimming sessions.

Rat hearts and skeletal muscles (*musculus quadriceps femoris*) were extracted, washed with ice-cold saline and frozen in liquid nitrogen until use.

Tissue homogenization. The hearts and skeletal muscles were homogenized in an Ultra-Turrax TP-18/10 homogenizer for 30 s. The homogenization medium contained 100 mM KCl and 10 mM Tris-HCl pH 7.5 at a tissue:medium ratio of 1:6 for the heart and 1:8 for skeletal muscles.

Measurements of activities of antioxidant enzymes. Catalase activity was measured by the method of Luck [1963] with allowance for modification in tissue homogenates. SOD activity was measured spectrophotometrically by the method of Beauchamp, Fridovich [1972] following the rate of inhibition of superoxide radical formation in a xanthine–xanthine oxidase system. The level of the superoxide anion was determined at 560 nm by formazan formation from tetranitrotetrazolium blue.

Measurements of Ca^{2+} transport. The rate of Ca^{2+} transport in the hearts and skeletal muscles was measured with the help of a Ca^{2+}-selective electrode (Model 93-20) of an Orion EA 940 ionomer (Orion Research, USA). The rate of Ca^{2+} uptake into SR vesicles with continuous computer registration of the dynamics of Ca^{2+} uptake as described previously [Meerson F.Z. et al., 1990] was measured. The rate of Ca^{2+} transport into SR was measured in an incubation medium which contained 100 mM KCl, 15 mM potassium oxalate, 20 mM HEPES pH 7.1, 4 mM $MgCl_2$ and 5 mM NaN_3 (37°C).

The calculations, statistical treatment and graphical presentation of the experimental results were carried out using a computer-aided program EXCEL.

The resistance to high level of Ca^{2+} of the Ca^{2+} transport system in the hearts and skeletal muscles was measured using 10 and 30 mM Ca^{2+} and under a standard level of other medium components.

Thermal inactivation of the SR Ca-pump. The activity of the Ca^{2+} transport system was determined in a thermal denaturation test [Sazontova, 1998] using thermostated cells and incubation in a soluble fraction medium which contained 10 mM Tris-HCl pH 7.5 (1:4) upon continuous stirring (41°C). After definite intervals of time (10, 20 and 30 min), aliquots of samples were withdrawn for measuring the rate of Ca^{2+} transport.

Resistance to ROS was studied *in vitro* in the Ca^{2+} transport system of the heart and skeletal muscles by following the oxidation in ROS-inducing systems in the presence of ascorbate (0.3 mM). Protein concentration did not exceed 3 mg/mg. After definite intervals of time (40,120 and 230 min for the heart and 10, 20 and 30 min for skeletal muscles) and at an equal level of a drop in the Ca^{2+} transport rate, aliquots were taken as describe previously for measuring the rate of Ca^{2+}-transport.

Protein concentration was determined from the amplitude of the fourth derivative of the absorption spectrum around 240-320 nm using the method of Padros et al. [1984].

Statistic treatment of experimental results was carried out on the basis of parametric and nonparametric statistic criteria (Microsoft Excel).

Results

These studies revealed significant differences in the effects of acute physical training and adaptation to training on the functional states of cardiac and skeletal muscle tissues.

Let us consider at first the situation with acute physical training. In our study, acute training was not exhaustive and represented a moderate exercise of 1-hr duration. However, in contrast to the heart where catalase and SOD activities did not diminish after acute physical load, in skeletal muscle tissue the activities of these enzymes decreased by 38% and 22%, respectively (Fig.1).

The rate of Ca^{2+}-transport to SR increased in both tissues – by 22% in the heart and by 46% in the skeletal muscle (Fig.2).

It is of note that the rate of Ca^{2+}-transport was measured under "ideal" conditions, viz., at optimal concentrations of ATP and Ca^{2+} and in the absence of damaging factors, such as free radical oxidation, proteases, high Ca^{2+} levels, etc. For this reason, we did not restrict ourselves to the measurements of the initial rates of the enzyme, but followed the changes in the enzyme resistance to damaging factors under acute conditions and during adaptation.

Thus, we studied the resistance of SR Ca^{2+}-transport to reactive oxygen species during *in vitro*-induced free radical oxidation. It was found that in cardiac tissue (Fig.3A) the resistance to reactive oxygen species did not decrease after a single physical training session, but even increased in

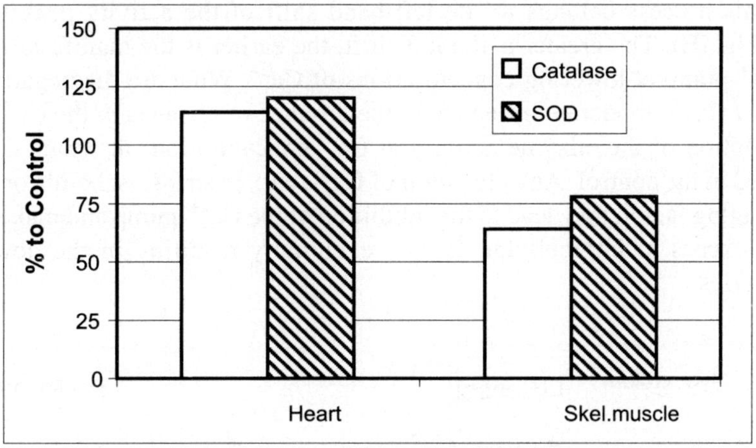

Fig. 1. Activities of antioxidant enzymes catalase and superoxide dismutase in heart and skeletal muscles after acute physical load (control – 100%).

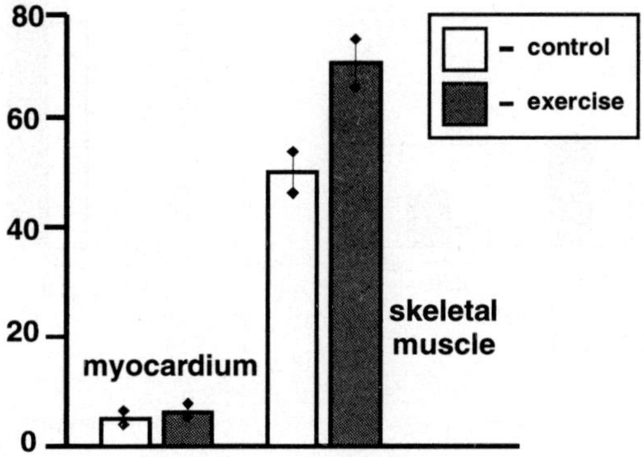

Fig. 2. Influence of acute physical load on the activity of Ca^{2+}-transporting system of the sarcoplasmic reticulum in the heart and skeletal muscle.

comparison with the control. These changes were especially well-pronounced in skeletal muscles (Fig.3B). Indeed, after 20-min oxidation, the rate of Ca^{2+} transport in control skeletal muscle was practically zero, but after acute physical load the enzyme activity was retained by 46%.

However, we still cannot assert that acute physical load has no negative effect on the activity of SR Ca^{2+}-pump, since physical training affects such an important parameter of the SR Ca^{2+}-pump activity as its resistance to high Ca^{2+} levels.

Under normal conditions, the dependence of enzyme activity on Ca^{2+} concentration can be described as follows. Initially, the rate of Ca^{2+} transport into the sarcoplasmic reticulum increases with an increase in Ca^{2+} concentration and gradually reaches a maximum and then a plateau. With a further rise in Ca^{2+} concentration, the activity of the system responsible for the removal of excess Ca^{2+} to intracellular depots (SR) begins to decrease. The maximum enzyme activity also decreases under the influence of acute factors, such as stress and hypoxia (Fig.4A).

A decrease in the maximum activity of the Ca^{2+}-pump is not critical in this particular case. The critical role in this process belongs to the left-hand shift of the activity peak towards lower Ca^{2+} concentrations (Fig.4B). The greater is the left shift, the earlier is the manifestation of the inhibiting effect on the Ca^{2+}-pump at lowering concentrations of Ca^{2+}. What are the negative consequences of this event? Even a single moderate influence in the absence of changes in the Ca^{2+}-pump activity can provoke the inhibition of the enzyme activity at Ca^{2+} concentrations at which Ca^{2+}-transport is not normally inhibited in the control. Any elevation of Ca^{2+}, e.g., in stress, ischemia or under the influence of any other damaging factor, may lead to the inhibition of the Ca^{2+}-pump and make the latter incapable to remove Ca^{2+} excess to intracellular depots, eventually resulting in the development of Ca^{2+}-mediated cell injuries.

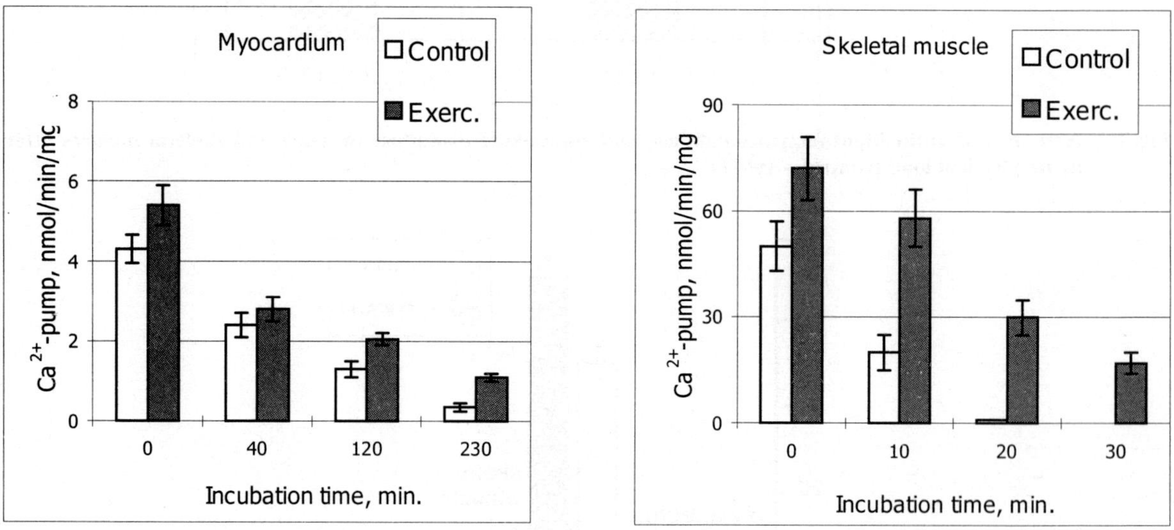

A B

Fig. 3. Resistance of Ca^{2+}-transporting system of the sarcoplasmic reticulum to free radical oxidation induced in vitro. A – heart; B – skeletal muscle. Inset shows the time of incubation in minutes.

And the third situation in the cell –if these two factors act simultaneously, the functional activity and resistance of the cell decrease (Fig.4C). This is exactly what takes place during acute physical training in the heart and, especially, in skeletal muscles where the resistance of Ca^{2+}-pump to high Ca^{2+} concentrations is decreased. Indeed, a 3-fold increase in Ca^{2+} concentration decreases the activity of the Ca^{2+}-pump in cardiac tissues (Fig.5A). In skeletal muscles, the decrease in the resistance of the Ca^{2+}-transport system to high Ca^{2+} levels after a single physical training is even more pronounced. In control samples, the rate of Ca^{2+} transport increases by 54% with a 3-fold increase in Ca^{2+} concentration. In contrast, after physical exercise the rate of Ca^{2+}-transport decreases by 26% (Fig.5B).

Moreover, acute physical load has a negative effect on the resistance of SR Ca^{2+}-pump to thermal inactivation. The resistance of Ca^{2+}-pump to thermal inactivation decreases after acute physical training even in more stable cardiac tissues (Fig.6). We failed to observe Ca^{2+}-transport in experimental samples after 10-min thermal inactivation, whereas in control samples rate of Ca^{2+}-transport was preserved after 10- and 20-min inactivation (by 46% and 23%, respectively).

These data suggest that acute physical training has a dual effect by increasing the activity of the Ca^{2+}-pump in cardiac and skeletal muscle SR and decreasing the resistance of the Ca^{2+}-pump. This indicates that under optimum conditions the activity of cardiac SR Ca^{2+}-pump is preserved and even increases after acute physical load. However, the change in environmental conditions and Ca^{2+}elevation under stress as well as ischemia, reperfusion and other pathological conditions where Ca^{2+} accumulation in SR is crucial for the cell all lead to a more rapid inhibition of the SR Ca^{2+}-pump

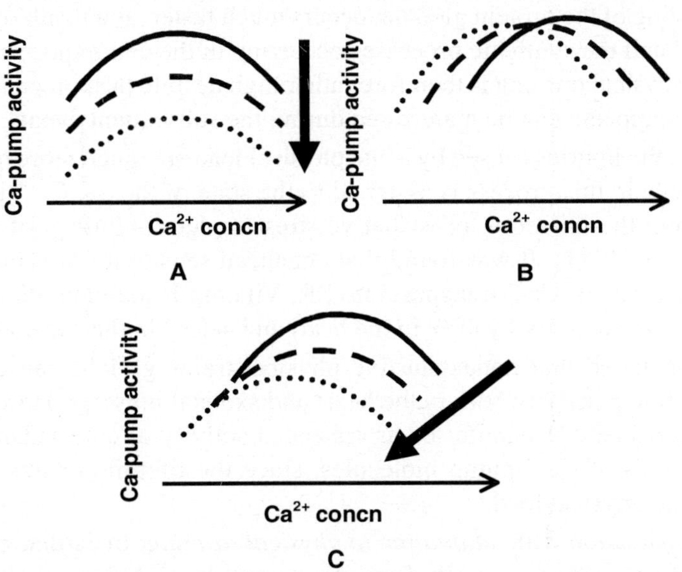

Fig. 4. Scheme of influence of damaging environmental factors to the effectivity of functioning of Ca-pump. Arrows indicate different shifts of Ca-dependence of Ca^{2+}-transporting system of the sarcoplasmic reticulum in the muscles:
A. Decrease of initial rate of Ca^{2+}-transport;
B. Increase in the sensitivity of Ca^{2+}-transport to high level of Ca^{2+};
C. Common effect of A + B.
Other explanations see in the text.

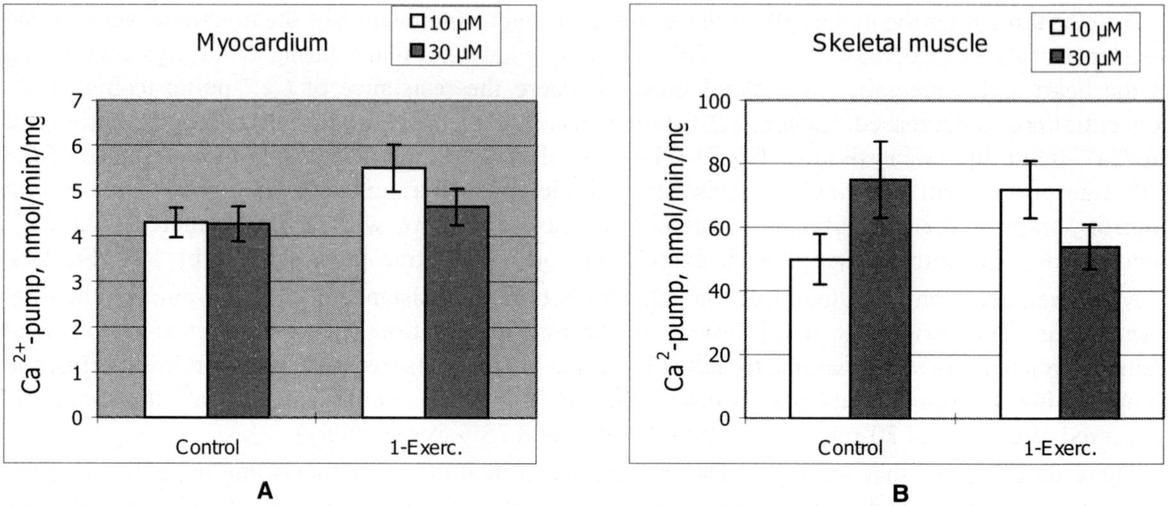

Fig. 5. Ca-pump resistance to high level of Ca^{2+} (from 10 to 30 ìM) in heart (A) and skeletal muscle (B) after acute physical load.

activity. Moreover, a marked increase in the rate of thermal inactivation of the enzyme testifies to noticeable changes in its native conformation which are close to denaturation. In this case denaturation, i.e., a complete unfolding of the protein globule, occurs much faster, as a result of which the lifetime of the enzyme decreases and the synthetic processes occurring in the cell require additional stimulation. The "price" of acute physical training is therefore rather high despite the compensatory response of the myocardial SR Ca^{2+}-pump and can be manifested during the subsequent events.

In skeletal muscles, the injuries caused by acute physical load are much more pronounced than in the heart. An important role in this process is assigned to the state of the SR Ca^{2+}-pump in the heart and skeletal muscles during the induction of oxidative stress under conditions of vitamin E deficiency [Àrkhipenko Yu.V. et al., 1987]. It was found that enhanced sensitivity of skeletal muscle tissues to ROS is reflected on the rate of Ca^{2+}-transport into SR. Vitamin E-deficient diets induce a significant decrease in the Ca^{2+}-pump activity by 40% in the heart and 4-fold in the skeletal muscle.

It may thus be concluded that nonexhaustive physical training (1 h) causes an urgent adaptive elevation of the Ca^{2+}-pump activity both in the heart and skeletal muscles. However, this elevation is concomitant with a considerable manifested as enhanced activity of antioxidant protection enzymes and enhanced resynthesis of Ca^{2+}-pump molecules, since the lifetime of this enzyme is decreased significantly after acute physical load.

Let us consider the situation with *adaptation to physical training*. In cardiac tissue, the activities of catalase and SOD did not differ essentially from the control level during all adaptation periods. The situation was quite different in skeletal muscles. At early stages of adaptation (4 – 11 sessions), the activities of these antioxidant enzymes are decreased by 35-42% in comparison with control.

The initial rate of heart Ca^{2+} transport into SR changes appreciably in the course of adaptation. The corresponding curves (Fig.7A) have a wavy shape: under acute physical training (1st exposure), the rate of Ca^{2+} transport in SR increased by 27% and approximated the control level after 4 days. After 11

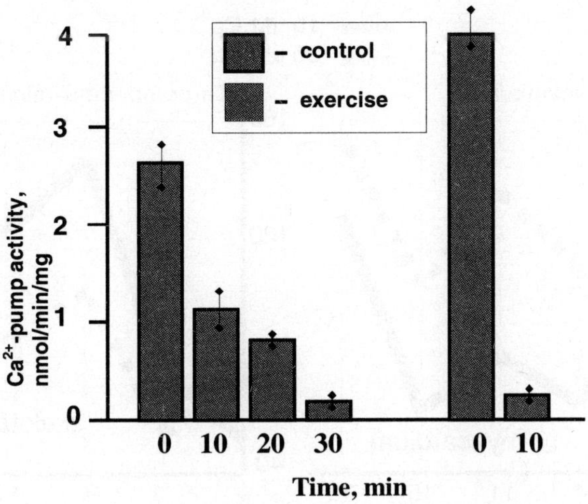

Fig. 6. Thermal resistance of myocardial Ca-pump (41°C) in control and after acute physical load.

days, it exceeded the control level and returned to it only by day 15. By the end of adaptation (day 30), it showed another significant increase, this time by 43%. This points to a gradual increase in the rate of cardiac Ca^{2+}-pump. These dates agree with enhanced activity of heart Ca^{2+}-ATPase after long-term adaptation of the rats to physical training (150 min, 5 days in a week, 7-8 weeks) by swimming (30-42%) [Penpargkul S. et al., 1977].

The situation in skeletal muscles is quite different: after four adaptation sessions, the rate of Ca^{2+} transport increased considerably (nearly 3-fold) in comparison with the control. By the 11th and 15th sessions, this activity decreased only slightly, but it still exceeded the control level more than 2-fold and returned to the control level only after 30 sessions (Fig.7B).

The resistance of the Ca^{2+}-transport system to high Ca^{2+} concentrations increased significantly in the heart at early adaptation stages (after 4 and 11 swimming sessions). After a 3-fold increase in Ca^{2+} concentration, the rate of Ca^{2+} transport increased significantly (by 26%), whereas that in control remained unchanged under identical conditions (Fig.7A).

In skeletal muscles, the resistance of the Ca^{2+}-transport system to high Ca^{2+} concentrations did not increase after 4 and 11 adaptation sessions in comparison with control. Contrariwise, the transport rate decreased (by 32 and 24%, respectively) (Fig.7B).

In the heart, the resistance of the Ca^{2+} transport system to thermal inactivation after 4 swimming sessions was even higher than in the control and significantly higher than after acute physical training (Fig.8). After acute physical training, Ca^{2+} transport was absent even after 10-min thermal inactivation, but after 4 training sessions the rate of Ca^{2+} transport reached 45% of the control. After 11 and 15 sessions, the resistance to thermal inactivation increased 2-fold.

In the heart, the resistance of the Ca^{2+} transport system to lipid peroxidation began to increase even after 4 sessions, but in skeletal muscles this was observed only after a period of 15 days, when the activity of Ca^{2+}-pump returned to the control level (Fig.9).

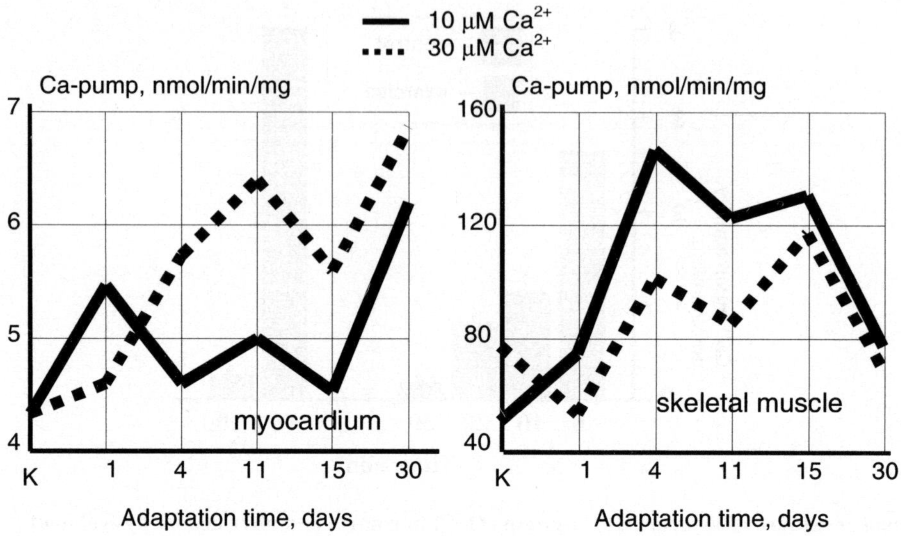

Fig. 7. Ca-pump resistance to high level of Ca^{2+} (from 10 to 30 μM) in heart (A) and skeletal muscle (B) during adaptation to physical load (1-4-11-15-30 days).

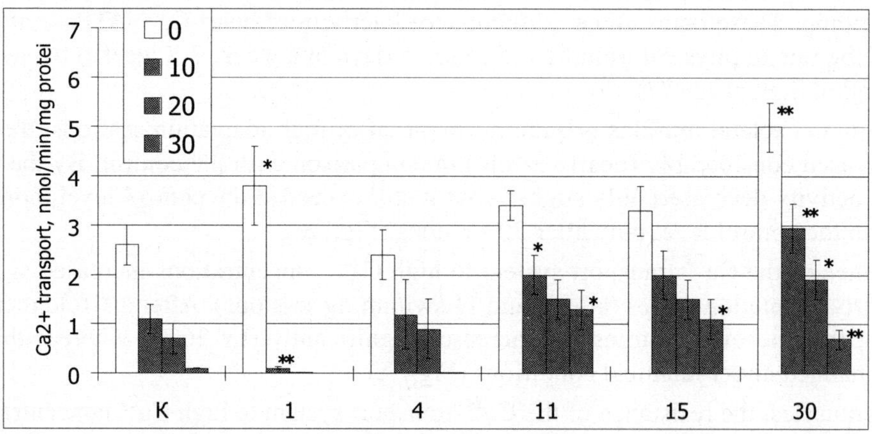

Fig. 8. Influence of adaptation to physical load on the thermal resistance of myocardial Ca-pump (41°C). Abscissa – time of adaptation, days. Inset shows the time of incubation in minutes.

Conclusion

In the heart, increased resistance of the Ca^{2+}-transport system to thermal inactivation, to high Ca^{2+} concentrations and to ROS was observed even at very early stages of adaptation – on the 4th or 11th day. The highest (1.5-2.0-fold) resistance was observed after 15-30 sessions.

In skeletal muscles, the increase in the resistance of the Ca^{2+} transport system was observed only in the case of long-term adaptation. It was manifested in a 2-fold decrease in Ca^{2+}-pump activity in comparison with the level observed after 15 days of adaptation. As a result, the resistance of the

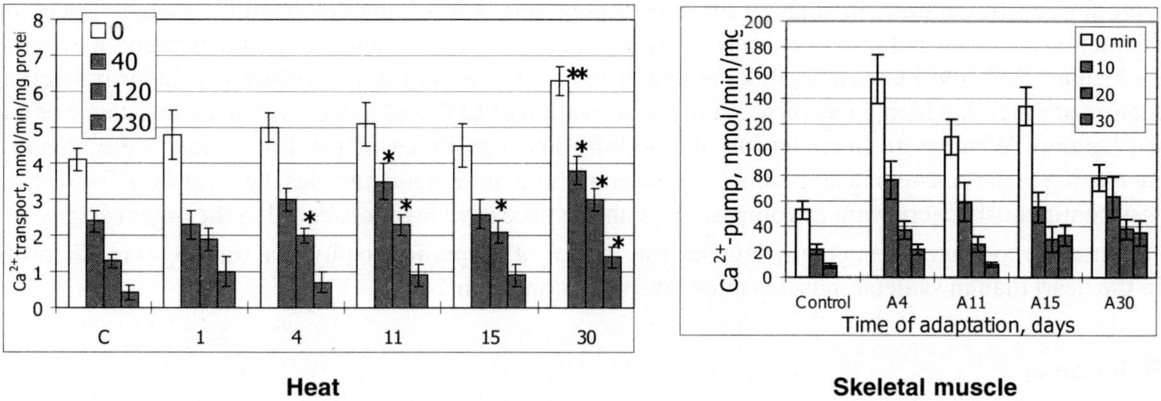

Fig. 9. Influence of adaptation to physical load on the resistance of heart and skeletal muscle Ca^{2+}-transporting system of the sarcoplasmic reticulum to free radical oxidation induced in vitro. Abscissa – time of adaptation, days. Insets show the time of incubation in minutes.

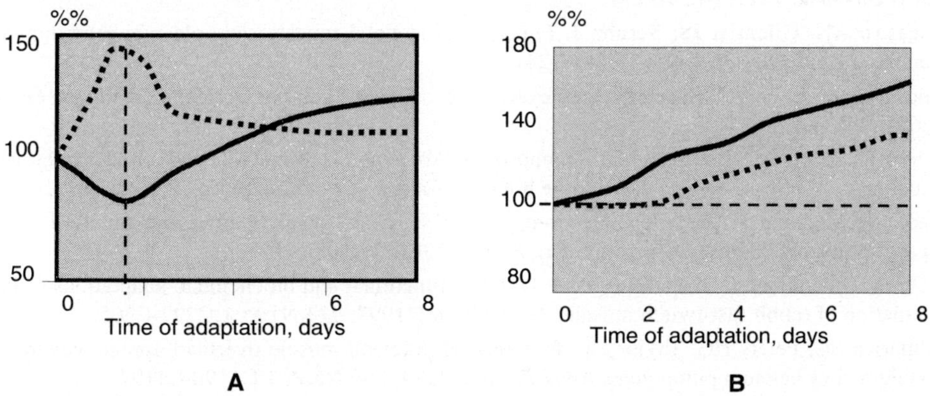

Fig. 10. Scheme. Ca-pump activity (dotted line) and resistance (continuous line) in dynamics of adaptation. Cases with drastic (A) and gradually (B) increase of Ca-pump activity at the early stages of adaptation are shown.

enzyme to damaging factors increased immediately: after 30 day-adaptation, the resistance to free radical oxidation exceeded that observed in the urgent and transition stages 1.5–2.7-fold and was 3.5 times higher in comparison with control.

It may thus be concluded that adaptation characterized by an initial increase in the resistance of the enzyme system was followed by an increase in the quantitative parameters (high activity or number of enzyme molecules after inducible *de novo* synthesis). If adaptation requires a sharp increase in the enzyme activity, this is followed by an immediate decrease of the enzyme resistance (Fig.10). This resistance can be restored only after a decrease in the activity to the control level. Our experiments have shown that this can be observed only at the terminal stage of adaptation, i.e., after 30 sessions.

A slight increase in the activity of the Ca^{2+}-pump and a significant increase in its resistance to endogenous damaging factors were observed even after the very first adaptation sessions. Thus, in myocardial tissues sharp fluctuations in the activity and other functional parameters of the Ca^{2+}-pump were absent. In contrast, in skeletal muscles urgent stages were characterized by a high "price" of adaptation, since all cell resources were mobilized to increasing the activity and the number of enzyme molecules. A 3-fold increase in this parameter led to the inhibition of synthesis of other protective factors of the cell, which, in its turn, led to the activation of LPO and a decrease in the resistance of the Ca^{2+}-pump. Whereas in heart tissues the activity and resistance of the Ca^{2+}-pump were steadily increasing in the course of adaptation to physical training, in skeletal muscles the rate of Ca^{2+}-transport was continuously decreasing in comparison with the excessive level observed in the urgent stages.

It may be concluded from these data that the "price" of adaptation to physical training is much lower in the heart than in skeletal muscles under identical conditions.

References

1. Arkhipenko YuV, Dzhaparidze LM, Gutkin DV, Rozhitskaya II, Spirichev VB, Comparative estimation of Vitamin E insufficiency influence to lipid peroxidation and Ca^{2+} transport in heart and skeletal muscle. *Vopr Med Khim.* 1987; 33:122-127.
2. Beauchamp C, Fridovich I. Superoxide dismutase: Improved assay and an assay applicable to acrylamide gels. *Analyt Biochem.* 1971; 44:276-287.
3. Belcastro AN, Gilchrist JS, Scrubb J. Function of skeletal muscle sarcoplasmic reticulum vesicles with exercise. *J Appl Physiol.* 1993; 75:2412-2418.
4. Bloor C, Leon A, Pasyk S. The effects of exercise on organ and cellular development in rats. *Lab Invest.* 1968; 19:675-680.
5. Favero TG, Zable AC, Bowman MB, Thompson A, Abramson JJ. Metabolic end products inhibit sarcoplasmic reticulum Ca^{2+} release and $[H^3]$ryanodine binding. *J Applied Physiol.* 1995; 78:1665-1672.
6. Guski H, Meerson F, Wassilew G. Comparative study of ultrastructure and function of the rat heart hypertrophied by exercise or hypoxia. *Exp Pathol.* 1981; 20:108-120.
7. Hicks A, Ohlendieck K, Gopel SO, Pette D. Early functional and biochemical adaptations to low-frequency stimulation of rabbit fast-twitch muscle. *Am J Physiol.* 1997; 273:N1:Pt 1:C297-C305.
8. Kandarian SC, Peters DG, Taylor JA, Williams JH. Skeletal muscle overload upregulates the sarcoplasmic reticulum slow calcium pump gene. *Am J Physiol.* 1994; 266:N5:Pt 1:C1190-C1197.
9. Leberer E, Timms BG, Campbell KP, MacLennan DH. Purification, calcium binding properties, and ultrastructural localization of the 53,000- and 160,000 (sarcolumenin) -Dalton glycoproteins of the sarcoplasmic reticulum. *J Biol Chem.* 1990; 265:10118-10124.
10. Leeuwenburgh C, Fiebig R, Chandwaney R, Ji LL. Aging and exercise training in skeletal muscle: Responses of glutathione and antioxidant enzyme systems. *Am J Physiol.* 1994; 267:¹2:Pt 2:R439-R445.
11. Luck H. Catalase. In: Bergmeyer HU, ed., *Methods of enzymatic analysis,* Verlag-Chemie Academic Press, New York, 1963:885-888.
12. Meerson FZ, Pshennikova MG. Adaptation to stress situations and physical load. Moscow, Meditzina, 1988, 256 p.
13. Meerson FZ, Sazontova TG, Arkhipenko YuV. Increased resistance of cardiac sarcoplasmic reticulum Ca-pump to autolysis after adaptation of rats to stress. *Biomed Sci.* 1990; 1:373-378.
14. Padros E, Dunach M, Morros A, Sabes M, Manosa J. 4-th-derivative spectrophotometry of proteins. *Trends Biochem Sci.* 1984; 9:508-510.
15. Penpargkul S, Repke DI, Katz AM, Scheuer J. Effect of physical training on calcium transport by rat cardiac sarcoplasmic reticulum. *Circ Res.* 1977; 40:134-148.
16. Piskova DM, Son'kin VD. In: Applied aspects of skeletal, heart and smooth muscle investigations. All-Russian Conference, Puschino, 1996:256.

17. Powers SK, Criswell D, Lawler J, Ji LL, Martin D, Herb RA, Dudley G. Influence of exercise and fiber type on antioxidant enzyme activity in rat skeletal muscle. *Am J Physiol.* 1994; 266:2:Pt 2:R375-R380.
18. Sazontova TG. Membrane adaptation in the development of resistance to environmental factors. Doctor of Science Thesis, Moscow, 1998.
19. Schluter JM, Fitts RH. Shortening velocity and ATPase activity of rat skeletal muscle fibers: effects of endurance exercise training. *Am J Physiol.* 1994; 266:6:Pt 1:C1699-C1673.
20. Yakovlev NN. Biochemical peculiarities of skeletal muscles. In: Ecological physiology of animals. *Manual of Physiology.* Part 2. Nauka, L., 1981:300-340.

Adaptation Biology and Medicine (Volume 4: Current Concepts)
Editors: A. Hargens, N. Takeda and P.K. Singal

10. Ingesting Only Glucose: Behavioral Adaptation to Lessen High Altitude Pulmonary Edema

H. T. Hammel, Ph.D., D.Sc.

Medical Sciences, Indiana University School of Medicine, Bloomington, IN 47405, USA.

Abstract

The rational for lessening high altitude pulmonary edema (HAPE) is based on an understanding of the role of diet in removing fluid from pulmonary alveoli. Extravasated fluid into the alveoli of the lungs is continuously removed to the pulmonary capillaries by the osmotic effect of CO_2 and bicarbonate ions diffusing within plasma from the arterial end toward the venous end of the capillaries. The diffusion of these ions within the capillary plasma drags on the water through which they diffuse. Plasma water in the capillary is altered like pure liquid water is altered by lowering the pressure applied to it an amount equal to the osmotic effect of the diffusing CO_2 and bicarbonate ions. Plasma water, altered this way, pulls fluid from the alveoli of the lungs continuously; and, thereby, prevents pulmonary edema. In the hypoxic environment of the mountain climber at high altitude, not only is too little oxygen available for oxidizing foodstuffs, too little carbon is oxidized and too little bicarbonate is carried in the plasma flowing through the pulmonary capillaries. For this reason, there may be insufficient diffusion of CO_2 and bicarbonate ions; and, therefore, insufficient removal of fluid from the pulmonary alveoli. Climbers ascending Mt. Everest may experience HAPE. HAPE, if untreated by inspiring oxygen or by immediate descent to a lower and less hypoxic altitude, can be fatal. However, the severity of HAPE may be lessened by: 1) eliminating all nitrogen bearing foodstuffs (meat and legumes) from the diet at high altitude, 2) maximizing the carbon content and maximizing the oxygen content in the high altitude diet, and 3) minimizing the hydrogen content in the diet. In other words, the high altitude diet should maximize the production of carbon dioxide and also require the least amount of inspired oxygen to metabolize carbon and hydrogen ingested as well as nitrogen from tissue. Depletion of carbohydrate reserves in the liver and other tissues should be minimized. Based on these considerations, an exclusive diet of pure glucose ($C_6H_{12}O_6$) and/or sucrose $C_{12}H_{24}O_{12}$ is recommended. Glucose has sufficient oxygen to metabolize half its carbon or all its hydrogen. The remaining carbon or hydrogen requires inspired oxygen. Any digestible carbohydrate with less hydrogen would be better still because it would require less oxygen to metabolize hydrogen and it would produce less metabolic water. Less metabolic water would allow a greater increase in CO_2 and HCO_3^- concentrations in plasma at the venous end of tissue capillaries, thereby, lessening tissue edema such as high altitude cerebral edema (HACE). Fats are less desirable because they have less oxygen per carbon in their molecules.

Introduction

The objectives for this article and others (4-11) are to persuade the reader that:

1. Osmosis and osmotic pressure are not caused by the diffusion of water from pure liquid water to a lower concentration of water in an aqueous solution.
2. Osmosis and osmotic pressure of water are caused by the pressure exerted by solute molecules reflected at all boundaries of the solution.
3. Solute pressure exerted at an unopposed boundary of a solution alters the internal tension in the forces bonding the water in the solution. Its altered internal tension lowers its vapor pressure and its chemical potential.
4. Solute molecules diffusing from a higher to a lower concentration of solute within a solution have an osmotic effect on the water equal to the difference between the osmotic pressures of the water at the differing solute concentrations, at the same temperature.

Consequently:

1. Proteins in plasma contribute nothing to fluid exchange between pulmonary capillaries and alveoli when blood flow is continuous and constant,
2. The diffusion of CO_2 and HCO_3^- from the arterial end to the venous end of a pulmonary capillary drag on the plasma through which they diffuse and have an osmotic effect to lessen extravasation of fluid into the alveoli and to return (pull) alveolar fluid into the capillary.
3. These assertions lead to the conclusion that ingesting glucose and/or sucrose can lessen High Altitude Pulmonary Edema (HAPE).

Objective I

With no exceptions, the water concentration theory of osmosis requires that the solute molecules lessen water concentration. There are at least eight reasons why water concentration does not cause osmosis. One reason is sufficient to be convincing. Figure 1 illustrates that adding solutes to water alters the water concentration in solutions. Dissolving Na_2SO_4 in water lessens the water concentration. However, dissolving NaF and in water increases, not decreases, water concentration. Nevertheless, osmosis, flow of water into the aqueous solution, occurs in these solutions as in all others when solute is added.

Objective II

Whenever a solute ion, atom or molecule is reflected at a boundary of a solution, it changes momentum. The time rate of change of momentum perpendicular to the reflecting surface of all the reflected particles (from protons to proteins) is a force. This force applied to a unit area of the reflecting surface is a pressure, the solute pressure. This solute pressure must be opposed. In Fig. 2A, the walls of the cylinder and the semi elastic, semipermeable membranes oppose the solute pressure. The pressure exerted by the solution must be attributed to the solute pressure and not to the water that entered the solution. Note that the internal tension in the water on either side of the membrane is the same, as is indicated by the yellow tint.

Objective III

When a boundary of a solution is unopposed, the solute molecules reflected at a unit area of that boundary exert a force that must be opposed by the force that binds the water molecules in the solution.

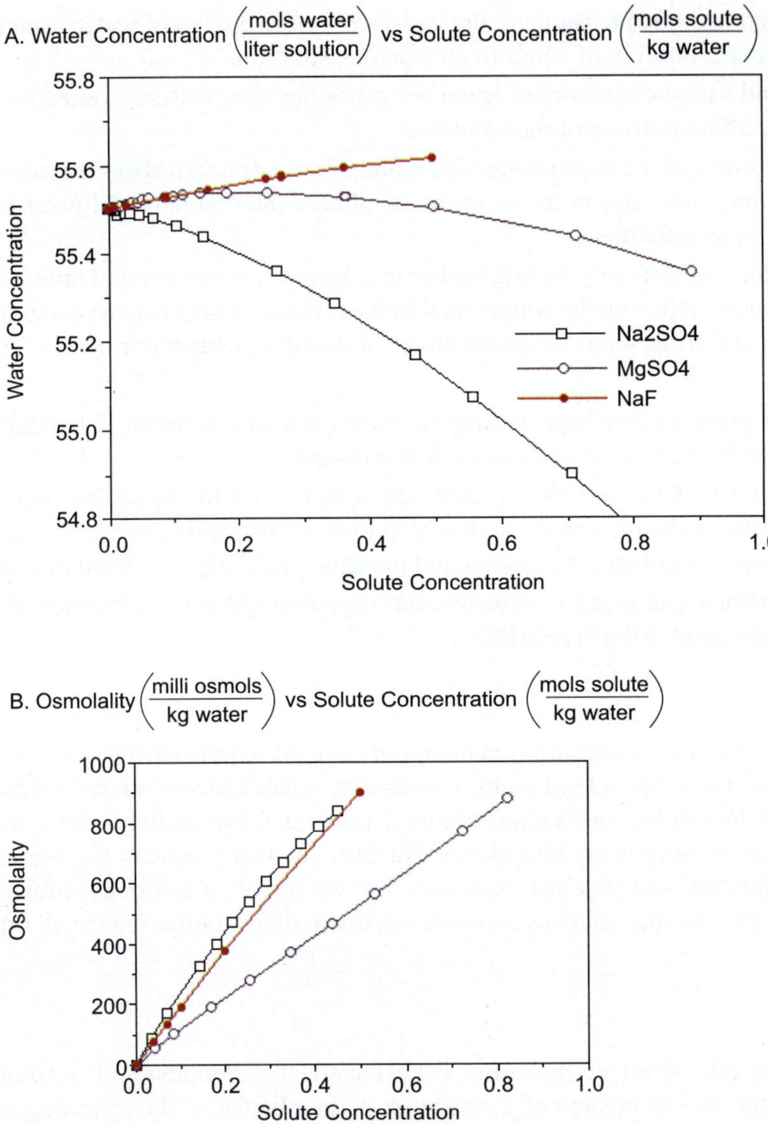

Fig. 1. Relationship between water concentration and solute concentration for three solutes, NaF, and Na_2SO_4 based on data by Millero and Knox (16). Reproduced from Hammel (Fig. 1, (9); and Fig. 2, (10).

This is Hulett's explanation of osmosis and osmotic pressure, as stated in 1903 (13). As illustrated in Fig. 3 for a 1.00 molal solution of dextrose, Hulett proved that the solute pressure exerted at the upper surface of the solution in Column I maintains that surface at 243.6 meters above 0. In Column II, pure liquid water is held against gravity at the same 243.6 meters. Due to gravity, the internal water tensions in both Columns I and II are altered the same amount, as indicated by the color tint from blue near the upper surfaces to yellow at the water surface at z = 0. The fact that the internal tensions in the water in both Columns I and II are altered by exactly the same amount insures that the vapor pressures of the

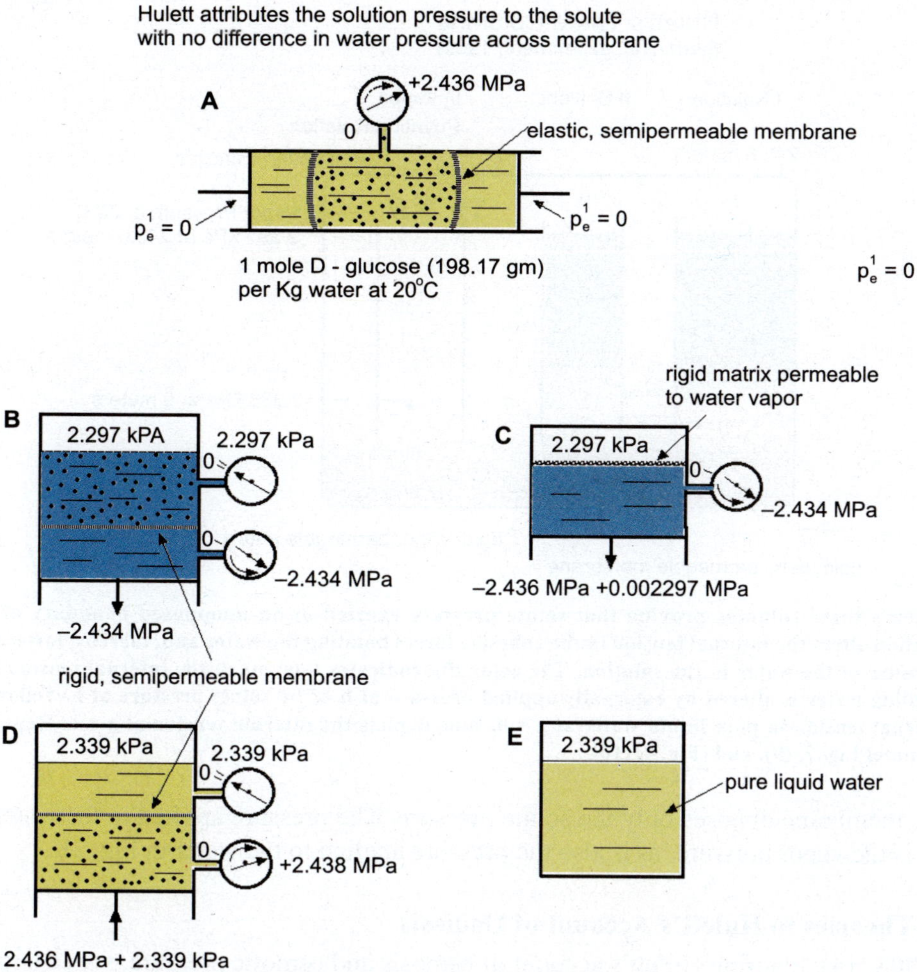

Fig. 2. Representation of Hulett's account of osmosis and osmotic pressure.

water at the two surfaces are exactly the same and are exactly the same at 243.6 meters in Column III. The vapor pressure at 243.6 meters in all three columns must be the same to insure that the Second Law of Thermodynamics is not violated.

Also, in Fig. 2B, the solute molecules exert a pressure of 2.436 MPa at the upper, unopposed surface of the solution. A negative pressure of -2.434 MPa must be applied to the water below the membrane. Since the water below the membrane is coupled to the water above the membrane, the negative pressure applied to the water below the membrane is the same as in the solution and it counters the pressure exerted by the solute molecules at the upper surface minus the vapor pressure. The solute pressure is also exerted against the membrane and is opposed by the rigid membrane. Note that the vapor pressure of water above the solution surface in Fig. 2B is the same as the vapor pressure of the liquid water in Fig. 2C to which the same negative pressure is applied. In Fig. 2D, the solution is below the membrane so the solute pressure plus the vapor pressure is opposed by the cylinder wall and the

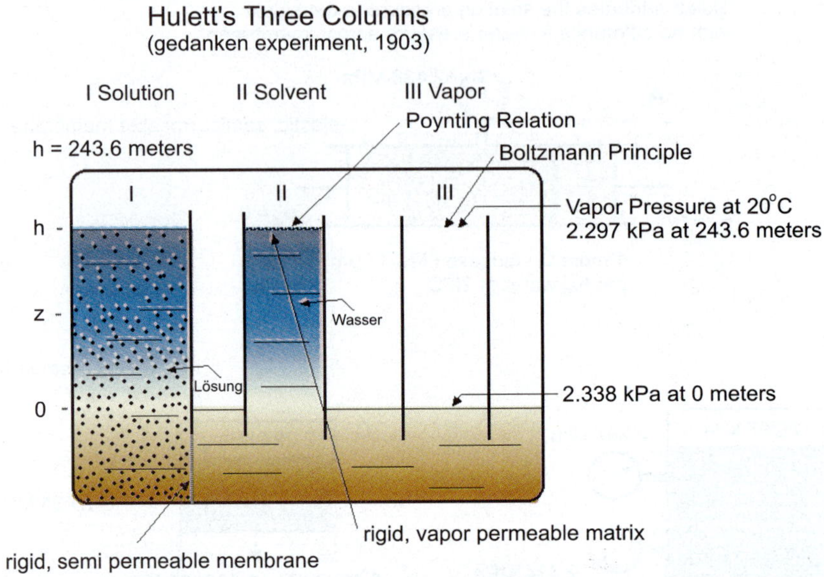

Fig. 3. Hulett's three columns proving that solute pressure exerted at an unopposed boundary of an aqueous solution alters the internal tension in the cohesive forces bonding the water and, thereby, lowering the vapor pressure of the water in the solution. The color tint indicates how much the internal tension in the forces bonding water is altered by externally applied pressure at h or by solute pressure at h. Yellow depicts the internal tension in pure liquid water at z = 0. Blue depicts the internal tension at z = h. Reproduced from Hammel Fig. 2, (9), and (Fig. 4, (10).

piston. The membrane opposes only the solute pressure. The pressure applied to the water above the membrane is the vapor pressure, as is also the pressure applied to the water in Fig. 2E.

Contrary Theories to Hulett's Account of Osmosis

Lewis in 1908 (14), ignoring Hulett's account of osmosis and osmotic pressure, stated another theory of osmosis. Lewis claimed that solute molecules lower the fugacity of water in an aqueous solution relative to the fugacity of pure liquid water. He defined activity of the water in the solution, $a^{l}_{H2O}(T,p^{l}_{e},x^{l}_{H2O})$, to be the ratio of the fugacity of the water in the solution to the fugacity of pure liquid water, i.e., $a^{l}_{H2O}(T,p^{l}_{e},x^{l}_{H2O}) \equiv \frac{f^{l}_{H2O}(T,p^{l}_{e},x^{l}_{H2O})}{f^{l*}_{H2O}(T,p^{l}_{e})}$, where T is the absolute temperature, p^{l}_{e} is the external pressure applied to the solution and to water and x^{l}_{H2O} is the mole fraction of the water in the solution. The superscript ^{l*} denotes pure liquid. Then, Lewis defined the activity of the water in the solution another way, namely, $\mu^{l}_{H2O}(T,p^{l}_{e},x^{l}_{H2O}) - \mu^{l*}_{H2O}(T,p^{l}_{e}) \equiv RT \ln a^{l}_{H2O}(T,p^{l}_{e},x^{l}_{H2O})$. That is, multiplying the natural log of activity by RT is an amount of available free energy identical with the difference between the chemical potentials of pure liquid water and the water in the solution. The activity of the water in the solution is a number (without dimensions) that is always ≥ 0 and ≤ 1. The chemical potential of the water in the solution is always less that the chemical potential of pure liquid water at the same temperature and applied pressure. For this reason, the natural log of activity is negative so that the activity of water in the solution must be less than 1. At no time did Lewis or any subsequent physical chemist explain how the solute molecules lower the fugacity or the activity of the water in the solution. For the same reason, they have never explained how the solute lowers the chemical potential of the water in the solution. Even more confusing was Lewis' failed attempt to reveal the physical meaning of fugacity. He said it was the "tendency of the water molecules to escape its liquid phase." Fugacity is like vapor pressure but it differs from vapor pressure for all real solvents. Only for the ideal solvent in an ideal solution are fugacity and vapor pressure the same, by the definition of an ideal solvent. Since vapor pressure is a physical property of all real solvents and is an exact measure of the "tendency to escape", fugacity cannot be what Lewis said it is. Some authors have recognized this flaw in Lewis' theory and have stated that fugacity is a corrected vapor pressure, as if a real physical property of a liquid needed correction by a term that has no physical meaning. The terms fugacity and activity are nothing more than defined, fictional terms without any physical meaning. Moreover, Lewis' theory of osmosis is misleading in that it implies that the solute molecules act on the water at the semipermeable membrane to lower its fugacity and activity, when the water in the solution is separated from pure water by a membrane that allows only water molecules to pass through it.

Biologists are mystified by the terms fugacity and activity. For this reason, they have supposed that solute dissolved in solvent always lowers the solvent concentration in the solution. Like Lewis, they suppose that water molecules diffuse through the semipermeable membrane from pure liquid water into the water in the solution and, thereby, increase the pressure in the water in the solution. Chemists suppose the lower fugacity and activity of the water in the solution causes the molecules to diffuse into the solution from the higher fugacity and activity of pure liquid water. Whereas, as stated, biologists suppose that the lower concentration of the water in the solution causes water molecules to diffuse from the higher to the lower water concentration. Both Lewis' theory and the water concentration theory attribute the pressure in the solution to the water that entered the solution by diffusion. As depicted in Fig. 4A, there is a pressure discontinuity in the water between the solution and pure liquid water at the membrane. This means that the internal tension in the water in the solution (depicted by red) differs from the internal tension in the liquid water (depicted by yellow). Likewise in Fig. 4B and 4D, the water pressures and the internal tensions in the water differ on the two sides of the membrane. Since the membrane is porous to water (and not to the solute) these conclusions based on Lewis' theory and the water concentration theory are not tenable. Moreover, they ignore the fact that it is the solute molecules that are reflected at the boundaries of the solution and they ignore the fact that this solute pressure must be opposed by an opposing external pressure at the boundary or by an opposing internal tension in the strong cohering force between water molecules, the hydrogen bond.

Objective IV

Solute-solvent drag

When solute particles diffuse from a higher to a lower concentration of solute within a solution, they drag on the water through which they diffuse. They alter the internal tension and the chemical potential of the water and, thereby, have an osmotic effect. This osmotic effect is illustrated in Fig. 5. After the right membrane in Fig. 5B was removed at time t = 0, water is pulled (does not diffuse) across the remaining membrane as the solute molecules in the solution diffuse into pure liquid water to the right

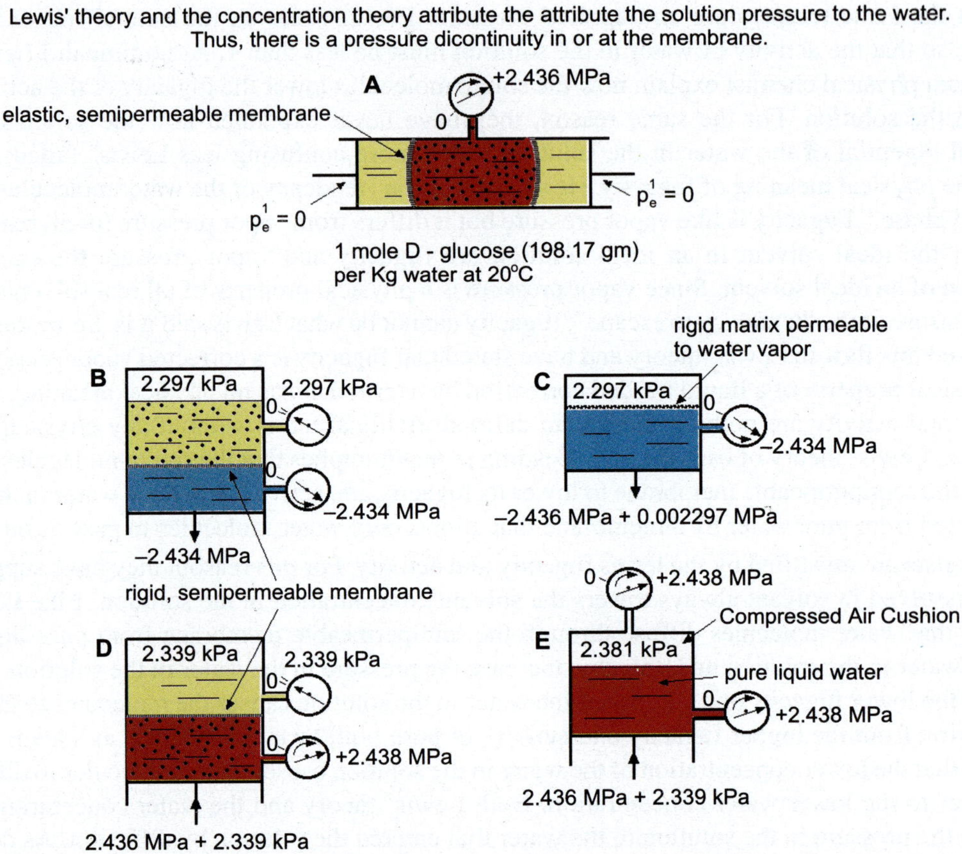

Fig. 4. Representation of Lewis' theory and the water concentration theory of osmosis.

of the missing membrane. But the rate of flow is much less than the rate of flow when pure liquid water pulls water across the membrane by a pressure difference of $-\pi^1_{H2O}(t \leq 0)$, as in Fig. 5C. The reason for the lesser rate of flow in Fig. 5B is that as water is pulled into the solution, solute molecules diffuse into the incoming water and exert a back pressure that retards the rate of flow of water into the solution. Note that the color in the solution grades into the color in the water into which the solute molecules are diffusing in Fig. 5 B. Note also that the membrane in Fig. 5C is distended much more to the right than is the membrane in Fig. 5B because the difference in water pressures across the membrane is much greater in Fig. 5C.

In Fig. 5A, the solute molecules exert a pressure 2.436 MPa against all boundaries of the solution, including the solution within the pressure gauge. The gauge reads this pressure. In Fig. 5D, both membranes were removed at time 0. Since no pressure is applied to the water into which the solute molecules are diffusing, the solute molecules drag on the water in the solution and pull on it in opposite directions by –2.436 MPa. Therefore, the gauge reads 0, i.e., the sum of the solute pressure and the negative pressure in the water in the solution. Note, however, that a negative pressure must be applied to the pure liquid water below the remaining rigid semipermeable membrane to prevent water from

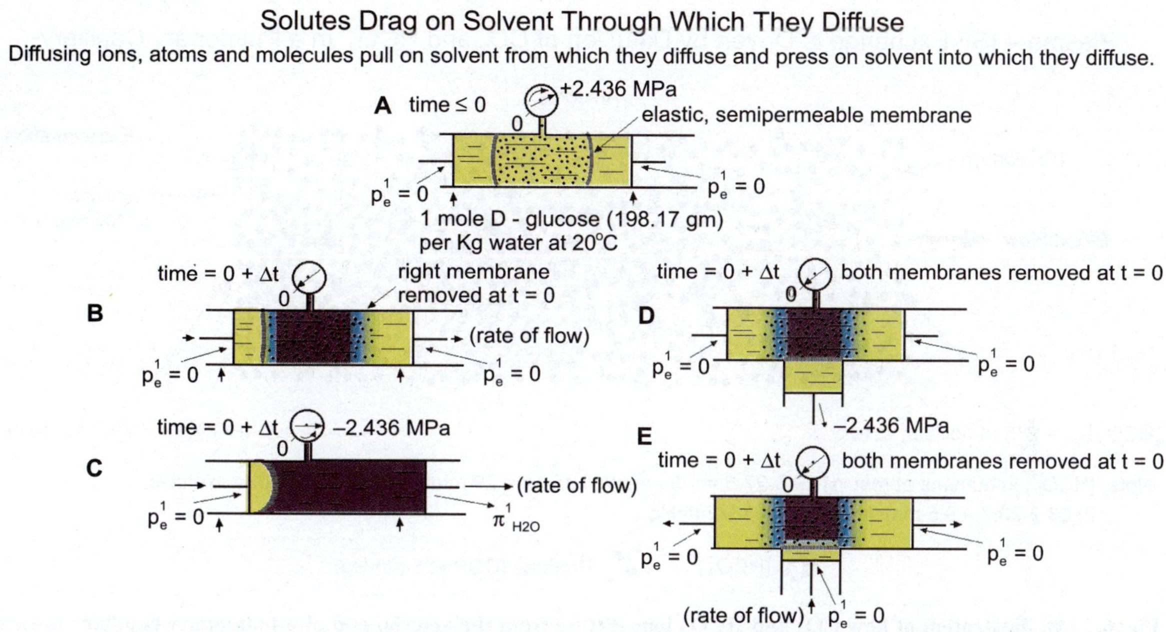

Fig. 5. A. Thought experiment illustrating how solute molecules in a 1.00 molal solution of dextrose at 20 °C distends the elastic, semipermeable membranes. B. Thought experiment illustrating how dextrose molecules diffuse into pure liquid water shortly after the right membrane was removed at time 0. The dextrose molecules press on the left side of the water into which they diffuse; the right piston applies no counter pressure so both pistons move to the right. C. Thought experiment illustrating how pure liquid water is pulled to the right by applying a pressure $-\pi^1_{H2O}$ to it. The rate of flow of water through the membrane in C exceeds the rate of flow of water in B. D. Thought experiment illustrating no flow of fluids after removal of the left and right membranes because $-\pi^1_{H2O}$ was applied to the pure water below the remaining membrane. E. Thought experiment illustrating flow of water into the solution shortly after removing left and right membranes when no pressure was applied to the water below the remaining membrane.

being pulled into the solution. In Fig. 5E, no pressure was applied to the water. Consequently, water flowed into the solution and the fluids in the cylinder flowed laterally.

Solute-solvent drag, as featured in Fig. 5, is an essential aspect of osmosis in biology. Without the osmotic effects of solute-solvent drag, it is not possible to explain fluid exchanges in biological fluids.

Consequently

1. The diffusion of CO_2 and HCO_3^- depicted in Fig. 6 from the arterial end to the venous end of a pulmonary capillary have an osmotic effect to lessen extravasation of fluid into the alveoli and to return alveolar fluid to the capillary. Note that the osmotic effects of the diffusing CO_2 and HCO_3^- increase with exercise, unlike the COP of protein in plasma that remains constant at about 25 mmHg in humans. When capillary flow is continuous and constant, the osmotic term in Starling's hypothesis cannot be attributed to plasma proteins, It must be attributed to the metabolites and CO_2 and HCO_3^-.

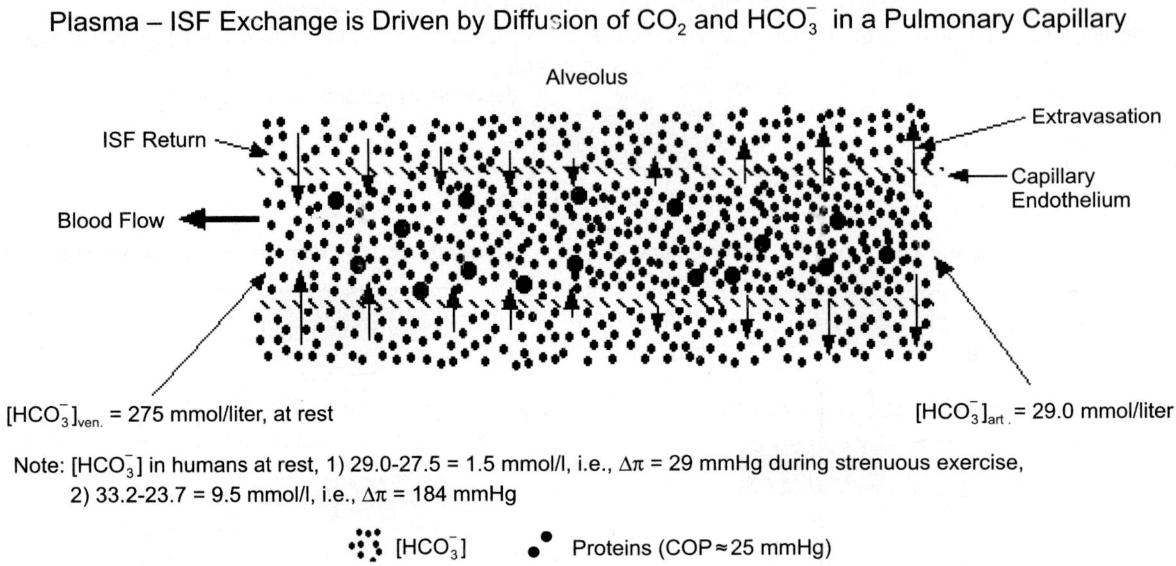

Fig. 6. **An illustration of how CO_2 and HCO_3^- ions diffuse from the arterial end of a pulmonary capillary toward the venous end of the capillary. By this diffusion they have an osmotic effect retarding extravasation of fluid from the arterial end and returning ISF to the capillary at the venous end. The diffusions of CO_2 and HCO_3^- ions are reversed in the systemic capillaries in metabolizing tissue so that extravasation of protein free plasma is retarded at the arterial ends and ISF is returned at the venous ends of the capillaries. Note that these rates of plasma-ISF exchange are much greater during strenuous exercise than at rest.**

2. For these reasons, to lessen the likelihood of HAPE in all climbers of Mt. Everest and to lessen the severity of HAPE when it occurs, climbers ought to ingest foodstuffs that yield the highest rate of CO_2 production and the lowest amount of metabolic water during their ascent to the highest altitudes and return. Glucose, $C_6H_{12}O_6$, and/or sucrose, $C_{12}H_{24}O_{12}$, are likely candidates for this purpose because they contain sufficient oxygen to oxidize half the carbon in these molecules. They require environmental oxygen for oxidizing the other half of the carbon and the hydrogen. Digestible foodstuffs with less hydrogen would be better still because less inhaled oxygen would be required to oxidize the hydrogen. Also, less metabolic water would allow the concentrations of CO_2 and HCO_3^- to increase more at the venous ends of systemic capillaries and, thereby, lessen tissue edema such as high altitude cerebral edema (HACE). Obviously, foodstuffs such as meat, legumes and fat should not be ingested during the few hours or the day of the ascent or even during the few days prior to the ascent and return when the climber is threatened with HAPE. Every effort must be made by the climber to minimize depletion of the carbohydrate reserves in the body, including glycogen in the liver. Ingesting glycogen would have no advantage over glucose. Although glycogen ($C_6H_{10}O_5$) has two less hydrogen, it also has one less oxygen than glucose. Note, these assertions do not claim that inappropriate foodstuffs are the sole cause of HAPE. Rather, they claim that ingesting sugar can lessen HAPE.

Discussion

As blood flows continuously through a capillary at a constant rate in a systemic or a pulmonary capillary, as assumed in Starling's (19) hypothesis, two pressures are applied to the endothelium of the elastic endothelium of the capillary, thereby, distending it. The proteins in plasma are reflected by the endothelium and exert a colloid osmotic pressure (COP) along the length of the capillary. The COP varies little along the length. For these reasons, a constant COP does not alter the volume of plasma in a capillary when flow is continuous. When blood is flowing, the hydrostatic pressure varies from end to end of the capillary. It is highest at the arterial end and least at the venous end. For this reason, the capillary is distended the most by hydrostatic pressure at the arterial end. The volume of the blood in a unit length of the capillary remains constant as the flow remains constant. That is, as fluid leaves and renters the capillary, the volume of the capillary remains constant as the rate of flow remains constant. The proteins can do nothing to effect the extravasation of fluid at the arterial end or the return of fluid at the venous end during a constant rate of blood flow. The proteins can only exert a pressure, the COP, as they are reflected by the endothelium; they do not attract ISF into the plasma and, although they may alter the water concentration of the plasma, this has no osmotic effect. For these reasons, the osmotic term in Starling's (19) hypothesis is not valid.

Only when flow is intermittent, as in resting muscle, can the constant COP of the proteins affect plasma-ISF exchange. When flow ceases, the hydrostatic pressure at the arterial end of the capillary falls to the hydrostatic pressure at the venous end. The distention of the capillary at the arterial end becomes less as the hydrostatic pressure falls to venous pressure. Thus, when flow stops, the volume of the capillary becomes less than when blood was flowing. The decrease in capillary volume, when flow ceases, depends on the magnitudes of the arterial hydrostatic pressure and the COP of the plasma. The decrease in capillary volume also depends on the elastic properties of the endothelium. Its elasticity (unit increase in volume per unit increase in pressure) is least when the pressures applied to it are great and its distension is the most. The endothelium is most elastic when the pressures are small and its distension is least. Therefore, when the COP of the plasma is high, the decrease in plasma volume of the capillary is low as flow ceases.

When a colloid is added to plasma, it increases the COP of the plasma and increases the total pressure applied to the endothelium. The volume of plasma in all capillaries increases regardless of whether the plasma is flowing or not. However, the increase in capillary volume is less when plasma is flowing than when plasma is not flowing. Thus, increasing the COP of plasma expands the plasma volume of all capillaries; but this increase in volume is somewhat more when plasma is not flowing. As mentioned above, when plasma stops flowing, as in many of the capillaries in resting muscle, the decrease in plasma volume in these capillaries is lessened by an amount depending inversely on the COP, i.e., the volume decreases less for the higher COP. The increase in plasma volume caused by adding colloid to the plasma in capillaries with intermittent flow is more than the increase in plasma volume when the colloid is added to plasma in capillaries with continuous flow.

On the other hand, when the protein concentration in plasma is too little, as in protein deficient disorders such as kwashiorkor, there are too few proteins in all capillaries to distend these capillaries. That is, the volume of all capillaries is less than normal and more ISF is retained in the interstitium, causing edema.

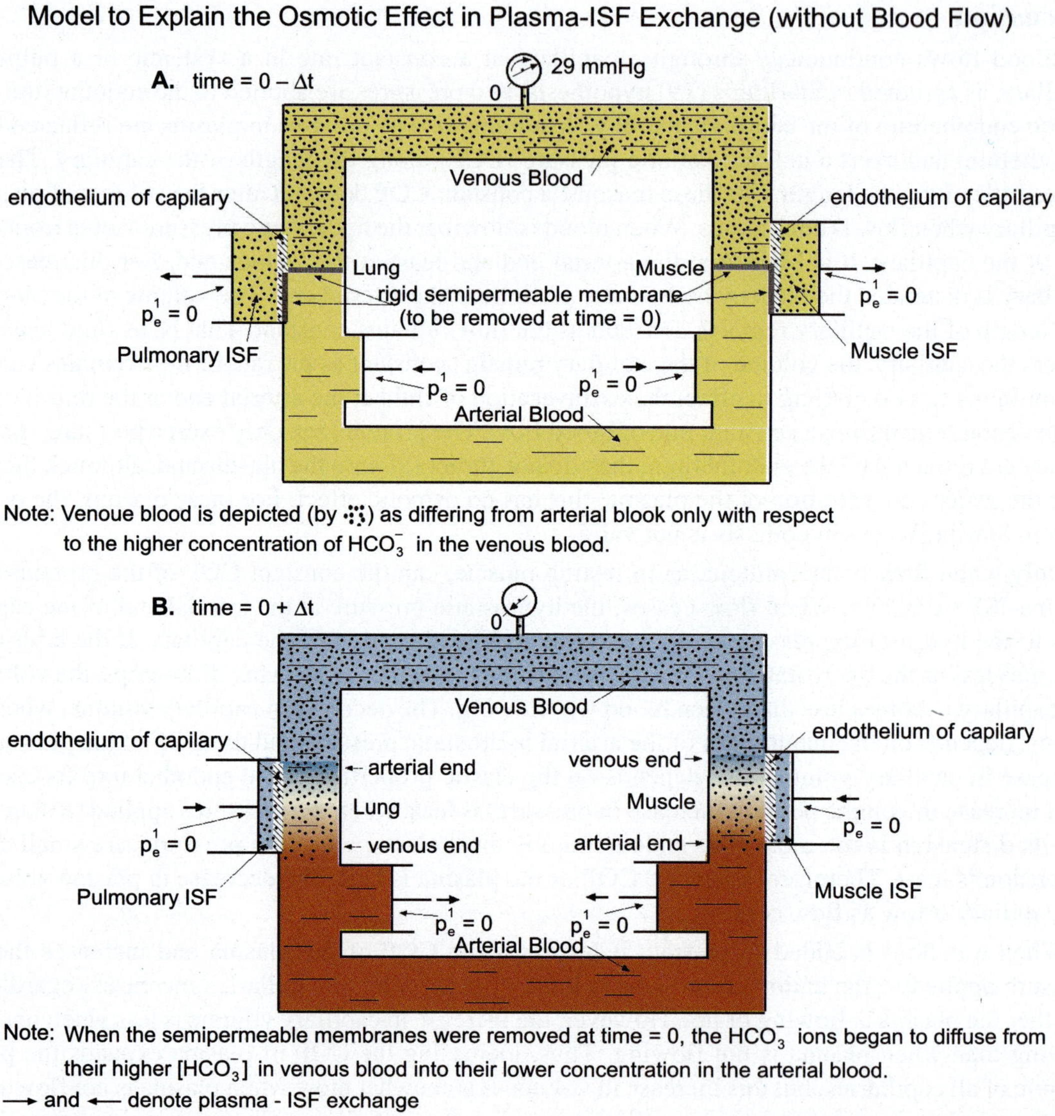

Fig. 7. As illustrated in B, HCO_3^- ions diffuse from venous plasma at the arterial ends of pulmonary capillaries toward arteralized plasma at the venous ends of these capillaries. This diffusion must be accompanied by diffusion of HCO_3^- ions from venous plasma at the venous ends of systemic capillaries toward arterialized plasma at the arterial ends of the systemic capillaries. Without these diffusions in opposite directions, arterial to venous ends in pulmonary capillaries and venous to arterial ends in systemic capillaries, ISF could not be returned to either pulmonary or systemic capillaries and increase the volume of arterial plasma. To explain these facts, artificial barriers (membrances impermeable to HCO_3^-) are positioned for a brief period, Δt, before time 0, in the pulmonary capillaries and in the systemic capillaries in A. At time 0, these barriers were removed so the HCO_3^- ions can diffuse from higher to lower concertrations within both pulmonary and systemic capillaries (from venous plasma to arteralized plasma in both). Note that in A and B, only the difference in HCO_3^- concentrations is depicted, i.e., in venous plasma only where the HCO_3^- concentration is higher by 1.5 mmol per liter.

In all tissues, elastic capillaries and plasma protein are essential for maintaining plasma volume. In tissues like muscle, intermittent blood flow also affects plasma volume. In addition, weakly acidic plasma proteins are also essential for accepting H^+ ions dissociated from H_2CO_3 when forming HCO_3.

Understanding the cause of osmosis and osmotic pressure, as stated by Hulett in 1903, and extending his account to include solute-solvent drag, is essential for understanding plasma-ISF exchange in systemic and pulmonary capillaries. The effects of environmental stresses on plasma-ISF exchange can be understood only when Hulett's explanation is applied to the studies of such stresses like microgravity, heat and cold stress, etc. Understanding the consequences of pathological stresses like congestive heart failure also require an understanding of the osmotic effects of solute-solvent drag. When a weakened left ventricle fails to maintain a low hydrostatic pressure in the pulmonary vein, excess fluid is extravasated into the alveoli and the diffusion of CO_2 and HCO_3^- is insufficient to remove all the fluid from the alveoli.

When blood flows through a systemic capillary, its osmolality must increase. Although oxygen required for metabolizing glucose, fatty acids, amino acids, etc. must diffuse through plasma, little (< 1 %) is dissolved in plasma. Thus, O_2 concentration in plasma changes little in plasma as plasma flows from end to end in the capillary. On the other hand, more than 90 percent of the metabolized carbon is dissolved in plasma, mostly as HCO_3^-. Necessarily then, the osmotic pressure of plasma must increase in systemic capillaries by about 33 mmHg (29 mmHg due to HCO_3^-) in humans at rest and nearly 500 mmHg (184 mmHg due to HCO_3^-) in strenuous exercise, McKenna, et al. (15). The solutes causing these changes in osmotic pressure in the plasma flowing through capillaries diffuse from the higher osmotic pressure toward the lower osmotic pressure. They drag on the plasma through which they diffuse. They retard extravasation of fluid into the interstitium at the arterial end and they pull ISF into the venous end of the capillary. The osmotic effect on plasma-ISF exchange depends, and must depend, on the metabolic rate of the tissue through which blood flows.

There is evidence of a behavioral preference for ingesting carbohydrates in response to hypoxia. Pugh (17) notes that climbers in the 1953 expedition to Mt. Everest preferred carbohydrates to fat. Singh et al. (18) noted that human volunteers brought to high altitude preferred sweets. Askew et al. (1) and Consolazio et al. (2) recommend high carbohydrate diets for reducing symptoms of acute mountain sickness. Dramise et al. (3) have shown that a high carbohydrate diet increases diffusion capacity of the lungs. During acclimatization to high altitude, Hansen et al. (12) found that alveolar and arterial oxygen pressures are improved and Young et al. (20) have shown that high carbohydrates in the diet improve endurance. Based on the role of carbohydrates in removing fluid from the alveoli by diffusion of CO_2 and HCO_3^- in pulmonary capillaries, it is not surprising that dietary sugar is preferred and recommended to lessen symptoms of mountain sickness.

References

1. Askew, EW (1989) Nutrition and performance under adverse environmental conditions. In Hickson, JF Jr, & Wolinsky, I (Eds) Nutri. Exer. Sports Boca Raton, FL. CRC Press, 367.
2. Consolazio, CF, Matoush, LO, Johnson, H., Krizywicki, HJ, Daws, TA & Isaac, GJ (1969) Effects of high-carbohydrate diets on performance and clinical symptomology after rapid ascent to high altitude. Fed. Proc. 28, 937.
3. Dramise JG, Inouye, CM, Christiansen, BM, Fults, RD, Canham, JE & Consolazia, CF (1975) Effects of a glucose meal on human pulmonary function at 1600 m and 4300 m altitudes. Avia. Space Envir. Med. 46, 365.

4. Hammel, HT (1976) Colligative properties of a solution: enhanced tension in the solvent gives rise to alteration in solution. Science 192, 748-757. (Note: the term "enhanced" should be replaced with "altered").
5. Hammel, HT and Scholander, PF (1976) Osmosis and Solvent Tension. Springer-Verlag, Berlin.
6. Hammel HT (1979) Forum on Osmosis. I. Osmosis: diminished solvent activity or altered solvent tension? Am. J. Physiol. 237, R95-R107.
7. Hammel, H. T. (1994) How solutes alter water in aqueous solutions. J. Physical Chem. 98, 4196-4204.
8. Hammel, HT (1995) Roles of colloidal molecules in Starling's hypothesis and in returning interstitial fluid to the vasa recta. Amer. J. Physiol. 268, H2133-2145.
9. Hammel, HT (1998) Replacing Lewis' theory of osmosis with Hulett's theory of altered chemical potentials of reacting constituents in solution. Recent Res. Devel. In Physical Chem. 2, 77-111.
10. Hammel, HT (1999). Evolving ideas about osmosis and capillary fluid exchange. FASEB J. 13, 213-23.
11. Hammel, HT (2002) Osmotic effects on solvent of solute diffusing in solution. In. Recent Res. Devel. Physical Chem. 6: 747-771. ISBN:81-7895-042-1
12. Hansen, JE, Hartley, LH, & Hogan, RP (1972) Arterial oxygen increase by high-carbohydrate diet at altitude. J. Appl. Physiol. 33, 441.
13. Hulett, G (1903) Beziehung zwischen negativem Druck und osmotischem Druck. Z. Phys. Chem. 42, 353-368.
14. Lewis, GN (1908) The osmotic pressure of concentrated solutions, and the laws of the perfect solution. J. Am. Chem. Soc. 30, 668-683.
15. McKenna, MJ, Heigenhauser, GJF, McKelvie, RS, MacDougal JD and Jones, NL (1997) Sprint training enhances ionic regulation during intense exercise in man. J. Physiol. 50, 687-702.
16. Millero, FG and JH Knox. (1973) Apparent molal volumes of aqueous NaF, Na_2SO_4, KCl, K_2SO_4, $MgCl_2$ and $MgSO_4$ solutions at 0 °C and 50 °C. J. Chem. Eng. Data 18, 407-411.
17. Pugh, LGCE (1954) Himalayan rations with special reference to the 1953 expedition to Mt. Everest. The Proceedings of the Nutrition Society 13, 60-69.
18. Singh, SB, Sharma, A, Yadav, DK, Tyagi, AK, Verma, SS, Srivastava, DN, Sharma, KN & Selvamurthy, W (1997) High altitude effects on human taste intensity and hedonics. Avia. Space Envir. Med. 68, 1123-1128.
19. Starling, EH (1896). On the absorption of fluids from connective tissue spaces. J. Physiol. London, 19, 312-326.
20. Young, AJ, Evans, WJ, Cymerman, A, Pandolf, KB, Knapik, JJ & Maher, JT (1982) Sparing effect of chronic high-altitude exposure on muscle glycogen utilization. J. Appl. Physiol. 52, 857-862.

Adaptation Biology and Medicine (Volume 4: Current Concepts)
Editors: A. Hargens, N. Takeda and P.K. Singal

11. Lower Body Negative Pressure Treadmill Exercise Counteracts Deconditioning of Lumbar Spine during 30 Days of Bed Rest

Shinji Kimura, M.D., Ph.D., Donald E. Watenpaugh, Ph.D.[#], Alan R. Hargens, Ph.D.

Department of Orthopaedics, University of California, San Diego,
350 Dickinson Street, 8894 San Diego, CA 92103-8894
Naval Submarine Medical Research Laboratory
Groton, CT 06349

Abstract

Objectives: To examine changes in spinal length, intervertebral angle, disc height and cross-sectional area of paraspinal muscle in the lumbar spine before and after 30 days bed rest (BR), and to determine whether or not LBNP treadmill exercise prevents deconditioning of the lumbar spine for 30 days BR.

Method: Six sets of identical twins (8 males and 4 females), 21-31 years old, were divided in two groups. One was a LBNP treadmill exercise (Ex) group, in which six subjects exercised supine in an LBNP chamber. Their brothers or sisters comprised the non-exercise, control (Cont) group. MRIs of the lumbar spine were taken to analyze the spinal length, disc height, intervertebral angle (L1/5) and cross-sectional area (CSA) of the psoas and spinal back muscle before and after 30 days BR. Axial load-dependent reductions of spinal length were analyzed using a MRI-compatible compression harness.

Results: The Cont group showed a significant increase in spinal length after 30 days BR as well as disc height at T12/L1, L1/2, L3/4 and L4/5, while the Ex group did not. Both groups showed a significant decrement in CSA of the spinal back muscle, but did not show any significant change in intervertebral angle and CSA of the psoas muscle. Axial load-dependent change in spinal length was not changed after 30 days in both groups.

Discussion: Our MRI data for the Cont group suggest that spinal lengthening after 30 days of BR results from the increase of disc height at multiple levels, without a change of intervertebral angle. Ex group, however, maintained spinal length, suggesting that the LBNP treadmill exercise is useful for preventing of spinal lengthening during 30 days BR. However, LBNP treadmill exercise has no significant effect on muscle atrophy during 30 days BR. The spinal compression data suggest that 30 days BR does not affect lumbar spine's ability to bear loads. However, more identical twins will be studied to test further our hypotheses.

Conclusion: LBNP treadmill exercise, in part, prevents lumbar physiological deconditioning of 30 days BR simulating space flight.

Introduction

Chronic bed rest (BR) or the microgravity of space flight reduces the integrity of structures adapted for accommodation of gravity, including the spine and paraspinal musculature[13,17]. Six degrees head-down BR simulates weightlessness in space flight[8]. Supine lower body negative pressure (LBNP) treadmill exercise provides integrated cardiovascular and musculoskeletal stimulation similar to that imposed by upright exercise in Earth gravity[1]. Supine treadmill exercise in a LBNP chamber, furthermore, maintains aerobic fitness and sprint speed during 15 days of BR[19]. Therefore, supine LBNP treadmill exercise may load the spine enough to prevent deconditioning effects, such as lumbar spinal lengthening and paraspinal muscle atrophy during long-term BR. We hypothesized that supine LBNP treadmill exercise maintains lumbar spinal length, intervertebral angle and paraspinal muscle volume during 30 days of BR. The objectives of this study were to examine changes in spinal length, intervertebral angle, disc height and cross-sectional area of psoas and spinal back muscle in the lumbar spine before and after 30 days BR, and to determine whether or not LBNP treadmill exercise prevents deconditioning in the lumbar spine during 30 days BR.

Methods

Subjects

Six sets of identical twins (8 males and 4 females), with a mean age of 25 (range: 21-31) years and body weight (BW) of 64 ± 4 kg, were randomly assigned to two groups. One was a LBNP treadmill exercise (Ex) group, in which six subjects exercised supine in a LBNP chamber for 40 minutes daily 6 days a week. Their brothers or sisters comprised the non-exercise, control (Cont) group.

LBNP treadmill exercise

LBNP treadmill exercise was described previously[7,19]. In brief, LBNP (52-63 mmHg) was applied to produce footward forces equivalent to those for upright running at 1.0-1.2 BW. On the basis of the result of the LBNP exercise familiarization and peak upright exercise measurements made before BR, we developed a linear regression for each subject that described the relationship between treadmill and Vo_2. Target speeds were then calculated for each of the desired training workloads. Treadmill grade remained set at 0% during LBNP exercise. Exercise training commenced on the first day of BR; predicted speeds were used, and these were adjusted later as necessary to achieve target Vo_2 at 1.0-1.2 BW of footward force and for subject tolerance. Subjects rated their perceived exertion on a 20-point scale before each change in workload[12]. Peak Vo_2 and submaximal treadmill exercise responses were quantified.

MRI study

MR imaging was conducted within a 1.5 Tesla system (Magnetom Symphony, Siemens, München, Germany) using a surface coil. All the subjects were investigated with sagittal and axial T1-weighted spin-echo (SE) sequence before and after BR. The parameters of MRI scanning were as follows: TR/TE: 450/15; FOV: 240X480 for 4 subjects, 512X512 (sagittal), 256X256 (axial) for remained 8 subjects; slice thickness: 4 mm. Sagittal MRIs were acquired at the center of the vertebral body as determined by frontal scout views of the lumbar spine. Axial MRIs were also acquired at the center of the intervertebral disc in parallel with the disc space at L3/4 and L4/5. Some parameters in the MR images were measured in each slice using a computer-linked digitizer (Numaris 3.5, Siemens, München, Germany), two-fold magnification was used for the measurement of disc height. To measure spinal length, a horizontal line was drawn at the anterior inferior corner of the T12 vertebral body; the other horizontal line was drawn at the anterior superior corner of the S1 vertebral body. Spinal length was then determined as the perpendicular distance between the two lines. In order to investigate an intervertebral angle, a straight line was drawn on the upper margin of each vertebral body at L1 and L5 (Fig. 1A, Line L1 and Line L5). The intervertebral angle at L1/L5 was then determined as an angle between Line L1 and Line L5[21]. Disc height was obtained from the average of anterior and posterior disc height according to Dabbs' method[3] (Fig. 1B). Supplemental cross lines were drawn between each corner of the vertebral body to determine the anterior and posterior corner of the vertebral body because the corner of the vertebral bodies was occasionally unclear on MRI views (Fig. 1B). The cross-sectional area (CSA) of the psoas (Fig. 1C, d,e) and spinal back muscle (rotatores, multifidus, spinalis, longissimus, iliocostalis, quadratus lumborum)[13,14,15] (Fig. 1C, f,g) were measured using axial views. The CSA of each muscle was determined as an average of bilateral CSA. Axial compression with 50 % of BW was applied using a MRI-compatible compression device as reported previously[6,10] before and after 30 days BR. MRI parameters were measured two times by one investigator and the mean values of the two measurements were used in this study.

Data Analysis

Data were expressed as mean ± standard error (SEM). Differences in all the data before and after 30 days BR were tested by Wilcoxon rank sum tests. Statistical significant was set at $p < 0.05$.

Results

The Cont group showed a significant increase in spinal length (before: 190 ± 8 mm, after: 195 ± 8 mm) before and after 30 days BR (Fig. 2) as well as disc height at T12/L1 (7.0 ± 0.4 mm, 8.1 ± 0.6 mm), L1/2 (8.2 ± 0.5 mm, 9.1 ± 0.6 mm), L3/4 (10.0 ± 0.6mm, 10.8 ± 0.5 mm) and L4/5 (11.1 ± 0.8 mm, 12.0 ± 0.8 mm) (Fig. 3), while Ex group did not. Both groups showed a significant decrease in CSA of the spinal back muscle at L3/4 (Cont group, before: 31.9 ± 3.8 mm^2, after: 29.1 ± 3.2 mm^2; Ex group, before: 30.3 ± 3.7 mm^2, after: 27.8 ± 3.2 mm^2) and L4/5 (Cont group, before: 28.1 ± 2.1 mm^2, after: 24.1 ± 1.7 mm^2; Ex group, before: 26.4 ± 2.3 mm^2, after: 23.5 ± 1.7 mm^2) (Fig. 4), but did not show any significant change in intervertebral angle (Fig. 5) and CSA of the psoas at L3/4 and L4/5 (Fig. 6). No significant change in axial load-dependent spinal length between pre-BR and post-BR was observed both in Cont and Ex group (Fig. 7).

Discussion

Lumbar spinal lengthening due to an increase in disc height, but not decrease in intervertebral angle in Cont group

Our data for the Cont group suggest that spinal lengthening after 30 days of BR is caused by an increase in disc height at T12/L1, L1/2, L3/4 and L4/5, but not a decrease of intervertebral angle. LeBlanc and his colleagues reported that disc height increases approximately 1 mm after 5 or 17 weeks of BR[12]. Our previous report[17] also demonstrated that total disc height at L4/5 plus L5/S1 increases 2.9

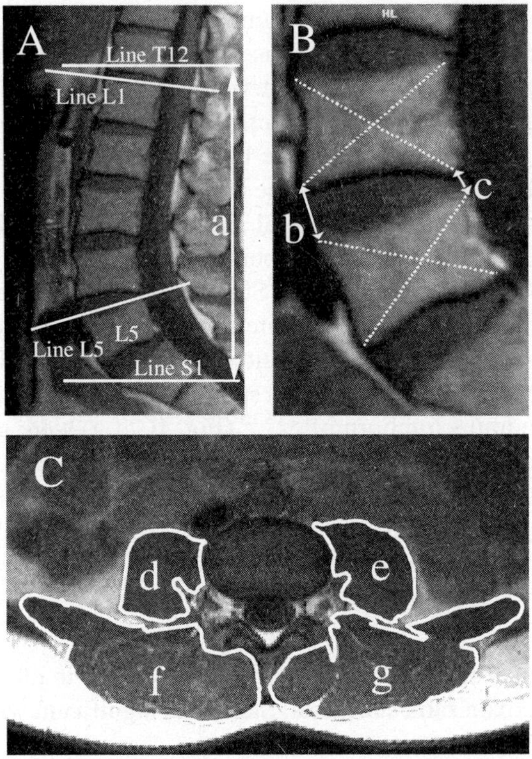

Fig. 1. Parameters measured in sagittal and axial MR image of the lumbar spine.
(A) Line T12: a horizontal line drawn at the antero-caudal corner of the twelfth thoracic vertebra. Line S1: a horizontal line drawn at the antero-cranial corner of the first sacral vertebra. a: spinal length between T12 and S1. Line L1 and L5: lines drawn along the cranial margin of the first and fifth lumbar vertebrae. Intervertebral angle at L1/5 is equal to that between Line L1 and Line L5. (B) Magnification of L4/5 intervertebral joint. b: anterior disc height, c: posterior disc height. Overall disc height: (b+c)/2. Dotted lines are used to determine corners of the vertebral body. (C) Axial MR image to measure cross-sectional areas (CSA) of psoas (d, e) and back muscle (f, g). The CSA of psoas and back muscles are determined using an average of these areas.

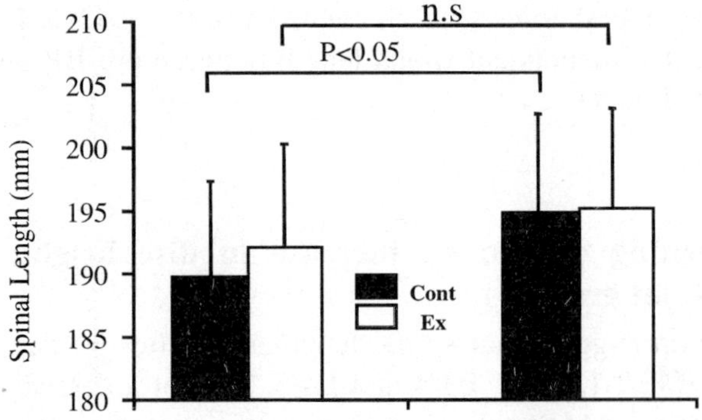

Fig. 2. Change in spinal length between pre- and post-bed rest in Cont and Ex group Pre: pre-bed rest, Post: post-bed rest. Data are expressed as mean ± SEM.of 6 subjects.

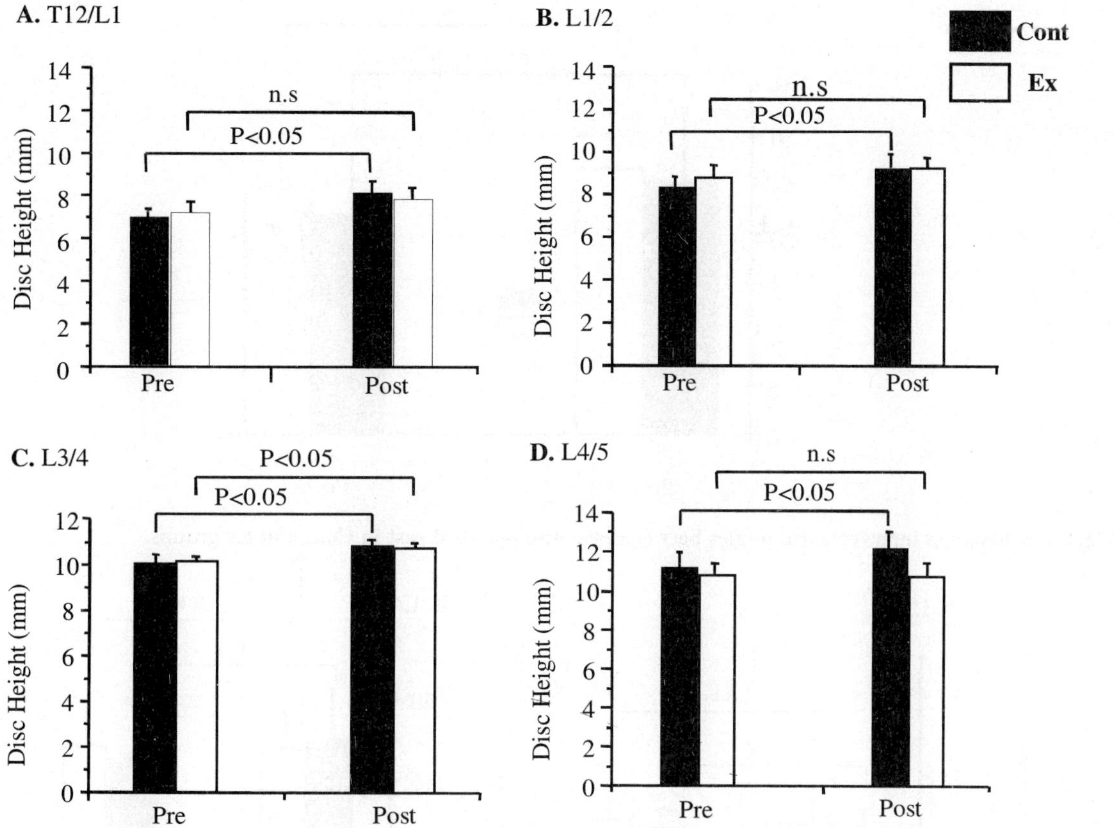

Fig. 3. Changes in disc height at T12/L1 (A), L1/2 (B), L3/4 (C) and L4/5 (D) between pre- and post-bed rest in Cont and Ex groups.

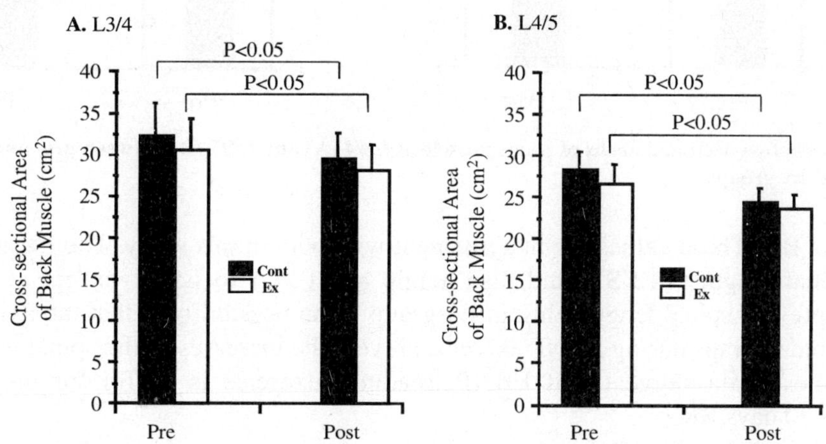

Fig. 4. Changes in cross-sectional areas of back muscle at L3/4 (A) and L4/5 (B) between pre- and post-bed rest in Cont and Ex groups.

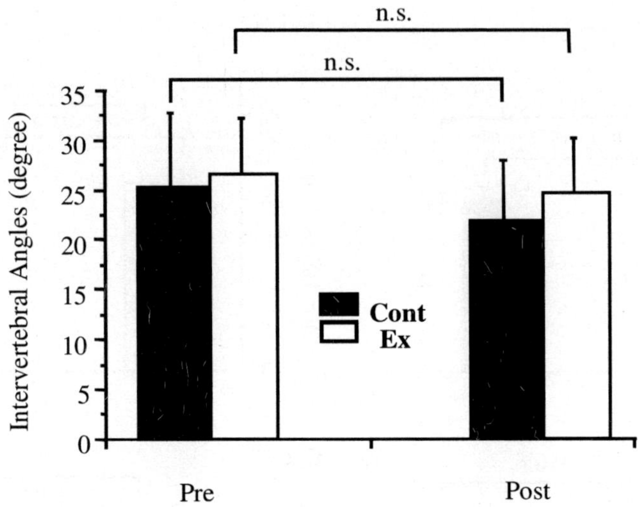

Fig. 5. Change in intervertebral angles between pre- and post-bed rest in Cont and Ex groups.

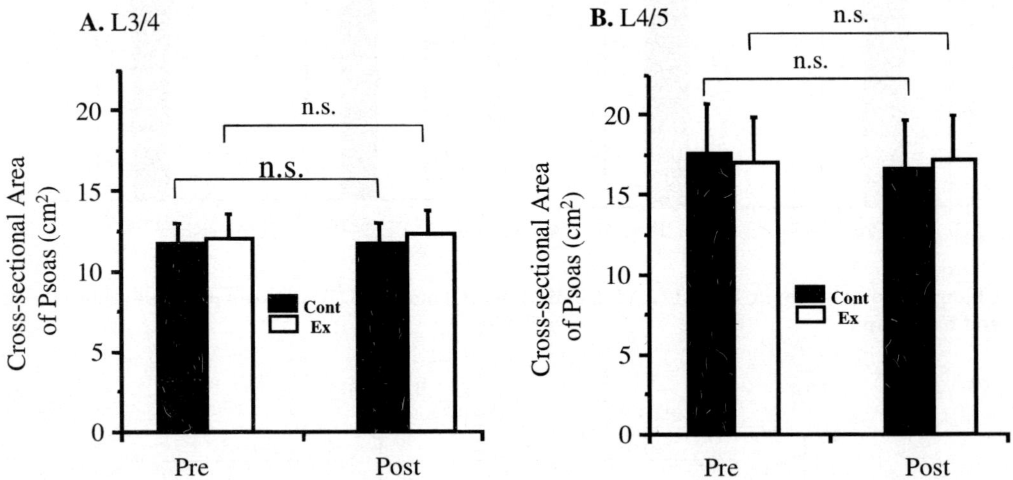

Fig. 6. Changes in cross-sectional areas of psoas muscle at L3/4 (A) and L4/5 (B) between pre- and post-bed rest in Cont and Ex groups.

mm after 3 days BR. These values are in agreement with ours in this study. The Ex group, however, maintained spinal length (T12-S1) and disc height at T12/L1 to L5/S1 except at L3/4. What is mechanism to prevent spinal lengthening in Ex group? One possibility is that the axial loads on the spine from shoulder straps during LBNP exercise prevent the increases of the spinal length as well as disc height. These data suggest that LBNP treadmill exercise is useful for preventing spinal lengthening for 30 days BR.

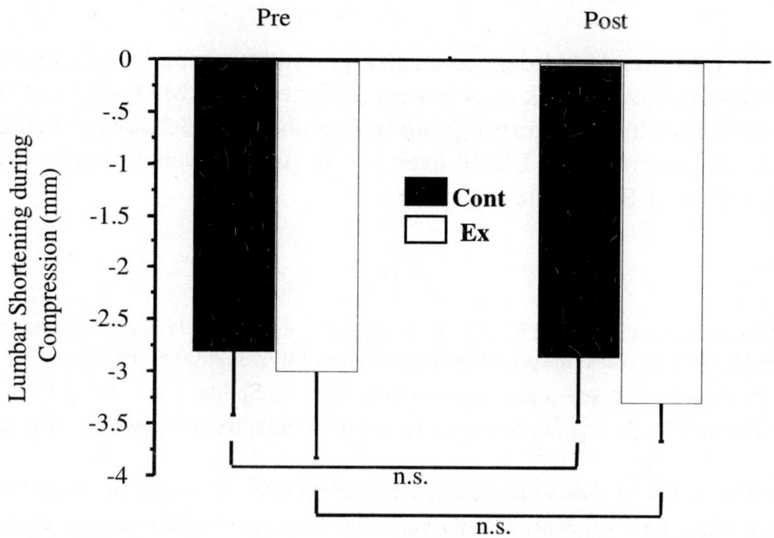

Fig. 7. Axial-load dependent change in lumbar shortening between pre- and post-bed rest in Cont and Ex groups.

LBNP exercise does not prevent spinal back muscle atrophy

Astronauts decrease CSA of back muscle by 10%, but did not decrease CSA of psoas muscle, after 8-day Shuttle flight[13]. In agreement with the previous study, our study showed that 1) Cont and Ex group decreased back muscle by 14 % and 11 % at L4/5, respectively, but did not decrease CSA of psoas muscle. We found no significant difference in back muscle atrophy between Cont and Ex groups, suggesting that LBNP treadmill exercise has no significant effect for spinal back muscle atrophy during 30 days BR. However, our previous report documented that LBNP exercise prevents spinal muscle atrophy only in men, but not women[7]. Therefore, more subjects are required to examine if LBNP exercise prevents spinal back muscle atrophy.

Axial compression study

An axial load of 50% body weight simulates upright weightbearing in the lumbar spine[10]. Willen and co-workers[20] report that axial loading of the lumbar spine reduces the cross-sectional area of the dural sac in patients with neurogenic intermittent claudication and/or sciatic pain. The new compression device helps understand the physiological changes in the upright lumbar spine. Many *in vivo* studies demonstrate that body height decreases 6.5-19.3 mm during an 8-hour period of normal upright activity[4,5,11,16,18]. Keller and Nathan[9] report an instantaneous loss of lumbar spine height of approximately 3.7 mm during quiet standing. Their data are consistent with ours, showing that axial compression of the lumbar spine (50% of body weight) produces 3.0 mm lumbar shortening. However, no significant change in axial load-dependent shortening between pre- and post-bed rest was observed in both groups (Fig. 7), These data suggest that 30 days BR does not affect lumbar spine's ability to bear loads.

Conclusions

Lumbar spinal length (plus axial load-dependent change), intervertebral angle, disc height and cross-sectional area of psoas muscle and back muscle were analyzed using MRI scans in Cont and Ex (lower body negative pressure treadmill exercise) group before and after 30 days of bedrest with 6° head-down tilt. Our data demonstrate that LBNP exercise, in part, prevents lumbar spine physiological deconditioning of 30 days of BR simulating space flight.

References

1. Boda WL, Watenpaugh DE, Ballard RE, Hargens AR. Supine lower body negative pressure exercise simulates metabolic and kinetic features of upright exercise. J Appl Physiol 2000;89:649-54.
2. Borg GAV. Psychological bases of physical exertion. Med Sci Sports Exerc 1982;14:377-381.
3. Dabbs VM, Dabbs LG. Correlation between disc height narrowing and low-back pain. Spine 1990;15:1366-1369.
4. Eklund JAE, Corlett EN. Shrinkage as a measurement of the effect of load on the spine. Spine 1984;9:189-194.
5. Goode JB, Theodore BM. Voluntary and diurnal variation in height and associated changes in spinal curves. Eng Med 1983;12:99-101.
6. Hargens AR, Hutchinson KJ, Ballard RE, Murthy G, Intervertebral Disc: Loaded on Earth and unloaded in space. In: Connective Tissue Biology: Integration and Reductionism, London, Portland Press, 1998.
7. Hargens AR, Groppo ER, Lee SMC, Watenpaugh DE, Schneider S, O'Leary D, Hughson RL, Shoemaker K, Smith SM, Steinbach GC, Tanaka K, Kawai Y, Bawa M, Kimura S, Macias B, Boda WL and Meyer RS. The gravity of LBNP exercise: preliminary lessons learned from identical twins in bed for 30 days. J Gravitational Physiology 2003;9:59-62.
8. Iwasaki K, Ring Z, Julie HZ, James AP, Benjamin DL. Effect of head-down-tilt bed rest and hypovolemia on dynamic regulation of heart rate and blood pressure. Am J Regul Integr Comp Physiol 2000;279:R2189-R2199.
9. Keller TS, Nathan M. Height change caused by creep in intervertebral discs: A sagittal plane model. J Spinal Disord 1999;12:313-324.
10. Kimura S, Steinbach G, Watenpauch D, et al. Lumbar spine disc height and curvature responses to an axial load generated by a compression device compatible with Magnetic Resonance Imaging. Spine 2001;26:2596-2600.
11. Krag MK, Cohen MC, Haugh LD, Pope MH. Body height change during upright and recumbent postures. Spine 1990;15:202-207.
12. LeBlanc A, Evans HJ, Schneider VS, Wendt RE 3rd, Hedrick TD. Changes in intervertebral disc cross-sectional area with bed rest and space flight. Spine 1994;19:812-817.
13. LeBlanc A, Rowe R, Schneider V, Evans H, Hedrick T. Regional muscle loss after short duration spaceflight. Aviat Space Environ Med 1995;66:1151-1154.
14. Peltonen JE, Taimela S, Erkintalo M, Salminen JJ, Oksanen A, Kujala UM. Back extensor and psoas muscle cross-sectional area, prior physical training, and trunk muscle strength -a longitudinal study in adolescent girls. Eur J Appl Physiol Occup Physiol. 1998;77:66-71.
15. Raty HP, Kujala U, Videman T, Koskinen SK, Karppi SL, Sarna S. Associations of isometric and isoinertial trunk muscle strength measurements and lumbar paraspinal muscle cross-sectional areas. J Spinal Disord 1999;12:266-270.
16. Rielly T, Tyrell A, Troup JDG. Circadian variation in human stature. Chronobiol Int 1984;1:121-126.
17. Styf JR, Ballard RE, Fechner K, Watenpaugh DE, Kahan NJ, Hargens AR. Height increase, neuromuscular function, and back pain during 6 degrees head-down tilt with traction. Aviat Space Environ Med 1997; 68:24-29.

18. Tyrell AR, Reilley T, Troup JDG. Circadian variation in stature and the effects of spinal loading. Spine 1985;10:161-164.
19. Watenpaugh DE, Ballard RE, Schneider SM, Lee SM, Ertl AC, William JM, Boda WL, Hutchinson KJ, Hargens AR. Supine lower body negative pressure exercise during bed rest maintains upright exercise capacity. J Appl Physiol 2000;89:218-227.
20. Willen J, Danielson B, Gaulitz A, et al. Dynamic effect on the lumbar spinal canal. Axially loaded CT-myelography and MRI in patients with sciatica and/or neurogenic claudication. Spine 1997;22:2968-2976.
21. Wood KB, Kos P, Schendel M, Persson K. Effect of patient position on the sagittal-plane profile of the thoracolumbar spine. J Spinal Disord 1996;9:165-169.

Adaptation Biology and Medicine (Volume 4: Current Concepts)
Editors: A. Hargens, N. Takeda and P.K. Singal

12. Activation of Protein Kinases and Cellular Redistribution of Inducible Hsp70 Protein in Chronically Hypoxic Infant Human and Rabbit Hearts: Role in Cardioprotection

Parvaneh Rafiee, Ph.D.[1], Yang Shi, Ph.D.[1], Kirkwood A Pritchard Jr., Ph.D.[1], James S Tweddell, M.D.[2,3], John E Baker, Ph.D., F.A.H.A.[1]

Divisions of Pediatric Surgery[1] and Cardiothoracic Surgery[2],
Medical College of Wisconsin, Milwaukee, WI 53226
and
Section of Cardiothoracic Surgery[3], Children's Hospital of Wisconsin,
Milwaukee, WI 53226

ABSTRACT

Many infants who undergo cardiac surgery have a congenital cyanotic defect where the heart is chronically perfused with hypoxic blood. However the signaling pathways by which infant hearts adapt to chronic hypoxia and resist subsequent surgical ischemia is unknown. We determined the role of two members of the heat shock protein 70 family, Hsp70i and Hsc70, in activation and translocation of protein kinase C (PKC) isoforms and mitogen activated protein kinases (MAP kinases) in human infants with cyanotic (SaO_2<85%) or acyanotic (SaO_2>95%) heart defects undergoing surgical repair and in rabbits raised from birth in a hypoxic (SaO_2<85%) or normoxic (SaO_2>95%) environment. In human infants with cyanotic heart defects PKCe, p38 MAP kinase and JUN kinase, but not p42/44 MAP kinase are activated and translocated from the cytosolic to the particulate fraction compared with acyanotic heart defects. In rabbit infants there is a parallel response for PKCe, p38 MAP kinase and JUN kinase similar to humans. In chronically hypoxic human and rabbit hearts message levels for Hsp70i were elevated 4-5 fold compared with normoxic hearts and Hsp70i protein was redistributed from the particulate to the cytosolic fraction. In normoxic infants Hsp70i protein was distributed almost equally between the cytosolic and particulate fractions. Hsc70 message and sub cellular distribution of Hsc70 protein were unaffected by chronic hypoxia. Protein kinases influence Hsp70i protein sub cellular distribution. In rabbit hearts SB203580 and chelerythrine reduced Hsp70i message levels while SB203580, chelerythrine and curcumin reversed the sub cellular redistribution of Hsp70i protein caused by chronic hypoxia, with no effect in normoxic hearts, indicating regulation of Hsp70i message and sub cellular distribution of Hsp70i protein in chronically hypoxic rabbit hearts is influenced by PKC and mitogen activated kinases, specifically p38 MAPK and JNK. In infant rabbit hearts inhibition of PKCe with chelerythrine, p38 MAP kinase with SB203580 and JUN kinase with curcumin abolished the cardioprotective effects of chronic hypoxia but had no effects on normoxic hearts. Infant human and rabbit hearts adapt to chronic hypoxia *via* activation of PKCe, p38 MAP kinase and JUN kinase signal transduction pathways which may control cellular distribution of Hsp70i. The response to oxygen deprivation between these two species is remarkably similar considering the origins of chronic hypoxia – a reduction in environmental oxygen levels with normal cardiac anatomy in the rabbit compared with normal oxygen levels in the human with an abnormal cardiac anatomy as a result of a congenital cyanotic defect. These protein kinases and molecular chaperones may be responsible for cardioprotection in the chronically hypoxic infant heart.

Introduction

Many infants who undergo cardiac surgery have a congenital cyanotic defect where the heart is chronically perfused with hypoxic blood. However the signaling pathways by which infant hearts adapt to chronic hypoxia and resist subsequent surgical ischemia are unknown.

By elucidating the impact that prolonged periods of hypoxia exert on resistance to subsequent ischemia, we should be able to improve cardioprotection in infants with congenital heart defects. Protein kinase C (PKC) family members are important mediators of hypoxia. In cardiomyocytes PKCa and PKCe translocate from soluble to particulate fractions of the cell in response to the stress of chronic hypoxia (1). The mitogen-activated protein kinases (MAP kinases) are ubiquitous signaling molecules activated by diverse stimuli and appear to mediate cellular responses including proliferation, differentiation, and adaptation to stress (2). Three major MAP kinase families have been characterized, including the extracellular signal-regulated kinases (ERK 1/2 or p42/44 MAPK), the c-Jun NH_2-terminal kinases (JUN kinase), and the p38 MAP kinases (p38 MAPKs)(2). ERKs are mainly involved in mediating anabolic processes such as cell division, growth, and differentiation, the JUN kinases and the p38 MAPK are generally associated with cellular response to diverse stresses. The clinical relevance of protein kinases in adult humans was recently demonstrated by an increased activity of JUN kinase and p38 MAPK in heart failure secondary to ischemic heart disease (3) and during cardiopulmonary bypass (4). However, the role of PKC and MAPKs in the mechanisms by which infant hearts adapt to chronic hypoxia and resist subsequent surgical ischemia is unknown.

Heat-shock proteins are self-protective proteins that maintain cell homeostasis against various forms of stress as an adaptive response (5). These proteins are induced by a wide variety of stressors and have broad cytoprotective functions. The 70-kDa family of heat shock proteins (Hsp70), in particular, plays a vital role in cellular protection and has been detected in various tissues subjected to stress (6, 7). The Hsp70 stress proteins exist as two isoforms in mammalian cells. Messenger RNA and protein for the cognate form of Hsp70, Hsc70, is constitutively expressed in the nonstressed cell, slightly inducible and functions as a molecular chaperone. However a slightly different form of Hsp70, Hsp70i, is highly inducible and quickly upregulates in response to stressful stimuli to enhance cellular chaperone activity. Hsp70 protein in unstressed cells is found in the cytoplasm and nucleus (8) but redistributes to the cytoplasm in response to stress. Overexpression of mRNA for Hsp70 using gene therapy translates to increased Hsp70 protein levels that are associated with increased cardioprotection, suggesting this stress protein plays an important role in mediating resistance to myocardial ischemia (9). Adaptation to the stress of chronic hypoxia also results in increased cardioprotection (10, 11). Thus adaptation to chronic hypoxia may result in increased expression of mRNA and sub cellular redistribution of Hsp70 protein that may confer cardioprotection. However the underlying mechanisms responsible for cellular redistribution of Hsp70 are unknown.

Hsp70 expression is controlled in part by protein kinases. Activation of PKC$_{\text{å}}$, p38 MAP kinase and JUN kinase signaling pathways appear to confer cardioprotection in infant rabbit hearts adapted to chronic hypoxia (10). However, the relationship of Hsp70 to these protein kinase signaling pathways following adaptation to chronic hypoxemia is unknown. Ohnishi *et al* (12) examined the involvement of protein kinases in the regulation of Hsp70i gene expression in the A-172 cell line with use of H-7, a potent inhibitor of PKC, PKA and PKG and have shown decreased Hsp70i expression. Treatment of rat hearts with chelerythrine, a PKC inhibitor, prior to heat shock increases infarct size compared to non heat shock treated animals (11). In addition, there was a marked increased in Hsp70i expression in the heat shock treated group. Pretreatment with chelerythrine failed to inhibit the expression of Hsp70i, suggesting that heat shock-induced ischemic tolerance is mediated *via* the PKC pathway and this protection does not appear to be directly related to the expression of Hsp70i in rat heart (11).

The MAPK family plays an important role in coordinating gene responses to various stresses. Induction of Hsp70 in the 9L rat is preceded by phosphorylation and activation of p38 MAPK and p42/44 MAPK. Specific inhibitors of p38 MAPK (SB203580) and p42/44 MAPK (PD98059) are known to eliminate Hsp70 induction (13). Phosphorylation and activation of Hsp27, a substrate for p38 MAP kinase, is present in chronically hypoxic infant hearts but not in normoxic hearts (10). Overexpression of Hsp27 in myocytes confers protection against simulated ischemia (14).

This chapter examines the role of these signaling pathways in adaptation to chronic hypoxia by the identification and characterization of PKC and MAPKs in hearts from human infants with cyanotic ($SaO_2 < 85\%$) or acyanotic ($SaO_2 > 95\%$) heart defects and in hearts from infant rabbits raised from birth in a hypoxic ($SaO_2 < 85\%$) or normoxic ($SaO_2 > 95\%$) environment. The contribution of PKC and MAPKs to cardioprotection in chronically hypoxic and normoxic infant rabbit hearts is also examined. Many of the protein kinase signaling mechanisms activated by chronic hypoxia in infant rabbits are identical to those activated by cyanotic heart defects in human infants. Furthermore protein kinases confer cardioprotection in the chronically hypoxic infant rabbit heart.

Chronic hypoxia represents a significant stress to the heart. However the role of heat shock proteins in mediating adaptation of the heart to chronic hypoxia is unknown. This chapter also examines the role of Hsp70 in adaptation to chronic hypoxia by identifying and characterizing message levels and sub cellular distribution of Hsp70i and Hsc70 protein in hearts from human infants with cyanotic ($SaO_2 < 85\%$) or acyanotic ($SaO_2 > 95\%$) heart defects and in hearts from infant rabbits raised from birth in a hypoxic ($SaO_2 < 85\%$) or normoxic ($SaO_2 > 95\%$) environment. PKC, p38 MAPK and JNK influence Hsp70 message expression and subcellular redistribution of Hsp70 protein in the signal transduction pathway activated by chronic hypoxia. Thus both infant human and rabbit hearts adapt to chronic hypoxia by increasing expression of message for Hsp70i but not Hsc70. Increased message for Hsp70i translates to altered sub cellular distribution of Hsp70i protein, with expression and sub cellular localization of Hsp70i influenced by protein kinases.

Methods

Humans

The use of human tissue was approved by the Human Research and Review Committee at Children's Hospital of Wisconsin and the Medical College of Wisconsin. Infants undergoing elective open-heart surgery for congenital heart defects were prospectively recruited. To determine whether protein kinases are activated by chronic hypoxia the patients were divided into cyanotic and acyanotic groups according to blood oxygen saturation (acyanotic, $SaO_2 > 95\%$, cyanotic, $SaO_2 < 85\%$). All cyanotic patients were stable with $SaO_2 < 85\%$ for 24 hours prior to surgery. There were no emergency operations performed on acutely hypoxic patients. Right atrial tissue (approximately 200mg) from infants with congenital acyanotic and cyanotic heart defects was harvested at the time of surgical repair. The tissue was immediately frozen in liquid nitrogen and processed for Western analysis as described previously (15). Pre-operative characteristics are summarized in Table 1.

Table 1. Patient characteristics.

		Cyanotic (n=7)	Acyanotic (n=8)
Age (months)			
	Mean	4.8 ± 0.9	5.8 ± 1.2
	Range	1 week-9 months	1 month-10 months
Body weight (kg)		3.9 ± 0.4	5.2 ± 0.5*
Sex (male/female)		4/3	4/4
Pathology†			
	CAVC	0	2
	VSD	0	2
	TOF	2	0
	AS	0	1
	DORV	1	0
	PAVC	0	3
	HLHS	4	0
Hemoglobin (g/dl)	15.6 ± 0.6	12.5 ± 1.3*	
Blood O_2 saturation (%)	73 ± 5	98 ± 1*	

†CAVC = complete atrio-ventricular canal, VSD = ventricular septal defect; TOF = tetralogy of Fallot; AVSD = atrio-ventricular septal defect; AS = aortic stenosis; DORV = double outlet right ventricle with transposition of the great arteries; ASD = atrial septal defect; PAVC = partial atrio-ventricular canal; HLHS = hypoplastic left heart syndrome.

* $p<0.05$ cyanotic vs. acyanotic

Rabbits

Animals were used in compliance with the "Guide for the Care and Use of Laboratory Animals" formulated by the National Research Council, 1996. Infant rabbits were maintained for 10 days in a hypoxic ($SaO_2 < 85\%$) or normoxic ($SaO_2 > 95\%$) environment as described previously (16).

Isolated heart perfusion

Isolated rabbit hearts (n=8/group) were perfused in a retrograde manner and instrumented as previously described (16).

Effect of PKC and MAPK inhibitors

Hearts from normoxic or chronically hypoxic rabbits were perfused in the Langendorff mode. Ventricular function and coronary flow were recorded under steady-state conditions (16). Hearts were then perfused for 15 minutes with vehicle, chelerythrine (1 μmol/L), SB203580 (15 μmol/L), curcumin (10 μmol/L) or PD98059 (10 μmol/L) prior to 30 minutes global normothermic (39°C) ischemia and 40 min reperfusion. The experimental protocol is described in Figure 1. Recovery of left ventricular developed pressure at 40 min reperfusion was used to assess resistance to ischemia. Results are expressed as the mean ± standard deviation.

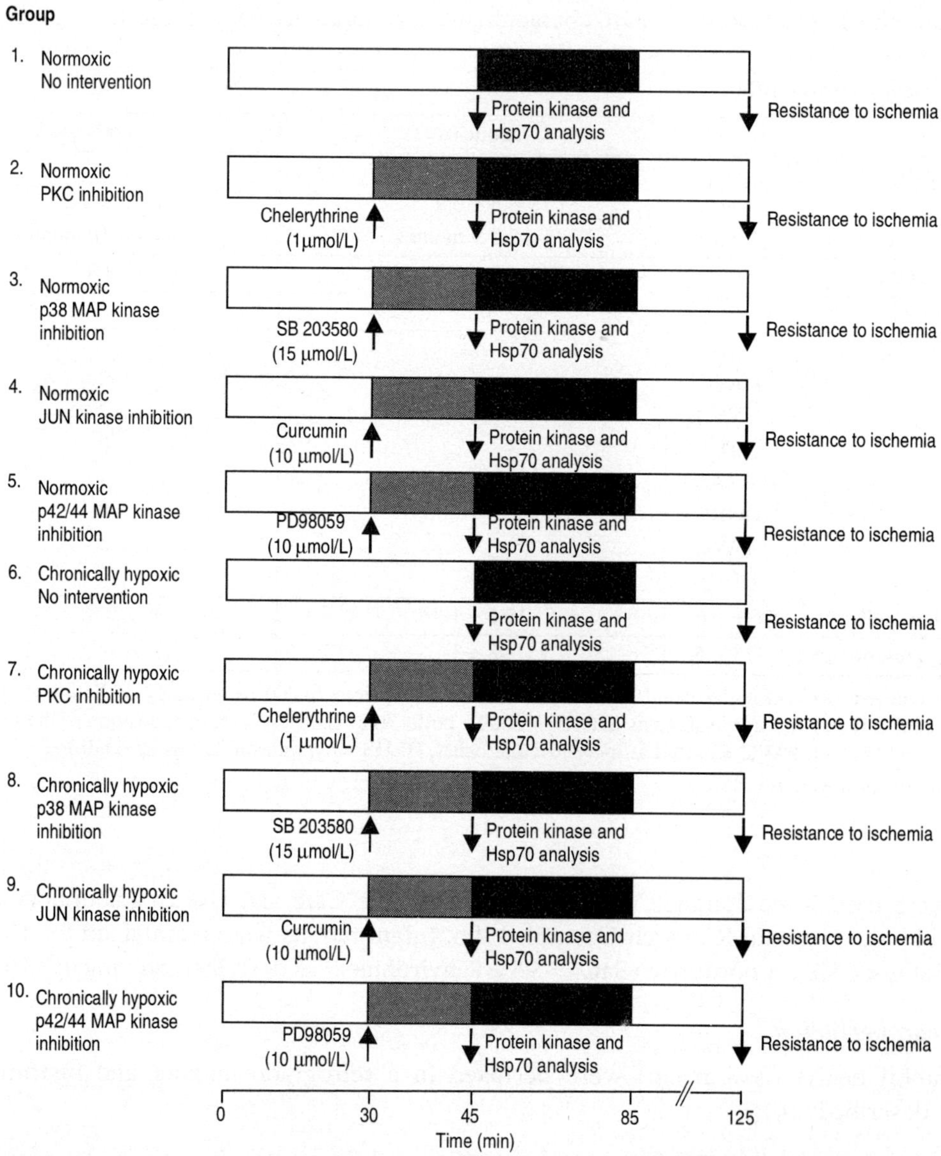

Fig. 1. Experimental protocol used to study the role of protein kinases in influencing Hsp70 mRNA expression and Hsp70i protein sub cellular distribution in normoxic and chronically hypoxic infant rabbit hearts and resistance to ischemia (n=10/group). Open boxes represent aerobic perfusion. Hatched boxes represent perfusion with protein kinase inhibitors. Solid boxes represent global ischemia.

To determine the effect of chelerythrine, SB203580 and curcumin on protein kinases and Hsp70 in chronically hypoxic and normoxic hearts, isolated hearts (n = 4-7/group) were aerobically perfused with these drugs for 15 minutes. The free wall of the left ventricle was then processed to obtain cytosolic and particulate fractions (17) for western analysis as described previously (15).

Hsp70 mRNA and protein analysis

Constitutive and inducible Hsp70 gene and protein expression was assessed in normoxic and chronically hypoxic hearts in infant human and rabbit hearts as described previously (18).

Results

Adaptation to chronic hypoxia

PKC and MAPK in human heart

The involvement of PKC and MAPKs in normoxic and hypoxic hearts was examined by SDS-PAGE and Western analysis in cytosolic and particulate fractions. Normoxic hearts contain multiple PKC isoforms (α, β, γ, ε, δ, and ζ) in the cytosolic fractions. However, adaptation to chronic hypoxia results only in the translocation of $PKC_{\text{å}}$ from cytosolic fraction to the particulate fraction (Figure 2). MAPK pathways also play a role in adaptation to chronic hypoxia. In normoxic hearts phospho-p38 MAPK is present in both cytosolic and particulate fractions, but chronic hypoxia results in an increase of phospho-p38 MAPK in the particulate fraction (Figure 2). Chronic hypoxia activates JUN kinase in human heart. Chronic hypoxia does not result in activation of phospho-p42/44 MAPK in human hearts. We confirmed that equal amounts of p38 and JNK proteins were analyzed by stripping and re-probing the same blots with control anti-p38 and anti-JNK antibodies (Figure 2).

Activation and translocation of $PKC_{\varepsilon,}$ p38 MAPK and JUN kinase was not related to the variability in clinical presentation of the two groups of patients studied (Table 1). In all hearts adapted to chronic hypoxia there was activation and translocation of protein kinases. In contrast, activation and translocation did not occur in any of the normoxic hearts. Thus in all cases changes in protein kinase activation and translocation were solely dependent on oxygen deprivation and not to the underlying clinical presentation responsible for the congenital defect.

p38 MAPK plays a protective role during adaptation to ischemic preconditioning by phosphorylating MAPKAPK-2 which in turn phosphorylates Hsp27 (19). Activation of this pathway is cardioprotective and overexpression of Hsp27 confers protection against ischemia in myocytes (14). This pathway is also present in human infants and is activated by adaptation to chronic hypoxia. Chronic hypoxia induces activation and translocation of both MAPKAPK-2 and Hsp27 from the cytosolic to the particulate fraction. Neither MAPKAPK-2 nor Hsp27 was activated in normoxic hearts (Figure 3).

p38 MAPK also transduces signals from the cytoplasm to the nucleus in response to cellular stress. ATF2 is a transcription factor phosphorylated by p38 MAPK (20). In hearts adapted to chronic hypoxia, phosphorylation of GST-ATF2 by p38 MAPK is present in hearts from chronically hypoxic but not in normoxic infants with phospho-p38 MAPK immunoprecipitates from chronically hypoxic hearts resulting in phosphorylation of GST-ATF-2 in the particulate fraction (Figure 3).

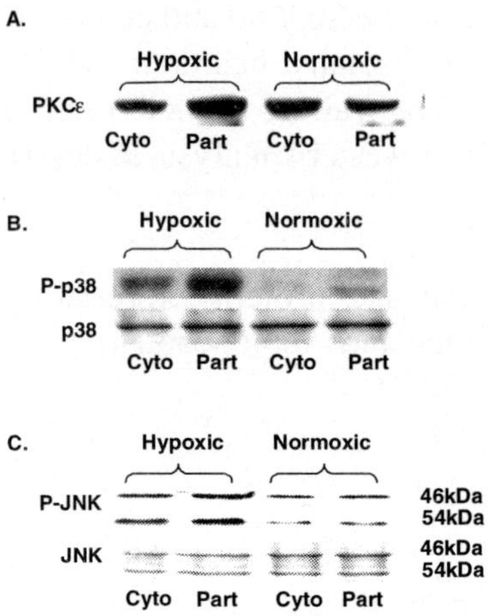

Fig. 2. Chronic hypoxia in infant human heart results in phosphorylation and translocation of PKCe, p38 MAP kinase and JUN kinase from cytosolic to particulate fraction. Cytosolic and particulate fractions were analyzed by Western blotting using phospho-specific antibodies against A), PKCe, B), p38 MAPK and C), JNK. Non phosphorylated antibodies were used to confirm equal loading of proteins for p38 MAPK and JNK. Cyto = cytosolic, Part = particulate.

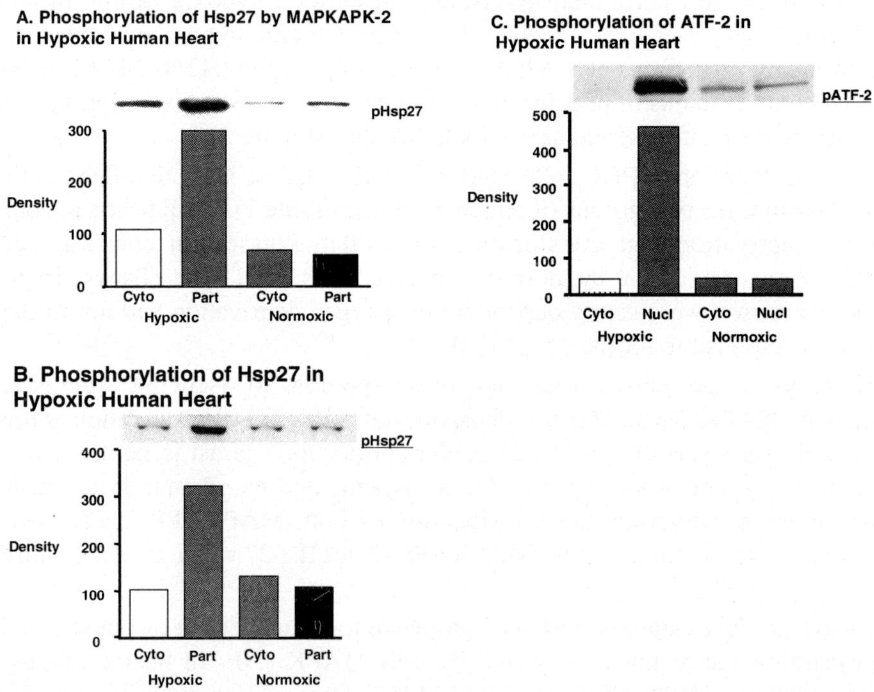

Fig. 3. Chronic hypoxia in infant human heart activates MAPKAPK-2, phosphorylates Hsp27 and ATF-2 (Thr 71). A), In vitro kinase assay shows phosphorylation of substrate Hsp27 by MAPKAPK-2 in particulate fraction. B), Chronic hypoxia-induced Hsp27 phosphorylation in particulate fraction. C), Chronic hypoxia results in ATF-2 (Thr 71) phosphorylation in nuclear fraction. Cyto = cytosolic, Part = particulate, Nucl = nuclear.

Hsp70i and Hsc70 mRNA expression in human hypoxic heart

If increased expression of mRNA and protein for Hsp70 confers protection against cardiac ischemic injury (9, 21) and adaptation to chronic hypoxia also confers cardioprotection (10, 16), then Hsp70 should play a role in adaptation of the infant human heart to chronic hypoxia. Thus we used semi-quantitative RT-PCR and their respective primers to examine inducible and constitutive levels of Hsp70 mRNA in normoxic and hypoxic human infant hearts. The levels of Hsp70 mRNA between chronically hypoxic and normoxic hearts were compared by densitometric analysis after normalization to β-actin, the internal control. Hsp70i mRNA expression was robustly increased 4-5 fold in chronically hypoxic hearts but minimally expressed in normoxic hearts (Figure 3). Hsc70 mRNA was expressed in both chronically hypoxic and normoxic hearts. However no detectable differences in the level of Hsc70 mRNA expression were detected between chronically hypoxic and normoxic hearts (Figure 4, upper panel). β-actin mRNA expression showed comparable density of bands for both normoxic and hypoxic conditions (Figure 4, lower panel). The amplified cDNA sizes for Hsp70i, Hsc70 and β-actin were 284-bp, 283-bp and 436-bp respectively. Thus infant human hearts adapt to the stress of chronic hypoxia by increasing expression of mRNA for Hsp70i but not Hsc70.

Hsp70i and Hsc70 protein expression in human hypoxic heart

If chronic hypoxia changes mRNA levels for Hsp70, we would expect this would be translated into similar changes for protein levels for Hsp70. Total cell lysates, cytosolic and particulate fractions from normoxic and hypoxic hearts were prepared. Protein content for constitutive and inducible Hsp70 was determined by SDS-PAGE and Western blot analysis using monoclonal antibodies specific for inducible and constitutive Hsp70. There were no changes in Hsp70i and Hsc70 protein levels in the total lysates obtained from chronically hypoxic and normoxic hearts (Figures 5 and 6). However analysis of the cytosolic and particulate fractions indicates that in chronically hypoxic human hearts, 80% of Hsp70i protein was localized in the cytosolic fraction with 20% of protein being in the particulate fraction. In normoxic human hearts, Hsp70i protein was distributed almost equally between

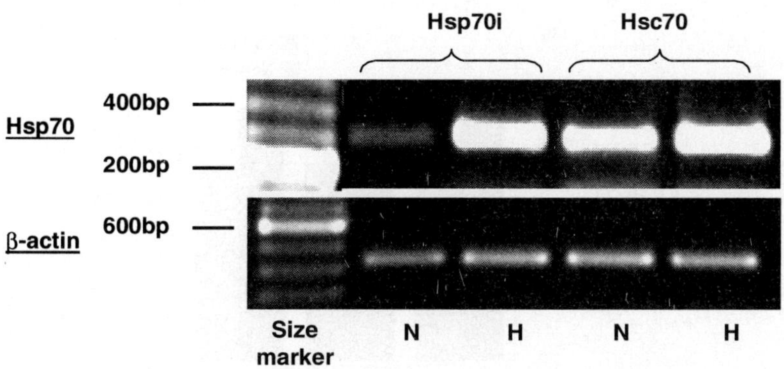

Fig. 4. mRNA levels for Hsp70i and Hsc70 in normoxic and chronically hypoxic infant human heart. RT-PCR using primers for inducible Hsp70 demonstrates that mRNA for Hsp70i was robustly expressed in chronically hypoxic hearts and minimally expressed in normoxic hearts. There were no changes in the level of Hsc70 in chronically hypoxic and normoxic hearts. β-actin served as an internal control. Data shown are representative of four hearts analyzed for each condition studied. N = Normoxic, H = Chronically hypoxic.

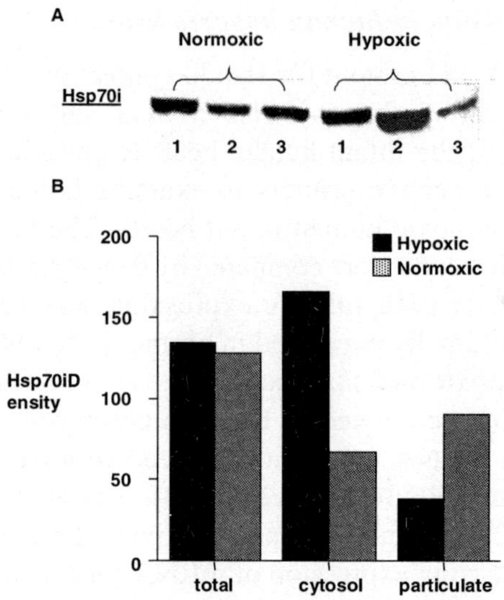

Fig. 5. Inducible Hsp70 protein levels in normoxic and chronically hypoxic infant human heart. Analysis of total lysate, cytosolic and particulate fractions was carried out as described in methods. A) Western blot demonstrates that in hypoxic heart 80% of inducible Hsp70 is localized in the cytosolic fraction with 20% localized in the particulate fraction. In normoxic hearts inducible Hsp70 protein was almost equally distributed between the cytosolic and particulate fractions. 1 = total lysate, 2 = cytosolic fraction, 3 = particulate fraction. B) Densitometric measurement of inducible Hsp70 protein in normoxic and hypoxic hearts representative of four experiments.

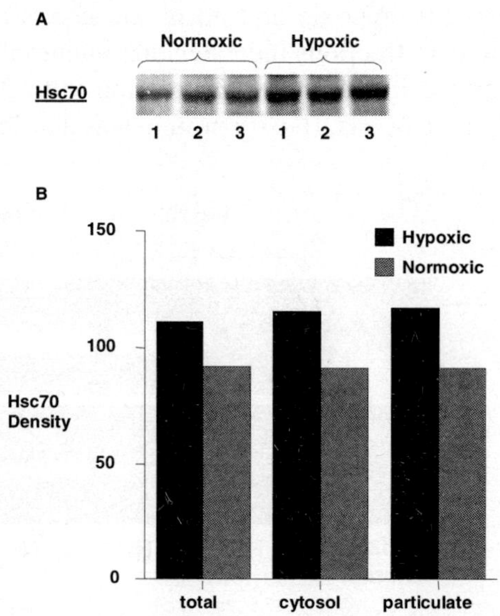

Fig 6 Constitutive Hsp70 protein levels in normoxic and chronically hypoxic infant human heart. Analysis of total lysates, cytosolic and particulate fraction was carried out as described in methods. A) Western blot demonstrates constitutive Hsp70 distributed equally in cytosolic and particulate fractions in chronically hypoxic and normoxic hearts. 1 = total lysate, 2 = cytosolic fraction, 3 = particulate fraction. B) Densitometric measurement of constitutive Hsp70 protein in normoxic and chronically hypoxic hearts representative of four experiments.

the cytosolic and particulate fractions (40% vs 60%) (Figure 5). In contrast, constitutive Hsc70 protein was equally distributed between the cytosolic and particulate fractions of chronically hypoxic and normoxic infant human hearts, with no detectable differences in the total lysates (Figure 6).

ATF-2 phosphorylation in nuclear fraction of hypoxic hearts

Transcriptional activity of ATF-2 can be stimulated by JNK and p38 MAPK. ATF-2 binds to both AP-1 and cAMP response element. Therefore, we examined whether chronic hypoxia phosphorylates and activates ATF-2. Adaptation to chronic hypoxia phosphorylates Thr71 of ATF-2 in the nuclear fraction (Figure 3), suggesting activation of this transcription factor. We confirmed that equal amounts of ATF-2 protein were analyzed by stripping and re-probing the same blots with control anti-ATF-2 antibody.

PKC and MAPK in rabbit heart

The pattern of activation for PKCe and MAPKs in isolated perfused hearts from rabbits adapted to chronic hypoxia is identical to that in human. Furthermore, chronic hypoxia induces activation of both MAPKAPK- 2 and Hsp27 in the particulate fraction similar to that present in human. This pattern of activation is also present in freshly excised rabbit hearts not subjected to perfusion prior to analysis. The relative upstream/downstream positions of PKCe, p38 MAPK and JUN kinase in the signal transduction pathway activated by chronic hypoxia was determined by perfusing hearts with specific inhibitors of PKC and p38 MAPK, followed by Western blot analysis of the heart lysates. Perfusion of isolated rabbit hearts with chelerythrine, an inhibitor of PKC, reversed the translocation of PKC_{ε}, p38 MAPK and JUN kinase in chronically hypoxic rabbits but had no effect in normoxic rabbits (Figure 7). Perfusion of hearts with SB203580, an inhibitor of p38 MAPK, also reverses the translocation of p38 MAPK but not PKC_{ε} or JUN kinase in chronically hypoxic hearts. SB203580 had no effect in normoxic rabbit hearts (Figure 8). These data suggest PKCe is an upstream kinase for activation of p38 MAPK and JUN kinase in chronically hypoxic rabbit hearts. SB20380 also prevented activation of ATF-2 by p38 MAPK in chronically hypoxic hearts. Clearly many of the protein kinase signaling mechanisms activated by chronic hypoxia in the infant rabbit heart do appear highly similar to the point of being essentially identical to the signaling mechanism in infant humans with cyanotic heart defects.

Hsp70i and Hsc70 mRNA expression in rabbit hypoxic heart

Using semi-quantitative RT-PCR and rabbit primers, the level of Hsp70 mRNA was determined in normoxic and hypoxic rabbit hearts. Transcripts for Hsp70i were elevated 4-5 fold in chronically hypoxic hearts compared with normoxic hearts (Figure 9). Hsc70 mRNA was robustly expressed in both chronically hypoxic and normoxic rabbit hearts. However, adaptation to chronic hypoxia had no effect on expression of Hsc70 message levels compared with normoxic hearts (Figure 9). Thus the adaptive response to chronic hypoxia in rabbit for Hsp70 mRNA was remarkably similar to that observed in human.

Hsp70i and Hsc70 protein expression in rabbit hypoxic heart

There was no change in Hsp70i protein levels in the total lysates obtained from chronically hypoxic and normoxic hearts (Figure 10). However in chronically hypoxic rabbit hearts, Hsp70i protein was mainly redistributed to the cytosolic fraction, whereas in normoxic rabbit hearts, Hsp70i was equally distributed between the cytosolic and particulate fractions (Figure 10). In chronically hypoxic and

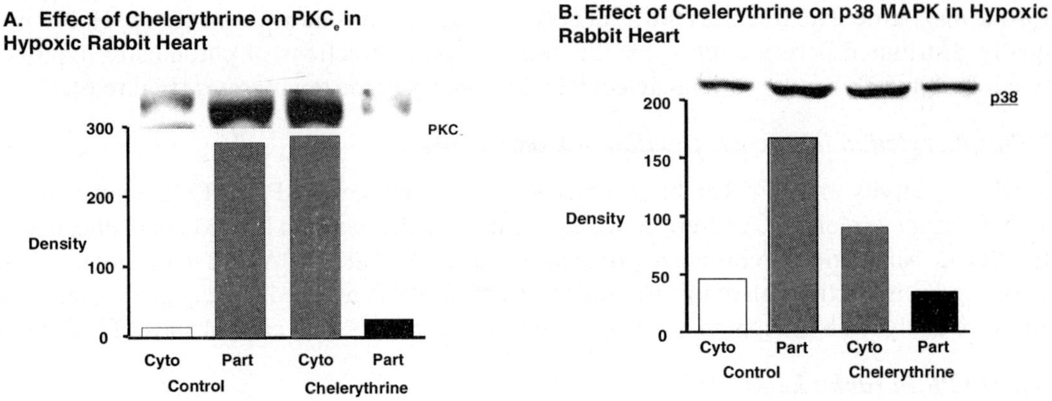

Fig. 7. **Effect of chelerythrine, a PKC inhibitor, on PKC_{ε} and p38 MAPK in chronically hypoxic rabbit heart. Cytosolic and particulate fractions were analyzed by Western blotting using specific antibodies against A), phospho-PKC_e and B), phospho-p38 MAPK. Chelerythrine signficantly inhibited translocation of both PKC_e and p38 MAPK from cytosolic to particulate fraction in hypoxic rabbit heart. Cyto = cytosolic, Part = particulate.**

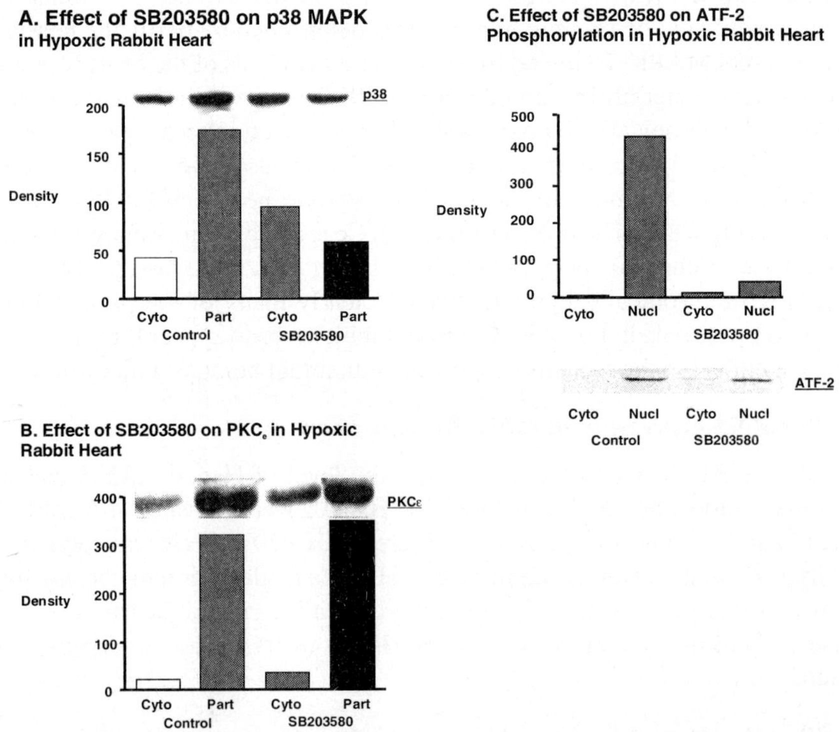

Fig. 8. **Effect of SB203580, a p38 MAPK inhibitor, on p38 MAPK, PKC_{ε} and ATF-2 in chronically hypoxic rabbit heart. Cytosolic, particulate and nuclear fractions were probed with specific antibodies against A), phospho-p38 MAPK, B), phospho-PKC_{ε}, C), phosphorylated and non phosphorylated ATF-2. SB203580 inhibits translocation of p38MAPK from cytosolic to particulate fraction in hypoxic rabbit heart but did not inhibit translocation of PKC_{ε}. SB203580 inhibits phosphorylated but not non phoshorylated ATF-2 in the nuclear fraction of hypoxic rabbit heart. Cyto = cytosolic, Part = particulate, Nucl = nuclear.**

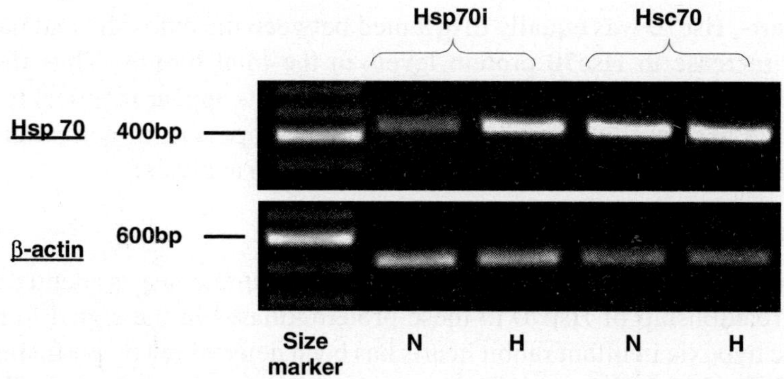

Fig. 9. mRNA levels for Hsp70i and Hsc70 in normoxic and chronically hypoxic infant rabbit heart. RT-PCR demonstrates inducible mRNA for Hsp70i robustly expressed in chronically hypoxic hearts and minimally expressed in normoxic hearts. mRNA levels for Hsc70 were unchanged in chronically hypoxic hearts compared with normoxic hearts. β-actin served as an internal control. Data shown are representative of four hearts analyzed for each condition studied. N = Normoxic, H = Chronically hypoxic

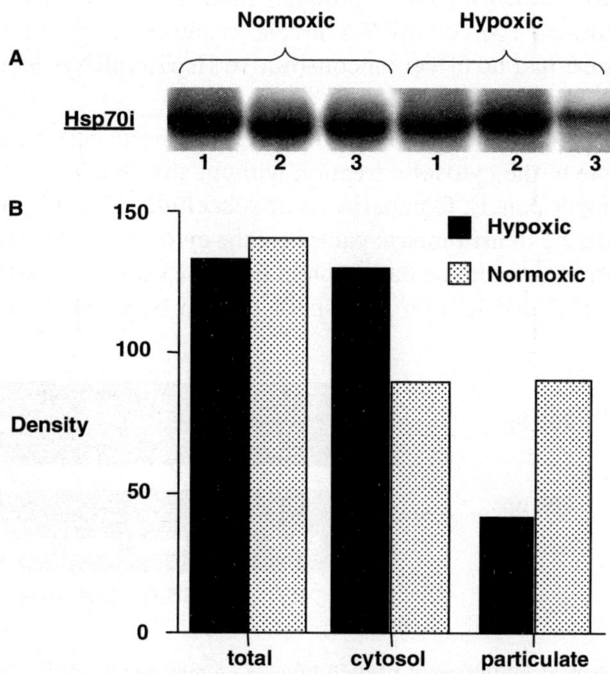

Fig. 10. Inducible Hsp70 protein level in normoxic and chronically hypoxic infant rabbit heart. Analysis of total lysate, cytosolic and particulate fractions was carried out as described in methods. A) Western blot demonstrates that in hypoxic heart 74% of Hsp70i protein is localized primarily in the cytosolic fraction with 26% localized in the particulate fraction. In normoxic hearts Hsp70i protein was equally distributed between the cytosolic fraction and particulate fractions. 1 = total lysate, 2 = cytosolic fraction, 3 = particulate fraction. B) Densitometric measurement of Hsp70i protein in normoxic and hypoxic hearts representative of four experiments.

normoxic rabbit hearts, Hsc70 was equally distributed between the cytosolic and particulate fractions, with no detectable increase in Hsc70 protein levels in the total lysates. Thus the Hsp70 signaling mechanisms activated by chronic hypoxia in infant rabbit hearts appear identical to those activated by cyanotic heart defects in infant human hearts. Moreover, this pattern of activation is also present in freshly excised rabbit hearts not subjected to perfusion prior to analysis.

Relationship between Hsp70 and protein kinases

The mechanisms by which Hsp70 expression are controlled in infant hearts adapted to chronic hypoxia are unknown. The relationship of Hsp70 to these protein kinases in the signal transduction pathway activated by chronic hypoxia in infant rabbit hearts has been determined by perfusing the isolated heart with inhibitors of PKC, p38 MAPK and JNK. Hearts were then examined for inducible and constitutive Hsp70 message levels by RT-PCR. Total cell lysates, cytosolic and particulate fractions were analyzed for distribution of constitutive and inducible Hsp70 protein by Western blot analysis.

Adaptation to chronic hypoxia results in increased message levels for Hsp70i (Figure 11). Perfusion of normoxic rabbit hearts with SB203580 (15 μmol/L), an inhibitor of p38 MAPK, had no effect on the message level for Hsp70i. However SB203580 decreased Hsp70i mRNA levels in chronically hypoxic hearts. The PKC inhibitor chelerythrine (1 μmol/L), had no effect on Hsp70i message levels in normoxic hearts, but reduced Hsp70i mRNA levels in chronically hypoxic hearts (Figure 10). SB203580 and chelerythrine had no effect on constitutive Hsp70 mRNA levels in either normoxic or chronically hypoxic hearts (Figure 12).

Furthermore adaptation to chronic hypoxia results in a shift in sub cellular redistribution for Hsp70i protein from the particulate to the cytosolic fraction without any changes in the protein level for total cell lysates (Figure 13, upper panel). Comparisons of subcellular Hsp70i protein distribution can be easily achieved by normalizing densitometric values for the cytosolic and particulate fractions, and can be seen in the relative distributions in the bar graph in Figure 13 (lower panel). These normoxic hearts have an approximately equal distribution of Hsp70i protein between the cytosolic and particulate

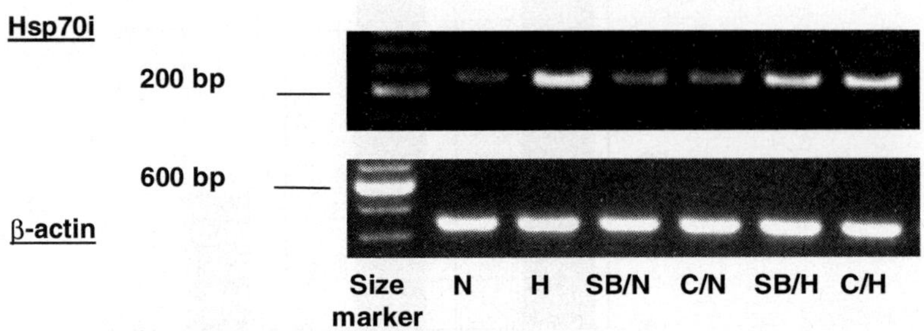

Fig. 11. Effect of pharmacological inhibition of protein kinases on message levels for inducible Hsp70 in normoxic and chronically hypoxic infant rabbit heart. RT-PCR using primers for Hsp70i demonstrates message levels 4-5 fold higher in untreated chronically hypoxic hearts compared with untreated normoxic hearts. β-actin served as an internal control. Message levels for Hsp70i were reduced in chronically hypoxic but not normoxic hearts following 15 minutes perfusion with SB30580 and chelerythrine. Data shown are representative of four hearts analyzed for each condition studied. N = Normoxic, untreated, H = Hypoxic, untreated, SB/N = Normoxic heart treated with SB203580, C/N = Normoxic heart treated with chelerythrine, SB/H = Hypoxic heart treated with SB203580, C/H = Hypoxic heart treated with chelerythrine.

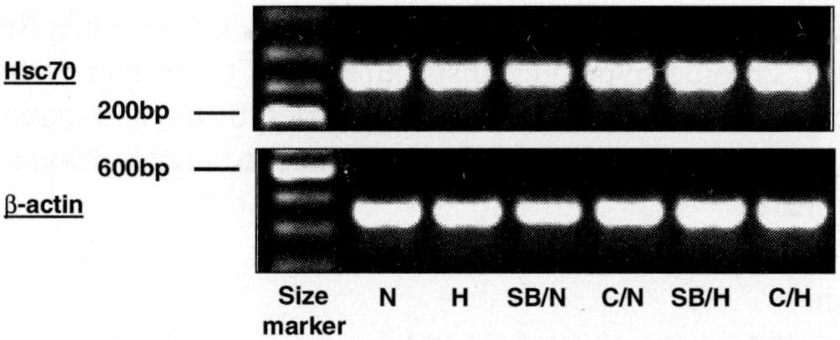

Fig. 12. Effect of pharmacological inhibition of protein kinases on message levels for constitutive Hsp70 in rabbit heart. RT-PCR using primers for Hsc70 demonstrate equal message levels for both normoxic and chronically hypoxic hearts. ®-actin served as an internal control. No changes present in Hsc70 message levels following SB203580 and chelerythrine treatment of normoxic and chronically hypoxic hearts. Data shown are representative of four hearts analyzed for each condition studied. N = Normoxic, H = Hypoxic, SB/N = Normoxic heart treated with SB203580, C/N = Normoxic heart treated with chelerythrine, SB/H = Hypoxic heart treated with SB203580, C/H = Hypoxic heart treated with chelerythrine. C/H = Chelerythrine/Hypoxic.

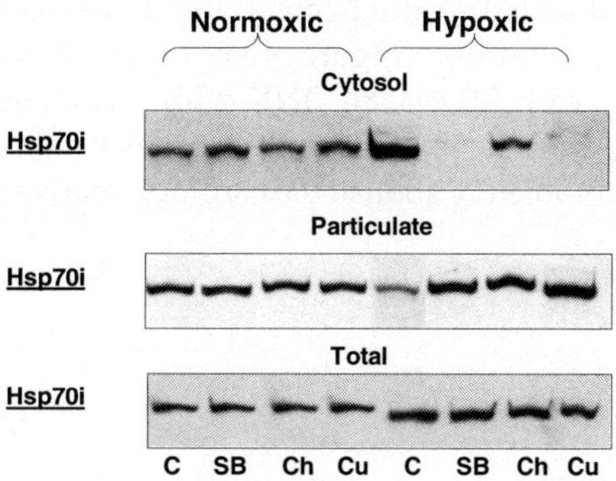

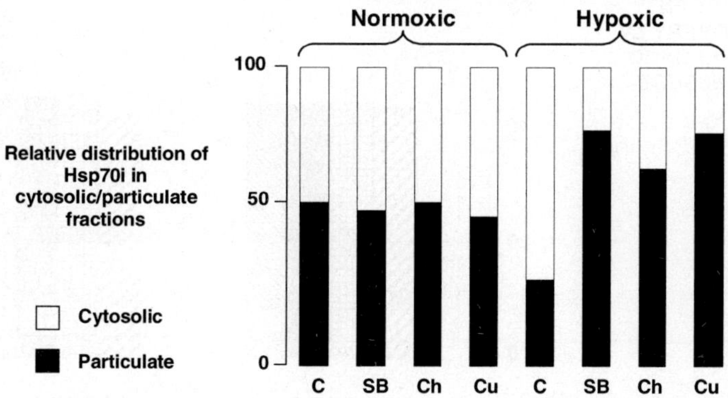

Fig. 13. Effect of pharmacologic inhibitors of protein kinases on inducible Hsp70 protein in rabbit heart total lysate, cytosolic and particulate fractions. Western blot shows that in hearts adapted to chronic hypoxia, Hsp70i translocates from the particulate to the cytosolic fraction. Pharmacologic inhibition of protein kinases had no effect on translocation of Hsp70i in normoxic hearts; however, in chronically hypoxic hearts SB203580, chelerythrine and curcumin reversed the sub cellular redistribution of Hsp70i protein caused by chronic hypoxia. C = Untreated control, SB = SB203580 treated, Ch = Chelerythrine treated, Cu = Curcumin treated.

fractions. Moreover this distribution was unaffected by perfusion with either SB203580, chelerythrine or curcumin. In contrast, chronic hypoxia redistributed Hsp70i protein from the particulate to the cytosolic fractions, which was reversed by SB20350, chelerythrine and curcumin (Figure 13, lower panel). Thus PKC, p38 MAPK and JNK appears to influence localization and redistribution of Hsp70i in chronically hypoxic hearts.

Resistance to ischemia

Cardiac function and the effects of protein kinase inhibitors on aerobic function prior to ischemia were determined in infant normoxic and chronically hypoxic rabbit hearts. Coronary flow rate was 18% higher in hypoxic hearts than normoxic controls as an adaptive response to increased oxygen delivery to the myocardium. Right ventricular developed pressure was higher in chronically hypoxic hearts than in normoxic hearts as a consequence of right ventricular hypertrophy. Chelerythrine (1 μmol/L), SB203580 (15 μmol/L), curcumin (10 μmol/L) and PD98059 (10 μmol/L) did not exert any affect on heart rate, coronary flow or developed pressure in left or right ventricle in normoxic or chronically hypoxic hearts prior to ischemia. Recovery of developed pressure in the left ventricle following ischemia in hearts not subjected to drug intervention was greater in chronically hypoxic hearts compared with normoxic controls (Figure 14). In normoxic hearts inhibition of PKC with chelerythrine, p38 MAPK with SB203580, JNK with curcumin and p42/44 MAPK with PD98059 prior to ischemia did not affect post-ischemic recovery of function. In contrast, chelerythrine, SB203580 and curcumin completely abolish the cardioprotective effects of chronic hypoxia. PD98059

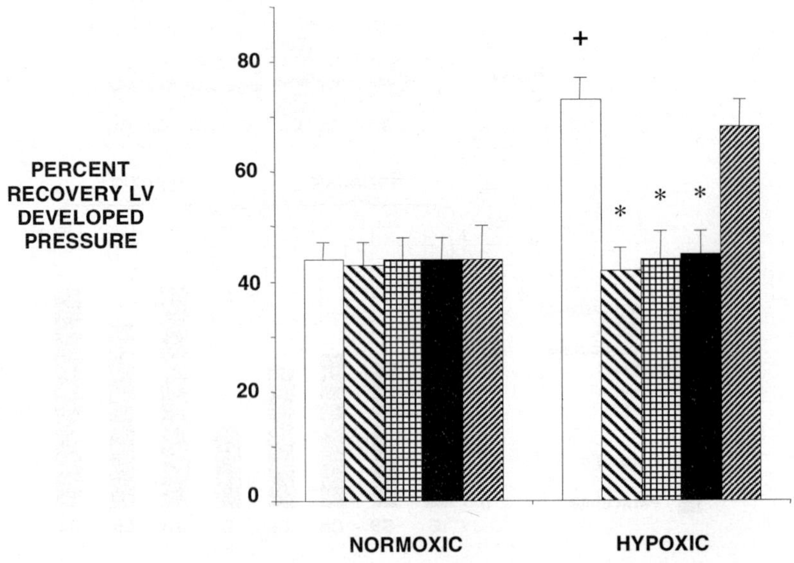

Fig. 14. Recovery of left ventricular developed pressure in infant rabbit heart following 15 min treatment with chelerythrine (1 μmol/L), SB203580 (15 μmol/L) curcumin (10 μmol/L) and PD98059 (10μmol/L) prior to 30 min global ischemia and 35 min reperfusion. □, control: ▧, chelerythrine: ▦, SB203580: ■, curcumin and ▨, PD98059. LV = left ventricle. Data are means ± SD (n=8 hearts/group). + = $p < 0.05$, normoxic vs. hypoxic, * = $p < 0.05$, drugs vs. control.

did not affect recovery of post-ischemic function in chronically hypoxic hearts. Recovery of post-ischemic function in the right ventricle for all drugs paralleled the change observed in the left ventricle.

Discussion

Although chronic hypoxia in infant rabbits increases resistance of the heart to global ischemia (16) the mechanisms by which hearts adapt to chronic hypoxia and resist subsequent ischemia remain unknown. Many of the signaling mechanisms activated by chronic hypoxia in infant rabbits are identical to those activated in infant humans. For example, infant human and rabbit hearts adapt to chronic hypoxia *via* PKC_{ε}, p38 MAPK and JUN kinase activation, but not p42/44 MAPK. Furthermore, activation of PKC_{ε}, p38 MAPK and JUN kinase but not p42/44 MAPK mediates cardioprotection in chronically hypoxic infant rabbits. Infant human hearts adapt to the stress of chronic hypoxia by increasing expression of Hsp70i message and redistributing Hsp70i protein from the particulate to the cytosolic fraction. In contrast, chronic hypoxia does not alter expression of Hsc70 message or sub cellular distribution of Hsc70 protein. Infant rabbit hearts also adapt to chronic hypoxia by increasing expression of Hsp70i message and sub cellular redistribution of Hsp70i protein. Thus the remarkably similar ways in which infant human and rabbit hearts adapt to chronic hypoxia suggest the rabbit may be useful to test adaptive mechanisms thought to occur in humans. Taken together, increased expression of Hsp70i message and sub cellular redistribution of Hsp70i protein are important adaptive responses to chronic hypoxia. Although the techniques for inducing chronic hypoxia in the infant rabbit are different from those present in infant humans with congenital defects, changes in cell signaling and chaperone function in the infant rabbit parallel the changes that take place in human infants with congenital birth defects.

Increased gene expression is often controlled by the sequential activation of cytoplasmic protein kinases. If activation of PKC and MAPK in hearts adapted to chronic hypoxia is related to Hsp70, then it would be expected that Hsp70i mRNA expression and sub cellular distribution of Hsp70i protein in chronically hypoxic infant rabbit hearts would be influenced by protein kinases, including PKC, p38 MAPK and JNK.

Adaptation to chronic hypoxia

Chronically hypoxic human infant and rabbit hearts demonstrate activation of PKCe which is evident by translocation of the PKC_{ε} isoform from the cytosolic to the particulate fraction. PKCe but not the α, β, δ, γ, and ζ isoforms of PKC were phosphorylated and translocated in hearts adapted to chronic hypoxia. PKC_{ε} is critical for cardiac myocyte protection by hypoxic preconditioning in a cell culture model (22). Changes in specific PKC isoforms located in the myocardium have been reported, particularly in ischemic preconditioning, ischemia-reperfusion, heart failure due to cardiomyopathy, and diabetes (17, 23-25). Thus activation of PKCe is an important adaptive response to chronic hypoxia.

Chronic hypoxia also results in activation of p38 MAPK and JUN kinase but not p42/p44 MAPK in both human and rabbit hearts. Phosphorylation and activation of Hsp27 a substrate for p38 MAPK is present in chronically hypoxic infant hearts but not in normoxic hearts. Chronic hypoxia also causes phosphorylation of Activating Transcription Factor ATF-2, a substrate for p38 MAPK. Thus activation of protein kinase signaling pathways occurs in infant human hearts in response to the stress of chronic hypoxia. In chronically hypoxic rabbit hearts inhibition of PKC_{ε} by chelerythrine prevents the activation and the translocation of PKC_{ε} and p38 MAPK but not p42/44 MAPK. Inhibition of p38 MAPK by SB203580 did not inhibit PKC_{ε} translocation in chronically hypoxic hearts. Thus in chronically hypoxic rabbit hearts PKCe appears upstream of the p38 MAPK pathway.

Adaptation to chronic hypoxia appears to stimulate phosphorylation of protein kinases to convert these signaling molecules from an inactive to an active state. Once activated protein kinases translocate from the cytosolic to the particulate fraction, where their presence is associated with increased cardioprotection. Inhibition of activated PKCe, p38 MAPK and JNK with the use of specific pharmacologic agents reverses chronic hypoxia-induced translocation of protein kinases resulting in the abolition of cardioprotection. One explanation for this may be that adaptation to hypoxia maintains protein kinases in a chronically active state with activation maintained by a mechanism involving continuous shuttling of protein kinases between the cytosolic and particulate fractions. These events would in turn maintain activation of nuclear transcription factors resulting in altered expression of target genes that confer cardioprotection.

Activation of PKC, p38 MAPK and JNK influences expression of mRNA for Hsp70i and sub cellular distribution of Hsp70i protein in hearts adapted to chronic hypoxia. This may lead to the synthesis of related proteins involved in cellular protection against injury or repair of injury. The finding that Hsp70i is regulated by protein kinases supports the work of Das *et al* (26) who demonstrated that stress induced by repeated cycles of ischemia and reperfusion in the heart results in activation of the p38 MAPK-MAPKAP2 pathway and induction of Hsp70, which is blocked by both genistein and SKF. There are no differences in either inducible or constitutive Hsp32 isoforms present in normoxic and chronically hypoxic hearts for both infant rabbit and human (18). These data suggest selective activation of some but not all small molecular weight Hsps in response to the stress of chronic hypoxia in infant human heart.

Perfusion of chronically hypoxic infant rabbit hearts with pharmacologic inhibitors of protein kinases for only 15 minutes results in reduced expression of Hsp70i message and a corresponding redistribution of Hsp70i protein from the cytosolic to the particulate fraction. Inhibition of protein kinases has no effect on expression of mRNA for Hsc70 or distribution of Hsc70 protein within the cell. The short time period required for inhibition of Hsp70i mRNA suggests a high turnover rate for Hsp70. SB203580, a selective p38 MAPK inhibitor, decreases Hsp70i message and redistributes Hsp70i protein in chronically hypoxic but not normoxic hearts. Thus p38 MAPK activity is essential for hypoxia-induced upregulation of Hsp70i which may contribute to subsequent cardioprotection and confirms previous findings in chronically hypoxic astrocytes where SB203580 attenuated the increase in Hsp70 message (27). Inhibition of p38 MAPK with SB203580 also abolishes the effect of Hsp70 on cytokine induced accumulation of NOS2 message (28). Furthermore, hypertonic induction of Hsp70 message in the kidney is inhibited by SB203580 (29). These findings suggest p38 MAPK activation is essential for adaptation to stress by induction of heat shock proteins. However, inhibition of Hsp70 by SB203580 may be the result of inhibition of HSF-1 phosphorylation. The effect of staurosporine, a potent PKC inhibitor, on HSF-HSE binding indirectly by heat in HT-29 cells was examined by Erdos and Lee (30). They demonstrated that staurosporine treatment did not alter heat-induced HSF-HSE binding ability and concluded that staurosporine did not inhibit HSF-1 phosphorylation. However staurosporine suppresses the accumulation of Hsp70 mRNA and Hsp70 in HT-29 cells induced by heat. A possible explanation is that Hsp70 mRNA suppression was the result of decrease in initiation and elongation activity of the Hsp70 gene. Similarly, general inhibitors of PKC, PKA and PKG (e.g. H-7 and H-8) suppress heat-induced accumulation of Hsp70 mRNA by (31) and suggest that protein kinases contribute to the synthesis of Hsp70 mRNA *via* HSF-1 phosphorylation without showing which protein kinase was involved. Regulation of HSF-1 phosphorylation *via* PKC and H-7 suppresses the DNA binding of HSF-1 (12). In addition to protein kinases, other genes have been shown to be important in regulating Hsp70 expression in response to stress. In an elegant study by Zhao *et al* on the role of the double-stranded RNA-dependent protein kinase gene (*pkr*), this gene was shown to be essential in the heat stress response and is involved in regulating expression of Hsp70 and other heat shock proteins through mRNA stabilization (32).

Amrani *et al* (9) and Okubo *et al* (21) have shown that introduction of exogenous mRNA for Hsp70 using gene transfer translates to an increase in Hsp70 protein content. However these studies performed on total cell lysates did not determine whether increased Hsp70 protein expression results in sub cellular redistribution of Hsp70 protein. Adaptation to chronic hypoxia results in an increase in endogenous mRNA for Hsp70i without a corresponding increase in protein content in total cell lysates. However there is a substantial change in the extent of sub cellular distribution for Hsp70i protein in chronically hypoxic hearts, with Hsp70i redistribution controlled by several protein kinases. Thus protein kinase-mediation of mRNA expression occurs that translates to sub cellular redistribution of Hsp70 protein in response to the stress of chronic hypoxia in the infant human and rabbit heart (18). Di *et al* (33) also have shown that in lymphocytes, Hsp70 undergoes a similar dynamic and reversible change in sub cellular distribution in response to heat stimuli. Furthermore, Hsp70 protein expression and distribution is controlled by PKC, which results in aggregation of Hsp70 with PKC, which is inhibitable by calphostin C. Thus Hsp70 mRNA expression and subcellular distribution of Hsp70i in chronically hypoxic infant rabbit hearts is influenced by protein kinases such as PKCe, p38 MAPK and JNK.

Resistance to myocardial ischemia

Rigorously controlled studies of resistance to myocardial ischemia can be performed in isolated hearts from rabbits, where a single experimental variable can be examind, but not in humans. Thus the rabbit heart has utility to study of mechanisms of cardioprotection that can be applied to humans, especially as many of the mechanisms responsible for adaptation to hypoxia in infant rabbit are identical to those in infant human. Perfusion of rabbit hearts prior to ischemia with inhibitors of PKC_{ε}, p38 MAPK and JUN kinase alone abolishes the cardioprotective effects of chronic hypoxia but has no effect in normoxic hearts. Inhibition of p42/44 MAPK by PD98059 prior to ischemia had no effect on cardioprotection in normoxic and chronically hypoxic hearts, which confirms that p42/44 MAPK does not play a role in the adaptation of infant hearts to hypoxia and resistance to subsequent ischemia.

Cardioprotection induced by adaptation to chronic hypoxia may involve changes in the actin cytoskeleton. Activation of p38 MAPK activates MAPKAP-2, which can in turn phosphorylate Hsp27 (34), an important regulator of actin dynamics that promotes polymerization of actin filaments, thus increasing the stability of the cytoskeleton (35). Activation of p38 MAPK prevents cytochalasin D-induced fragmentation of actin filaments, thus preserving cell viability (35, 36). Furthermore, overexpression of Hsp27 in isolated rat ventricular myocytes confers protection against simulated ischemia (14). Because prolonged ischemia is known to cause cytoskeleton disruption, activation of the MAPKAPK-2/Hsp27 pathway and preservation of the actin filaments may explain some of the cardioprotective effects of adaptation to chronic hypoxia. In addition, phosphorylated Hsp27 interacts with Daxx, a mediator of Fas-induced apoptosis, preventing the interaction of Daxx with both Ask1 and Fas to block Daxx-mediated apoptosis (37). Cardioprotection by adaptation to chronic hypoxia is also associated with activation of sarcolemmal and mitochondrial K_{ATP} channels (38). PKC activates the sarcolemmal K_{ATP} channel by phosphorylation of the pore forming Kir6.2 subunit (39). Thus activation of PKC by chronic hypoxia may mediate cardioprotection by regulating K_{ATP} channel function.

Myocardial ischemia and reperfusion injury is an important problem in the clinical setting. Surgical intervention, pharmacological therapy and physical exercise have been prescribed for the treatment of patients with cardiovascular disease. To demonstrate the importance of Hsp70 in cardioprotection, Hsp70-transgenic mice have been generated (40). In these mice, the rat Hsp70 gene is placed under control of an hCMV-IE enhancer and β-actin promoter, resulting in strong constitutive expression of Hsp70 in cardiac muscle, skeletal muscle, and brain. These mice display resistance against several models of heart ischemic injury (40-42). Also by means of adenoviruses, the protecting capacity of Hsp70 against myocardial ischemia was demonstrated (43). Another argument for a cytoprotective role of Hsp70 was provided by the construction of HSF-1 knockout mice (44). HSFs regulate the stress-inducible synthesis of HSPs (45). HSF-1 knockout mice show an increased sensitivity to LPS-induced toxicity and lethality (46). Finally, there are numerous reports clearly demonstrating a cytoprotective role of Hsp70 *in vitro* by means of heat shock induction or Hsp70 overexpression (47-49) against toxicity induced by several cytokines. Recently however, attention has focused on gene-based therapies with Hsp70 to confer cardioprotection in the setting of surgical ischemia (9, 11, 50). Thus exploitation of the Hsp70 signaling pathway may afford cardioprotection to human infants undergoing repair of congenital heart defects.

Infant human and rabbit hearts adapt to chronic hypoxia *via* activation of PKCe, p38 MAPK and JUN kinase which may control the cellular distribution of Hsp70i. These pathways may be responsible for cardioprotection in the chronically hypoxic infant rabbit heart. The response to oxygen deprivation between these two species is remarkably similar considering the origins of chronic hypoxia – a reduction in environmental oxygen levels with normal cardiac anatomy in the rabbit compared with normal oxygen levels in the human with an abnormal cardiac anatomy as a result of a congenital cyanotic defect. Protection of the infant human heart during surgical repair of congenital heart defects remains incomplete (51). As infant rabbit and human hearts adapt to chronic hypoxia by remarkably similar mechanisms, the infant rabbit heart can be used to test cardioprotective strategies that can be applied to protect the infant human heart. Exploitation of one or more of these protein kinase signaling pathways may afford increased cardioprotection to human infants undergoing repair of cyanotic as well as acyanotic congenital heart defects.

References

1. Goldberg M, Zhang HL, Steinberg SF. Hypoxia alters the subcellular distribution of protein kinase C isoforms in neonatal rat ventricular myocytes. *J Clin Invest.* 1997;99(1):55-61.
2. Sugden PH, Clerk A. "Stress-responsive" mitogen-activated protein kinases (c-Jun N-terminal kinases and p38 mitogen-activated protein kinases) in the myocardium. *Circ Res.* 1998;83(4):345-52.
3. Cook SA, Sugden PH, Clerk A. Activation of c-Jun N-terminal kinases and p38-mitogen-activated protein kinases in human heart failure secondary to ischaemic heart disease. *J Mol Cell Cardiol.* 1999;31(8):1429-34.

4. Talmor D, Applebaum A, Rudich A, Shapira Y, Tirosh A. Activation of mitogen-activated protein kinases in human heart during cardiopulmonary bypass. *Circ Res.* 2000;86(9):1004-1007.
5. Snoeckx LH, Cornelussen RN, Van Nieuwenhoven FA, Reneman RS, Van Der Vusse GJ. Heat shock proteins and cardiovascular pathophysiology. *Physiol Rev.* 2001;81(4):1461-97.
6. Ang D, Liberek K, Skowyra D, Zylicz M, Georgopoulos C. Biological role and regulation of the universally conserved heat shock proteins. *J Biol Chem.* 1991;266(36):24233-6.
7. Benjamin IJ, McMillan DR. Stress (heat shock) proteins: molecular chaperones in cardiovascular biology and disease. *Circ Res.* 1998;83(2):117-32.
8. Gething MJ, Sambrook J. Protein folding in the cell. *Nature.* 1992;355(6355):33-45.
9. Amrani M, Corbett J, Allen NJ, O'Shea J, Boateng SY, May AJ, et al. Induction of heat-shock proteins enhances myocardial and endothelial functional recovery after prolonged cardioplegic arrest. *Ann Thorac Surg.* 1994;57(1):157-60.
10. Rafiee P, Shi Y, Kong X, Pritchard Jr K, Tweddell J, Litwin S, et al. Activation of protein kinases in chronically hypoxic infant human and rabbit hearts: role in cardioprotection. *Circulation.* 2002;106:239-45.
11. Kukreja RC, Qian YZ, Okubo S, Flaherty EE. Role of protein kinase C and 72 kDa heat shock protein in ischemic tolerance following heat stress in the rat heart. *Mol Cell Biochem.* 1999;195(1-2):123-31.
12. Ohnishi K, Wang X, Takahashi H, Ohnishi T. The protein kinase inhibitor, H-7, suppresses heat induced activation of heat shock transcription factor 1. *Mol Cell Biochem.* 1999;197(1-2):129-135.
13. Hung JJ, Cheng TJ, Lai YK, Chang MD. Differential activation of p38 mitogen-activated protein kinase and extracellular signal-regulated protein kinases confers cadmium-induced HSP70 expression in 9L rat brain tumor cells. *J Biol Chem.* 1998;273(48):31924-31.
14. Martin JL, Mestril R, Hilal-Dandan R, Brunton LL, Dillmann WH. Small heat shock proteins and protection against ischemic injury in cardiac myocytes. *Circulation.* 1997;96:4343-4348.
15. Shi Y, Pritchard Jr K, Holman P, Rafiee P, Griffith O, Kalyanaraman B, et al. Chronic myocardial hypoxia increases nitric oxide synthase and decreases caveolin-3. *Free Radic Biol Med.* 2000;29:695-703.
16. Baker JE, Holman P, Gross GJ. Preconditioning in immature rabbit hearts: role of KATP channels. *Circulation.* 1999;99(9):1249-54.
17. Ping P, Zhang J, Qiu Y, Tang XL, Manchikalapudi S, Cao X, et al. Ischemic preconditioning induces selective translocation of protein kinase C isoforms epsilon and eta in the heart of conscious rabbits without subcellular redistribution of total protein kinase C activity. *Circ Res.* 1997;81(3):404-14.
18. Rafiee P, Shi Y, Pritchard KA, Jr., Ogawa H, Eis AL, Komorowski RA, et al. Cellular redistribution of inducible Hsp70 protein in the human and rabbit heart in response to the stress of chronic hypoxia: role of protein kinases. *J Biol Chem.* 2003;278(44):43636-44.
19. Maulik N, Watanabe M, Zu Y, Huang C, Cordis G, Schley J, et al. Ischemic preconditioning triggers the activation of MAP kinases and MAPKAP kinase 2 in rat hearts. *FEBS Letters.* 1996;396(2-3):233-237.
20. Seko Y, Takahashi N, Tobe K, Kadowaki T, Yazaki Y. Hypoxia and hypoxia/reoxygenation activate p65PAK, p38 mitogen- activated protein kinase (MAPK), and stress-activated protein kinase (SAPK) in cultured rat cardiac myocytes. *Biochem Biophys Res Commun.* 1997;239(3):840-4.
21. Okubo S, Wildner O, Shah MR, Chelliah JC, Hess ML, Kukreja RC. Gene transfer of heat-shock protein 70 reduces infarct size in vivo after ischemia/reperfusion in the rabbit heart. *Circulation.* 2001;103(6):877-81.
22. Gray MO, Karliner JS, Mochly-Rosen D. A selective epsilon-protein kinase C antagonist inhibits protection of cardiac myocytes from hypoxia-induced cell death. *J Biol Chem.* 1997;272(49):30945-51.
23. Bowling N, Walsh RA, Song G, Estridge T, Sandusky GE, Fouts RL, et al. Increased protein kinase C activity and expression of Ca2+-sensitive isoforms in the failing human heart. *Circulation.* 1999;99(3):384-91.
24. Strasser RH, Simonis G, Schon SP, Braun MU, Ihl-Vahl R, Weinbrenner C, et al. Two distinct mechanisms mediate a differential regualtion of protein kinase C isozymes in acute and prolonged myocardial ischemia. *Circ Res.* 1999;85:77-87.

25. Inoguchi T, Battan R, Handler E, Sportsman JR, Heath W, King GL. Preferential elevation of protein kinase C isoform beta II and diacylglycerol levels in the aorta and heart of diabetic rats: differential reversibility to glycemic control by islet cell transplantation. *Proc Natl Acad Sci U S A.* 1992;89(22):11059-63.

26. Das DK, Maulik N, Engelman RM, Rousou JA, Deaton D, Flack 3rd JE. Signal transduction pathway leading to Hsp27 and Hsp70 gene expression during myocardial adaptation to stress. *Ann NY Acad Sci.* 1998;851:129-138.

27. Uehara T, Kaneko M, Tanaka S, Okuma Y, Nomura Y. Possible involvement of p38 MAP kinase in HSP70 expression induced by hypoxia in rat primary astrocytes. *Brain Res.* 1999;823(1-2):226-30.

28. Bellmann K, Burkart V, Bruckhoff J, Kolb H, Landry J. p38-dependent enhancement of cytokine-induced nitric-oxide synthase gene expression by heat shock protein 70. *J Biol Chem.* 2000;275(24):18172-9.

29. Sheikh-Hamad D, Di Mari J, Suki WN, Safirstein R, Watts BA, 3rd, Rouse D. p38 kinase activity is essential for osmotic induction of mRNAs for HSP70 and transporter for organic solute betaine in Madin-Darby canine kidney cells. *J Biol Chem.* 1998;273(3):1832-7.

30. Erdos G, Lee YJ. Effect of staurosporine on the transcription of HSP70 heat shock gene in HT-29 cells. *Biochem Biophys Res Commun.* 1994;202(1):476-83.

31. Lee YJ, Berns CM, Erdos G, Corry PM. Effect of isoquinolinesulfonamides on heat shock gene expression during heating at 41 degrees C in human carcinoma cell lines. *Biochem Biophys Res Commun.* 1994;199(2):714-9.

32. Zhao M, Tang D, Lechpammer S, Hoffman A, Asea A, Stevenson MA, et al. Double-stranded RNA-dependent protein kinase (pkr) is essential for thermotolerance, accumulation of HSP70, and stabilization of ARE-containing HSP70 mRNA during stress. *J Biol Chem.* 2002;277(46):44539-47.

33. Di Y, Repasky E, Sujeck J. Distribution of HSP70, protein kinase C, and spectrin is altered in lymphocytes during a fever-like hyperthermia exposure. *J Cell Physiol.* 1997;172(1):44-54.

34. Freshney NW, Rawlinson L, Guesdon F, Jones E, Cowley S, Hsuan J, et al. Interleukin-1 activates a novel protein kinase cascade that results in the phosphorylation of Hsp27. *Cell.* 1994;78(6):1039-49.

35. Guay J, Lambert H, Gingras-Breton G, Lavoie JN, Huot J, Landry J. Regulation of actin filament dynamics by p38 map kinase-mediated phosphorylation of heat shock protein 27. *J Cell Sci.* 1997;110(Pt 3):357-68.

36. Huot J, Houle F, Spitz DR, Landry J. HSP27 phosphorylation-mediated resistance against actin fragmentation and cell death induced by oxidative stress. *Cancer Res.* 1996;56(2):273-9.

37. Charette SJ, Lavoie JN, Lambert H, Landry J. Inhibition of Daxx-mediated apoptosis by heat shock protein 27. *Mol Cell Biol.* 2000;20(20):7602-12.

38. Kong X, Tweddell J, Gross G, Baker J. Sarcolemmal and mitochondrial K(ATP) channels mediate cardioprotection in chronically hypoxic hearts. *J Mol Cell Cardiol.* 2001;33:1041-1045.

39. Light PE, Bladen C, Winkfein RJ, Walsh MP, French RJ. Molecular basis of protein kinase C-induced activation of ATP-sensitive potassium channels. *Proc Natl Acad Sci U S A.* 2000;97(16):9058-63.

40. Marber MS, Mestril R, Chi SH, Sayen MR, Yellon DM, Dillmann WH. Overexpression of the rat inducible 70-kD heat stress protein in a transgenic mouse increases the resistance of the heart to ischemic injury. *J Clin Invest.* 1995;95(4):1446-56.

41. Hutter JJ, Mestril R, Tam EK, Sievers RE, Dillmann WH, Wolfe CL. Overexpression of heat shock protein 72 in transgenic mice decreases infarct size in vivo. *Circulation.* 1996;94(6):1408-11.

42. Trost SU, Omens JH, Karlon WJ, Meyer M, Mestril R, Covell JW, et al. Protection against myocardial dysfunction after a brief ischemic period in transgenic mice expressing inducible heat shock protein 70. *J Clin Invest.* 1998;101(4):855-62.

43. Mestril R, Giordano FJ, Conde AG, Dillmann WH. Adenovirus-mediated gene transfer of a heat shock protein 70 (hsp 70i) protects against simulated ischemia. *J Mol Cell Cardiol.* 1996;28(12):2351-8.

44. McMillan DR, Xiao X, Shao L, Graves K, Benjamin IJ. Targeted disruption of heat shock transcription factor 1 abolishes thermotolerance and protection against heat-inducible apoptosis. *J Biol Chem.* 1998;273(13):7523-8.

45. Morimoto RI, Santoro MG. Stress-inducible responses and heat shock proteins: new pharmacologic targets for cytoprotection. *Nat Biotechnol.* 1998;16(9):833-8.

46. Xiao X, Zuo X, Davis AA, McMillan DR, Curry BB, Richardson JA, et al. HSF1 is required for extra-embryonic development, postnatal growth and protection during inflammatory responses in mice. *Embo J.* 1999;18(21):5943-52.

47. Jaattela M, Saksela K, Saksela E. Heat shock protects WEHI-164 target cells from the cytolysis by tumor necrosis factors alpha and beta. *Eur J Immunol.* 1989;19(8):1413-7.

48. Larrick JW, Wright SC. Cytotoxic mechanism of tumor necrosis factor-alpha. *Faseb J.* 1990;4(14):3215-23.

49. Margulis BA, Sandler S, Eizirik DL, Welsh N, Welsh M. Liposomal delivery of purified heat shock protein hsp70 into rat pancreatic islets as protection against interleukin 1 beta-induced impaired beta-cell function. *Diabetes.* 1991;40(11):1418-22.

50. Li F, Hayes JK, Wong KC. Gene therapy: a novel method for the treatment of myocardial ischemia and reperfusion injury—mini-review. *Acta Anaesthesiol Sin.* 2000;38(4):207-15.

51. Imura H, Caputo M, Parry A, Pawade A, Angelini GD, Suleiman MS. Age-dependent and hypoxia-related differences in myocardial protection during pediatric open heart surgery. *Circulation.* 2001;103(11):1551-6.

Adaptation Biology and Medicine (Volume 4: Current Concepts)
Editors: A. Hargens, N. Takeda and P.K. Singal

13. Hypoxic Therapy of Cardiovascular Diseases

V.I. Potievskaya

Institute General Pathology & Pathophysiology, RUSSIA

By the present time cardiovascular diseases have firmly established themselves as a primary cause of mortality. More than 30 millions have been suffering from hypertension and ischemic heart disease in Russia (1). Russia takes one of the first places in cardiovascular morbidity in Europe. (2). That is why management and especially prevention of cardiovascular diseases is one of the primary tasks of contemporary medical science.

There are many methods and medications in the cardiovascular therapeutics at present, but all drugs have negative side effects. Besides all medicines must be taking permanently. All mentioned above lowers compliance and efficacy of the drug treatment. It has been reported that the efficacy of the treatment is only 17.5% for females versus 5.7% for males in Russia.

The method of adaptation to intermittent normobaric hypoxia (INH) has been invented in Russia by R.B.Strelkov and A.Ya.Chizhov (3, 4, 5). The method was perfected in 1970. INH has been using in health care since 1973. The development and perfection of this method has led to its current highly effective application to increase bodily resistance to adverse environmental agents, physical and mental stresses and fatigue, and also to treat patients with various common internal diseases.

This method involves the inhalation of gaseous mixtures with reduced oxygen content in accordance with various schemes. Curative and rehabilitative effect of INH on cardiovascular diseases is connected with the influence of hypoxia on the main pathological mechanisms (6).

Adaptation to hypoxia has been shown to reduce aldosteron production and stimulate release of bradykinin. Bradykinin has a vasodilatator effect resulting from the stimulation of the receptors on endothelial cells and release of nitric oxide, prostacyclin and the endothelium derived hyperpolarizing factor (7).

Completed adaptation to hypoxia has been proven to reduce activity of sympathetic nervous system (8).

It has been also reported that adaptation to hypoxia stimulates organization of new microvessels and reduction in structural component of peripheral vascular resistance (9).

This study was aimed towards estimation of INH influence on health conditions, clinical and functional parameters in patients with cardiovascular diseases, i.e. hypertension and ischemic heart disease.

Materials and methods

137 patients with hypertension (mean age 46.3±0.2 years, 70 male and 67 female) have been followed up. 18 patients had also ischemic heart disease. A half of the patients (66, or 48.2%) have been suffering from cardiovascular diseases more than 10 years, 22 (16.1%) – 6 – 10 years, 40 (29.2%) – 1 – 5 years, 9 (6.6%) – less than 1 year. Recrudescence of the disease occurred less than once a year in 28 (20.4%) patients, 1- 2 times a year – in 67 (48.9%), 3 times a year and more – in 42 (30.7%). In 90 (65.7%) hypertension was hereditary determined. 84 (61.3%) patients have been treated only by the INH method. 53 (38.7%) patients received multimodality therapy with INH and drugs. The study have been performed comparing the INH therapy versus placebo. Placebo group consisted of 59 patients with hypertension and ischemic heart disease. The sessions of treatment have been imitated by inhaling atmospheric air through apparatus "Elbrus-10A" without connection with nitrogenous balloons. The placebo group did not differ from the experimental group by composition of diagnosis and age.

63 healthy persons formed the control group.

Hypoxic therapy was held under the inhaling gaseous hypoxic mixture (GHM), containing 10% oxygen and 90% nitrogen in intermittent regimen. GHM-10 was created in the apparatus for INH "Elbrus-10A". According to the methodics patients were given GHM-10 for 3 - 5 minutes, then had a rest for 3 - 5 minutes, that formed one cycle. One session of the treatment included from 4 to 10 cycles of this type. The course of INH treatment consisted of 15 - 30 sessions. All the patients of placebo group have received the course of "treatment" consisting from 10 to 20 sessions.

Computerized system "ESKIZ" was used to evaluate health reserves of the patients. "ESKIZ" has been invented by I.A.Gundarov in Scientific Research center for Preventive Medicine of Russian Academy of Medical Science. "ESKIZ" is based on the long term follow up thousands of patients (10). The examination was performed in the morning before meals or 2 hours after light breakfast. Patients were to avoid psychoemotional stresses, intensive physical exercises, alcohol excesses and other unusual situations. Smoking was prohibited one hour before the examination. The examination was not carried out during acute diseases, one month after recuperation and if the body temperature had been increased. The examination included inquiry, measurement of height, weight, blood pressure and heart rate. The questionnaire consisted of following chapters:

A. Chest pain.

   This chapter included the standard questionnaire of World Health Organization for angina pectoris.

B. Neurological questionnaire.

   This chapter included the standard questionnaire for initial signs of cerebral circulation insufficiency. This questionnaire has been worked out using criterions of Scientific Research Institute of Neurology of Russian Academy of Medical Science.

C. Smoking (regular or not, anamnesis).

D. Cough, sputum.

   This chapter included the questionnaire of the London School for Hygiene and Tropic Diseases for revealing symptoms of chronic bronchitis.

E. Anamnesis.

This chapter consisted of questions revealing myocardial infarction or stroke in anamnesis.

F. Self-evaluation of the health quality.

This chapter included self-evaluation of health, life in general and psychoemotional condition last time.

G. Psysiological parameters.

Height - measurement was carried out without shoes with precision up to 0.5 sm.

Weight - measurement was carried out without shoes and warm clothes with precision up to 100g.

Blood pressure - measurement was carried out with precision up to 1 mm Hg.

Pulse rate had been measuring during 1 minute patient's hand lying on a table. The measurement was carried out once.

Age.

Area of residence for the last 2 years.

All the results of the questionnaire were written down in the special form and afterwards in the computer program.

By means of the "ESKIZ" program the health index was calculated and health reserve determined. There were 5 groups varied from very small to very large health reserves. The program also determined probability of favourable prognosis for the nearest 8 years (from less than 70% to more than 99%) and the part of potential mortality in the groups for the nearest 8 years (from every 3rd to every 100th). Cerebral vascular tone has been evaluated by the program. This parameter allowed revealing signs of cerebral circulation insufficiency.

The program also calculated the Kettle index (weight in kg and body surface in square meters ratio) and indicated signs of diseases and risk factors.

All these data were included in the standard conclusion.

To assess general working capacity exercise test PWC has been performed. The first exercise was determined according to the weight: 0.5 Wt/kg for male and 0.25 Wt/kg for female. Physical exercise had been performing for 5 minutes, then patients had a rest for 3 minutes. The equation for assessing the second exercise is:

$N_2 = N_1 + F - f_1 x17/10$ for male and

$N_2 = N_1 + F - f_1 x17/15$ for female.

N_1 – the first physical exercise capacity;

F – submaximal heart rate for appropriate age group;

f_1 – heart rate at the last 30 seconds of physical exercise.

The second exercise had been performing for 5 minutes, then patients had a rest for 5 minutes. ECG was registered in the leads dorsalis, anterior and inferior before the exercise test, at the 2nd and 5th minutes of each exercise and at the end of each period of rest.

PWC was calculated using the equation:

$PWC = N_1 + (N_2 - N_1)xF - f_1/f_2 - f_1$ (kgm/min).

f_2 – heart rate at the last 30 seconds of physical exercise.

Maximal oxygen consumption was calculated using the equation:

$MOC = 1.7 \times PWC + 1240$ (ml/min) (11).

Systemic hemodynamics was assessed by Kubicek's pletismography method in modification of Yu.T.Pushkar et al. (12). The following parameters have been assessed: heart rate (HR), systolic blood pressure (SBP), diastolic blood pressure (DBP), mean blood pressure (MBP), stroke index (SI) ml/m^2, cardiac index (CI) l/m^2, specific peripheral vascular resistance (SPVR), CI and proper CI (PCI) ratio, SPVR and proper SPVR (PSPVR) ratio. Proper values were calculated:

PCI = PCO/S,

PCO – proper cardiac output, S - body square.

PCO = PBM/422,

PBM – proper basal metabolism (11).

PSVR = MBP/PCI.

Hyperkinetic type of systemic hemodynamics was determined when CI>PCI and SPVR<PSPVR, eukinetic type - when CI>PCI and SPVR> or = PSPVR, hypokinetic - when CI< PCI and SPVR>PSPVR.

To assess kinetics of oxygen metabolism (KOM) transcutaneous polarography method has been used (oxygen monitor TCM-1, FRG). Evaluation of KOM is widely used in clinical practice as an objective and comfortable test for assessment of tissue respiration intensity. In normoxic gaseous medium in apparently healthy adults the correlation ratio $TcPO_2/PO_2$ is within the range 0.7 - 0.98. The correlation ratio remains high and relatively constant in considerable fluctuations of hematocrit and arterial blood pressure. Hence, the tendency of $TcPO_2$ alterations in normal barometric pressure reliably reflects the dynamics of PO_2. The body is an open reactive system where the processes of O_2 consumption are balanced by the processes of delivery thereof. Consequently, the value $TcPO_2$ is an integral one (i.e. is formed by oxygen delivery by the cells and the rate of oxygen consumption and cannot therefore reflect the presence of tissue hypoxia and the degree of its severity. A relatively high level of PO_2 in tissues of the body corresponds to this stationary condition. It is necessary to transfer the body into a special condition to study the dynamics of oxygen consumption by the bodily tissue (13).

To measure the process of oxygen consumption the local ischemia has been created by overpressing brachial artery with a cuff under 200 mm Hg; in a case when BP is higher - under 20 - 25 mm higher than BP. After a hand of a patient was overpressed, $TcPO_2$ falls down to the zero level. When the air from the cuff is let out, $TcPO_2$ will be returned to the primary level (figure 1).

During the period of the local ischemia the processes of oxygen consumption have been assessed. After the local ischemia had been stopped, we assessed processes of oxygen delivery during the period of restoration of blood circulation.

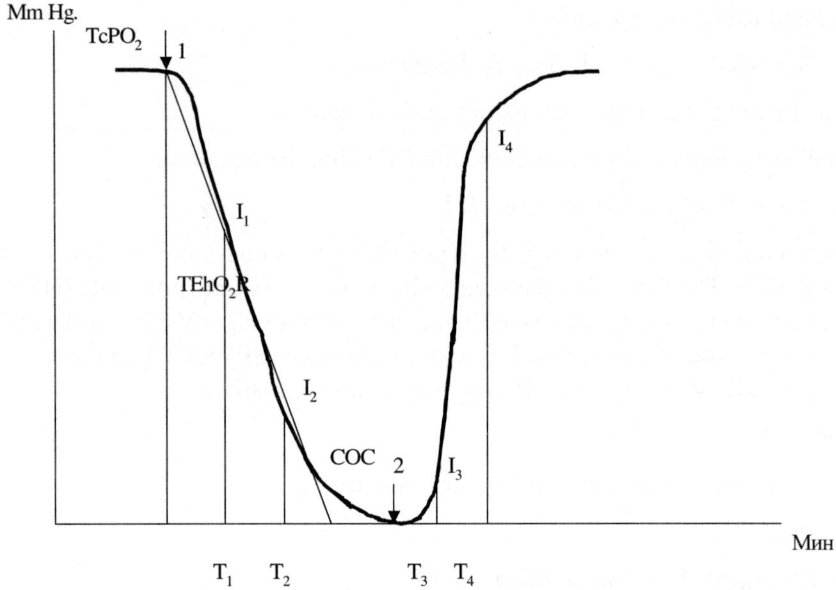

Fig. 1. Assessment of kinetics of oxygen metabolism by means of trancutaneous polarography
1 – creation of local ischemia
2 – stoppage of local ischemia

The following parameters have been evaluated: transcutaneous oxygen partial pressure in arteriolized blood (TcPO2), time of the exhaustion of oxygen reserve (TEO_2R), time of exhaustion of a half of oxygen reserve ($TEhO_2R$), constant of the speed of oxygen absorption (CSO_2A), constant of the speed of oxygen restoration (CSO_2R), CSO_2R/CSO_2A ratio, time of aerobic processes (TAP), time of anaerobic processes (TAnP), TAnP/TAP ratio, critical oxygen concentration (COC) (14).

The hypoxic test has been performed in 37 patients. The patients inhaled GHM-10 in intermittent regimen: 5 - 7 minutes of breathing with GHM-10 alternated with 5 - 7 minutes of breathing with atmospheric air (one complete cycle). The followed patients have been given 4 - 5 cycles per a session. KOM was assessed before and after the hypoxic test in this group of the patients. The polarographic curve had been recording continiously during the hypoxic test. The scheme of hypoxic treatment has been calculated by the computer program and included the time of GHM-10 inhaling, the time of breathing with atmospheric air and a number of cycles per a session. The time of GHM-10 inhaling has been determined as a maximal time needed for 50% $TcPO_2$ reduction. The time of breathing with atmospheric air has been determined as a time needed for $TcPO_2$ complete restoration.

It is known that a precise assessment of efficacy of any therapy in hypertensive patients requires the 24-hour BP monitoring (15, 16). 62 hypertensives have been examined using this method. 32 patients received multimodality treatment including INH and drug therapy (ACE-inhibitors, b-blockers, calcium antagonists and diuretics). 30 patients received only drug therapy. BP monitoring was performed using the apparatus "Meditech" ABPM-02" (Hungary). Following indices have been assessed: maximal, minimal and mean SBP, DBP, MBP and HR; SBP and DBP variability - VSBP and VDBP; daily index (DI) - mean diurnal and nocturnal BP ratio (%); time index, representing %

increased BP measurements (normal readings—not more than 140/90 for diurnal BP and not more than 120/80 for nocturnal BP); square index (SI), representing duration of a period of increased BP and a degree of BP elevation.

The Shtange's test (measurement of maximal time of delay of breathing on inspiration) has been performed in all the patients.

All the patients have been examined twice: before and after the course of INH.

The following examinations have been performed in placebo group: BP and HR measurements, PWC test and MOC calculation, Shtange's test, assessment of systemic hemodynamics. All the data have been obtained twice—before and after the course imitating hypoxic therapy.

Results and discussion

Significant positive effect of the hypoxic therapy has been achieved in the most of the patients (99 persons or 80.5% of total number). Slight improvement of general condition and decrease of BP level has been observed in 20 patients (16.2%). There was no any clinical effect in 4 patients (3.3%). None of the patients has demonstrated change for the worse or increase in BP level. Clinical symptoms have been eliminated in the most of the patients, general condition improved (figure 2).

Temporary BP elevations have been observed in 46 patients (37.4%). The periods of BP elevation were short and were not accompanied by any clinical symptoms. The final result of hypoxic therapy has been good enough in all 46 patients without exceptions. This fact gave ground to infer that it was only a reaction of temporary exacerbation. The reaction of exacerbation occurred in different periods of the INH course: from the 2nd to the 16th session, in average—at 7.5±0.8 session. Most frequently the recrudescence was observed between the 5th and 10th sessions of the INH therapy.

Improvement in general condition and BP decrease have been observed from the 2nd to the 25th sessions in different patients (mean 9.5±0.8 session). Patients with mild form of hypertension demonstrated the improvement earlier—at 7.8±0.7 INH session in average ($p<0.05$). There was no difference between patients with moderate and severe forms of hypertension (the improvement was revealed at 13.3±3.5 and 11.5±1.2 sessions accordingly). The encouraging results of the INH therapy permitted to discontinue the drug therapy in 38 patients (79.2%) and reduce the dosage in 10 (20.8%) patients of those had being received multimodality treatment in average at 9.9±1.2 session (varied from the 2nd to the 18th sessions in different persons).

The obtained results support the idea that the clinical effect of the INH treatment increases in the prolonged courses of hypoxic therapy. The information about this can clearly be set out in a table as follows (table 1).

The data show that patients demonstrate lower percentage of improvement after 21 - 25 sessions than after 16 - 20 sessions of the INH therapy. This fact can be explained by following preposition. The prolonged course of treatment (21 - 25 sessions) has been prescribed patients with more serious forms of diseases: moderate and severe hypertension, duration of the disease more than 10 years, the third functional class of angina pectoris, myocardial infarction or stroke in anamnesis. The results support the idea that such patients need a long-term INH treatment, because the effect of hypoxic therapy increased in the group of patients received 26 - 30 sessions. All aforesaid leads to the conclusion that patients with mild form of hypertension, stable angina pectoris I - II functional classes, suffering from

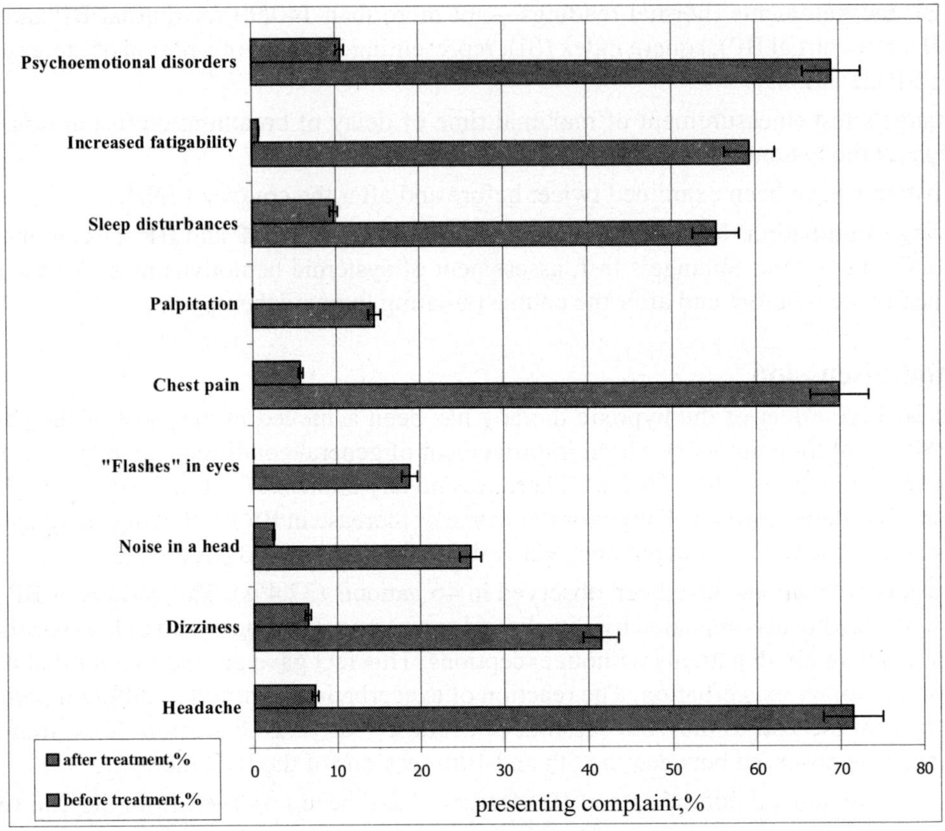

Fig. 2. Effect of INH on the main clinical symptoms in patients with with cardiovascular diseases

Table 1. Clinical effect INH depending on duration of the course

Quantity of sessions	Number of patients	% total number of patients	Significant positive effect of treatment	
			Number of patients	% total number of patients
< 15	26	21.1	18	69.2
16 – 20	56	45.5	48	85.7
21 – 25	24	19.5	18	75.0
26 – 30	17	13.8	15	88.2

cardiovascular diseases less than 10 years are recommended to undergo 16 - 20 sessions of INH. Patients with severe forms of hypertension and coronary artery disease with cardiovascular events in anamnesis need prolonged INH courses—up to 26 - 30 sessions.

Statistically reliable decrease of SBP, DBP and HR has been observed after the course of the INH treatment (table 2).

34 patients with cardiovascular diseases have been examined by 'ESKIZ" system for assessment quantity and quality of health. 7 patients have been suffering from mild hypertension, 9 - moderate

Table 2. Effect of INH therapy on blood pressure and heart rate in patients with cardiovascular diseases

	Before treatment	After treatment	P
Systolic BP	165.0±2.1	132.7±1.4	<0.001
Diastolic BP	100.3±1.1	82.8±1.0	<0.001
Mean BP	121.9±1.3	99.3±1.1	<0.001
Heart rate	61.8±0.9	57.8±0.8	<0.05

hypertension, 18 - ischemic heart disease. According to the obtained results more than a half of the followed up demonstrated low health reserve (18, or 52.9%). The examination has revealed high risk for such major ischemic events as myocardial infarction, stroke and also tumours. The calculated risk of these events was more than 30% in 10 (29.4%) patients, 16 - 30% - in 8 (23.5%), 6 - 15% - in 6 (17.6%), 1 - 5% - in 9 (26.4%) and only one patient had a potential risk less than 1%. In average potential general mortality the next 8 years could be 174 cases for each 1000 persons according to the program calculations (table 3). Such unfavourable prognostic situation is closely related to high rate of cardiovascular diseases and risk factors in general population. 15 patients (44.1%) had increased BP, 11 (32.3%) - stable angina pectoris, 21 (61.8%) - insufficiency of cerebral circulation. Chronic bronchitis has been revealed only in 3 patients (8.8%), because of the prevalence of cardiovascular diseases in this group of patients. 7 (20.6%) were smokers, 12 (35.3%) had overweight. More than a half of the patients demonstrated low quality of health. Low self-evaluation of health has been revealed in 17 (50%) persons, low social self-evaluation - in 21 (61.8%), low level of psychoemotional condition - in 23 (67.3%) - table 3.

Table 3. Summary assessment of health parameters in patients with cardiovascular diseases before and after the INH course.

		Before treatment		After treatment		P
I.	Average health parameters: health index, balls		49.0±1.3		54.0±1.4	<0.05
	potential mortality the next 8 years for 1000 persons		174±6.5		145±6.0	<0.05
	self-evaluation of health, balls		61.0±3.0		66.0±2.4	>0.05
	social self-evaluation, balls		60.0±4.2		64.0±3.9	>0.05
	psychoemotional condition, balls		57.0±2.4		67.0±3.6	<0.05
II.	Rate of different health levels	Number of the patients	%	Number of the patients	%	
	High health reserve	16	47.1±8.2	25	73.5±7.2	<0.05
	Low health reserve	18	52.9±8.2	9	26.5±7.2	<0.05
III.	Rate of diseases and risk factors:					
	Hypertension, %		44.1±8.1		8.8±4.9	<0.05
	Angina pectoris, %		32.3±7.7		5.8±3.6	<0.05
	Chronic bronchitis, %		8.8±4.9		4.0±2.7	>0.05
	Insufficiency of cerebral blood circulation, %		61.9±7.9		29.4±7.5	<0.05
	Smoking, %		20.6±6.4		26.6±6.4	>0.05
	Overweight, %		35.3±7.9		32.3±7.3	>0.05
IV.	Rate of disturbances of health quality:					
	low self-evaluation of health, %		50.0±8.2		50.0±8.2	>0.05
	low social self-evaluation, %		61.8±7.9		52.0±8.6	>0.05
	low level of psychoemotional condition, %		67.6±7.7		45.0±8.1	<0.05

Information about SBP, DBP, pulse rate, cerebral vascular tone and Kettle index can clearly be set out in the table 4.

Table 4. Effect of the INH course on functional parameters characterizing health level in patients with cardiovascular diseases.

	Before treatment	After treatment	P
SBP, mm Hg	155.9±4.1	140.8±3.7	<0.05
DBP, mm Hg	91.2±1.4	85.0±1.5	<0.05
Pulse rate, per minute	70.0±1.3	64.3±1.5	<0.05
Cerebral vascular tone, % normal	204.2±9.0	176.6±8.4	<0.05
Kettle index, kg/m^2	27.6±4.1	27.8±3.9	>0.05

Before the INH course mean BP was at the level of borderline hypertension, cerebral vascular tone was significantly elevated and reflected disturbances of cerebral blood circulation. The results obtained after the INH course have revealed the significant improvement of health quantity and quality parameters. The INH therapy resulted in increase in the main integral health parameter, i.e. health index. The results have revealed the following evidence: hypoxic therapy conferred increase in the number of patients with high health reserve and 2 times reduction in the number of patients with low health reserve. The INH treatment resulted in a significant reduction in the risk of myocardial infarction, stroke and malignant tumours. It was also observed that more than 30% potential morbidity was revealed only in 17.6% of the patients versus 29.4% before the treatment. Potential mortality the next 8 years has been reduced from 174 to 145 cases per 1000 persons.

Clinical symptoms of hypertension, angina pectoris and insufficiency of cerebral circulation have been significantly reduced (table 3). However, no changes have been observed in the number of the smokers and persons with overweight in spite of F.S.Meerson data (8). Some possible explanations for this fact can be discussed. Probably there were no adequate motives for the change of the life style.

The examination has shown positive changes of health quality in all the patients. General mood and psychological condition have been improved. INH conferred reduction in the number of persons with low health quality (P<0.05). However, there was no impact observed on social self-evaluation of the patients. It can be explained by excessive attention of the patients to their health condition because of the examination procedure and revealing a number of diseases and risk factors (so-called intervention phenomenon).

Hypoxic stimulation also resulted in SBP and DBP reduction to normal level. INH normalizing effect on hemodynamics also manifested in slowing down heart rate. Hypoxic therapy effect can be compared with physical exercise, because both the trainings lead to economical function of cardiovascular system. The followed up persons demonstrated reduction in cerebral vascular tone and, consequently, improvement of cerebral blood circulation.

The obtained results demonstrate benefits of the INH therapy in reduction of risk factors and potential mortality.

Hypoxic therapy resulted in 25.9% increase in PWC (P<0.001) and 9.8% increase in MOC (P<0.01), thereby suggesting elevation of physical training reserves (table 5).

Table 5. Effect of the INH treatment on physical working capacity and maximal oxygen consumption in patients with cardiovascular diseases.

	Before treatment	After treatment	P
PWC, kg/m/min	800.0±34.10	1007.59±35.92	<0.001
MOC, l/min	2.684±0.060	2.948±0.060	<0.01

These findings correlate with data obtained for the other groups of the persons (17). A.Ya.Chizhov and R.B.Strelkov (14) also observed increase in PWC and MOC after adaptation to hypoxia. These results support the idea that adaptation to hypoxia results in increase in possibilities of aerobic energetic metabolism due to more effective work of oxygen transport. These findings are supported by the studies of F.Z.Meerson and M.G.Pshennikova (18). The authors have shown that the hypoxic training contribute to increase in the number of mitochondrias in the cells and, consequently, increase in efficacy of oxygen metabolism.

To assess systemic hemodynamics 93 examined patients have been divided into 3 groups: I - hyperkinetic type (74 cases, or 79.6%), II - eukinetic type (11 cases, or 11.8%), hypokinetic type (8 cases, or 8.6%) - table 6.

SBP and DBP reduction was observed in all three groups of the patients, but hemodynamic changes took different ways. Group II demonstrated 29.4% SPVR reduction (P<0.05) and moderate increase in CI and SI (24.9% and 13.0%, P <0.05). More significant CI and SI elevation (29.0% and 30.3%,

Table 6. Effect of INH on systemic hemodynamics in patients with cardiovascular diseases

	Before treatment	After treatment	P
Hyperkinetic type n=74			
Stroke index, ml/m^2	68.09±2.60	69.36±2.85	>0.05
Cardiac index, l/min/m^2	4.203±0.148	3.970±0.177	>0.05
Specific peripheral vascular resistance (SPVR)	26.91±1.12	26.32±1.26	>0.05
Cardiac index/Proper cardiac index	2.036±0.073	1.910±0.075	>0.05
SPVR/Proper SPVR	0.626±0.025	0.613±0.027	>0.05
Eukinetic type n=11			
Stroke index, ml/m^2	44.05±3.4	55.03±3.1	<0.05
Cardiac index, l/min/m^2	2.734±0.107	3.090±0.091	<0.05
Specific peripheral vascular resistance (SPVR)	49.48±3.05	37.91±4.30	<0.05
Cardiac index/Proper cardiac index	1.283±0.054	1.478±0.055	<0,05
SPVR/Proper SPVR	1.200±0.063	0.918±0.093	<0,05
Hypokinetic type n=8			
Stroke index, ml/m^2	29.56±2.08	38.13±3.4	<0.05
Cardiac index, l/min/m^2	1.768±0.030	2.304±0.192	<0.05
Specific peripheral vascular resistance (SPVR)	59.72±1.24	45.34±4.82	<0.05
Cardiac index/Proper cardiac index	0.818±0.031	1.108±0.136	<0.05
SPVR/Proper SPVR	1.468±0.029	1.095±0.133	<0.05

P<0.05) was observed in group III. SPVR was also reduced in group III (24.1%, P<0.05). Ratios CI/PCI and SPVR/PSPVR were normalized after the course of the INH treatment in groups II and III.

However, there were no certain changes in group I in despite of BP reduction. It was suggestful that group I consisted of patients with different reactive types. To reveal mechanism of BP reduction we have divided group I into 3 subgroups (A, B and C) depending on SI and SPVR changes. We have taken in consideration that BP reduction can be resulted in SI or SPVR fall or simultaneous SI and SPVR reduction. The patients of subgroup A (26 cases or 35.2%) showed SI elevation and SPVR reduction, the patients of subgroup B (37 cases, or 50%) - SI reduction without certain changes of SPVR, the patients of subgroup C (11 cases, or 14.8%) - SI and SPVR reduction.

These results lead to the conclusion that BP was most frequently decreased in the patients with hyperkinetic type of hemodynamic by SI reduction. Evidence was gathered that this mechanism was most optimal for patients with hyperkinetic type because they were characterized by increased cardiac output. SI reduction was due to decrease in CI (14%, P<0.05) and HR (7.0%, P<0.05). The data support the idea that increase in cardiac output in these patients is connected with individual peculiarities of cardiovascular regulation. The patients of the subgroup C demonstrated SI (16.0%, P<0.05) and SPVR (13.1%, P<0.05) reduction. SI decrease was due to HR (9.7%, P<0.05) fall without CI changes.

Thus, BP reduction took different ways in all three hemodynamic groups of the patients, but in all cases deflected hemodynamic parameters drew near to the proper ones after the course of hypoxic treatment.The study has revealed some peculiarities of kinetics of oxygen metabolism in hypertensives differing from healthy persons of the control group (table 7).

Table 7. Kinetics of oxygen metabolism in patients with hypertension and healthy persons

	Patients with hypertension n=137	Healthy persons n=63	P
ÒñÐO_2, mm Hg.	63.3±1.4	70.1±2.1	<0.01
TEO_2R, sec	137.8±4.2	109.9±4.9	<0.001
TehO_2R, sec	38.3±1.0	32.1±2.2	<0.05
CSO_2A, sec^{-1}	0.0326±0.0012	0.0484±0.0022	<0.001
CSO_2R, sec^{-1}	0.0983±0.0011	0.0910±0.0050	>0.05
CSO_2R/CSO_2A	3.37±0.12	2.25±0.20	<0.001
COC, mm Hg	9.93±0.40	5.86±0.37	<0.001
TAP, sec	69.0±1.6	63,8±3.1	>0.05
TAnP, sec	68.7±3.3	39.4±4.1	<0.01
TAP/TAnP, sec	1.02±0.05	0.68±0.09	<0.001

TcPO_2, TEO_2R, TEhO_2R and CSO_2A usually appeared to be reduced in the hypertensive patients. These results lead to the conclusion that tissue respiration is depressed in these patients (19). Disturbances in tissue respiration may be related to microcirculation changes in systemic hypertension. Rarefication of microvessels results in reduction of oxygen delivery (20). Lowered oxygen delivery leads to tissue hypoxia and depression of tissue respiration. Increased ratio CSO_2R/CSO_2A has been observed invariably in hypertensive patients due to CSO_2A reduction. CSO_2R has been the same as in healthy persons of the control group. However, $TcPO_2$ has not been elevated, because significant oxygen metabolic disturbances have been observed in hypertension. The studies have reported that following disorders usually are revealed in systemic hypertension: malfunction of external breathing (reduction of respiration power and index of oxygen consumption), shift of HbO_2 dissociation curve to the right and downward, disturbances in diffusion through alveolar membranes due to enlarged distance from alveolas to capillaries (21).

Our study has also revealed elevation of COC in hypertensives ($P<0.001$). Consequently, these patients have showed oxygen metabolism depression during the test of regional ischemia under higher $TcPO_2$ than the patients of the control group. The results support the idea that functional energetic reserves are reduced in hypertension.

After the course of the INH treatment significant improvement of kinetics of oxygen metabolism was observed (table 8).

Table 8. Effect of the INH treatment on kinetics of oxygen metabolism in patients with hypertension

	Before treatment	After treatment	P
$TcPO_2$, mm Hg.	68.3±1.4	62.9±0.9	>0.05
TEO_2R, sec	137.8±4.2	117.4±2.7	<0.01
$TehO_2R$, sec	38.3±1.0	35.0±0.8	<0.05
CSO_2A, sec^{-1}	0.0326±0.0012	0.0447±0.0022	<0.001
CSO_2R, sec^{-1}	0.0983±0.0011	0.0977±0.010	>0.05
CSO_2R/CSO_2A	3.37±0.12	2.60±0.11	<0.001
COC, mm Hg	9.93±0.40	6.75±0.23	<0.001
TAP, sec	69.0±1.6	65.6±1.5	>0.05
TAnP, sec	68.7±3.3	51.5±1.7	<0.001
TAP/TAnP, sec	1.02±0.05	0.79±0.02	<0.01

Positive changes in kinetics of oxygen metabolism appeared to be closely related to improvement of clinical condition of the patients. Some improvement of kinetics of oxygen metabolism was revealed after the 5th session (TEO_2R was reduced, $P<0.05$). These changes were accompanied by the first signs of clinical improvement. There were no significant changes comparing the initial data after the 10th INH session (the period of clinical recrudescence). Moreover, some changes for the worse were observed comparing at the 5th INH session. It is suggestful that activity of the sympathetic nervous system increases on initial stages of adaptation to hypoxia. Increased sympathetic activity refers to BP elevation, centralization of the blood circulation and increase in oxygen delivery to the organs and systems of vital importance. Deterioration of microcirculation results in temporary inhibition of oxygen metabolism. Significant improvement of the most KOM indices was observed after the 15th INH session (table 8). CSO_2A reduction ($P<0.001$) represents improvement of cell oxygen absorption due to stimulation of tissue respiration. CSO_2R/CSO_2A ratio has been decreased. However, no significant $TcPO_2$ changes have been observed. These findings stimulate speculation about normalization of all mentioned above processes of oxygen metabolism (external breathing, diffusion through alveolar membranes, HbO_2 dissociation curve et al.) after the course of hypoxic therapy. The

INH course resulted in reduction of COC ($P<0.001$). This fact represents increase in functional energetic cell reserves and enlargement of dimensions and quantity of mitochondrias per unit of a cell. This process is to be called systemic structural trace (8). Therefore energy supply increases in a cell. The hypoxic test has demonstrated KOM inhibition after the first INH session. Following changes of parameters have been observed: 43.3% TEO_2R elevation ($P<0.05$), 84.6% CSO_2R/CSO_2A ($P<0.01$), 108.5% COC ($P<0.01$), 68.1% TAnP ($P<0.05$) and 50% TAnP/TAP ($P<0.05$) increase, 27.9% CSO_2A reduction ($P<0.05$). These changes are more significant than in the control group.

After the course of hypoxic therapy activation of compensatory reactions occurred after the hypoxic test. Increase in COC was evidently less than after the first session (97.1% versus 108.2%, $P<0.01$). However, the most important achievement of the INH treatment appeared to be acceleration of oxygen delivery processes after the hypoxic test. It was represented by 7.7% increase in CSO_2R ($P<0.05$).

The obtained results give ground to infer that hypoxic therapy contributes to enlargement of functional reserves of oxygen metabolism due to activation of oxygen transport. These findings support the view of V.B.Koshelev (22) concerning organization of new microvessels and decrease in structural component of vascular resistance. These changes result in improvement of microcirculation and increase in oxygen delivery.

Our study has also revealed some peculiarities of polarographic curve in patients with cardiovascular diseases representing $TcPO_2$ deflections during the hypoxic test. After the first INH session increase in amplitude of polarographic curve has been observed from cycle to cycle. It was accompanied by increase in $TcPO_2$ at the end of the hypoxic test (12.8% in average, $P<0.05$). Some possible explanations for these changes may be discussed. Most probably hypoxia stimulates processes of oxygen delivery to cover oxygen insufficiency. Minimal $TcPO_2$ during inhaling GHM-10 has been decreased from 42.9±1.2 to 38.9±1.3 mm Hg ($P<0.05$). Increase in $TcPO_2$ after the hypoxic test in the controls (healthy persons) was 12.3% ($P<0.05$). However, no decrease in $TcPO_2$ has been observed from cycle to cycle at the first session in the controls. There was also a difference in a degree of $TcPO_2$ fall during inhalation of hypoxic mixture between the patients and the controls. The $TcPO_2$ reduction was 31% ($P<0.01$) in the patients and 66% in the controls ($P<0.001$). It is suggestful that tissue hypoxia is present in patients with cardiovascular diseases and so they have been already adopted to hypoxia.

We observed waves of $TcPO_2$ deflections in 85.7% hypertensive patients after hypoxic inhalations during periods of breathing with atmospheric air. One of the possible explanations of this fact is stimulation of changes in vascular tone by hypoxia. These deflections may be referred to disturbances of autonomic nervous system in hypertensives.

Moreover, a paradoxal reaction on hypoxic stimulation has been evidenced in 23.8% hypertensives: $TcPO_2$ was decreased more significantly during the period of breathing with atmospheric air than during the inhalation of hypoxic mixture. After this fall $TcPO_2$ was quickly restored. The $TcPO_2$ drop may be explained by temporary spasm of microvessels due to increase in PO_2 in the inhaling air. This reaction appeared to be compensative preventing tissue injury in the reoxygenation period.

According to the results of the hypoxic test the scheme of INH treatment has been determined for patients with cardiovascular diseases. Average time of the inhaling of hypoxic mixture was 3.6±0.2 min (215±13 sec) and average time of breathing with atmospheric air was 5.9±0.4 min (352±26 sec) for the first INH session. At the end of the INH course the recommended time of GHM-10 inhaling has not been changed, however, the time of breathing with atmospheric air has been enlarged to 6.7±0.2 min (404±10 sec).

No statistical significant BP changes have been observed in the placebo group (table 9).

Table 9. BP in the patients of placebo group before and after the course imitating hypoxic therapy.

BP, mm Hg	Before the course	After the course	P
SBP	155±4.8	150.8±3.6	>0.05
DBP	96.2±3.7	93.5±3.6	>0.05

Heart rate, Shtange's test, MOC and PWC have not been also changed in the placebo group (table 10).

Table 10. Some functional parameters in the placebo group before and after the course imitating hypoxic therapy.

	Before the course	After the course	P
HR, per minute	73.2±2.1	76.3±3.3	>0.05
Time of delay of breathing on inspiration, sec	47.8±2.9	41.3±2.1	>0.05
MOC, ml/kgxmin	34.8±4.5	32.1±2.0	>0.05
PWC, kgm/min	601.6±30.3	621.5±29.6	>0.05

The study has shown no statistical significant improvement in the systemic hemodynamics in the placebo group (table 11).

Table 11. Effect of the course imitating hypoxic therapy on systemic hemodynamics in the placebo group.

	Before the course	After the course	P
SI, ml/min/m^2	52.3±2.9	55.4±2.4	>0.05
CI, l/min/m^2	4.570±0.115	4.378±0.323	>0.05
SPVR	35.6±7.5	34.7±6.8	>0.05
SI/PSI	0.826±0.111	0.897±0.098	>0.05
SPVR/PSPVR	1.211±0.078	1.219±0.086	>0.05

Thus, the results of the INH treatment significantly differ from the results of placebo.

24 hour BP monitoring showed the following results in hypertensive patients (tables 12 and 13).

The obtained results give ground to infer that all patients of the INH group and the group of the drug treatment showed improvement. However, no certain decrease has been observed in diurnal mean DBP, diurnal maximal DBP and MBP and nocturnal maximal DBP and MBP in the group of the drug treatment. These indices appeared to be diminished in the INH group. The patients of the INH group showed more significant decrease in maximal peaks of daily SBP, in mean diurnal DBP and maximal diurnal and nocturnal DBP. Thus, new evidence was uncovered that multimodality therapy appeared to be more effective in the treatment of BP elevation episodes. This fact stimulates speculation about beneficial effects of INH on cardiovascular events. Simultaneous using of INH and drug therapy contributed to more significant reduction in minimal daily BP (14.6% SBP, 11.7% DBP and 17.6% MBP decrease in the main group versus 9.7% SBP, 15.4% DBP and 14.4% MBP decrease in the group of the drug therapy, P<0.05) . INH also resulted in more significant elevation of daily index (85.3% SBP and 61.5% DBP increase in the INH group versus 31.5% SBP and 21% increase in the group of the drug therapy, P<0.05). Normalization of 24 hour BP profile was accompanied by increase in the number of patients with adequate BP reduction in the night. After the INH course the patients demonstrated more significant reduction in duration of episodes of BP elevation: 76% lowering of square index was observed for SBP and 78.2% - for DBP comparing with 56.2% for SBP and 65.7% for DBP in the group of the drug treatment. Multimodality treatment resulted in reduction in hypertension load lower than 25%. These changes appeared to be more significant than those after the drug therapy (tables 12 and 13).

Table 12. Effect of INH therapy on 24-hour BP profile in hypertensive patients

	Before treatment			After treatment		
	24 hour	day	night	24 hour	day	night
Mean SBP, mm Hg	133.4±6.8	137.5±8.2	125.2±4.3	120.7±2.5*	126.0±3.2*	107.7±1.8*
Mean DBP, mm Hg	78.2±5.9	84.5±6.9	72.9±2.2	70.9±3.0*	76.4±3.1*	61.1±3.2*
SBP max, mm Hg	166.8±6.6	169.3±8.7	148.1±9.5	153.0±3.9*	156.8±4.3*	129.7±1.2*
DBP max, mm Hg	100.0±3.1	104.3±6.6	85.5±6.8	94.3±1.8*	98.8±4.6*	79.5±2.8
SBP min, mm Hg	104.4±6.6	110.6±2.8	107.0±2.9	89.2±1.8*	94.0±3.7*	89.0±5.1*
DBP min, mm Hg	53.5±5.2	62.0±2.1	57.2±3.8	44.1±1.4*	52.1±2.9	46.2±4.1*
TISBP, %	31.2±2.6	34.5±6.8	35.3±3.2	19.4±2.8*	17.8±9.1*	25.7±4.1*
TIDBP, %	23.0±3.2	24.9±4.2	23.5±6.8	13.6±1.1*	15.6±3.8*	8.1±3.2*
DISBP,%	6.8±2.1			12.6±3.4*		
DIDBP, %	10.4±2.8			16.8±3.2*		

· p<0.05 comparing with data before the INH treatment

Table 13. Effect of INH therapy on 24 hour BP profile in hypertensive patients

	Before treatment			After treatment		
	24 hour	day	night	24 hour	day	night
SBP mean, mm Hg	137.7±3.6	140.7±3.6	127.6±3.8	124.8±3.3*	128.7±3.6*	112.2±1.8*
DBP mean, mm Hg	81.5±3.9	83.8±3.8	73.5±4.3	72.5±4.2*	75.5±4.3	62.3±3.0*
SBP max, mm Hg	174.4±6.1	174.2±3.4	149.3±6.1	161.2±2.9*	161.2±4.2*	135.5±2.2*
DBP max, mm Hg	105.2±2.2	105.2±6.1	87.1±3.7	96.1±2.9*	97.0±3.0	81.6±5.2
SBP min, mm Hg	104.8±2.6	108±2.8	110.1±3.5	92.5±3.1*	98.5±3.1*	94.0±3.7*
DBP min. mm Hg	56.8±3.4	60.7±2.2	59.5±4.2	46.6±2.8*	52.2±3.1*	48.8±2.9*
TISBP, %	59.1±8.0	56.2±12.1	67.4±11.4	25.2±1.7*	24.8±11.2*	28.0±4.6*
TIDBP, %	39.1±8.5	41.1±10.1	41.7±12.2	16.6±1.6*	18.5±3.3*	10.1±4.0*
DISBP,%	9.5±1.4			12.5±1.5		
DIDBP, %	13.8±2.1			16.7±2.7		

*** p<0.05 comparing with data before the INH treatment**

Before the INH course 50% hypertensive patients were “non-dippers”, 18.8% - “over-dippers”, 12.4% - “night-peakers” and only 18.8% - “dippers” according the BP profile. After the INH course “night-peakers” were not revealed, 40.6% were “dippers”, the number of “over-dippers” was the same and the number of “non-dippers” was reduced.

Improvement of BP profile has been also observed in the group of the drug treatment. No “night-peakers” were registered, the number of “non-dippers” was reduced due to increase in the number of “dippers”. However, the number of “over-dippers” appeared to be increased in this group from 10 to 30%.

Therefore the obtained results have revealed reduction in the number of “non-dippers” in the both groups. This findings support the idea that the INH course improves BP daily rhythms, restores the periods of nocturnal BP decrease and eliminates BP night peaks. However, increase in the number of “over-dippers” is unfavourable in the group of the drug treatment. Excessive nocturnal BP decrease may contribute to reduction in cerebral and coronary blood flow and increase in the risk of cardiovascular events. It is suggestful that the INH course prevents excessive nocturnal BP decrease.

The study strongly supports the concept that the main functional parameters of human body can be normalized by means of adaptation to INH. According to our findings they are: physical working capacity, maximal oxygen consumption, systemic hemodynamics, kinetics of oxygen metabolism, 24 hour BP profile.

The obtained results give ground to infer that hypoxic therapy improves clinical condition of the patients with cardiovascular diseases. The INH treatment appeares to be effective in BP reduction in hypertensive patients.

Hypoxic therapy increases quantity and quality of health and results in reduction of risk factors, morbidity and mortality in the patients with hypertension and ischemic heart disease.

Thus, the INH method can be recommended for treatment, prevention and rehabilitation in patients with cardiovascular diseases.

References

1. Gogin E.E. *Hypertension.* Medicine, Moscow, 1997: 10 – 28.
2. The Guidelines for Prevention, Diagnosis and Treatment of Arterial Hypertension. *Arterial Hypertension.* 2001; 7:1 - 16.
3. Strelkov R.B. *The method for protection of mammalia of influence of ionizing radiation.* Author’s certificate 389549, USSR, 1971.
4. Chizhov A.Ya., Karash Yu.M., Filimonov V.G., Strelkov R.B. *The method of increase in compensatory possibilities of human body.* Author’s certificate 950406, USSR, 1981.
5. Strelkov R.B. *Normobaric hypoxic therapy.* Guidelines of Ministry of Health of Russia, PAIMS, Moscow, 2001: 1 - 16.
6. Meerson F.Z. *Adaptation, stress and prophylaxis.* Medicine, Moscow, 1981: 106 – 110..
7. Bachatti T. Is bradykinin important for the clinical outcome? *Dialogues in cardiovascular medicine.* 2000; 5(2): 87 - 92.
8. Meerson F.Z. *Adaptive Medicine: mechanisms and protective effects of adaptation.* Medicine, Moscow, 1993: 47 – 49.
9. Koshelev V.B. *Structural rebuilding of circulation bed in experimental arterial hypertension and adaptation to hypoxia: mechanisms and regulatory consequences.*Thesis of doctor of biological sciences, Moscow, 1990.

10. Gundarov I.A. How can be health measured? *Vrach.* 1992; 26: 31-33.

11. *Instrumental methods of assessment of cardiovascular system.* Edited by T.S.Vinogradova, Medicine, Moscow, 1986: 404.

12. Pushkar Yu.T., Bolshov V.M., Elizarova N.A. et al. Assessment of cardiac output by means of tetrapolar chest pletismography and its measurement possibilities. *Cardiology,* 1977; 7: 85 - 91.

13. Epstein I.M. Life assessment of constant of the speed of oxygen tissue absorbtion. In: *Mitochondrias. Structure and functions in norm and pathology*, Medicine, Moscow, 1971: 3 - 8.

14. Chizhov A.Ya., Strelkov R.B. *Normobaric hypoxia in treatment, prophylaxis and rehabilitation,* edition 2nd, Uralskiy rabochiy, Ekaterinburg, 2001: 353.

15. White W.B., Morgenroth J. Usefulness of ambulatory monitoring of blood pressure in assessing antihypertensive therapy. *Amer. J. Cardiol.* 1989; 63: 94 - 98.

16. Olbiskaya L.I., Martinov A.I., Hapayev B.A. *Monitoring of blood pressure in cardiology,* Russkiy Vrach, Moscow, 1998: 1 - 99.

17. Krasnikov N.N. *Influence of hypoxic and hypoxic-hypercapnic mixtures on cardiorespiratory systems and physical working capacity in human beings.* Thesis of Ph.D. in biological sciences, Moscow, 1982: 1 – 23.

18. Meerson F.Z., Pshennikova M.G. *Adaptation to stress situations and physical exercises*, Medicine, Moscow, 1988: 21 – 35.

19. Chizhov A.Ya. Kinetics of oxygen methabolism in patients with chronic salpingoophoritis under using of normobaric hypoxic treatment. *Akusherstvo and gynecology*, 1987; 11:29 - 32.

20. Koshelev V.B., Markov H.M. , Pikalina V.G. et al. Hypoxic factor in pathogenesis of experimental arterial hypertension. *Thesises of reports of IV Congress of pathophysiologists*, Kishinev, 1989; Vol.3: 18 -20.

21. Smirnov I.P. Diffusion of oxygen in lungs in patients with hypertension. *Vrach. delo*, 1975; 6: 17 - 19.

22. Koshelev V.B., Rjasina T.V., Krushinsky A.L., Kuznetsova L.M. Adaptation to hypoxia - method for prevention of experimental stroke. *Papers of VII Russian symposium "Ecologo-physiological problems of adaptation*, Moscow, 1994: 129.

Adaptation Biology and Medicine (Volume 4: Current Concepts)
Editors: A. Hargens, N. Takeda and P.K. Singal

14. Autoimmunity and Risk Factors in Atherosclerosis

N.K. Ganguly*, K. Kaur, D. Kumar, H. Lou and P.K. Singal

Institute of Cardiovascular Sciences and Department of Physiology,
St Boniface Research Center, Faculty of Medicine, University of Manitoba, Winnipeg, Canada.

Abstract

Chronological events for coronary atherosclerosis, a multifactorial disease, remain an enigma. Hyperlipidemia and oxidation of low-density lipoproteins (LDL) in the subendothelial region initiate a cascade of events, which also attracts cells of the immune system such as T cells, macrophages and platelets. The cross talk among different cellular elements such as endothelial cells, smooth muscle cells (SMC) and cells of the immune system, through cytokines, growth factors, adhesion molecules and complement activation, promotes the progression of plaque formation. Different risk factors such as hypertension, cigarette smoke, obesity, diabetes and endotoxins play an important role in the initiation as well as progression of atherosclerosis. The whole process appears to be an organ specific autoimmune disease preceded by oxidation of LDL, both of which have a humoral and delayed hypersensitivity component. Further details of crosstalk at the molecular level within a single pathway as well as converging pathways involving aspects of immune processes are required to fully describe the pathogenesis of coronary atherosclerosis for an optimization of its management.

Introduction

Atherosclerosis is no longer considered to be an inert mass of lipids, matrix proteins, fibrous tissue and necrotic material. It is rather a highly active compendium of a variety of immunocompetent cells, which play a major role in its evolution as well as progression. With the advent of recent cell biology and molecular biology techniques, we are now beginning to understand the crosstalk among different cells and/or components as well as their significance in the pathogenesis of this disease.

Although important data has been added to unravel the pathophysiology of coronary artery disease, one of the vexing points have been the wide incubation period of hyperlipidemia and oxidation of LDL emphasizing the importance of different host factors in atherosclerosis (Ross and Glomset, 1976; Chakravarti et al., 1991). A wider incubation period is a clear indication of adaptive-maladaptive response at these sites. Role of host-factors has been generally under-rated in relation to other factors such as environment influence, hyperlipidemia, hypertension, smoking, diabetes, obesity, high insulin

* Visiting Professor, Director General ICMR, New Delhi, India

levels and homocystenemia (Chakravarti et al., 1991; Munro and Cotran, 1988; Steiner, 1981; Newman et al., 1986; Gotto and Farmer, 1988). However, there has always been an endeavor towards finding out the triggers for the lesion which has been listed as mechanical, toxic, immunological, viral and metabolic (Munro and Cotran, 1988; Benditt et al., 1983; Hansson et al., 1989; Libby and Hansson, 1991; Wick et al., 1995).

In the prevailing view about the inciting stimulus, a strong emphasis has been on the denudation of the endothelium as the first event. Frequent formation of the plaque at lesions appearing in vascular areas subjected to hemodynamic pressure or turbulence exerted by blood flow or at lesion sites created experimentally by balloon catheters provided evidence in favor of the denudation theory (Ross and Glomset, 1976; Ku et al., 1985). Next event is considered to be an increased sticking of platelets and macrophages to the denuded site, each producing a host of cytokines and growth factors followed by cellular proliferation. Endothelial cells, smooth muscle cells, macrophages, T-cells and platelets are considered essential in the progression of the atherosclerotic process (Faggiotito et al., 1984; Aqel et al., 1985; Davies, 1986; Jonasson et al., 1985, 1986; Munro et al., 1987; Bevilacqua et al., 1985). Although current evidences strongly indicate that atherosclerosis is an immune mediated process, the precise nature of the development of this disease still remains to be elucidated. The presence of antibodies and immune complexes, cytokines and lymphocytes infiltration in the atherosclerotic plaque further supports immune-mediated pathogenesis of the disease.

In this review, the major emphasis is to describe the pertinent autoimmune changes associated with atherosclerosis. Involvement of risk factors in the process of atherosclerosis has been analyzed (Figure 1). Role of oxidative stress and oxidation of low density lipoprotein (LDL) in atherosclerosis and heart diseases has been subject of other reviews (Chakravarti et al., 1991; Kaul et al 1993)

Auto-Immunity in Atherogenesis

General concepts

The possible role of immunity in human atheromatous process has been examined using immunocytochemical techniques which showed the presence of T-cells and platelets in fatty streaks, fibro fatty lesions, necrotic atheromas and in intimal thickening in close apposition to each other (Xu et al., 1990). In experimental hyperlipidemia, both T-cells and macrophages stick to endothelium as early as seven hours and infiltrate intima within 17 hours (Xu et al., 1990). In humans also the infiltration of T-cells has been observed in all of the atheromatous processes, right from the fatty streak to the atheromatous plaque (Munro et al., 1987; Van der Wal et al., 1989; Emerson and Robertson, 1988). Twenty percent of total cells in fatty streak and fibro fatty lesions were T-cells; however their number diminished as the process advanced towards necrotic lesions (Table 1). In junctional areas, the T-cell number constituted 40% of the cell population. Similarly high numbers of monocytes/ macrophages and foam cells were seen at the various nascent as well as advanced lesions. Polymorphonuclear cells have been shown to be sticking to the endothelium very early, during high cholesterol feeding of the animal (Muller and Weigl, 1992). T-cells have also been shown sticking to the endothelium following ischemia and reperfusion which also accords these cells some role in the biology of atherogenesis and ischemic heart diseases (Salomon et al., 1991). In advanced lesions, T-cells concentrate in the shoulder and the rim of the advanced atherosclerotic plaques (Xu et al., 1990). The majority of the foam cells in atherosclerotic lesions are of monocyte/macrophage origin and very small proportion is of smooth muscle cell origin (Munro and Cotran, 1988).

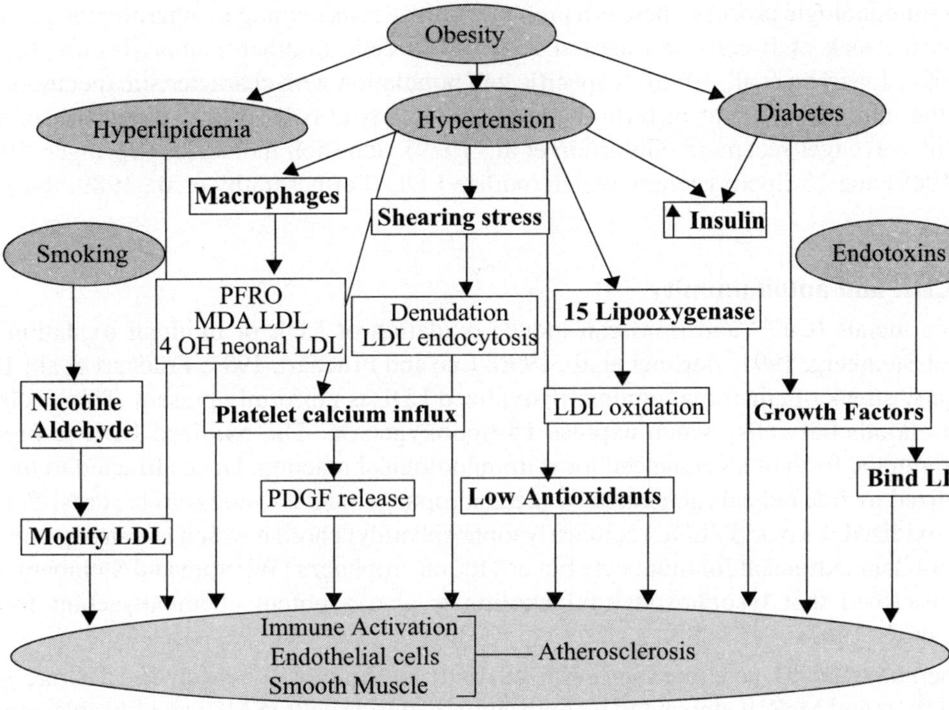

Fig 1. Risk factors acting as trigger or promoter of atherosclerosis by triggering immunological response, activation of endothelial cells and smooth muscle cells.

Table 1. Cell Distribution In Young (16-30 Yrs)^{Y} And Aged Plaque (Above 60 Yrs)^{A} In Different Regions Of The Plaque

Cell Type	Diffuse Intimal Thickening	Transition Zone		Fatty Streak		Fibrous Plaque
T-cells %	Few	40 (Y)	9 (A)	32 (Y)	10 (A)	21
Macrophages %	Few	20 (Y)	18 (A)	39 (Y)	29 (A)	9
$T_H : T_S$ (Ratio)	Few	3:2 (Y)	4:2 (A)	1:1 (Y)	4:1(A)	1:1
SMC%	Rare	4 (Y)	10 (A)	5 (Y)	16 (A)	30
HLA- DR Cells %	?	70%		70%		70%
	Distribution of M and T-cells in Different Regions of Fibrous Plaque					
	Intima	**Shoulder**		**Lipidcore**		**Fibrous Cap**
Macrophages %	9	78		60		24
T-cells %	8	22		2		18

Transition zone refers to the area between intimal and foam cell core of the fatty streak. Young and Aged comparison is given only for the transition zone and fatty streak. HLA- DR, Human leukocytes antigen expressing MHC (major histocompatability complex) class II cells. For details please see the text.

Like any immunologic process, there is a pre-selection of cells coming to atheromatous areas which may explain the lack of B-cells and natural killer (NK) cells in atheromatous lesions (Libby and Hansson, 1991; Jonasson et al., 1986). A specific cell population with characteristic metabolic activity may enter the endothelium and in turn acquires characteristic cell surface properties particularly expression of scavenger receptors (Goldstein et al., 1979), adhesion molecules (Springer, 1990; Yiä-Herttuala, 1989) and 15-lipooxygenase which oxidize LDL (Parthasarathy et al., 1989; Rankin et al., 1991).

Oxidized LDL and autoimmunity

Various trace metals (Cu^{++4} and iron) can induce oxidation of LDL or minimal oxidation of LDL (Wiztum and Steinberg, 1991; Berliner et al., 1990; Luc and Fruchart, 1991; Fruchart et al., 1989). At the site of fatty streak of atheroma, minimally oxidized LDL is uniformly present. This could be also oxidized in endothelial cells, which express 15-lipooxygenase. The oxidized LDL is products of inflammation in the form of an enhanced local immunological reaction. Once attracted to the site, the LDL is oxidized by free radicals generated by the macrophages and a vicious circle starts. These lipids (LDL in its oxidized form or βVLDL) contain lysophosphatidyl choline which is a strong endocellular proliferation-chemoattractant for monocyte but not for macrophages (Witztum and Steinberg, 1991). It has been described that lysophosphatidyl choline is also a potent chemoattractant for T-cells (McMurray et al., 1993).

Other chemoattractants generated by oxidized LDL and minimally oxidized LDL are secretory products. McP1α and McP1β elaborated by both smooth muscle cells (SMC) and fibroblasts are found in atherosclerotic plaques. McP1 is a strong chemoattractant for monocytes but not for granulocytes (Leonard and Yoshimura, 1990). Recently there has been some debate that T lymphocytes in the presence of small number of monocytes can also elaborate McPI. Another chemoattractant JE for monocytes is produced through oxidized LDL as well as minimally oxidized LDL under the stimulation from endothelial cells. This gene product in-fact is similar to McP1 in mass, cationic charge and its inability to attract neutrophils (Leonard and Yoshimura, 1990).

Another dimension to local reactions is endothelial cell toxicity through oxidized LDL which also results in local denudation, thereby promoting the sticking of macrophages, T-cells, and platelets (Rosenfeld et al., 1990; Steinbrecher etal, 1990; Steinberg, 1991). After the initiation of these events, the scenario changes to a local delayed type of immune response in that the same oxidized LDL, which attracted monocytes, does not allow the macrophages to leave the site (Quinn et al., 1987). Now a chain of events starts wherein interleukin 8 (IL8), a product of inflammation, is generated which is also a chemoattractant to T-cells (Libby and Hansson, 1991; Dejana et al., 1987).

Other growth factors elaborated by T-lymphocytes, particularly basic fibroblast growth factor (bFGF), heparin binding endothelial growth factor (HBEGF) and vascular endothelial growth factor (VEGF) induce release of large number of other chemoattractants. The list includes smooth muscle cells colony stimulating factor (SMCSF) generated by SMC (Valente et al., 1984), granulocyte-macrophage colony stimulating factor (GMCSF) elaborated by T-lymphocytes and macrophage colony stimulating factor (mCSF) elaborated by smooth muscle and endothelial cells. bFGF and VEGF by themselves are also chemoattractant. Platelet derived growth factor (PDGF) elaborated by platelets, macrophages and endothelial cells (Blotnick et al., 1994; Peoples et al., 1995; Libby and Hansson,

1991) and TGFβ secreted by T-lymphocytes, macrophages, platelets and endothelial cells are also chemoattractants (Rains and Ross, 1996). All of these factors by their interaction with each other not only accumulate the monocyte/macrophage and T-lymphocytes but also induce the proliferation and/or activation of smooth muscle cells, endothelial cells, and macrophages (Ross, 1995). Some of these processes are summarized in Figure 2.

Antibodies and autoimmunity

Initiation of another cascade of events which helps in the expression of different factors could be called true immunologic phenomena. Peroxidation of apo B100 (Witztum and Steinberg, 1991) or unsaturated fatty acids and products like MD LDL or 4 hydroxy nonenal generates auto antibodies to LDL (Palinski et al., 1990). Similarly antibodies to LDL heparin complex, complexes with various glycosaminoglycans (Iverius, 1972) and chondroitin (Witztum and Koschinsky, 1989; Curtiss et al., 1985). Different antibodies against several necrotic material of the plaque, including DNA material, have also been described in coronary artery disease (Libby and Hansson, 1991). There is also a shift in collagen content from Type III to Type I elaborated by SMC triggered by growth factors. Anticollagen antibodies as well as antifibronectin antibodies (Hansson et al., 1979, 1980) have been described in coronary artery disease. Antibodies are also formed to HSP 70 which is expressed in the ischemic vessels (Kauffmann, 1990; Minota et al., 1988; Parnam, 1989). All these antibodies form antigen-antibody complexes, also accumulate at the site (Minick etal, 1978). Antigens are unique in atheromatous area and are capable of fixing complement (Vlaicu etal, 1985). The complement is

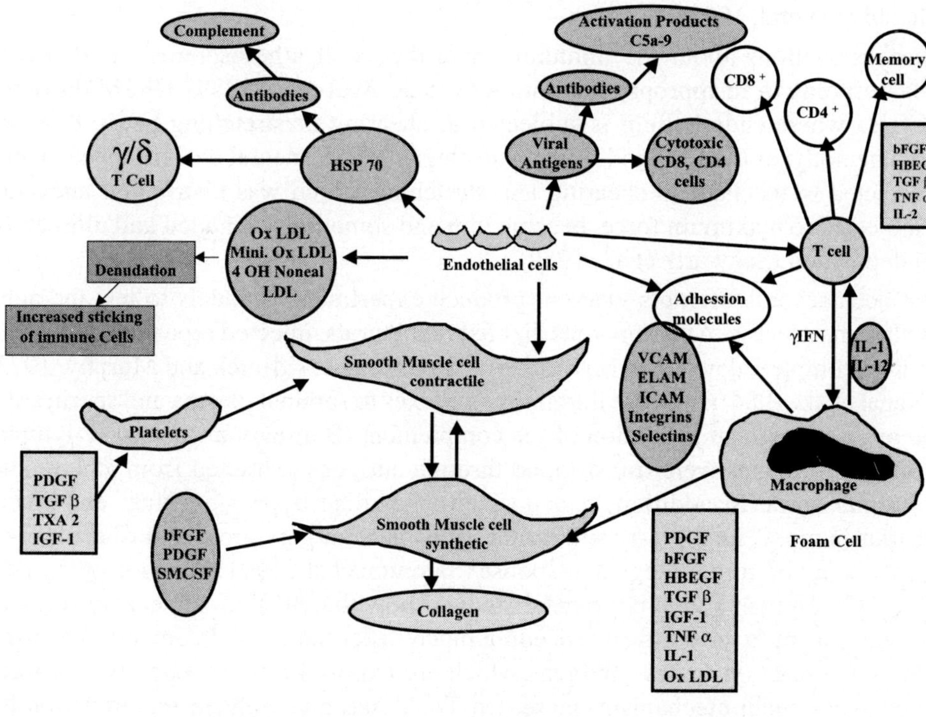

Fig 2. Downstream effects of immune cell activation and cross talk with endothelial and smooth muscle cells.

activated through the classical pathway involving the generation of C5a, which is a strong chemoattractant to neutrophils and monocytes. Circulating immune complexes (Vlaicu etal., 1985), and C5a C9 deposits have been demonstrated in atheromatous plaques (Vlaicu et al., 1985; Xu et al., 1990).

Evidence supporting the role of LPS and endotoxin in T-cell activation is also available. Small amounts of endotoxins circulate in human blood when people get infected by bacteria. Normally Kupffer cells degrade endotoxins. However, endotoxin can form complexes particularly with LDL and can then activate both macrophages and T-cells through the induction of interferon γ (IFNγ) and TNFα. Endotoxin could also lift off endothelial cells and can directly act on these cells as agonist (Libby and Hansson, 1991). Blood samples collected from coronary sinus during ischemic and reperfusion phase of bypass surgery showed that endotoxin could activate monocyte and macrophages through PKC (protein kinase C). Simultaneously, T-lymphocytes produced more IFN, IL4 and TFNα. All of these events further demonstrated that ischemic process with hyperlipidemia could change $CD4^+/CD8^+$ ratio and could activate T-cells.

The monocytes of atheromatous plaque are functionally abnormal e.g. they secrete 1.5 to 3 times more prostaglandin E_2 and 6 ketoprostaglandin $F_1\alpha$ in response n-formyl-methionyl, leucil or calcium ionophore A 23187. These differences were never normalized even when plasma cholesterol levels in these patients became normal as shown by decreased low density lipoproteins through apheresis (Navab et al., 1994; Bath et al., 1991; Stragliotto, 1993). Although these macrophages showed better adhesion to glass, expression of scavenger receptors did not occur in the activated macrophages. However, there is a strong possibility of an intimate interaction between T-cells and macrophages in this event (Hershkoviz etal, 1993).

The serious reservations about the immunological theory of atherosclerosis is that it is a local immunological response to an appropriate stimulus (Van der Wal et al., 1989). One of the obvious local factors is the area where endothelium is subjected to shearing or stretching because of anatomical lesions through hemodynamics of blood flow. In an elegant experimental design, sheets of endothelial cells were subjected to mechanical shearing and stretching which was distributed unevenly. Areas, which were subjected to maximum force, became thin and sometimes denuded and ultimately became sites for lipid deposition (Schwartz et al., 1989).

There have been several attempts made to produce experimental models to test the autoimmune hypothesis with some success. Atheromatous diet fed rabbits/rats, injected repeatedly with serum, BSA and BSA immune complex, developed early atheromatous plaque (Minick and Murphy, 1973; Minick et al., 1978; Nagal et al., 1984). Specific immune complexes to seminal plasma and sperm antigen were formed in the primates with an activation of the complement (Bansal et al., 1986). T-lymphocytes of atherogenic diet fed primates were transformed through antigens extracted from atheromatous aorta and not the normal aorta. In addition, restenosis after cardiac bypass-grafting, endartectomy and percutaneous transhumoral angioplasty and cardiac transplant surgery provide further strong evidence of a direct involvement of immunological response (Salomon et al., 1991; Hansson et al., 1989; Libby and Hansson, 1991). Human and experimental studies show that 40% of subjects develop restenosis and atheroma subsequent to the surgical procedure much faster than seen in any other condition. Host versus graft immune reaction to new antigens which are exposed through operative procedure have been postulated as the main mechanism. Increased T-cell and macrophage accumulation has been a common feature of the above conditions (Ross, 1993). Balloon angioplasty of rat carotid artery caused increased activity of PDGF and FGF leading to intimal thickening 7-21 days after injury (Ferns et al., 1991; Fingerle et al., 1989; Lindner and Reidy, 1991). The antibodies to FGF and PDGF reduce the thickening (Lindner and Reidy, 1991). Similarly, cyclosporin-A, a strong T-cell modulator also reduces the intimal thickening and atheromatous lesions in rat (Jonasson et al., 1988).

Above events have shown that there could be specificity in immunological activation of T-cells. Another important facet of autoimmune reaction is the presence of $\gamma\delta$ T-cells at the fibrous plaque and atheromatous plaque sites. These are strong immunomodulators elaborating certain growth factors, which are known to proliferate keratinocytes in the skin and crypt cells in the intestine (Heng and Heng, 1994). Their presence in atheromatous vessels is novel.

Association of viral infections has been detected for the development of atheromatous plaque (Yamashiroya et al., 1988; Benditt et al., 1983; Minnick et al., 1979 Hendrix et al. 1990). In coronary atherectomy, 79% of the specimens had evidence of chlamydia within atheromatous tissue. In contrast only 4% of nonatherosclerotic coronary artery specimen had evidence of viral infection (Muhelstein et al., 1996). Thus viral theory remains an interesting possibility but a clear cut evidence is lacking except for the data on chlamydia.

Another important pre-requisite for an immunologically mediated process will be a definite recognition system, which could escape tolerance. It has been shown that T-cells of atheromatous plaque express HLA DR antigen and have increased IL2 receptor expression (Hansson et al., 1989b) where as both SMC and endothelial cells express, HLA class II antigen (Xu, 1990; Hansson et al., 1986, 1988; Pober et al., 1982; Warner et al., 1989). This expression is enhanced by the action of cytokine IFN ã (Libby et al., 1989; Stemme et al., 1990). All of these are important recognition systems for immune cells.

Immunocompetent Cells In Atherogenesis

In a normal endothelium there are only a few T-cells and macrophages but in fatty streak their numbers increase. At this time overall number of $CD3^+$ cells are roughly 20% and in transition zone it approaches 40%. Both $CD4^+$ and $CD8^+$ cells are present, though $CD8^+$ cells are much more initially and $CD4^+$ are more abundant later (Emeson and Robertson, 1988). However, ultimately the ratio of $CD4^+$: $CD8^+$ is 3:2 in young and 4:2 in aged plaques (Table 1). Macrophage cells are also present in abundance during this phase. In both types, 70% of these cells are HLA-DR positive and activate macrophages with Mac1 expression. In the transition zone, some SMC are also HLA-DR^+, suggesting that the inflammatory process is very active in this area. In the fatty streak, CD11c macrophages predominate in lesions of both young and aged plaques. These accumulate in the core of the lesion in the form of foam cells. $CD3^+$ cells on the other hand are found in sub-endothelium and occasionally in the core, scattered with CD11c positive cells. At this position MHC class II expression of endothelium and SMC are similar to that seen in transition zone.

Atherosclerotic plaques could be divided into fibrous cap, shoulder (transition zone) and atheromatous core. Foam cells are not found in the core but border the core towards lumen and plaque shoulder. These cells in the shoulder and cap areas demonstrate CD11C expression and most of them also express HLA-DR. Number of $CD3^+$ T-lymphocytes decrease in this area compared to their population in the fatty streak. Few neutrophils are also visible but they are not present in normal intima or fatty streak. Most of SMC are in the cap and subendothelial zone and 30-40% in the cap are HLA-

DR^+. Since they also show invariant expression of HLA-DR^+, they may proliferate during the atherosclerotic process. T-cells of the atherosclerotic lesion bear both αβTcR and γδTcR. About 9.7 % of T-cells in the transition zone carry γδTcR and the number decreases to 6.6 and 4.3% in fatty streak and atheromatous plaques (Kleindienst, 1993). Thus the whole scenario in atherosclerotic process suggests an immunologically dominated chronic inflammation of localized nature (Hansson et al., 1989; Xu et al., 1990; Libby et al. 1991; Wick et al., 1995)

In hypercholesteremic animals, the attachment of clusters of T-lymphocytes and endothelial cells has been reported. The T-helper cells secrete IFN γ, which leads to the development of MHC Class II molecules on endothelial cells. Adhesion molecules and IL8, attract T-cells, which are increased in this process. These T-cells, macrophages and endothelial cells interact. In the process, macrophages get activated and express two kinds of scavenger receptors which internalize low density lipoproteins (LDL) including endothelial cell modified LDL and form foam cells. By this time, these cells have migrated to the subendothelium. These activated macrophages elaborate PDGF like factor with chemoattractant and proliferative properties for smooth muscle cells, which in turn elaborate IL1 and TNFα recruiting more monocytes. Macrophages present antigen to T-lymphocytes through MHC class II recognition, leading to its activation. These cells express mCSF and later help in the recruitment of more monocytes elaborating IFNγ and TNFα. This results not only in macrophage activation but also imparts both endothelial and SMC with new characteristics including antigen expression and regulation of lipoprotein metabolism.

The direct action of T-cells on the SMC is also through HLA-DR expression. $CD4^+$ cells transport HB EGF to smooth muscle cells, which is only effective when transported to close vicinity as they lack the secretary signal peptide. The latter is 22 KDa heparin binding growth factor and is a homologous member of EGF family. It is also a potent chemoattractant factor for SMC and fibroblasts but not for endothelial cells. It has much more proliferative activity over SMC compared to EGF. Because TGFβ is able to bind to heparin sulfate proteoglycan on the SMC surface, it facilitates the binding of heparin to EGF receptor. This activity provides SMC with mesenchymal cell property so that they lay down important matrix proteins, which are hallmark of an atherosclerotic plaque. HBEGF is also involved in SMC hyperplasia in pulmonary hypertension.

Both $CD4^+$ and $CD8^+$ cells synthesize and export bFGF, a 18KDa heparin binding mitogen that can proliferate fibroblasts, SMC and endothelial cells. It is also an angiogenesis factor. This could be effectively transported only by T-cell, since secretary signal peptide is present in T-cells, is lacking in other bFGF producing cells (Blotnick et al., 1994; Peoples et al., 1995; Folkman and Klagsbrun, 1987; Burgess and Maciag, 1989). This is responsible for SMC proliferation following intra-arterial injury. It is possible that T-cell bFGF is a homologous gene product and it has obtained a signal peptide by alternative splicing or has been post-translationally modified to facilitate export (Blotnick et al., 1994). T-lymphocytes, isolated from atherosclerotic plaque have recently been shown to produce HBEGF and bFGF. Their role in angiogenesis of atheromas is also undisputed (Peoples et al., 1995). This may be the initial response but at a later stage, PDGF, PDGF-like mitogen, TNFα, VEGF, TGFβ and TGFα are produced by a multitude of cells e.g. platelets, macrophages, endothelial cells and SMC can further augment the process (Figure 2). Overall immune response could be intended as a defensive adaptation wherein T-lymphocytes exert a feed-back mechanism by which IFNγ and TGFβ act as growth antagonists (Raines et al., 1989; Battegay, 1990; Hajjar, 1987). Similarly macrophages may also have a beneficial effect by not only taking back the esterified lipids and oxidized LDL from the fatty streak site but also by elaborating IL1 which is also a growth antagonist (Libby et al., 1989 b).

On certain areas of plaque, only $CD4^+$ and $CD8^+$ cells have been seen. It is conceivable that in autoimmune or chronic inflammatory process $CD4^+$ with Class II recognition and array of cytokines they generate play an important role (Van der wal, 1989; Hansson et al., 1989; Jonasson et al., 1985; Stemme, 1990). Some SMC and endothelial cells express class I antigen which are also recognized by $CD8^+$ cells (Libby et al., 1991).

Signal Transduction in Atherogenesis

Growth factors, cytokines, including PDGF (Hart et al., 1988; Heldin et al., 1990), bFGF (Burgess and Maciag, 1989), HBEGF (Klagsburn and Edelman, 1989; Higashiyama et al. 1991), insulin like growth factor (IGF) (Banskota et al., 1989), IL1 (Libby et al., 1989), TNFα (Old, 1985) and TGFα (Moses et al., 1987, 1990; Roberts et al., 1990) initiate and regulate cell recruitment, migration, proliferation and laying down of matrix proteins as well as lipid biosynthesis during atheromatous process. These cytokines and growth factors are generally implicated in immunity and inflammation in atherosclerosis. The same factors act as inflammatory as well as growth regulators by inducing/inhibiting proliferation as well as acting as chemoattractant. Some of the important cell proliferation molecules are not present in normal artery but are present in atheromatous vessels (Ross et al., 1993). All of these can also cause smooth muscle cell proliferation and are up regulated in atheromatous vessels. The chemoattractants are as necessary in atherosclerosis as in restenosis and angioplasty events. They not only bring new cells to intima and subendothelium but also bring SMC from media to intima of blood vessels. CSF, McP1, Oxy LDL and TGFβ can cause monocyte chemotaxis and endothelial cell transmigration (Ross, 1993). PDGF and IGF1 are chemoattractants for SMC and bFGF is proliferative for SMC and proliferative as well as chemoattractant for endothelial cells (Folkman et al., 1988). HBEGF is a strong mitogen for SMC and comes in very early in the entire chain of events. IL8 (Libbey and Hansson, 1991) and oxidized LDL are also important T-cell chemoattractants (Steinbrecher et al., 1990; Rosenfeld et al. 1990; Steinberg, 1991). These cytokines IL1, TNFα, IFN γ and IL2 with various CSF are strong immunomodulators and play a considerable role in local immunologic reactions (Amento et al., 1991). Two other important modulators are IL6 and IL4. The latter has been shown to be increasingly expressed by lymphocytes of coronary sinus obtained during ischemic and reperfusion state. Whereas IL6 with its signal transduction arm is utilized in atherogenic process when majority of the other cytokines lack this effect (Libby and Hansson, 1991).

Signal transduction during an atheromatous process is important in networking one molecule to induce expression of another molecule in a target cell, which in turn can be stimulated through an autocrine or paracrine process. For example oxidized LDL induces secretion of IL1 or TNFα from macrophage. These products with TGFβ express PDGF AA gene in SMC (Battegay, 1990) which intern can result in the proliferation of SMC. Endothelial cells when exposed to IL1 (Raines et al., 1989), TNFα (Hajjar et al., 1987; Libby et al., 1988) and TGFβ (Battegay etal, 1990) through an underlying activated macrophages, express PDGF BB gene. The gene product is secreted and in turn activates and proliferates an underlying smooth muscle cell. An excess of IL1, TNFα and TGFβ can then down regulate PDGFAA and PDGF receptors thereby inhibiting proliferation, having a negative feedback effect (Battegay et al., 1990).

There are other regulators in the plasma as well as in the cells taking part in atheromatous process. One of the principle ones is α2 macroglobulin which can bind and metabolize PDGF, TGFβ, IL1, IL2, IL6 and bFGF (Raines et al., 1992). Some connective tissue molecules e.g. heparin can bind and sequester HB EGF, bFGF and PDGF and it can release TGFβ from a carrier protein. Heparin along with fibronectin and lamelin can also have effects on smooth muscle cell phenotype, conferring an ability to these cells to respond to antigens or chemoattractants (McCaffrey, 1989; Raines et al., 1992). Thus adherence to other cells, matrix proteins and integrins have a profound effect on cell to cell interaction leading to altered cell regulatory activity and transmission of cell signals.

There is a good evidence of interaction of cytokine and growth factors in atheromatous cells (Clinton, 1992) and integration of cytokines, growth factors, signal transduction with eicosanoid network (Hajjar et al., 1992). bFGFs role in angiogenesis, where channel like structures are formed, is very important in the ultimate ulceration and thrombus formation in the lesions (Klagsburn and Edelman, 1989; Davies et al., 1984). TGFβ produced by platelets can activate serum proteases e.g. plasmin or trypsin which in turn are potent stimulators of matrix proteins e.g. collagen type I, II, IV and V as well as fibronectin, proteoglycans and glycosaminoglycan (Sporn et al., 1987; Roberts et al., 1990). GMCSF and mCSF are important for proliferation of macrophages, which have entered the arteries in S phase. mCSF lowers plasma cholesterol by up-regulating scavenger receptors (Rosenfeld and Ross, 1990; Gordon et al. 1990; Shimano et al. 1990).

Adhesion molecules and atherogenesis

Another important aspect of the immunologic process is the cell-cell interaction through cell adhesion molecules. Several substances can increase the adhesion of monocyte and lymphocytes. Oxidized LDL stands out very prominently in this regard (Berliner et al., 1990; Esterbauer et al., 1990). Growth factors bFGF, HBEGF and PDGF can all increase stickiness of monocytes and T-lymphocytes. Growth factor VEGF also increases adhesion of monocytes to endothelial cells and it also stimulates them to produce more partially reduced form of oxygen (PRFO). Action of VEGF on monocytes from atherogenic animals is greater than those obtained from normal animals. These interactions have an important role in immunologic mechanisms (Munro and Cotran, 1988; Ross, 1993,1995; Navab et al., 1994).

Some of these adhesion molecules are ICAM I and ICAM II which are constitutively present in endothelium but their expression increases because of the activation of endothelial cells by TNFα and IL1. These dock lymphocyte function associated antigen 1 (LFA1) which is a β integrin (Marlin et al., 1987). Monocytes also express a β integrin known as Mac1, which is an important molecule for their adhesion and transmigration (Miller et al., 1987; Bevilaqua, 1993; Butcher, 1991). ICAM 1 has been shown to be increasingly expressed in human atherosclerotic plaques and ICAM 2 which is an integral part of membrane protein can also bind to both LFA1 and Mac1 (Printseva et al., 1992; Poston et al., 1992; Faruqi et al. 1993). Inflammatory cytokines also induce vascular cell adhesion molecule I (VCAM1) which could bind to monocytes through very late antigen-4 (VLA-4). This adhesion pathway has also been implicated in atherosclerosis (Osborn et al. 1992).

Selectin P and E are adhesion molecules, which bind through carbohydrate ligand. P selectin is present on platelets and endothelial cells and presents itself on the surface when stimulated by endotoxin, phorbolesters, thromboxin, IL1 and TNFα. It is a part of an endothelial Weible-Palade body and when activated, is quickly translocated to plasma membrane (Bonfanti et al., 1989; Hattori et al.,

1989; Yeo et al., 1989). The lymphocyte molecule L selectin, which manifests only on activation, is important for lymphocytes for their early adhesion. This is ultimately shed leading to detachment, but important for transmigration (Shimizu et al., 1992; Picker and Butcher, 1992; Pober and Cotran, 1991). Platelet-endothelial cellular adhesion molecule I, which is a member of leucin rich proteins is known as Cd-14 which participates in response to lipopolysaccharides. Its monoclonal antibody inhibits monocyte adhesion to IL1 activated endothelial monolayers. Large body of evidence has accumulated from the experimental induction of adhesion molecule in baboons injected with lipopolysaccharide. This could also be induced through the injection of TNFα (Ferrero et al., 1990; Wright, 1991; Munro et al. 1991).

Athero ELAM which has structural similarities to VCAM1 is induced in human coronary artery plaque as well as in rabbit atherosclerotic plaque (Li et al., 1993). Certain substances e.g. lactose-I, maltose-I phosphate (DiCorleto et al., 1989), cytokine IL8 (Wheeler et al., 1988; Gimbrone et al., 1989), IL4 and a leucin derivative leumidin which tightly bind to LDL and HDL, inhibit leukocyte adhesion as well as enterotoxic shock. (Burch et al., 1991; Navab et al., 1993). Similarly probucol (Faruqi and Dicorleto, 1992, 1993), vitamin E, nitric oxide and L-arginine inhibit adhesion thereby reducing atherosclerotic lesions in experimental animals (Tsao et al., 1993; Cooke et al., 1992).

Transmigration of the leukocyte after being attracted to the site through various chemoattractants already cited, occurs through interaction of β integrin with adhesion molecule and selectin. Particularly CD11/CD18 complex present on monocytes interact with ICAM 1 of endothelial cells. Thus they protrude pseudopodia and quickly make tight junction and rapidly transmigrate to endothelial cell layer (Muller and Weigl, 1992). T lymphocyte adhere to VCAM1 through a CD-18 independent mechanism (perhaps lysophotadilcholine) and this complex, besides being a chemoattractant, also helps in adherence and transmigration (Navab et al., 1994).

Risk Factors and Autoimmunity

Several risk factors such as hypertension, hyperlipidemia, smoking, obesity and diabetes have been identified as triggers or promoters of atherosclerosis. There is a significant body of knowledge on each of the risk factors. It is impossible to cover all risk factors in any greater detail in a single paper. Following is a brief description with some pertinent references to direct readers for further information.

Hypertension, which is one of the important risk factors for coronary artery disease, might add to the shearing stress on the endothelial cells at particular anatomical sites which may lead to a chain of events. This has been amply demonstrated in elegant experiments carried on cultured endothelial cells exposed to steady state fluid mechanical shear by putting stress of 30-35 dynes/cm^2. This leads to elongation and orientation of the cells in the direction of flow, as well as increased cell stiffness because of reduced cellular compliance and increased negative intracellular potential. Enhanced receptor mediated LDL endocytosis with increased number of LDL (B/E) receptors increased phosphatidylionositide and decreased membrane fluidity (Schwartz et al., 1989). The enhanced prostaglandins, through 15-lipooxygenase pathway, could further facilitate LDL oxidation (Parthsarathy et al., 1989) which could promote the immune activation (Rankin et al, 1991). Hence there is recognition of shear stress system and the oxidized LDL being generated may also provide the first immunologic trigger. The hypertension might also trigger platelet calcium transport and activation, thereby releasing PDGF which could also trigger immunologic processes (Gulati et al.,

1992). In hypertension, lowering of antioxidant and increased generation of PRFO by macrophages have been reported which is linked to the severity of the disease that could induce oxidized LDL, MDALDL, 4OH nonenal, LDL and apo β adducts which could themselves be immunogenic and could trigger immunologic responses (Sagar et al., 1992). Higher insulin levels in hypertension may also modulate the immunologic interaction of various cell populations by modifying the signaling system.

Hyperlipidemia, which is also a risk factor, seems to be an important part of all the immunologic events we see in experimental atherosclerosis. Hence it seems to be an important adjunct and is clearly interwoven with immunologic hypothesis (Dhawan, 1990). Role of hyperlipidemia and Oxy LDL have been discussed in detail in the prevailing pages of this review

Obesity is strongly linked in the lipid abnormality and hypertension and could in a similar fashion modulate the events (Steinberg et al., 1987). Diabetes through lipid abnormality, hypertension and abnormalities in growth factor expression and insulin levels can modify immunologic responses. A lot of experimental data is now available suggesting that in diabetes the immunological responses are altered (Gordon et al., 1981).

Cigarette smoking leads to high nicotine levels which could modify LDL, generate more PRFO and nitric oxide, all of which interfere with immunologic triggers as well as processes after LDL oxidation (Harats et al., 1990). Another factor in cigarette smoke that has recently been identified is aldehyde generated from sugar, which is added during cigarette making. Aldehyde modifies LDL and could modulate the immune system (Halfon et al., 1982; Janoff, 1985;).

Conclusions

It will be too simplistic to give too much importance to any one mechanism in the pathophysiology of atherosclerotic process,which is multifactorial. However, a consensus holistic approach is being advocated where proper dietary control (control of lipids), exercise (control of obesity), antioxidants, anti-inflammatory and immunologic strategies could be used as preventive or therapeutic means of reversing atherosclerotic process. A global approach is necessary to understand the pathogenesis of atherosclerotic plaque formation. The approach must analyze all the cross talk within a single pathway as well as among different converging pathways involving aspects of autoimmune processes playing an important role in atherosclerosis.

Acknowledgments

Ms Kuljeet Kaur and Ms Huiquan Lou received studentship from the Faculty of Graduate Studies, University of Manitoba. Grant from the Canadian Institute for Health Research is also greatly acknowledged.

References

Amento EP, Ehsani N, Palmer H, Libby P. Cytokines and growth factors positively and negatively regulate interstitial collagen gene expression in human vascular smooth muscle cells. Arterioscler Thromb. 1991; 11: 1223-1230.

Aqel NM, Ball RY, Waldmann H, Mitchinson MJ. Identification of macrophages and smooth muscles cells human atherosclerosis using monoclonal antibodies. J Pathol. 1985; 146: 197-204

Bansal N, Majumdar S, Ganguly NK, Chakravarti RN. Long term effect of vasectomy on experimental athrosclerosis in rhesis monkey. Aust J Exp Biol Med Sci. 1986; 64: 527- 533.

Banskota NK, Taub R, Zellner K, King GL. Insulin, insulin-like growth factor I and platelet-derived growth factor interact additively in the induction of the protooncogene c-myc and cellular proliferation in cultured bovine aortic smooth muscle cells. Mol Endocrinol. 1989; 3:1183-1190.

Bath PM, Hassal DG, Gladwin AM, Palmer RM, Martin JF. Nitric oxide and prostacyclin. Divergence of inhibitory effects on monocyte chemotaxis and adhesion to endothelium *in vitro*. Arterioscler Thromb. 1991; 11: 254-260.

Battegay EJ, Raines EW, Seifert RA, Bowen-Pope DF, Ross R. TGF-beta induces bimodal proliferation of connective tissue cells via complex control of an autocrine PDGF loop. Cell. 1990; 63: 515-524.

Benditt EP, Barrett T, McDougall JM. Viruses in the etiology of atherosclerosis. Proc Natl Acad Sci USA. 1983; 80: 6386-6389.

Berliner JA, Territo MC, Sevanian A, Ramin S, Kim JA, Bamshad B, Esterson M, Fogelman AM. Minimally modified low density lipoprotein stimulates monocyte endothelial interactions. J Clin Invest. 1990; 85: 1260-1266.

Bevilacqua MP. Endothelial-leukocyte adhesion moleucles. Annu Rev Immunol. 1993;11:767-804.

Blotnick S, Peoples GE, Freeman MR, Eberleins TJ, Klagsbrun M. T lymphocytes synthesize and export heparin-binding epidermal growth factor-like growth factor and basic fibroblast growth factor, mitogens for vascular cells and fibroblasts: Differential production and release by $CD4^+$ and $CD8^+$ T cells. Proc Natl Acad Sci USA. 1994; 91: 2890-2894.

Bonfanti R, Furie BC, Furie B, Wagner DD. PADGEM (GMP140) is a component of Weibel-Palade bodies of human endothelial cells. Blood. 1989; 73:1109-1112.

Burch RM, Weitzberg M, Blok N, Muhlhauser R, Martin D, Farmer SG, Bator JM, Connor JR, KoC, Kuhn H. N-(fluroenyl-9- methoxycarbonyl) amino acids, a class of antiinflammatory agents with a different mechanism of action. Proc Natl Acad Sci Usa. 1991; 88:355-359.

Burgess WH, Maciag T. The heparin-binding (fibroblast) growth factor family of proteins. Annu Rev Biochem. 1989; 58:575-606.

Butcher EC. Leukocyte-endothelial cell recognition: three (or more) steps to specificity and diversity. Cell. 1991; 67:1033-1036.

Chakravarti RN, Kirshenbaum LA, Singal PK. Atherosclerosis: its pathophysiology with special reference to lipid peroxidation. J App Cardiol. 1991; 6:91-112.

Clinton SK, Libby P. Cytokines and growth factors in atherogenesis. Arch Pathol Lab Med. 1992; 116:1292-1300.

Cooke JP, Singer AH, Tsao P, Zera P, Rowan RA, Billingham ME. Antiatherogenic effects of L-arginine in the hypercholesterolemic rabbit. J Clin Invest. 1992; 90:1168-1172.

Curtiss LK, Witztum JL. Plasma apolipoproteins AI, AII, B, CI, and E are glucosylated in hyperglycemic diabetic subjects. Diabetes. 1985; 34:452-461.

Davies MJ, Thomas A. Thrombosis and acute coronary-artery lesions in sudden cardiac ischemic death. N Engl J Med. 1984; 310:1137-1140.

Davies PF. Vascular cell interactions with special reference to the pathogenesis of atherosclerosis. Lab Invest. 1986; 55: 5-24.

Dejana E, Ji-Ming W, Mantovani A. The recruitment of leukocytes and their interaction with the vessel wall: the role of interleukin-1 and tumor necrosis factor. Scand J Rheumatol. 1987; 66(Suppl):19-25.

Dhawan V, Sharda N, Majumdar S, Ganguly NK, Chakravarti RN. Platelet aggregability and serum thrombos level in hypercholesteremic atheroslcerotic monkeys. Med Sci Res. 1990; 18:149-151.

DiCorleto PE, De La Motte CA. Role of cell surface carbohydrate moieties in monocytic cell adhesion to endothelium *in vitro*. J Immunol. 1989; 143:3666-3672.

Emeson EE, Robertson AL. T lymphocytes in aortic and coronary intimas: Their potential role in atherogenesis. Am J Pathol. 1988; 130:369-376.

Esterbauer H, Striegl G, Puhl H, Rotheneder M. Continuous monitoring of *in vitro* oxidation of human low density lipoprotein. Free Radical Res Commun. 1990; 6:67-75.

Faggiotto A, Ross R, Harker L. Studies of hypercholesteremia in the nonhuman primate. I. Changes that lead to fatty streak formation. Arteriosclerosis. 1984; 4:323-340.

Faruqi RM, DiCorleto PE. Inhibition of moncyte adhesion to human umbilical vein endothelial cells (EC) by α-tocopherol (α-tcp). FASEB J. 1992; 6:A1592.

Faruqi RM, DiCorleto PE. Mechanisms of monocyte recruitment and accumulation. Br Heart J. 1993; 69:S19-29.

Ferns GAA, Raines EW, Sprugel KH, Motani AS, Reidy MA, Ross R. Inhibition of neointimal smooth muscle accumulation after angioplasty by an antibody to PDGF. Science. 1991; 253:1129-1132.

Ferrero E, Hsieh CL, Francke U, Goyert SM. CD14 is a member of the family of leucine-rich proteins and is encoded by a gene syntenic with multiple receptor genes. J Immunol. 1990; 145:331-336.

Fingerle J, Johnson R, Clowes AW, Majesky MW, Reidy MA. Role of platelets in Smooth muscle cell proliferation and migration after vascular injury in rat carotid artery. Proc Natl Acad Sci USA. 1989; 86:8412-8416.

Folkman J, Klasbrun M. Angiogenic factors. Science. 1987; 235: 442-447.

Folkman J, Klagsbrun M, Sasse J, Wadzinski M, Ingber D, Vlodavsky I. A heparin-binding angiogenic protein—basic fibroblast growth factor—is stored within basement membrane. Am J Path. 1988; 130: 393-400.

Fruchart JC, Sauzieres J, Clavey V, Plancke MO. Antioxidant therapy and uptake of human oxidized LDL by macrophage. Ann NY Acad Sci. 1989; 570:447-448.

Gimbrone MA Jr, Obin MS, Brock AF, Luis EA, Hass PE, Hebert CA,Yip YK, Leung DW, Lowe Dg, Kohr Wj, Darbonne WC, Bechtol KB, Baker JB. Endothelial interleukin-8: A novel inhibitor of leucocyte-endothelial interactions. Science. 1989; 246:1601-1603.

Goldstein JL, Ho YK, Basu SK, Brown MS. Binding site of macrophages that mediates uptake and degradation of actylated low density lipoprotein, producing massive cholesterol deposition. Proc Natl Acad Sci USA. 1979; 76:333-337.

Gordon D, Guyton JR, Karnovsky MJ. Intimal alterations in rat aorta induced by stressful stimuli. Lab Invest. 1981; 45:14-27.

Gordon D, Reidy MA, Benditt EP, Schwartz SM. Cell proliferation in human coronary arteries. Proc Natl Acad Sci USA. 1990; 87:4600-4604.

Gotto AM Jr, Farmer JA. Risk factors for coronary artery disease. In: Braunwald E, ed. Heart Disease. Philadelphia, London: WB Saunders Co.; 1988: p. 1153.

Gulati S, Khullar M, Sargar S, Ganguly NK, Sharma BK. Ca^{+2} transport in unstimulated platelets of essential hypertensives and their blood relatives. J Hypertens. 1992; 37:1213-1219.

Hajjar KA, Hajjar DP, Silverstein RL, Nachman RL. Tumor necrosis factor-mediated release of platelet-derived growth factor from cultured endothelial cells. J Exp Med. 1987; 166:235-245.

Hajjar DP, Pomerantz KB. Signal transduction in atherosclerosis: integration of cytokines and the eicosanoids network. FASEB J. 1992; 6:2933-2941.

Halfon ST, Kark JD, Baras M, Friedlander Y, Eisenberg S. Smoking, lipids and lipoproteins in Jerusalem 17-year-olds. Israel J Med Sci. 1982; 18:1150-1157.

Hansson GK, Bondjers G, Nilsson LA. Plasma protein accumulation in injured endothelial cells. Immunofluorescentlocalization of IgG and fibrinogen in the rabbit aortic endothelium. Exp Mol Pathol. 1979; 30: 12-26.

Hansson GK, Bondjers G, Bylock A, Hjalmarsson L. Ultrastructural studies on the localization of IgG in the aortic endotheliumand subendothelial intima of atherosclerotic and nonatherosclerotic rabbits. Exp Mol Pathol. 1980; 33: 302-315.

Hansson GK, Jonasson L, Holm J, Claesson-Welsh L. Class II MHC antigen expression in the atherosclerotic plaque: smooth muscle cells express HLA-DR, HLA-DQ and the invariant gamma chain. Clin Exp Immunol. 1986; 64:261-268.

Hansson GK, Jonasson L, Lojsthed B, Stemme S, Kocher O, Gabbiani G. - Localization of T lymphocytes and macrophages in fibrous and complicated human atherosclerotic plaques. Atherosclerosis. 1988; 72:135-141.

Hansson GK, Holm J, Jonasson L. Detection of activated T lymphocytes in the human atherosclerotic plaque. Am J Pathol. 1989; 135:169-175.

Hansson GK, Jonasson L, Seifert PS, Stemme S. Immune mechanisms in atherosclerosis. Arteriosclerosis. 1989; 9: 567-578.

Harats D, Ben-Naim M, Dabach Y, Hollander G, Havivi E, Stein O, Stein Y. Effect of vitamin C and E supplementation on susceptibility of plasma lipoproteins to peroxidation induced by acute smoking. Atherosclerosis. 1990; 85:47-54.

Hart CE, Forstrom JW, Kelly JD, Seifert RA, Smith RA, Ross R, Murray MJ, Bowe-pope DF. Two classes of PDGF receptor recognize different isoforms of PDGF. Science. 1988; 240:1529-1531.

Hattori R, Hamilton KK, Fugate RD, McEver RP, Sims PJ. Stimulated secretion of endothelial Von Willebrand factor is accompanied by rapid redistribution to the cell surface of the intracellular granule membrane protein GMP-140. J Biol Chem. 1989; 264: 7768-7771.

Heldin C-H, Westermark B. Platelet-derived growth factor: mechanism of action and possible in vivo function. Cell Reg. 1990; 1:555-566.

Hendrix MG, Salimans MM, van BCP, Bruggeman CA. High prevalence of latently present cytomegalovirus in arterial walls of patients suffereing from grade III atherosclerosis. Am J Pathol. 1990; 136:23- 28.

Heng MK, Heng MCY. Heat-shock protein 65 and activated γ/δ T cells in injured arteries. Lancet. 1994; 344:921-923.

Hershkoviz R, Gilat D, Miron S, Mekori YA, Aderka D, Wallach D, Vlodavsky I, Cohen IR, Lider O. Extracellular matrix induces tumour necrosis factor-alpha secretion by an interaction between resting rat CD4+ T cells and macrophages. Immunology. 1993; 78: 50-57.

Higashiyama S, Abraham JA, Miller J, Fiddes JC, Klagsbrun M. A Heparin-binding growht factor secreted by macrophage like cells that is related to EGF . Science. 1991; 251:936-939.

Iverius PH. The interaction between human plasma lipoproteins and connective tissue glycosaminoglycans. J Biol Chem. 1972; 247:2607-2613.

Janof A. Elastases and emphysema. Current assessment of the protease-antiprotease hypothesis. Am Rev Respir Dis. 1985; 132:417-433

Jonasson L, Holm J, Skalli O, Gabbiani G, Hansson GK. Expression of class II transplantation antigen on vascular smooth muscle cells express in human atherosclerosis. J Clin Invest. 1985; 76:125-131.

Jonasson L, Holm J, Skalli O, Bonders G, Hansson GK. Regional accumulations of T cells, macrophages, and smooth muscle cells express in the human atherosclerotic plaque. Arterioscleriosis. 1986; 6:131-138.

Jonasson L, Holm J, Hansson GK.Smooth muscle cells express express Ia antigens during arterial response to injury. Lab Invest. 1988; 58:310-315.

Kaufmann SH. Heat shock proteins and the immune response. Immunol Today. 1990; 11:129-136

Kaul N, Siveski-Iliskovic N, Hill M, Slezak J, Singal PK. Free radicals and the heart. J Pharmacol Toxicol Methods. 1993; 30: 55-67.

Klagsbrun M, Edelman ER. Biological and biochemical properties of fibroblast growth factors. Implications for the pathogenesis of atherosclerosis. Arteriosclerosis. 1989; 9:269-278.

Kleindienst R, Xu Q, Willeit J, Waldenberger FR, Weimann S, Wick G. Immunology of atherosclerosis. Demonstration of heat shock protein 60 expression and T lymphocytes bearing α/β or γ/δ receptor in human atherosclerotic lesions. Am J Pathol. 1993; 142:1927-1937.

Ku DN, Giddens DP, Zarins CK, Glagov S. Pulsatile flow and atherosclerosis in the human carotid bifurcation. Positive correlation between plaque location and low oscillating shear stress. Arteriosclerosis. 1985; 5: 293-302.

Leonard EJ, Yoshimura T. Human monocyte chemoattractant protein-1 (MCP-1). Immunol Today. 1990; 11:97-101.

Li H, Cybulsky MI, Gimbrone MA Jr, Libby P. An atherogenic diet rapidly induces VCAM-1, a cytokine-regulatable mononuclear leukocyte adhesion molecule, in rabbit aortic endothelium. Arterioscler Thromb. 1993; 13:197-204.

Libby P, Warner SJC, Salomon RN, Birinyi LK. Production of platelet-derived growth factor-like mitogen by smooth-muscle cells from human atheroma. N Engl J Med. 1988; 318:1493-1498.

Libby P, Friedman GB, Salomon RN. Cytokines as modulators of cell proliferation in fibrotic disease. Am Rev Resp Dis. 1989; 140:1114-1117.

Libby P, Salomon RN, Payne DD, Schoen FJ, Pober JS. Functions of vascular wall cells related to the development of transplantation-associated coronary aeriosclerosis. Transplantation Proc. 1989; 21:3677-3684.

Libby P, Hansson GK. Biology of disease. Involvement of the immune system in human atherogenesis. Current knowledge and unanswered questions. Lab Invest. 1991; 64:5-15.

Lindner V, Reidy MA. Proliferation of SMCafter vascular injury is inhibited by an antibody against basic fibroblast growth factor. Proc Natl Acad Sci USA. 1991; 88:3739-3743.

Luc G, Fruchart J-C. Oxidation of lipoproteins and atherosclerosis. Am J Clin Nutr. 1991; 53:206S-209S.

Marlin SD, Springer TA. Purified intercellular adhesion molecule-1 (ICAM-I) is a lipid for lymphocyte function associated antigen 1 (LFA-I). Cell. 1987; 51:813-819.

McCaffrey TA, Falcone DJ, Brayton CF, Agarwal LA, Welt FG, Weksler BB. Transforming growth factor-beta activity is potentiated by heparin via dissociation of the transforming growth factor-beta/alpha 2-macroglobulin inactive complex.. J Cell Biol . 1989; 109:441-448.

McMurray HF, Parthasarathy S, Steinberg D. Oxidatively modified low density lipoprotein is a chemoattractant for human T lymphocytes. J Clin Invest. 1993; 92:1004-1008.

Miller LJ, Bainton DF, Borregaard N, Springer TA. Stimulated mobilization of monocyte Mac-1 and p150,95 adhesion proteins from an intracellular vesicular compartment to the cell surface. J Clin Invest. 1987; 80:535-544.

Minick CR, Alonso DR, Rankin L. Role of immunologic arterial injury in atherogenesis. Thromb Haemost. 1978; 39:304-311.

Minick CR, Fabricant CG, Fabricant J, Litrenta MM. Atheroarteriosclerosis induced by infection with a herpesvirus. Am J Pathol. 1979; 96:673-706.

Minick CR, Murphy GE. Experimental induction of arteriosclerosis by the synergy of allergic injury to arteries and lipid-rich diet. II. Effect of repeatedly injected foreign protein in rabbits fed a lipid-rich, cholesterol-poor diet. Am J Pathol. 1973; 73:265-300.

Minota S, Cameron B, Welch WJ, Winfield JB. Autoantibodies to the constitutive 73-kD member of the hsp70 family of heat shock proteins in systemic lupus erythematosus. J Exp Med. 1988; 168:1475-1480.

Moses HL, Yang EY, Pietenpol JA. TGF-beta stimulation and inhibition of cell proliferation: new mechanistic insights. Cell. 1990; 63: 245-247.

Moses HL, Coffey RJ Jr, Leof EB, Lyons RM, Keski-Oja J. Transforming growth factor beta regulation of cell proliferation. J Cell Physiol. 1987;(Suppl 5):1-7.

Muhlestein JB, Hammond EH, Carlquist JF, Radicke E, Thomson MJ, Karagounis LA, Woods ML, Anderson JL. Increased incidence of Chlamydia species within the coronary arteries of patients with symptomatic atherosclerotic versus other forms of cardiovascular disease. J Am Coll Cardiol. 1996; 27: 1555-1561.

Muller WA, Weigl SA. Monocyte-selective transendothelial migration: dissection of the binding and transmigration phases by an *in vitro* assay. J Exp Med. 1992; 176:819-828.

Munro JM, van der Walt JD, Munro CS,Chalmers JAC, Cox EL. An immunohistochemical analysis of human aortic fatty streaks. Human Pathol. 1987; 18:375-380.

Munro JM, Cotran RS. Biology of disease. The pathogenesis of atherosclerosis: atherogenesis and inflammation. Lab Invest. 1988; 58:249-261.

Munro JM, Pober JS, Cotran RS. Recruitment of neutrophils in the local endotoxin response: association with *de novo* endothelial expression of endothelial leukocyte adhesion molecule-1. Lab Invest. 1991; 64:295-299.

Navab M, Hama SY, van Lenten BJ, Drinkwater DC, Laks H, Fogelman AM. A new antiinflammatory compound, leumedin, inhibits modification of low density lipoprotein and the resulting monocyte transmigration into the subendothelial space of cocultures of human aortic wall cells. J Clin Invest. 1993; 91:1225-1230.

Navab M, Hama SY, Nguyen TB, Fogelman AM. Monocyte adhesion and transmigration in atherosclerosis. Coron Artery Dis. 1994; 5:198-204.

Newman WP, Freedman DS, Voors AW, Gard PD, Srinivasan SR, Cresanta JL, Williamson GD, Webber LS, Berenson GS. Relation of serum lipoprotein levels and systolic blood pressure to early atherosclerosis. N Engl J Med. 1986; 314:138-144.

Old LJ. Tumor necrosis factor (TNF). Science. 1985; 230:630-632.

Osborn RM, Vassalo C, Benjamin CD. Activated endothelium bind lymphocytes through a novel binding site in the alternatively sliced domain of vascular cell adhesion molecule-1. J Exp Med. 1992; 176:99-107.

Palinski W, Ylä-Herttuala S, Rosenfeld ME, Butler SW, Socher SA, Parthasarathy S, Curtiss LK, Witztum JL. Antisera and monoclonal antibodies specific for epitopes generated during oxidative modification of low density lipoprotein. Arteriosclerosis. 1990; 10:325-335.

Parham P. MHC molecules. A profitable lesson in heresy (news). Nature (London). 1989; 340:426-428.

Parthasarathy S, Wieland E, Steinberg D. A role for endothelial cell lipoxygenase in the oxidative modification of low density lipoprotein. Proc Natl Acad Sci Usa. 1989; 86:1046-1050.

Peoples GE, Blotnick S, Takahashi K, Freeman MR, Klagsbrun M, Eberlein TJ. T lymphocytes that infiltrate tumors and atherosclerotic plaques produce heparin-binding epidermal growth factor-like growth factor and basic fibroblast growth factor: a potential pathologic role. Proc Natl Acad Sci U S A. 1995; 92: 6547-6551.

Picker LJ, Butcher EC. Physiological and molecular mechanisms of lymphocyte homing. Annu Rev Immunol. 1992;10:561-591.

Pober JS, Gimbrone MA Jr. Expression of Ia-like antigens by human vascular endothelial cells is inducible *in vitro*: demonstration by monoclonal antibody binding and immunoprecipitation. Proc Natl acad Sci USA. 1982; 79:6641-6645.

Pober JS, Cotran RS. Immunologic interactions of T lymphocytes with vascular endothelium. Adv Immunol. 1991; 50:261-302.

Poston RN, Haskard DO, Coucher JR, Gall NP, Johnson-Tidey RR. Expression of intercellular adhesion molecule-1 in atherosclerotic palques. Am J Pathol. 1992; 140:665-673.

Printseva OYU, Peclo MM, Gown AM. Varios cell types in human atherosclerotic lesions express ICAM-1. Further immunocytochemical and immunochemical studies employing monoclonal antibody 10F3. Am J Pathol. 1992; 140:889-896.

Quinn MT, Parthasarathy S, Fong LG, Steinberg D. Oxidatively modified low density lipoproteins: a potential role in recruitment and retention of moncyte/macrophages during atherogenesis. Proc Natl Acad Sci USA. 1987; 84:2995-2998.

Raines EW, Dower SK, Ross R. Interleukin-1 mitogenic activity for fibroblasts and smooth muscle cells express is due to PDGF-AA . Science. 1989; 243:393-396.

Raines EW, Ross R. Compartmentalization of PDGF on extracellular binding sites dependent on exon-6-encoded sequences. . J Cell Biol. 1992; 116:533-543.

Raines EW, Ross R. Multiple growth factors are associated with lesions of atherosclerosis:specificity or redundancy? Bioessays. 1996; 18: 271-282.

Rankin SM, Parthasarathy A, Steinberg D. Evidence for a dominant role of lipoxygenase(s) in the oxidation of LDL by mouse peritoneal macrophages. J Lipid Res. 1991; 32:449-456.

Roberts AB, Sporn MB. The transforming growth factors in Handbook of Experimental Pharmacology: Peptide Growth Factors and Their Receptors I (eds. Sporn. M.B. and Roberts, AB) 419-472 (Springer, Berlin, 1990).

Rosenfeld ME, Khoo JC, Miller E, Parthasarathy S, Palinski W, Witztum JL. Macrophage-derived foam cells freshly isolated from rabbit atherosclerotic lesions degrade modified lipoproteins, promote oxidation of low density lipoproteins, and contain oxidation specific lipid protein adducts. J Clin Invest. 1990; 87:90-99.

Rosenfeld ME, Ross R. Macrophage and smooth muscle cell proliferation in atherosclerotic lesions of WHHL and comparably hypercholesterolemic fat-fed rabbits. Arteriosclerosis. 1990; 10:680-687.

Rosenfeld ME, Palinski W, Yla-Herttuala S, Carew TE. Macrophages, endothelial cells, and lipoprotein oxidation in the pathogenesis of atherosclerosis. Toxicol Path. 1990; 18: 560-571.

Ross R, Glomset JA. The pathogenesis of atherosclerosis (First of two parts). N Engl J Med. 1976; 295:369-377.

Ross R. The pathogenesis of atherosclerosis: a perspective for the 1990s. Nature. 1993; 362:801-809.

Ross R. Cell biology of atherosclerosis. Annu Rev Physiol. 1995; 57:791-804.

Sagar S, Ganguly NK, Koicha M, Sharma BK. Immunopathogenesis of Takayasu arteritis. Heart Vessels. 1992; 7:85-90.

Salomon RN, Hughes CC, Schoen FJ, Payne DD, Pober JS, Libby P. Human coronary transplantation-associated arteriosclerosis. Evidence for a chronic immune reaction to activated graft endothelial cells. Am J Pathol. 1991; 138:791-798.

Schwartz CJ, Kelley JL, Nerem RM, Sprague EA, Rozek MM, Valente AJ, Edwards EH, Prasad AR, Kerbacher JJ, Logan SA. Pathophysiology of the atherogenic process. Am J Cardiol. 1989; 64: 23G-30G

Shimano H, Yamada N, Ishibashi S, Harada K, Matsumoto A, Mori N, Inaba T, Motoyoshi K, Itakura H, Takaku F. Human monocyte colony-stimulating factor enhances the clearance of lipoproteins containing apolipoprotein B-100 via both low density lipoprotein receptor-dependent and -independent pathways in rabbits. J Biol Chem. 1990; 265:12869-12875.

Shimizu Y, Newman W, Tanaka Y, Shaw S. Lymphocyte interactions with endothelial cells. Immunol Today. 1992; 13:106-112.

Sporn MB, Roberts AB, Wakefield LM, de Crombrugghe B. Some recent advances in the chemistry and biology of transforming growth factor-beta. J Cell Biol. 1987; 105:1039-1045.

Springer TA. Adhesion receptors of the immune system. Nature. 1990; 346:425-434.

Steinberg D. Current theories of the pathogenesis of atherosclerosis. In Hypercholesterolemia and Athrosclerosis. Pathogenesis and Prevention, edited by Steinberg D, Olefsky JM, p 5. New York, Churchill/Livingstone, 1987.

Steinberg D. Antioxidants and atherosclerosis. A current assessment. Circulation. 1991; 84: 1420-1425.

Steinbrecher UP, Zhang HF, Lougheed M. Role of oxidatively modified LDL in atherosclerosis. Free Radical Biol Med. 1990;9;155-168.

Steiner G. Diabetes and atherosclerosis: an overview. Diabetes. 1981; 30: 1-7.

Stemme S, Fager G, Hansson GK. MHC class II antigen expression in human vascular smooth muscle cells express is induced by interferon-gamma and modulated by tumor necrosis factor and lymphotoxin. Immunology. 1990; 69:243-249.

Stragliotto E, Camera M. Postiglione A, Sirtori M, Di Minno G, Tremoli E. Functionally abnormal monocytes in hypercholesterolemia. Arterioscler Thromb. 1993; 13:944-950.

Tsao PS, McEvoy LM, Drexler H, Butcher EC, Cooke JP. Endothelial-monocyte interaction in hypercholesterolemia is abrogated by an NO precursor. Circulation. 1993; 88:I251A.

Valente AJ, Fowler SR, Sprague EA, Kelley JL, Suenram CA, Schwartz CJ. Initial characterization of a peripheral blood mononuclear cell chemoattractant derived from cultured arterial smooth muscle cells. Am J Pathol. 1984; 117:409-417.

Van der Wal AC, Das PK, Bentz van de Berg D, van der Loos CM, Becker AE. Atherosclerotic Lessions in Humans. In sity immunophenotypic analysis suggesting an immune mediated response. Lab Invest. 1989; 61:166-170

Nagal V, Ganguly NK, Chakravarti RN. Immune complex mediated cardiac lesions in rats. Indian J Med Res. 1984; 79:250-259.

Vlaicu R, Niculescu F, Rus HG, Cristea A. Immunohistochemical localization of the terminal C5b-9 complement complex in human aortic fibrous plaque. Atherosclerosis. 1985; 57:163-177.

Warner SJC, Friedman GB, Libby P. Regulation of major histocompatibility gene expression in cultured human vascular smooth muscle cells. Arteriosclerosis. 1989; 9:279-288.

Wheeler ME, Luscinskas FW, Bevilacqua MP, Gimbrone MA Jr. Cultured human endothelial cells stimulated with cytokines or endotoxin produce an inhibitor of leucocyte adhesion. J Clin Invest. 1988; 82:1211-1218.

Wick G, Schett G, Amberger A, Kleindienst R, Xu Q. Is atherosclerosis an immunologically mediated disease? Immunology Today. 1995; 16:27-33.

Witztum JL, Koschinsky T. Metabolic and immunological consequences of glycation of low density lipoproteins. Prog Clin Biol Res. 1989; 304:219-234.

Witztum JL, Steinberg D. Role of oxidized low density lipoprotein in atherogenesis. J Clin Invest. 1991; 88:1785-1792.

Wright SD. Multiple receptors for endotoxin. Curr Opin Immunol. 1991; 3:83-90.

Xu Q, Oberhuber G, Gruschwitz M, Wick G. Immunology of atherosclerosis: cellular composition and major histocompatibility complex class II antigen expression in aortic intima, fatty streaks, and atherosclerotic plaques in young and aged human specimens. Clin Immunol and Immunopathol. 1990; 56:344-359.

Yamashiroya HM, Ghosh L, Yang R, Robertson AL. Herpesviridae in coronary vessels and aorta of young trauma victims. Am J Pathol. 1988; 130:71-79.

Yeo E, Furie BC, Furie B. PADGEM protein in human erythroleukemia cells. Blood. 1989; 73:722-728.

Yla-Herttuala S, Palinski W, Rosenfeld ME, Parthasarathy S, Carew TE, Butler S, Witztum JL, Steinberg D. Evidence for the presence of oxidatively modified low density lipoprotein in atherosclerotic lesions of rabbit and man. J Clin Invest. 1989; 84:1086-1095.

Adaptation Biology and Medicine (Volume 4: Current Concepts)
Editors: A. Hargens, N. Takeda and P.K. Singal

15. Prospects for Using Methods of Adaptive Medicine in Alzheimer's Disease

Manukhina E.B., #Wiegant F.A.C., Goryacheva A.V., Khomenko I.P., Kruglov S.V., Mashina S.Yu., Pokidyshev D.A., Popkova E.V., Pshennikova M.G., Vlasova M.A., Zelenina O.M., Malyshev I.Yu.[1]

Institute of General Pathology and Pathophysiology, Moscow, Russia
#Utrecht University, Utrecht, The Netherlands

Introduction

Alzheimer's disease (AD) is a neurodegenerative disease of the central nervous system characterized by progressive memory loss and other cognitive disorders. This disease affects from 5 to 10% of people older than 65 years. The incidence almost doubles every 5 years for people between 65 and 80 years old. The etiology of AD is multi-factorial involving a multitude of genetic and environmental factors [44].

AD is characterized by the formation of toxic senile plaques and neurofibrillary tangles in hippocampus and brain cortex. The senile plaques are generated by an extra- and intracellular deposition of the b-amyloid peptide (Aβ). The neurofibrillary tangles are formed inside neurons and consist of hyperphosphorylated tau proteins. Many research groups have provided evidence to show that Aβ is centrally involved in the pathogenesis of AD via a number of mechanisms. Deposition of the aggregated Aβ becomes the initiating factor for multiple neurotoxic pathways, which may include excitotoxicity, Ca^{2+} homeostasis disruptions, free radical production, and neuro-inflammation [21, 22].

Glutamate is the major excitatory neurotransmitter in the corticocortical system, and the glutamatergic pathway has been implicated in excitotoxic events including AD. Excessive glutamatergic activation of the NMDA and AMPA/kainate receptors leads to pathological Ca^{2+} influx.

[1] To whom correspondence should be sent:
Igor Yu. Malyshev; PhD., MD., Prof.
Head, Department of Adaptive Biology and Medicine,
Institute of General Pathology and Pathophysiology, RAMS
Baltijskaya str.8, 125315 Moscow, Russia
tel.: +7(095) 155-4748; +7(095) 766-2440
e-mail: igor.malyshev@mtu-net.ru

The resulting increase in intraneuronal Ca^{2+} concentration induces the activation of a variety of neurotoxic compounds that compromise neuronal viability [25].

Accumulation of oxidative damage occurs in the non-demented brain [14], similar or more severe oxidative insults are likely to play a significant role in AD pathogenesis. [56]. Aβ, by inducing free radical formation, induces membrane oxidation leading to the subsequent impairment of Na^+/K^+ ATPase and Ca^{2+} ATPase, which are responsible for maintaining cytoplasmic Ca^{2+} at a low resting level [75]. The resultant increase in intraneuronal Ca^{2+} concentration produces further radical formation by activating NO synthase (NOS) and phospholipases, as well as by adversely altering mitochondrial function [28]. This positive feedback mechanism further disturbs Ca^{2+} homeostasis and neuronal integrity [56].

In the AD brain, numerous immunoproteins and cytokines are produced by neurons, astrocytes, and microglia [81]. It has been hypothesized that an ongoing chronic inflammation process is occurring in the AD brain [38]. It appears that Aβ is one of the factors responsible for the activation of astrocytes and microglia [40, 105], the two major cell types that participate in immune function in AD to produce a variety of potentially neurotoxic compounds including superoxide, glutamate and nitric oxide (NO) In addition to its vasoactive properties, NO has significant neurophysiological functions. However, NO alone or in cooperation with superoxide anion and peroxynitrite can also be neurotoxic, primarily due to its free radical properties, and it has been implicated in AD-related neurodegeneration. At the same time release of NO from cerebral endothelial cells plays a key role in vascular tone, blood pressure regulation and vascular homeostasis and acts to inhibit platelet and leukocyte adhesion to the endothelium, a process that may down-regulate pro-inflammaroty events [51, 92].

Structural microvessel pathology, which is frequently observed in AD, results in endothelial dysfunction and dysregulation of NO, primarily in the hippocampus and entorhinal cortex. Constitutively reduced cerebrovascular NO production leads to cerebral hypoperfusion due to impaired vasodilation responses, and diminished capacity to remove respiratory waste products and toxins from the extracellular space due to reduced capillary permeability [89].

Therefore excitotoxicity, Ca^{2+} homeostasis disruptions, oxidative stress, neuro-inflammation, disturbed synthesis of NO and impaired cerebral circulation are the key pathogenetic factors of Alzheimer's disease.

Pharmacological past and adaptation future in treatment of Alzheimer's disease

The almost centenary history of pharmacologist fighting against Alzheimer's disease has demonstrated rather modest potentialities of drug therapy and prevention of this disease. The drug therapy slowing the rate of cognitive decline is mainly symptomatic and provides only moderate savings of about 1,500 EUR per patient [80]. In addition, development and use of drugs that aim at positively influencing the cognitive decline in patients with AD raises many ethical questions such as the significance of these drugs for the well-being and quality of life of patients [10]. Most pharmacological approaches used in Alzheimer's disease have been based on a simple «compensatory» or «inhibitory» principle. However many pathogenetic mechanisms of this disease have a «dual» nature, i.e., some of them can paradoxically activate neuronal defense. For example, elevated production of neurotoxic Aβ is postulated to represent a major event in the development of AD [22]. Under certain conditions, however, this is just Aβ that chelates copper ions and thereby restricts their pro-oxidant effect on brain neurons [50]. It is also well known that the increased production of proinflammatory cytokines (IL-1, IL-6) and TNFα results in neuroinflammation, NO overproduction and apoptosis in AD. However the same cytokines activate phagocytosis of Aβ to restrict its proinflammatory and other neurotoxic effects [43]. Another example. Increased glutamate concentrations can, on the one hand, provoke exitotoxicity and neuron death [25], but, on the other hand, can improve the cognitive function decline in AD [6]. Drugs may reduce glutamate receptor sensitivity [6, 126] to enhance neuron resistance but at the same time they may reduce cognitive functions. It is difficult to predict, which aspect of a pathogenetic factor will be stronger affected by the drug.

By the present time several classes of drugs have been developed and used for therapy of AD including acetylcholine esterase inhibitors, drugs influencing NMDA and glutamate receptors, drugs affecting synthesis of Aβ and formation of neurofibrillar tangles, anti-inflammatory drugs, etc. [6]. However efficacy of these drugs is limited by the facts that 1) each drug influences only a single step of the AD pathogenesis and 2) the drugs affect both damaged and normal cells. Cell-selective drug delivery is theoretically possible but such studies are yet at their very beginning.

At the same time it is clear already now that AD progression can be restricted by brain self-defense systems for a long time after the disease onset. These systems include those of antioxidants, heat shock proteins (HSPs), NO and other so-called stress-limiting systems [62, 68, 82]. These systems represent most sensitive sensors of intra- and extracellular adverse alterations and the first responders to the changes induced at the earliest stages of AD. These protective factors may be induced in the appropriate place and at the appropriate time. This is virtually impossible for pharmacological drugs. In addition, self-defense factors are regulated by the negative feedback mechanism, which prevents them from excessive accumulation. Drugs lack this property as well. Already now, available data allow development of a new trend in treatment of AD, the search for approaches to activation of self-defense to restrict neurodegenerative disorders.

The brain is subjected to multiple factors that result in damage of its cellular constituents, the neuron and supporting cells, and the neural networks that form the bases of cognitive ability. Like other systems, the brain has remarkable capacity to repair that damage and to adapt or compensate for the loss of neurons and the disruption of the neural architecture. Brain aging and dementia can be conceptualized as a balance between neuronal injury and repair. This balance can be affected not only by genetic and age-related factors but also by multiple environmental factors. The latter includes many factors, such as education, nutrition, exercise, socialization, and stress. These factors can be modified through lifestyle choices. By altering the balance between neuronal injury and repair, it is possible to delay the expression and progression of the neurodegenerative processes of brain aging, AD, and related dementias [7].

Recently Heininger [39] has put forward an interesting hypothesis that disorders of memory and other cognitive functions in Alzheimer's disease result from exhaustion of adaptive reserves in brain (Fig. 1).

Brain of elderly people tries to adapt actively to progressive substrate deprivation by decreasing general metabolism, enhancing oxidative stress and restricting cholinergic neurotransmission. These rearrangements are aimed at decreasing the substrate demands, enhancing the oxidative utilization of ketone bodies and preserving glucose. In this process Aβ plays a role of a metabolic switch, which inhibits the glucose utilization and stimulates the oxidative utilization of ketone bodies [39].

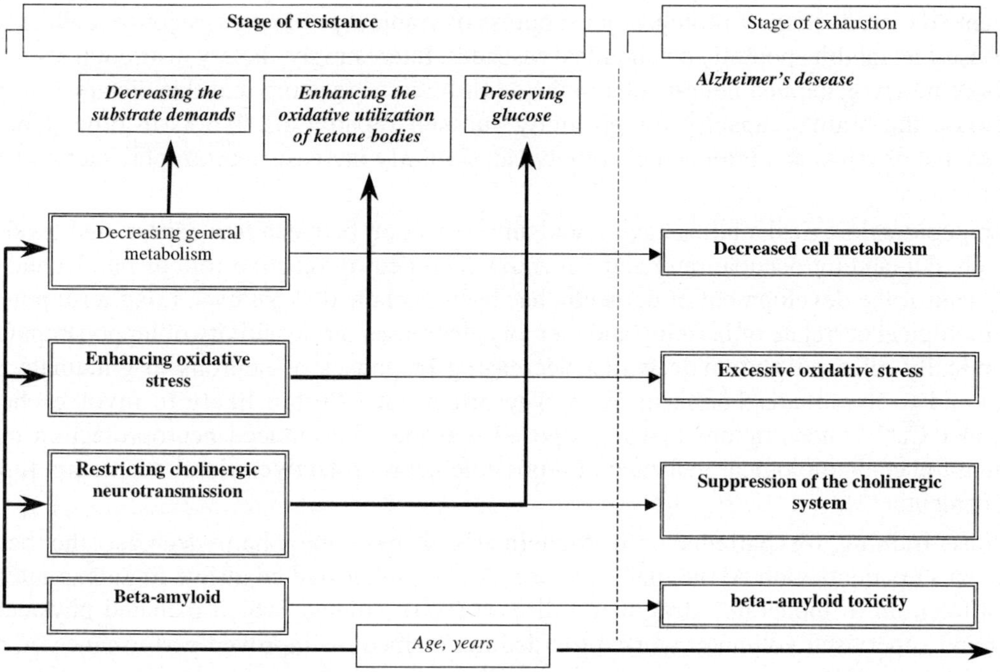

Fig. 1. Exhaustion of adaptive reserve in brain as a factor of Alzheimer's disease. For explanation see text.

Furthermore, as already mentioned, Aβ can bind copper ions and thereby prevent excessive oxidative stress [50]. This adaptive program provides functioning of an aging brain in the conditions of substrate deprivation.

However the adaptive program already contains risk factors for neurodegeneration, such as Aβ toxicity, decreased cell metabolism, oxidative stress and suppression of the cholinergic system. According to the hypothesis by Heininger [39], normal aging and AD represent two successive stages: stage of resistance and stage of exhausted adaptive reserves in brain. The hypothesis allows believing that methods of adaptive medicine aimed at increasing the adaptive reserve of the organism might help to combat AD.

Indeed, at present a major attention is paid to the means that may enhance adaptive potential and mobilize self-defense systems of the organism, such as natural adaptogens; among adaptogens ginkgo biloba is being extensively tested for its efficacy in improving neuropsychological parameters (trail-making speed, digit memory span, verbal learning, geriatric symptoms, depressive mood, memory status, etc.) [3, 26].

Available data suggest that adaptation to dietary restriction, physical and mental activity or mild stress exposure may reduce both the incidence and severity of neurodegenerative disorders in humans.

It was demonstrated that dietary restriction (reduced calorie intake) can increase the resistance of neurons in the brain to dysfunction and death in experimental models of AD. The mechanism underlying the beneficial effects of dietary restriction involves stimulation of the expression of HSPs and neurotrophic factors. The neurotrophic factors induced by dietary restriction may protect neurons by inducing the production of proteins that suppress oxyradical production, stabilize cellular calcium homeostasis and inhibit apoptotic biochemical cascades. Interestingly, dietary restriction also increases numbers of newly-generated neural cells in the adult brain suggesting that this dietary manipulation can increase the brain's capacity for plasticity and self-repair [76]. Works in other laboratories suggested that physical and intellectual activity can similarly increase neurotrophic factor production and neurogenesis.

Several epidemiological studies have found an association between low educational level (or low cognitively demanding occupations) and dementia. The neuroprotective role of intellectual activity training against the development of dementia has been explained as follows. Long-term potentiation (LTP, a biological correlate of learning and memory) increases the sensitivity of hippocampal neurons to synaptically released glutamate whilst decreasing responses of neurons to glutamate receptor agonists and to hypoxia/ischemia in vitro. The effects of LTP are likely to involve changes in intracellular Ca^{2+} concentration. It was proposed that the LTP-induced neuroprotection may help explaining the epidemiological evidence of a possible neuroprotective role of adaptation to learning against dementia [2].

Exercise training for patients with Alzheimer's disease may help decrease the behavioral impairment in patients with Alzheimer's disease. A comprehensive cognitive-linguistic intervention program for mild to moderate Alzheimer's disease (AD) patients, which included physical fitness training and supervised volunteer work, provided maintained or improved performance on multiple discourse outcome measures, preserving communicative function, slowing down of cognitive decline and improvement of mood [60, 117]. Data from the 1991-1992 Canadian Study of Health and Aging, a prospective cohort study of dementia, showed that compared with no exercise, physical activity was associated with lower risks of cognitive impairment, Alzheimer's disease, and dementia of any type. [55]. Therefore regular physical activity can represent an important and potent protective factor for cognitive decline and dementia in elderly persons.

Neuroprotective mechanisms of adaptation to environmental factors

Adaptation of the organism to environment is characterized by gradual attenuation of the stress response associated with formation of protective effects [82, 83]. It was demonstrated that the NMDA-mediated neurotoxic brain damage is potentiated by chronic administration of high doses of corticosterone, a major stress hormone, whereas administration of low-dose corticosterone mimicking adaptation to moderate stress attenuated the NMDA-triggered neurodegeneration [1]. It is attractive to direct the development of therapeutic strategies toward stimulation of metabolic rate/neuronal activity to improve cognition and other symptoms in AD. Studies have shown that stimulation of neurons through different mechanisms may protect those cells from the deleterious effects of aging and AD and, to a certain degree, restore several aspects of cognition and other central functions. For instance, the circadian system, which controls the sleep/wake cycle, may be stimulated in AD patients by exposing them to more light or transcutaneous nerve stimulation [114], the procedure, which has been used to induce adaptation to mild stress [83].

Protective effects of adaptation to hypoxia on the central nervous system have been demonstrated with respect to injuries and diseases of the cardiovascular system, immune system, and respiratory system [83]. Potentialities of adaptation to hypoxia for prevention of CNS disorders are less studied. It was shown that adaptation to intermittent hypobaric hypoxia produced in an altitude chamber exerted a protective effect in experimental epilepsy [87]; adaptation to high altitude hypoxia in mountains improved formation and retention of conditioned reflex in mice [82]. In patients, adaptation to hypobaric hypoxia has been used for treatment of schizophrenia and alcohol abuse [83]. Finally, adaptation to normobaric hypoxia proved efficient for prevention of behavioral disorders associated with neurodegenerative processes in experimental Parkinson disease [36]. It may be hypothesized that the adaptive resistance of nerve cells to Aβ toxicity may be partially due to an enhanced flux of glucose through both the glycolytic pathway and the hexose monophosphate shunt. These changes in glucose metabolism are due to the activation of the transcription factor hypoxia inducible factor 1 (HIF-1) [112], which is most efficiently expressed in adaptation to hypoxia [90].

In our experiments we mimicked Alzheimer's disease in rats by bilateral injection of Aβ peptide (25-35) into *n. basalis magnocellularis*. Prior to the β-amyloid treatment, a part of animals was exposed to a course of adaptation to intermittient hypobaric hypoxia (simulated altitude 4,000 above sea level; 4 hours daily for 14 days) in a hypobaric chamber. Cognitive function of animals was evaluated using the passive shock-avoidance conditioned response test [138] and the extrapolation escape task, which characterizes the rate of problem solution in stressful situations [101].

For the passive shock-avoidance conditioned response test in the training trial, the rats were placed in an illuminated chamber and the latency to step into the dark chamber was recorded. Upon entry into the dark chamber a foot shock was delivered until the rat escaped the dark chamber. In the retention trial, retesting was performed 24 hours later, and the latency to step into the dark chamber was recorded again. The better was memory of a rat the greater was the difference between latencies of the pre-shock and post-shock tests.

After the Aβ treatment, the change in latency of entry into the dark chamber was 30% less than in control (Fig.2). This fact represented worsening of retention, a marker sign of AD. Adaptation to hypoxia itself increased changes in post-shock latency and completely prevented the memory disorders induced by Aβ.

In the extrapolation escape task, a rat was placed in a glass cylinder plugged in water. In order to escape from this stressful situation, the rat should have to dive under the cylinder edge. The following parameters were recorded: the total latency of the motor reaction reflecting the quickness of decision-making onset; the number of abortive attempts to escape reflecting the efficiency of problem solution; and the latency of an escape reaction reflecting the quickness of problem solution in stressful situations.

It was shown that Aβ significantly increased almost twofold the latency of motor reaction and latency of escape, that is, worsened the cognitive function necessary to find a way out in an acute stress situation. Adaptation itself decreased the latency of motor reaction and prevented the Aβ-induced increase in this parameter. It means that adaptation to hypoxia increased the quickness of decision-making onset in stressful situation and prevented impairment of this function in animals treated with Aβ (Fig. 3).

Table 1 shows key mechanisms of neurodegeneration in AD and potential neuroprotective mechanisms of adaptation to hypoxia.

Thus, oxidative stress and increased Ca^{2+} influx in neurons can be restricted by adaptive activation of antioxidant enzymes [84] and Ca^{2+} transport systems [100, 106]. Adaptation to hypoxia is able to restrict both NO overproduction by iNOS and nNOS and deficient activity of eNOS [70], the processes

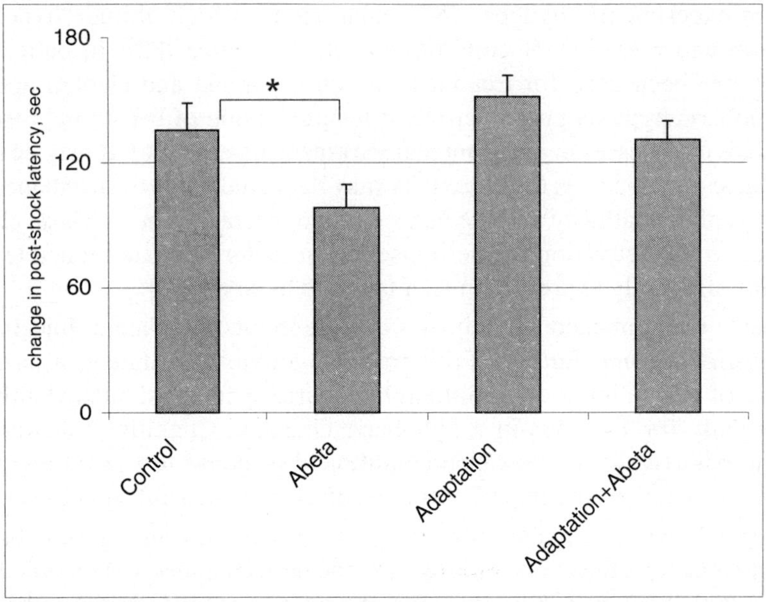

Fig. 2. Effect of adaptation to hypoxia on the retention ability of rats (Aβ-induced change in the latency of entry into the dark chamber in the passive shock avoidance conditioned response test.) *Significant differences, p<0.05.

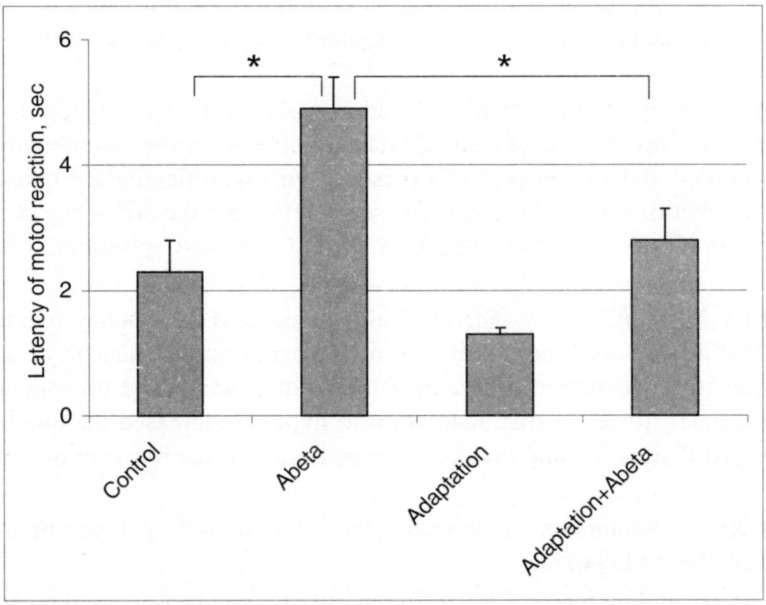

Fig. 3. Effect of adaptation to hypoxia on the Aβ-induced change in parameters of extrapolation escape task. *Significant differences, p<0.05.

Table 1. Potential Neuroprotective Mechanisms of Adaptation to Hypoxia

Mechanisms of neurodegeneration in Alzheimer's disease	Protective mechanisms of adaptation to hypoxia
Excessive oxidative stress	Increased activity of antioxidant enzymes *(Meerson et al., 1992)*
Increased calcium entry in neurons	Increased activity of calcium transport systems *(Sazontova et al., 1995)*
Disturbed NO synthesis (increased activity of *iNOS* and depressed activity of *eNOS*)	Restricted NO overproduction and compensation for NO deficiency by NO binding to and release from NO stores, respectively *(Manukhina et al., 2002).*
Neurodegeneration	Activated synthesis of the neuroprotective proteins HSP70 *(Malyshev et al., 1999)*
Disturbed cerebral circulation	Stimulated synthesis of the vasodilator NO and increased density of vascular network in brain. *(Manukhina et al., 1982)*

involved in vasculopathy and disorders of cerebral circulation in AD [120]. This type of modulation cannot be achieved by pharmacological means. Finally, adaptive stimulation of HSP70 synthesis [62, 85, 100] may restrict neurodegeneration in AD.

This hypothesis is supported by data of literature and results of our own experiments.

Adaptive restriction of free-radical oxidation for protection of brain against neurodegeneration

Involvement of free radicals in pathogenesis of AD is supported by the fact that neurons are extremely sensitive to attacks by destructive free radicals. Furthermore, lesions are present in the brains of AD patients that are typically associated with attacks by free radicals (eg, damage to DNA, protein oxidation, lipid peroxidation, and advanced glycosylation end products), and metals (eg, iron, copper, zinc, and aluminum) that have catalytic activity to produce free radicals. Beta-amyloid is aggregated and produces more free radicals in the presence of free radicals; beta-amyloid toxicity is eliminated by free radical scavengers [21].

Treatment with antioxidants is a promising approach for slowing disease progression to the extent that oxidative damage may be responsible for the cognitive and functional decline observed in AD. Although not a uniformly consistent observation, a number of epidemiological studies have found a link between antioxidant intake and a reduced incidence of dementia, AD and cognitive decline in elderly populations. In AD clinical trials molecules with antioxidant properties such as vitamin E and *Ginkgo biloba* extract have shown modest benefit. A clinical trial with vitamin E is currently ongoing to determine if it can delay progression to AD in individuals with mild cognitive impairment. Combinations of antioxidants might be of even greater potential benefit for AD, especially if the agents worked in different cellular compartments or had complementary activity (e.g. vitamins E, C and ubiquinone). Naturally-occurring compounds with antioxidant capacity are available and widely marketed (e.g. vitamin C, ubiquinone, lipoic acid, beta-carotene, creatine, melatonin, curcumin) and synthetic compounds are under development by industry. Nevertheless, the clinical value of these agents for AD prevention and treatment is ambiguous [35].

Effect of intermittent hypoxia on antioxidant enzymes activity was investigated in patients with dyscirculatory encephalopathy in the presence of arterial hypertension. After a 10-day hypoxic training (60 min daily atmospheric air breathing alternated with 9-10 V% O_2 hypoxic mixture breathing), total oxidant activity and thiobarbituric acid reactive substances (TBARS) were decreased whereas activities of superoxide dismutase, catalase, glutathione peroxidase in erythrocytes were increased. The treatment resulted in reduction of peak systolic and peak diastolic blood flow rate in the middle cerebral artery, decrease in frequency of headache episodes and in improvement of nighttime sleep and short-term memory. The results demonstrated a possibility for correction of disturbed oxidative homeostasis in patients with dyscirculatory encephalopathy using adaptation to hypoxia [29].

Experiments on the rats showed that a 7-hour exposure to 10% hypoxic gas mixture left unaffected the Fe^{2+}-induced chemiluminescence and rate of accumulation of TBARS in plasma, brain and other tissues. Two-week adaptation to intermittent hypoxia induced some activation of free-radical oxidation and a more pronounced potentiation of the endogenous antioxidant system. These changes in the free-radical oxidation system and antioxidant defense appear relevant for the mechanism of the well-established preventive and curative effects of intermittent hypoxia [9].

Adaptation to intermittent hypoxia in the altitude chamber increased activities of antioxidant enzymes in rat heart, liver and brain while the content of peroxidation products remained at the baseline level; this effect correlated with adaptive protection of rat heart against reperfusion arrhythmias [84].

Finally, adaptation to hypoxia may stimulate synthesis of melatonin, which is deficient in approximately 45% of AD patients. Melatonin is widely used as an antioxidant and also for treatment of sleep disorders and sundowning agitation in AD [17].

Melatonin has been shown to be highly effective in reducing oxidative damage in the central nervous system; this efficacy derives from its ability to directly scavenge a number of free radicals and to function as an indirect antioxidant. In particular, melatonin detoxifies the highly toxic hydroxyl radical as well as the peroxyl radical, peroxynitrite anion, nitric oxide, and singlet oxygen, all of which can damage macromolecules in brain cells. Additionally, melatonin stimulates a variety of antioxidative enzymes including superoxide dismutase, glutathione peroxidase and glutathione reductase [103]. Besides the direct scavenging properties and indirect antioxidant actions of melatonin, its ability to protect neurons probably also stems from its antiamyloidogenic properties [96].

A study by Kaur et al. [45] examined the effects of high-altitude exposure on the pineal gland, the main source of production of melatonin. It was surmised that hypoxia experienced at high altitude, caused by decreased oxygen tension in the ambient air, might lead to some structural alterations in the pineal gland and, hence, affect its melatonin production. The plasma melatonin level showed a steady increase following altitude exposure peaking at 7 days and returned to control levels thereafter.

Therefore there is abundant indirect evidence that adaptation to hypoxia may be beneficial for prevention of AD-related disorders due to restriction of free radical processes. However studies demonstrating this effect have been absent up to the present.

In our experiments oxidative stress was evaluated in Aβ-treated rats by TBARS in different brain structures including the cortex, cerebellum and hippocampus.

Table 2 shows that Aβ selectively induced oxidative stress in the hippocampus. Adaptation to hypoxia alone did not affect the level of TBARS but, at the same time, it restricted the increase in TBARS induced by Aβ. As it has been mentioned above, adaptation to hypoxia efficiently prevented cognitive disorders in Aβ-treated rats. This is the first demonstration of the fact that one of the cognition-protective mechanisms of adaptation to hypoxia may be related with restriction of oxidative stress in the hippocampus.

Table 2. Effect of adaptation to hypoxia on Abeta-induced oxidative stress in brain structures.

	Thiobarbituric acid reactive substances (MDA), nmol/g tissue		
	Cortex	Cerebellum	Hippocampus
Control	57.6 ± 4.6	56.8 ± 5.4	53.8 ± 2.2
Abeta	56.7 ± 4.7	52.7 ± 2.8	63.1 ± 2.7 *
Adaptation	55.3 ± 7.2	57.7 ± 4.5	54.7 ± 3.5
Adaptation + Abeta	61.2 ± 4.9	54.6 ± 2.8	56.1 ± 2.1

Adaptive modulation of disturbed NO synthesis for protection of brain against neurodegeneration

NO acts as a neuromodulator in the CNS and participates in the regulation of diverse physiological process including cerebral circulation, brain development, pain perception, neuronal plasticity, memory and behavior. All three isoforms of NOS are found in the brain. NNOS is expressed in highly ramified neurons throughout the brain including cerebellum, cerebral cortex, hippocampus, amygdala, and substantia nigra [122]; eNOS is primarily localized in endothelial cells although it has been detected in small populations of neurons; iNOS is not found in healthy tissues but can be expressed after brain insult in astrocytes, neurons and endothelial cells. When produced in excessive amount, NO switches from a physiological neuromodulator to a neurotoxic effector. Overproduction of NO may occur from nNOS following persistent stimulation of excitatory amino acid receptors mediating glutamate toxicity and/or from iNOS after its induction by diverse stimuli including Aβ in microglial cells and cytokine-activated astrocytes. The predominant mechanism, by which NO promotes neuronal death implicates the reaction of NO with superoxide anion to generate cytotoxic peroxynitrite. NO can directly impair by nitrosylation the function of essential proteins containing iron-sulphur clusters and thiol residues. Neuronal death either by apoptosis and/or necrosis occurs by inhibition of key enzymes of the tricarbonic acid cycle, the mitochondrial respiratory chain, mitochondrial calcium metabolism, or DNA damage with subsequent activation of the energy-consuming pathway involving poly(ADP-ribose) synthase (PARS). In this cascade, mitochondria, which are very sensitive to the noxious effects of NO and peroxynitrite, appear to play a pivotal role in the development of neurodegenerative disorders [19].

On the other hand, NO can be regarded as a protective factor in AD. A diminished capacity of vascular endothelium to generate NO may be associated with increased risk of AD. Vascular NO has the potential to enhance the membrane polarization of cerebral neurons by increasing the open probability of calcium-activated potassium channels; this may protect neurons from the excessive calcium influx, potentiated by Abeta that is thought to mediate neuronal damage in AD [78]. Indeed, astrocytic and epithelial cells, that produce more nitrite/nitrate are better protected against the NO toxicity than the less nitrite/nitrate producing neuronal cell lines [33].

In patients with AD, the intrathecal levels of nitrate were significantly and inversely correlated to the degree of intellectual impairment [116]. This study demonstrated an inverse correlation between the intrathecal levels of nitrate and the degree of cognitive impairment in patients with AD, suggesting a neuroprotective effect of NO in AD. This neuroprotective effect of NO may be due to its role in regulating the cerebral circulation. Alternatively, the neuroprotective effect of NO may be due to its role as neurotransmitter. Interestingly, an increasing body of evidence suggests that NO participates in the long-lasting enhanced synaptic efficacy after high-frequency firing of excitatory synapses in the cerebral cortex and hippocampus called long-term potentiation, on which phenomenon certain forms of learning are believed to depend. Böhme et al. [11] have shown that a NOS inhibitor blocks long-term potentiation, whereas an NO donor induces a long-lasting enhancement in synaptic efficacy. In AD patients with a higher constitutive capacity to produce NO, long-term potentiation may be facilitated, ameliorating the learning ability of these subjects.

Vasculopathy in AD was correlated with reduced levels of eNOS expression in cerebral vessels. The low levels of cerebrovascular eNOS were associated with increased levels of the pro-apoptosis gene product, p53 in smooth muscle and endothelial cells, suggesting a role for altered eNOS expression in AD-associated vascular degeneration. Constitutively reduced cerebrovascular eNOS expression and NO production could also lead to cerebral hypoperfusion due to impaired vasodilation responses, and diminished capacity to remove respiratory waste products and toxins from the extracellular space due to reduced capillary permeability [88]. Evidence indicates that AD is to a considerable extent a vascular disorder with neurodegenerative consequences. The clinical convergence of advanced ageing in the presence of a chronic, pre-morbid vascular risk factor, can contribute to an endotheliopathy involving basal NO deficit, to the degree where regional metabolic dysfunction leads to cognitive meltdown and to progressive neurodegeneration characteristic of AD [119].

NO is involved in the organism self-defence not only due to its direct participation in major physiological processes but also due to its ability to activate synthesis of protective HSPs. It was shown by our studies that both endogenous and exogenous NO can induce synthesis of HSP70 [61, 63]. Moreover the NO-dependent HSP70 synthesis was demonstrated to be an integral part of adaptation of the organism to environmental factors such as hypoxia, exercise training, heat, emotional stress, etc. [62]. Endogenous NO and NO donors were reported to increase heme oxygenase (HSP32) activity and NOS mRNA level in cell culture [46]. On the other hand, sodium nitroprusside reduced heme oxygenase activity and a NOS inhibitor increased it in homogenates of rat brain [127]. These reports suggested and further experiments confirmed that the NO/HSP32 system may function in concert in the brain and that various types of cells in the brain are able to increase the HSP32 expression in response to NO [115]. The NO-induced HO activation may provide cells with biliverdin and bilirubin, two reactive oxygen species scavengers [24]. This is why NO and HSPs are considered as interrelated components of a united self-defense system, and the studies directed to this system in AD may bring much benefit to the problem of AD. Indeed, it was shown that promotion of endothelial NO activity may decrease risk for age-related neurodegeneration [78].

Therefore excessive NO is neurotoxic and contributes to development and progression of AD while deficient production of endothelial NO precipitates and aggravates AD-related disorders mediating cerebral hypoperfusion and insufficiency of NO-inducible protective mechanisms. This is why it would be reasonable to seek for the means capable of "bidirectional" modulation of NO production. Chronic non-drug stimulation of endogenous NO production can be produced most efficiently by special diets [18, 98] or adaptation to environmental factors such as hypoxia, exercise, cold, stress, heat, etc. [67]. The most efficient stimulation of NO production was obtained in adaptation to hypoxia and exercise training, the two types of adaptation most generally employed in experimental and clinical setting [62, 65, 66]. Both types of adaptation appear to stimulate NO production primarily due to increased eNOS activity and expression [18, 37, 54, 109, 111, 131]. This effect may contribute to the well-established preventive and curative effect of these adaptations in cardiovascular diseases associated with endothelial dysfunction [67]. At the same time, while stimulating endothelial NO synthesis, adaptation to environmental factors efficiently prevented NO overproduction and restricted excessive endothelium-dependent vasodilation and hypotension induced by acute myocardial infarction [70], heat shock [64, 71] and anaphylactic shock [74].

There are two possible mechanisms, which might underlie the simultaneous adaptive protection against NO overproduction and deficiency. First, NO overproduction is restricted by NO itself through the negative feedback [5] and, therefore, the prior increase in NO synthesis induced by adaptation may contribute to the adaptive prevention of NO overproduction. Second, various types of adaptation are consistently associated with formation of so-called NO stores (NO-containing complexes) in vascular wall [72, 121]. Physiological experiments have demonstrated that formation of NO stores is apparently an adaptive response, which can protect the organism against toxic effects of excessive NO; at the same time NO stores can serve as an additional non-enzymic source of NO to compensate for its deficiency [70, 72]. Figure 4 shows the dynamics of NO production and formation of NO stores in the course of adaptation to hypoxia. In this process, plasma levels of the stable NO metabolites nitrite and nitrate was significantly correlated with the size of NO stores [69].

In our experiments adaptation to hypoxia limited the decrease in NO production induced by Aβ apparently due to potentiation of NO synthesis and release of NO from NO stores. Aβ significantly reduced by 40% the plasma level of nitrite and nitrate in rats. Behavioral experiments demonstrated that the NOS inhibitor L-NNA considerably potentiated the adverse effect of β-amyloid on the retention ability of rats. Adaptation to hypoxia improved the cognitive function in rats and prevented the decrease in plasma nitrite and nitrate induced by Aβ. Therefore the decreased NO production in the organism might predetermine a higher vulnerability of cognitive functions to the adverse effect of β-amyloid whereas the mechanism of adaptive protection may be related with restriction of the Aβ-induced decrease in NO production.

Adaptive improvement of cerebral circulation for protection of brain against neurodegeneration

Vasculopathic lesions or chronic hypoperfusion characteristic of AD may deprive brain cells of vital nutrients that can result in metabolic and physiological changes leading to neuronal death pathways. To treat such a state, promotion of endogenous neoangiogenesis may be beneficial [118]. A number of techniques have been proposed for creation of new blood vessels in peripheral tissues including intra-arterial infusion of recombinant fibroblast growth factor-2 [57], basic fibroblast growth factor [97, 108], plasmid delivery of vascular endothelial growth factor [59, 120], «seeding» of endothelial cells cultured from endothelial progenitor cells [12, 130], and, finally, controlled puncture of very small

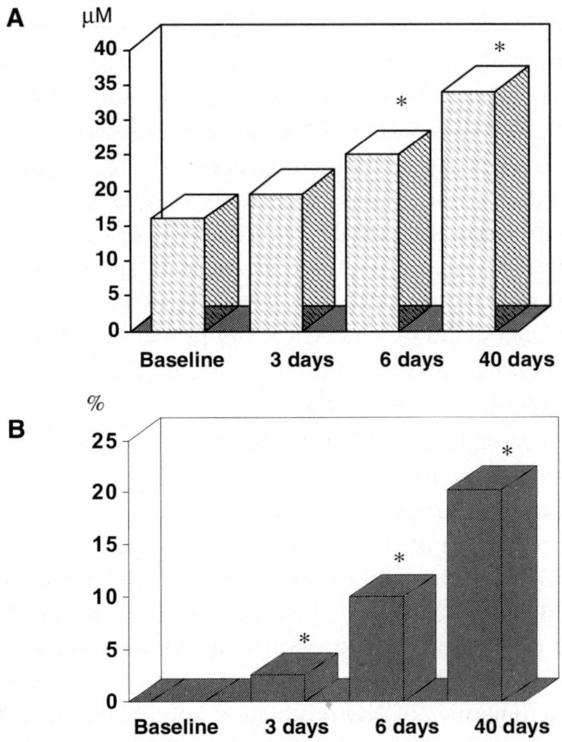

Fig. 4. Effect of adaptation to hypoxia on NO production and storage in rats.
A: Plasma concentration if nitrite and nitrate (µM).
B: Volume of NO stores in the isolated aorta from rats adapted to hypoxia. NO stores were revealed using the relaxation response of noradrenaline-precontracted aorta to diethyldithiocarbamate (DETC), which released NO from NO stores. The response to DETC was expressed as per cent of the aorta contractile response to noradrenaline.
***Significant difference from baseline value, $p<0.05$.**

holes in tissue using laser energy, which induced rapid formation of new blood vessels [89]. However the brain presents many problems not encountered in more readily accessible organs like the heart, and these techniques will require sophisticated development and adjustment.

Improvement of cerebral blood flow represents one of protective effects of adaptation to hypoxia. This effect is based not only on stimulation of NO synthesis but also on the increased density of vascular network, which was observed in adaptation to hypobaric hypoxia in different organs including skeletal muscles [99], placenta [137], and brain [73]. The neovascularization is attributed to hypoxia-induced activation of HIF-1, which upregulates expression of genes involved in the adaptation of higher organisms to hypoxic conditions, caused by high altitude, anemia, wound healing or during development. Examples of these oxy-genes include erythropoietin, a hormone regulating erythropoiesis and hence the oxygen transport capacity, and vascular endothelial growth factor, a potent inducer of angiogenesis leading to increased blood capillary density [124].

Role of HSP70 in the protection of brain against neurodegeneration

HSP70 is now considered as a molecular 'chaperone' and a cell-protective agent. The expression of these proteins is closely related to that of amyloid precursor protein (APP). HSPs have been reported to regulate the apoptotic pathway, suppress oxyradical production, stabilize cellular calcium homeostasis and play a critical role in protein conformational diseases such as AD [13, 96, 104].

The HSP70 mRNA levels in brain of patients with AD are significantly lower than those from patients with vascular dementia and nondemented controls. It was suggested that the lower levels of constitutive HSP70 mRNA in AD play an important role in developing AD and that the measurement of HSP70 mRNA may be useful for the diagnosis of AD [123]. Getchell et al. [32] showed that an age-dependent decrease in HSP70 in olfactory receptor neurons of older subjects and those with Alzheimer's disease might be attributable to their greater susceptibility to stress.

The dysregulated processes of HSPs synthesis that lead to disturbed self-defense in AD are not completely known. However, after studying the morphology, evolution, and distribution of HSPs in AD it was suggested that these proteins could represent a defensive response to various stressful stimuli, either endogenous or exogenous. The hypothesis was confirmed by many studies that showed stress response in AD brain [110].

In AD, stress proteins play, first of all, a neuroprotective role [8, 92]. At least 7 mechanisms are known, which may underlie this neuroprotection: 1) restriction of apoptosis; 2) restriction of NO overproduction; 3) disaggregation of extracellular Aβ aggregates; 4) enhancement of Aβ elimination from intercellular space; 5) restriction of tau-protein hyperphosphorylation; 6) protection of neurons from glutamate toxicity; and 7) restriction of intracellular Aβ cytotoxicity. Each of these mechanisms is discussed below in more detail (Fig.5).

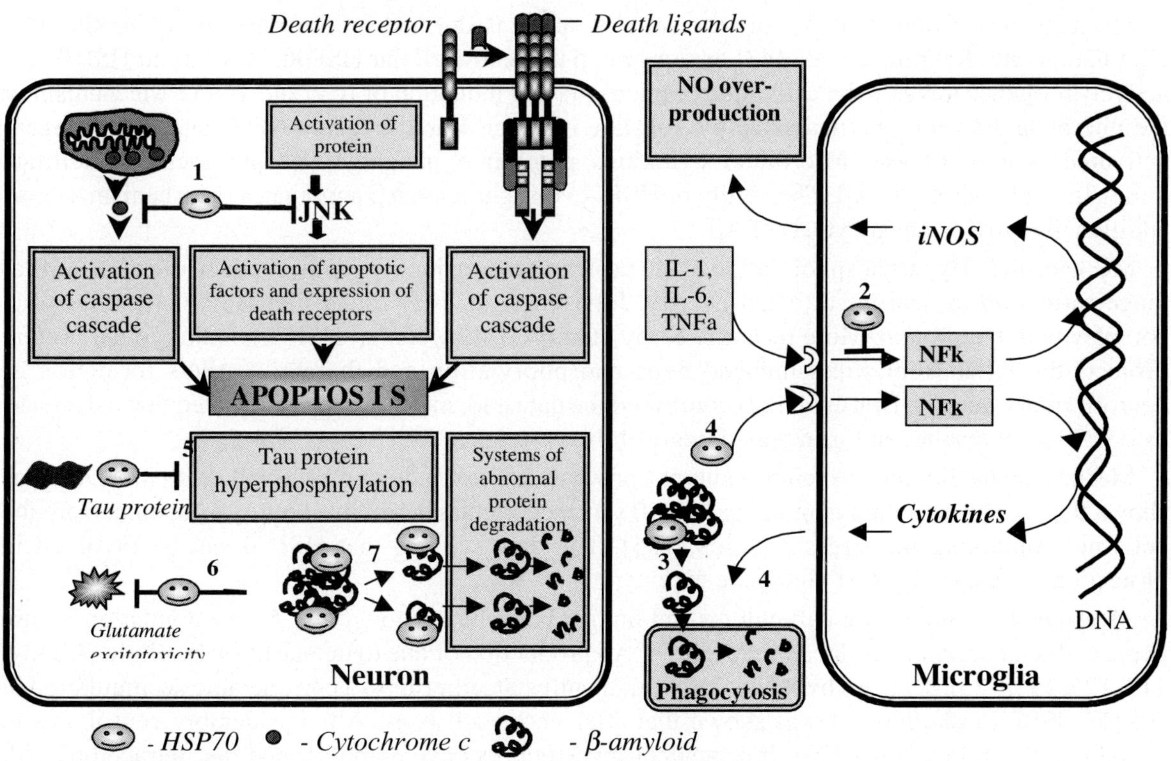

Fig. 5. Tentative neuroprotective effects of HSPs in Alzheimer's disease. 1-7: Neuroprotective mechanisms of HSPs. For explanation see text.

Mechanism 1. Death of neurons in AD is mediated primarily by the apoptotic pathway. Initiation of apoptosis involves receptor- and mitochondria-dependent pathways. In receptor-dependent apoptosis, extracellular death ligands, such as TNF-α, induce trimerization of cell surface active death receptors [4]. The increased amount of death receptors and activation of some intracellular proapoptotic factors can occur due to activation of stress-inducible protein kinase JNK (c-Jun–N-terminal kinase) [107]. The trimerized receptor complex activates caspases, which, in their turn, selectively split cell proteins. The mitochondria-dependent apoptotic pathway is triggerred by the apoptosis-inducing factor (AIF) [16, 58] and cytochrome *c,* which is released from mitochondria to activate the caspase cascade together with ATP and the protein Apaf-1 [49, 134]. It appeared that HSP70 can inhibit apoptosis by inhibiting the release of cytochrome *c* from mitochondria [48], inactivation of Apaf-1 and AIF [102]. In addition, HSP70 may interrupt transmission to the apoptotic signal at the level of JNK [31].

Mechanism 2. The NO overproduction induced by cytokines affecting glial cells substantially contributes to pathogenesis of inflammatory responses in AD. It was shown that HSPs can restrict NO overproduction and thus alleviate neuroinflammation [15]. This is due to the fact that HSP70 inhibits activation of NFkB and thereby inhibits expression of cytokine and iNOS genes [136].

Mechanism 3. It is accepted that the pronounced accumulation of amyiloid plaques is one of the most important triggers of neurodegenerative process. Kudva et al. [52] demonstrated that low molecular weight stress proteins can prevent formation of Aβ aggregates *in vitro* due to chaperonic properties of stress proteins. While such experiments have not been performed with respect of HSP70, the latter may also be involved in this process with a high extent of probability.

Mechanism 4. Content of Aβ in extracellular space is defined by the ratio of Aβ production/elimination rate. Kakimura et al., [43] demonstrated that extracellular HSP90, HSP70 and HSP32 can actively influence this ratio by activation of microglia and induction of IL-6 and TNFα. Mechanism of the microglia activation is medicated by Toll-like receptor 4 and involves NFkB and p38 mitogen-activated protein kinase. Microglial cytokines potentiate phagocytosis and thereby facilitate elimination of neurotoxic Aβ. The ability of HSPs to disaggregate Aβ aggregates (Mechanism 4) may additionally provide phagocytosis of Aβ.

Mechanism 5. Hyperphosphorylation of tau protein is the major trigger mechanism of neurofibrillar tange formation in neurons affected by AD. Johnson et al. [41] found that HSP70 form a stable complex with tau protein. More recently, Kirby et al. [47] showed that HSP70 binding to tau protein protects the latter from stress-induced hyperphosphorylation and thereby restricts formation of neurofibrillary tangles. Dou et al. [27] confirmed the data and, moreover, demonstrated that a decrease in HSP70 level resulted in formation of neurofibrillary tangles.

Mechanism 6. Glutamate excitotoxicity is known as a factor inducing neuronal death in AD. It was shown that a cell population containing HSP70 survived glutamate-induced injury as distinct from the cells not containing the stress proteins [135]. The data suggest that HSP70 can be involved in protection of neurons against glutamate toxicity.

Mechanism 7. Studies on cell culture and human brain have shown that Aβ accumulation within nerve cells can occur either due to intracellular Aβ production or due to uptake of extracellular Aβ [34, 113, 125, 126, 133]. This is why Aβ toxicity can manifest itself prior to a considerable accumulation of Aβ [53, 129]. Furthermore it was shown that after nerve cell lysis, Aβ considerably contributes to formation of senile plaques [23]. Independent investigators have demonstrated that intracellular Aβ

forms complexes with several proteins, many of which possess chaperonic activity [30, 132]. The most specific interaction was observed for intracellular Aβ and HSP70 [30]. To reveal the implication of HSP70 interaction with Aβ for formation of the pathological degenerative cell phenotype, Fonte et al. [30] enhanced the shaperonic function of HSP70 using the dsRNAi technology in transgenic *C. elegans* overproducing intracellular human Aβ. The enhanced chaperonic function of HSP70 appeared to suppress completely the formation of intracellular Aβ induced degenerative phenotype of *C. elegans.* The data suggest that the chaperon system of cell including HSP70 recognizes intracellular Aβ as an abnormal protein. In result, HSP70, probably together with other chaperon proteins actively rearrange Aβ metabolism from the secretory mode to the alternative mode of disaggregation and degradation of the abnormal protein through the lysosomal [20] or ubiquitine-dependent pathway [77].

Taken together available data of literature suggest that stress proteins HSP70 represent an important endogenous system protecting neurons in AD. This protection is realized at several levels of the molecular mechanism of this disease.

In recent decade it was clearly demonstrated that adaptation to hypoxia or hypoxic preconditioning induced HSP70-dependent resistance of brain to hypoxia and glucose deprivation, the factors implicated in AD. Thus, hypoxic tolerance induced by preconditioning was demonstrated using the maintenance of cerebral glucose metabolic rate as a neuronal viability index. In addition, profiling of gene expression using an Atlas Rat Stress Array suggested the involvement of the expression of HSPs in hypoxic tolerance induction [93]. Direct evidence was obtained that selective overexpression of HSP70 enhances the survival of astrocytes challenged with oxygen-glucose deprivation [94]. Our experiments showed that adaptation to intermittent hypobaric hypoxia induced resistance of rats to acute sublethal hypoxia. This protective effect was accompanied by accumulation of HSP70 in brain. The NOS inhibitor L-NNA abolished both the adaptive protection and HSP70 induction; this fact indicated involvement of increased NO synthesis in HSP70 accumulation in adaptation to hypoxia [65].

Therefore the evidence is available that in Ab injury, the adaptive protection of cognitive functions may be due to restriction of oxidative stress, prevention of impaired NO production, accumulation of protective HSPs, and improvement of cerebral circulation.

Theoretically, there are three possible approaches to activation of endogenous defense systems: i) a pharmacological approach, which implies certain intrinsic drawbacks such as side effects, individual intolerance, cell non-specificity, etc.; ii) a molecular biological approach, which may be potentially the most efficient but is very complicated for application, especially in clinical setting; and iii) an adaptation approach, which seems very promising for clinical application. The latter approach implies that activation of self-defense systems will be achieved due to adaptation of the organism to moderate periodic influence of environmental factors such as hypoxia, heat or exercise. In this review we have selectively crystallized data that point to adaptation as a possible non-drug means for prevention of AD to provide a break-through in clinics of this disease.

Acknowledgements

The study was supported by NWO (grant 047.011.2001.010) and the Russian Foundation for Basic Research (grant 03-04-49065).

References

1. Abraham, I., Harkany, T., Horvath, K.M., Veenema, A.H., Penke, B., Nyakas, C., Luiten, P.G. Chronic corticosterone administration dose-dependently modulates Abeta(1-42)- and NMDA-induced neurodegeneration in rat magnocellular nucleus basalis. J. Neuroendocrinol. 12: 486-494, 2000.
2. Addae, J.I., Youssef, F.F., Stone, T.W.. Neuroprotective role of learning in dementia: a biological explanation. J. Alzheimers Dis. 5: 91-104, 2003.
3. Ahlemeyer, B., Krieglstein, J. Pharmacological studies supporting the therapeutic use of Ginkgo biloba extract for Alzheimer's disease. Pharmacopsychiatry 36 Suppl 1: S8-14, 2003.
4. Ashkenazi, A. and Dixit, V.M. Death receptors: signaling and modulation. Science 281: 1305-1308, 1998.
5. Assreuy, J., Cunha, F.Q., Liew, F.Y., Moncada, S. Feedback inhibition of nitric oxide synthase activity by nitric oxide. Br. J. Pharmacol. 108: 833-837, 1993.
6. Bachurin, S.O. Medical chemistry of targeted search for drugs for treatment and prevention of neurodegenerative diseases as exemplified by Alzheimer's disease. Neurodegenerative Diseases and Aging. Zavalishin, I.A., Yakhno, N.N., Gavrilova S.I., Eds. Moscow, 2001, 399-454 (in Russian).
7. Ball, L.J., Birge, S.J.. Prevention of brain aging and dementia. Clin. Geriatr. Med. 18: 485-503, 2002.
8. Behl, C., Schubert, D. Heat shock partially protects rat pheochromocytoma PC12 cells from amyloid beta peptide toxicity. Neurosci. Lett. 154: 1-4, 1993.
9. Belykh, A.G., Gukasov, V.M., Chukaev, S.A. State of the free-radical oxidation system in normobaric hypoxia. Fiziol. Zh. 38: 73-76, 1992 (in Russian).
10. Berghmans, R.L. Anti-Alzheimer drugs: ethical aspects of research and practice. Tijdschr. Gerontol. Geriatr. 31:100-106, 2000.
11. Böhme, G.A., Bon, C., Stutzmann, J.-M., Doble, A., Blanchard, J.-C. Possible involvement of nitric oxide in long-term potentiation. Eur. J. Pharmacol. 199: 379-381, 1991.
12. Boyer, M., Townsend, L.E., Vogel, L., Falk, J., Reitz-Vick, D., Trevor, K. Isolation of endothelial cells from human peripheral blood. J. Vasc. Surg. 31: 181-189, 2000.
13. Brown, I.R., Gozes, I.. Stress genes in the nervous system during development and aging diseases. Ann. N. Y. Acad. Sci. 851:123-128, 1998.
14. Butterfield, K.A., Howard, B., Yatin, S., Koppal, T., Drake, J., Hensley, K., Aksenov M., Aksenova, M., Subramaniam, R., Varadarajan, S., Harris-White, M.E., Pedigo Jr., N.M., Carmey, J.M. Elevated oxidative stress in models of human brain aging and Alzheimer's disease. Life Sci. 65: 1883-1892, 1999.
15. Calabrese, V., Bates, T.E., Stella, A.M. NO synthase and NO-dependent signal pathways in brain aging and neurodegenerative disorders: the role of oxidant/antioxidant balance. Neurochem. Res. 25: 1315-1341, 2000.
16. Cande, C., Cohen, I., Daugas, E., Ravagnan, L., Larochette, N., Zamzami, N., Kroemer, G. Apoptosis-inducing factor (AIF): a novel caspase-independent death effector released from mitochondria. Biochimie. 84: 215-122, 2002.
17. Cardinali, D.P., Brusco, L.I., Liberczuk, C., Furio, A.M. The use of melatonin in Alzheimer's disease. Neuroendocrinol. Lett. Suppl. 1: 20-23, 2002.
18. Cellermajer, D.S. Endothelial dysfunction: Does it matter? Is it reversible? J. Am. Coll. Cardiol. 30: 325-353, 1997.
19. Charbrier, P.-E., Demerlé-Pallardy, C., Auguet, M. Nitric oxide synthases: targets for therapeutic strategies in neurological diseases. Cell Mol. Life Sci. 55: 1029-1035, 1999.
20. Chiang, H.L., Terlecky, S.R., Plant, C.P., Dice, J.F. A role for a 70-kilodalton heat shock protein in lysosomal degradation ofintracellular proteins. Science 246: 382-385, 1989.
21. Christen, Y. Oxidative stress and Alzheimer disease. Am J Clin Nutr. 71: 621S-629S, 2000.
22. Clippingdale, A.B., Wade, J.D., Barrow. C.J. The amyloid-beta peptide and its role in Alzheimer's disease. J. Pept. Sci. 7: 227-249, 2001.

23. D'Andrea, M.R., Nagele, R.G., Wang, H.Y., Peterson, P.A., Lee, D.H. Evidence that neurons accumulating amyloid can undergo lysis to form amyloid plaques in Alzheimer's disease. Histopathology 38: 120-134, 2001.

24. Datta, P.K., Lianos, E.A. Nitric oxide induces heme oxygenase-1 gene expression in mesangial cells. Kidney International 55: 1734-1739, 1999.

25. Dodd, P.R. Excited to death: different ways to lose your neurons. Biogerontology 3: 51-56, 2002.

26. Dongen van, M.C., Rossum van, E., Kessels, A.G., Sielhorst, H.J., Knipschild, P.G. The efficacy of ginkgo for elderly people with dementia and age-associated memory impairment: new results of a randomized clinical trial. J. Am. Geriatr. Soc. 48: 1183-1194, 2000.

27. Dou, F., Netzer, W.J., Tanemura, K., Li, F., Hartl, F.U., Takashima, A., Gouras, G.K., Greengard, P., Xu, H. Chaperones increase association of tau protein with microtubules. Proc. Natl. Acad. Sci. USA 100: 721-726, 2003

28. Dykens, J.A. Isolated cerebral and cerebellar mitochondria produce free radicals when exposed to elevated Ca^{2+} and Na^{+}: implication for neurodegeneration. J. Neurochem. 63: 584-591, 1994.

29. El'chaninova, S.A., Koreniak, N.A., Smagina, I.V., Pinegin, L.E., Varshavskii, B.Ia. Intermittent hypoxia in the treatment of dyscirculatory encephalopathy. Zh. Nevrol. Psikhiatr. Im. S. S. Korsakova 102: 29-32, 2002 (in Russian).

30. Fonte, V., Kapulkin, V., Taft, A., Fluet, A., Friedman, D., Christopher D. Interaction of intracellular β amyloid peptide with chaperone proteins. Proc. Natl. Acad. Sci. USA 99:9439-9444, 2002.

31. Gabai, V.L., Meriin, A.B., Yaglom, J.A., Volloch, V.Z., Sherman, M.Y Role of Hsp70 in regulation of stress-kinase JNK: implications in apoptosis and aging. FEBS Lett. 438: 1-4, 1998.

32. Getchell, T.V., Krishna, N.S., Dhooper, N., Sparks, D.L., Getchell, M.L. Human olfactory receptor neurons express heat shock protein 70: age-related trends. Ann. Otol. Rhinol. Laryngol., 104: 47-50, 1995.'

33. Ghosh, C., Lahiri, D.K. Increased vulnerability of neuronal cell lines to sodium nitroprusside-mediated toxicity is caused by the decreased level of nitric oxide metabolites. J. Mol. Neurosci. 13: 77-92, 1999.

34. Gouras, G. K., Tsai, J., Naslund, J., Vincent, B., Edgar, M., Checler, F., Greenfield, J. P., Haroutunian, V., Buxbaum, J. D., Xu, H., Greengard, P., Relkin, N.R. Intraneuronal Abeta42 accumulation in human brain. Am. J. Pathol. 156: 15-20, 2000.

35. Grundman, M., Grundman, M., Delaney, P. Antioxidant strategies for Alzheimer's disease. Proc. Nutr. Soc. 61: 191-202, 2002.

36. Gulyaeva, N.V., Stepanichev, M.V., Onifriev, M.V., Sergeev, I.V., Mitrokhina, O.S., Moiseeva, Yu.V., Tkatchouk, E.N. Interval hypoxia trainig prevents oxidative stress in striatum and locomotor disturbances in a rat model of parkinsonism. Progress in Alzheimer's and Parkinson's Diseases. Fisher, A., Hanln, I., Yoshida, M. Plenum Press, New York, 1998, 717-723.

37. Hampl, V., Cornfield, D.N., Cowan, N.J., Archer, S.L. Hypoxia potentiates nitric oxide synthesis and transiently increases cytosolic calcium level in pulmonary artery endothelial cells. Eur. Resp. J. 8: 515-522, 1995.

38. Hauss-Wegrzyniak, B., Dobrzanski, P., Stoehr, J.D., Wenk G.L. Chronic inflammation in rats reproduces components of the neurobiology of Alzheimer's disease. Brain Res. 780: 294-303, 1998.

39. Heininger, K. A unifying hypothesis of Alzheimer's disease. IV. Causation and sequence of events. Rev. Neurosci. 11: 213-328, 2000.

40. Hu, J., Akama, K.T., Krafft, G.A., Chromy, B.A., Van Eldik, L.J. Amyloid-beta peptide activates cultured astrosytes: morphological alterations, cytokine induction and nitric oxide release. Brain Res. 785: 195-206, 1998.

41. Johnson. G., Refolo, L.M., Wallace, W. Heat-shocked neuronal PC12 cells reveal Alzheimer's disease—associated alterations in amyloid precursor protein and tau. Ann. N.Y. Acad. Sci. 695: 194-197, 1993.

42. Kakimura, J., Kitamura, Y., Takata, K., Umeki, M., Suzuki, S., Shibagaki, K., Taniguchi, T., Nomura, Y., Gebicke-Haerter, P.J., Smith, M.A., Perry, G., Shimohama, S. Microglial activation and amyloid-beta clearance induced by exogenous heat-shock proteins. FASEB J 16:601-603, 2002.

43. Kakimura, J., Kitamura, Y., Takata, K., Umeki, M., Suzuki, S., Shibagaki, K., Taniguchi, T., Nomura, Y., Gebicke-Haerter, P.J., Smith, M.A., Perry, G., Shimohama, S. Microglial activation and amyloid-beta clearance induced by exogenous heat-shock proteins. FASEB J. 16: 601-603, 2002.

44. Katzman, R., Kawas, C. The epidemiology of dementia and Alzheimer's disease. In: Terry, R.D., Katzman, R., Bick K.L., Eds., Alzheimer disease. New York, Raven Press, 1994.

45. Kaur, C., Srinivasan, K.N., Singh, J., Peng, C.M., Ling, E.A. Plasma melatonin, pinealocyte morphology, and surface receptors/antigen expression on macrophages/microglia in the pineal gland following a high-altitude exposure. J. Neurosci. Res. 67: 533-543, 2002.

46. Kim, Y.-M., Bergonia, H.A., Muller, C., Pitt, B.R., Watkins, W.D., Lancaster, J.R. Loss and degradation of enzyme bound heme induced by cellular nitric oxide synthesis. J. Biol. Chem. 270: 5710-5713, 1995.

47. Kirby, B.A., Merril, C.R., Ghanbari, H., Wallace, W.C. Heat shock proteins protect against stress-related phosphorylation of tau in neuronal PC12 cells that have acquired thermotolerance. J. Neurosci. 14: 5687-5693, 1994.

48. Klein, S.D., Brune, B. Heat-shock protein 70 attenuates nitric oxide-induced apoptosis in RAW macrophages by preventing cytochrome c release. Biochem. J. 362 (Pt 3): 635-641, 2002.

49. Kluck, R.M., Bossy-Wetzel, E., Green, D.R., Newmeyer, D.D. Mitochondrial control of apoptosis: the role of cytochrome c. Science 275: 1132-1143, 1997

50. Kontush, A. Amyloid-beta: an antioxidant that becomes a pro-oxidant and critically contributes to Alzheimer's disease. Free Radic. Biol. Med. 31: 1120-1131, 2001.

51. Kubes, P., Kanwar S., Niu, X.F. Nitric oxide synthesis inhibition induces leukocyte adhesion via superoxide andmust cells. FASEB J. 7: 1293-1299, 1993.

52. Kudva, Y.C., Hiddinga, H.J., Butler, P.C., Mueske, C.S., Eberhardt, N.L. Small heat shock proteins inhibit in vitro A beta(1-42) amyloidogenesis. FEBS Lett. 416: 117-121, 1997.

53. Kumar-Singh, S., Dewachter, I., Moechars, D., Lubke, U., De Jonghe, C., Ceuterick, C., Checler, F., Naidu, A., Cordell, B., Cras, P., van Broeckhoven, C., van Leuven, F. Behavioral disturbances without amyloid deposits in mice overexpressing human amyloid precursor protein with Flemish (A692G) or Dutch (E693Q) mutation. Neurobiol. Dis. **7:** 9-22, 2000.

54. Laughlin, M.H. Endothelium-mediated control of coronary vascular tone after chronic exercise training. Med. Sci. Sports Exerc. 27: 1135-1144, 1995.

55. Laurin, D., Verreault, R., Lindsay, J., MacPherson, K., Rockwood, K. Physical activity and risk of cognitive impairment and dementia in elderly persons. Arch. Neurol. 58: 498-504, 2001.

56. Law, A., Gauther, S., Quirion, R. Say NO to Alzheimer's disease: the putative link between nitric oxide and dementia of the Alzheimer's type. Brain Res. Rev. 35: 73-96, 2001.

57. Lederman, R.J., Mendelson, F.O., Anderson, R.D., Saucedo, J., Tenaglia, A., Hermiller, J. Therapeutic angiogenesis with recombinant fibroblast growth factor-2 for intermittent claudication (the TRAFFIC study): a randomized trial. Lancet 359: 2948-2050, 2002.

58. Lorenzo, H.K., Susin, SA., Penninger, J., Kroemer, G. Apoptosis inducing factor (AIF): a phylogenetically old, caspase-independent effector of cell death.Cell Death Differ. 6: 516-524, 1999.

59. Losordo, D.W., Vale, P.R., Symes, J.F., Dunnington, C., Esakof, D. Gene therapy for myocardial angiogenesis: initial clinical results with direct myocardial injection of phVEGF165 as sole therapy for myocardial ischemia. Circulation 98: 2800-2804, 1998.

60. Mahendra, N., Arkin, S. Effects of four years of exercise, language, and social interventions on Alzheimer discourse. J. Commun. Disord.. 36: 395-422, 2003.

61. Malyshev, I.Yu., Malugin, A.V., Golubeva, L.Yu., Zenina, T.A., Manukhina, E.B., Mikoyan, V.D., Vanin, A.F. Nitric oxide donor induces HSP70 accumulation in the heart and in cultured cells. FEBS Lett. 391: 21-23, 1996
62. Malyshev, I.Yu., Manukhina, E.B. Stress, adaptation and nitric oxide. Adaptation Biology and Medicine (Vol. 2). Pandolf, B.B., Takeda, N. Singal, P.K., Eds. Narosa Publ. House, New Delhi, 1999, 375-392.
63. Malyshev, I.Yu., Manukhina, E.B., Mikoyan, V.D., Kubrina, L.N., Vanin, A.F. Nitric oxide is involved in heat-induced HSP70 accumulation. FEBS Lett. 370: 159-162, 1995.
64. Malyshev, I.Yu., Trifonov, A.I., Mikoyan, V.D., Kubrina, L.N., Vanin, A.F., Manukhina, E.B. Cross-talk between NO and HSP70 in the antihypotensive effect of adaptation to heat. Physiol. Pes. 49: 99-105, 2000.
65. Malyshev, I.Yu., Zenina, T.A., Golubeva, L.Yu., Saltykova, V.A., Manukhina, E.B., Mikoyan, V.D., Kubrina, L.N., Vanin, A.F. NO-dependent mechanisms of adaptation to hypoxia. - Nitric Oxide 3: 105-113, 1999.
66. Manukhina, E.B., Lapshin, A.V., Meerson, F.Z., Mikoyan, V.D., Kubrina, L.N., Vanin, A.F. Effect of adaptation to exercise on endothelium-dependent reponses of isolated blood vessels and NO production in rat. Fiziol. Zh. Im. I.M. Sechenova 82: 54-60, 1996 (in Russian).
67. Manukhina, E.B., Malyshev, I.Yu. Role of nitric oxide in protective effects of adaptation. Adaptation Biology and Medicine (Vol. 3). J.Moravec, N.Takeda, P.K.Singal, eds. Narosa Publishing House, New Delhi, 2002, 312-327.
68. Manukhina, E.B., Malyshev, I.Yu. Stress-limiting system of nitric oxide. Rossijskij Fiziologicheskij Zhurnal, 86: 1283-1292, 2000 (in Russian)
69. Manukhina, E.B., Malyshev, I.Yu., Smirin, B.V., Mashina, S.Yu., Saltykova, V.A., Vanin, A.F. Production and storage of nitric oxide in adaptation to hypoxia. - Nitric Oxide 3: 393-401, 1999.
70. Manukhina, E.B., Mashina, S.Yu., Smirin, B.V., Lyamina, N.P., Senchikhin, V.N., Vanin, A.F., Malyshev, I.Yu. Role of nitric oxide in adaptation to hypoxia and adaptive defense. Physiol. Res. 49:. 89-97, 2000.
71. Manukhina, E.B., Pokidyshev, D.A., Malyshev, I.Yu., Mashina, S.Yu., Wiegant, F., Mikoyan, V.D., Kubrina, L.N., Vanin, A.F. Prevention of NO overproduction by adaptation to stress exposure. Biology Bull. 25: 243-246, 1998.
72. Manukhina, E.B., Smirin, B.V., Malyshev, I.Yu., Stoclet, J.-C., Muller, B., Solodkov, A.P., Shebeko, V.I., Vanin, A.F. Nitric oxide stores in the cardiovascular system. Izvestiya AN 5: 585-596, 2002 (in Russian).
73. Manukhina, E.B., Sokolova, I.A., Rodionov, I.M. Changed density of the vascular network on brain surface in rats with experimental hypertension and adaptation to high altitude. Kardiologia 10: 118-119, 1982 (in Russian).
74. Marcovic, B.M., Dordevic, I.L.J., Lazarevic, M., Sporcic, Z., Duric, V.J., Jankovic B.D. Chronic stress and anaphylactic shock in the rat. Period. Biol. 92: 69, 1990.
75. Mark, R.J., Hensley, D.A., Butterfield, D.A., Mattson, M.P. Amyloid beta-peptide impairs ion-motive ATPase activities: evidence for a role in loss of neuronal Ca2+ homeostasis and cell death. J. Neurosci. 15: 6239-6249, 1995.
76. Mattson, M.P. Neuroprotective signaling and the aging brain: take away my food and let me run. Brain Res. 886: 47-53, 2000.
77. Mayer, R.J., Arnold, J., Laszlo, L., Landon, M., Lowe, J. Ubiquitin in health and disease. Biochim. Biophys. Acta 1089: 141-157, 1991.
78. McCarty, M.F. Vascular nitric oxide may lessen Alzheimer's risk. Med. Hypotheses 51: 465-476, 1998.
79. McCarty, M.F. Vascular nitric oxide, sex hormone replacement, and fish oil may help to prevent Alzheimer's disease by suppressing synthesis of acute-phase cytokines. Med. Hypotheses 53: 369-374, 1999.
80. McDonnell, J., Redekop, W.K., van der Roer, N., Goes, E., Ruitenberg, A., Busschbach, J.J., Breteler, M.M., Rutten, F.F. The cost of treatment of Alzheimer's disease in The Netherlands: a regression-based simulation model. Pharmacoeconomics 19: 379-390, 2001.
81. McGeer, E.G., McGeer, P.L. Inflammatory cytokines in the CNS. CNS Drugs 7: 214-287, 1997.

82. Meerson, F.Z. Adaptation, Stress and Prophylaxis. Springer-Verlag, Berlin, 1984
83. Meerson, F.Z. Essentials of Adaptive Medicine: Protective Effects of Adaptation. Hypoxia Medical LTD. Moscow, 1994.
84. Meerson, F.Z., Arkhipenko, I.V., Rozhitskaia, I.I., Didenko, V.V., Sazontova, T.G. Opposite effects on antioxidant enzymes of adaptation to continuous and intermittent hypoxia. Biull. Eksp. Biol. Med. 114: 14-15, 1992.
85. Meerson, F.Z., Malyshev, I.Yu., Zamotrinsky, A.V. Differences in the development of the phenomenon of adaptive stabilization of structures during adaptation to stress and adaptation to hypoxia are related with the differential accumulation of hsp70 isoforms. Mol. Cell. Biochem. 111: 87-95, 1992.
86. Meerson, F.Z., Manukhina, E.B., Lapshin, A.V. Adaptation to short-term stress prevents postinfarction hyperactivation of the endothelium and decrease in blood pressure in rats. Biomed. Sci. 2: 580-586, 1991.
87. Meerson, F.Z., Pinelis, V.G., Koshelev, V.B., Golubeva, L.Iu., Riasina, T.V., Arsen'eva, N., Krushinskii, A.L., Storozhevykh, T.P. Adaptation to periodic hypoxia restricts subdural hemorrhages in audiogenic epileptiform convulsions in rats. Biull Eksp Biol Med. 116: 572-574, 1993.
88. Monte de la, S.M., Lu, B.X., Sohn, Y.K., Etienne, D., Kraft, J., Ganju, N., Wands, J.R. Aberrant expression of nitric oxide synthase III in Alzheimer's disease: relevance to cerebral vasculopathy and neurodegeneration. Neurobiol. Aging 21:309-319, 2000
89. Mueller, X.M., Tevaearai, H., Chaubert, P., Genton, C.Y., Sergesser, L. Mechanism of action of transmyocardial revascularization. Schweiz. Med. Wochenschr. 129: 1889-1892, 1999.
90. Neubauer, J.A. Physiological and pathophysiological responses to intermittent hypoxia. J. Appl. Physiol. 90: 1593-1599, 2001.
91. Niu,X.F., Smith, C.W., Kubes, P. Intracellular oxidative stress induced by nitric oxide synthesis inhibition increases endothelial cell adhesion to neutrophils. Circ. Res. 74: 1133-1140, 1995.
92. Ohtsuka, K.. Suzuki, T. Roles of molecular chaperones in the nervous system. Brain Res. Bull. 53: 141-146, 2000.
93. Omata, N., Murata, T., Takamatsu, S., Maruoka, N., Wada, Y., Yonekura, Y., Fujibayashi, Y. Hypoxic tolerance induction in rat brain slices following hypoxic preconditioning due to expression of neuroprotective proteins as revealed by dynamic changes in glucose metabolism. Neurosci Lett. 329: 205-208, 2002.
94. Papadopoulos, M.C., Sun, X.Y., Cao, J., Mivechi, N.F., Giffard, R.G. Over-expression of HSP-70 protects astrocytes from combined oxygen-glucose deprivation Neuroreport. 7: 429-432, 1996.
95. Pappolla, M.A., Chyan, Y.J., Poeggeler, B., Frangione, B., Wilson, G., Ghiso, J., Reiter, R.J. An assessment of the antioxidant and the antiamyloidogenic properties of melatonin: implications for Alzheimer's disease. J. Neural Transm. 107: 203-231, 2000.
96. Pappolla, M.A., Sos, M., Omar, R.A., Sambamurti, K. The heat shock/oxidative stress connection. Relevance to Alzheimer disease. Mol. Chem. Neuropathol. 28: 21-34, 1996.
97. Pecher, P., Schumacher, B.A. Angiogenesis in ischemic human myocardium: clinical results after 3 years. Ann. Thorac. Surg. 69: 1414-1419, 2000.
98. Pedrazachaverri, J., Tapia, E., Medinacampos, O.N., Granados, M.D., Franco, M. Garlic prevents hypertension induced by chronic inhibition of nitric oxide synthesis. Life Sci. 62: PL71-PL77, 1998.
99. Prewitt, R.L., Cardoso, S.S., Wood, W.B. Prevention of arteriolar rarefaction in the spontaneously hypertensive rat by exposure to simulated high altitude. J. Hypertens. 4: 735-740, 1986.
100. Pshennikova M.G., Manukhina E.B., Sazontova T.G., Prodius P.A., Golantsova N.E., Malyshev I.Yu. Molecular mechanisms of adaptation to environmental factors: New achievements of the Meerson school. In: Adaptation Biology and Medicine (Vol. 2). Pandolf, B.B., Takeda, N., Singal, P.K. (eds.) Narosa Publ. House, New Delhi, 1999, 199-213.
101. Rayevsky, K.S., Bondarenko, N.A., Kudrin, V.S., Miroshnichenko, I.I. Cognitive deficiency induced by the acute stress in rats: a possible role of brain catecholaminergic systems. Ann. Ist. Super Sanita 26: 25-29, 1990.

102. Ravagnan, L., Gurbuxani, S., Susin, S.A., Maisse, C., Daugas, E., Zamzami, N., Mak, T., Jaattela, M., Penninger, J.M., Garrido, C., Kroemer, G. Heat-shock protein 70 antagonizes apoptosis-inducing factor. Nat. Cell Biol. 3: 839-843, 2001.
103. Reiter, R.J., Cabrera, J., Sainz, R.M., Mayo, J.C., Manchester, L.C., Tan, D.X. Melatonin as a pharmacological agent against neuronal loss in experimental models of Huntington's disease, Alzheimer's disease and parkinsonism. Ann. N.Y. Acad. Sci. 890: 471-485, 1999.
104. Renkawek, K., Bosman, G.J., Gaestel, M. Increased expression of heat-shock protein 27 kDa in Alzheimer disease: a preliminary study. Neuroreport 5: 14-16, 1993.
105. Sasaki, A., Yamaguchi, H., Ogawa, A., Sugihara, S., Nakazato, Y. Microglial activation in early stages of amyloid beta protein deposition. Acta Neuropathol. (Berl.) 94: 316-322, 1997.
106. Sazontova, T.G., Arkhipenko, Iu.V., Meerson, F.Z. Adaptation to periodic hypoxia and diet with omega-3 polyunsaturated fatty acids increases the stability of myocardial sarcoplasmic reticulum Ca^{2+} transport to free radical oxidation. Biull. Eksp. Biol. Med. 120: 42-45, 1995 (in Rusian).
107. Schulze-Osthoff, K., Ferrari, D., Los, M., Wesselborg, S., Peter, M.E. Apoptosis signaling by death receptors. Eur. J. Biochem. 254: 439-459, 1998.
108. Schumacher, B., Pecher, P., von Specht, B, Stegman, Th. Induction of neogenesis in ischemic myocardium by human growth factors. Circulation 97: 645-650, 1998.
109. Sessa, W.C., Pritchard, K., Seyedi, N., Wang, J., Hintze, T.H. Chronic exercise in dogs increases coronary vascular nitric oxide production and endothelial cell nitric oxide synthase gene expression. Circ. Res. 74: 349-353, 1994.
110. Shanavas, A., Papasozomenos, S.Ch. t tkinases in the rat heat shock model: Possible implications for Alzheimer disease. Proc. Natl. Acad. Sci. USA 97: 14139-14144, 2000.
111. Shen, W.Q., Zhang, X.P., Zhao, G., Wolin, M.S., Sessa, W., Hintze, T.H. Nitric oxide production and NO synthase gene expression contribute to vascular regulation during exercise. Med. Sci. Sports Exerc. 27: 1125-1134, 1995.
112. Soucek, T., Cumming, R., Dargusch, R., Maher, P., Schubert, D. The regulation of glucose metabolism by HIF-1 mediates a neuroprotective response to amyloid beta peptide. Neuron 39: 43-56, 2003.
113. Sun, X., Cole, G.M., Chu, T., Xia, W., Galasko, D., Yamaguchi, H., Tanemura, K., Frautschy, S. A., Takashima, A. Intracellular Abeta is increased by okadaic acid exposure in transfected neuronal and non-neuronal cell lines. Neurobiol. Aging 23: 195-203, 2002.
114. Swaab, D.F., Dubelaar, E.J., Scherder, E.J., Van Someren, E.J., Verwer, R.W. Therapeutic strategies for Alzheimer disease: focus on neuronal reactivation of metabolically impaired neurons. Alzheimer Dis. Assoc. Disord. 17: S114-S122, 2003.
115. Takahashi, K., Hara, E., Suzuki, H., Sasano, H., Shibahara, S. Expression of heme oxygenase isozyme mRNAs in the human brains and induction of heme oxygenase-1 by nitric oxide donors. J. Neurochem. 67: 482-489, 1996.
116. Tarkowski, E., Ringqvist, A., Blennow, K., Wallin, A., Wennmalm, A. Intrathecal release of nitric oxide in Alzheimer's disease and vascular dementia. Dement. Geriatr. Cogn. Disord. 11: 322-326, 2000.
117. Teri, L., Gibbons, L.E., McCurry, S.M., Logsdon, R.G., Buchner, D.M., Barlow, W.E., Kukull, W.A., LaCroix, A.Z., McCormick, W., Larson, E.B. Exercise plus behavioral management in patients with Alzheimer disease: a randomized controlled trial. JAMA. 290: 2015-2022, 2003.
118. Torre de la, J.C. Alzheimer's disease: How does it start? J. Alzheimer's Dis. 4: 497-512, 2002.
119. Torre de la, J.C., Stefano, G.B. Evidence that Alzheimer's disease is a microvascular disorder: the role of constitutive nitric oxide. Brain Res. Rev. 34: 119-136, 2000.
120. Tsunumi, Y., Takeshita, S., Chen, D., Keaney, M., Rossow, S. Direct intramuscular gene transfer of naked DNA encoding vascular endothelial growth factoe augments collateral development and tissue perfusion. Cirulation 94: 3281-3290, 1996.

121. Vanin, A.F. Dinitrosyl iron complexes and S-nitrosothiols are two possible forms of nitric oxide stabilization and transport in biosystems. Biochemistry (Moscow) 63: 924-938, 1998.

122. Vincent, S.R., Kimura, H. Histochemical mapping of nitric oxide synthase in the rat brain. Neuroscience, 46: 755-784, 1992.

123. Wakutani, Y., Urakami, K., Shimomura, T., Takahashi, K. Heat shock protein 70 mRNA levels in mononuclear blood cells from patients with dementia of the Alzheimer type. Dementia, 6: 301-305, 1995.

124. Wenger, R.H., Gassmann, M. Oxygen(es) and the hypoxia-inducible factor-1. Biol. Chem. 378: 609-616, 1997.

125. Wertkin, A. M., Turner, R. S., Pleasure, S. J., Golde, T. E., Younkin, S. G., Trojanowski, J. Q., Lee, V. M. Human neurons derived from a teratocarcinoma cell line express solely the 695-amino acid amyloid precursor protein and produce intracellular beta-amyloid or A4 peptides. Proc. Natl. Acad. Sci. USA 90: 9513-9517, 1993.

126. Wild-Bode, C., Yamazaki, T., Capell, A., Leimer, U., Steiner, H., Ihara, Y., Haass, C. Intracellular generation and accumulation of amyloid beta-peptide terminating at amino acid 42. J. Biol. Chem. 272: 16085-16088, 1997.

127. Willis, D., Tomlinson, A., Frederick, R., Paul-Clark, M.J. Modulation of heme oxygenase activity and rat brain and spleen by inhibitors and donors of nitric oxide. Biochem. Biophys. Res. Commun. 214: 1152-1156, 1995.

128. Winblad, B., Mobius, H.J., Stoffler, A. Glutamate receptors as a target for Alzheimer's disease—are clinical results supporting the hope? J. Neural. Transm. Suppl. (62): 217-25, 2002.

129. Wirths, O., Multhaup, G., Czech, C., Blanchard, V., Moussaoui, S., Tremp, G., Pradier, L., Beyreuther, K., Bayer, T. A. Intraneuronal Abeta accumulation precedes plaque formation in beta-amyloid precursor protein and presenilin-1 double-transgenic mice. Neurosci. Lett. 306: 116-120, 2001.

130. Wissink, M.J., Beernink, R., Poot, A.A., Engbers, G., Beugeling, T. Improved endothelization of vascular grafts by local release of growth factors from heparinized collagen matrices. J. Controlled Release 64: 103-114, 2000.

131. Woodman, C.R., Muller, J.M., Laughlin, M.H., Price, E.M. Induction of nitric oxide synthase mRNA in coronary resistance arteries isolated from exercise-trained pigs. Am. J. Physiol. 273: H2575-H2579, 1997.

132. Yan, S. D., Fu, J., Soto, C., Chen, X., Zhu, H., Al-Mohanna, F., Collison, K., Zhu, A., Stern, E., Saido, T., Tohyama M, Ogawa S, Roher A, Stern D. An intracellular protein that binds amyloid-beta peptide and mediates neurotoxicity in Alzheimer's disease. Nature 389: 689-695, 1997.

133. Yang, A. J., Chandswangbhuvana, D., Margol, L., Glabe, C. G. Loss of endosomal/lysosomal membrane impermeability is an early event in amyloid Abeta1-42 pathogenesis. J. Neurosci. Res. 52: 691-698, 1998.

134. Yang, J., Liu, X., Bhalla, K., Kim, C.N., Ibrado, A.M., Cai, J., Peng, T.I., Jones, D.P., Wang, X. Prevention of apoptosis by Bcl-2: release of cytochrome c from mitochondria blocked. Science 275: 1129-1132, 1997.

135. Yee, W.M., Frim, D.M., Isacson, O. Relationships between stress protein induction and NMDA-mediated neuronal death in the entorhinal cortex Exp. Brain Res. 94(2):193-202, 1993.

136. Yoo, C.G., Lee, S., Lee, C.T., Kim, Y.W., Han, S.K., Shim, Y.S. Anti-inflammatory effect of heat shock protein induction is related to stabilization of I kappa B alpha through preventing I kappa B kinase activation in respiratory epithelial cells. J. Immunol. 164: 5416-5423, 2000.

137. Zamudio, S. The placenta at high altitude. High Alt. Med. Biol. 4: 171-191, 2003.

138. Zee van der, E.A., Douma, B.R., Bohus ,B., Luiten, P.G. Passive avoidance training induces enhanced levels of immunoreactivity for muscarinic acetylcholine receptor and coexpressed PKC gamma and MAP-2 in rat cortical neurons. Cereb. Cortex 4:376-390, 1994.

Adaptation Biology and Medicine (Volume 4: Current Concepts)
Editors: A. Hargens, N. Takeda and P.K. Singal

16. Adaptation to Radiation and Combined Impacts

Igor B. Ushakov
State Scientific Research Testing Institute of Military Medicine, Moscow, Russia

Studying of the combined influence of environment factors is the important medical and biological problem. In life practically there are no situations of the isolated influence of the factor, there is only its quantitative prevalence over this or that situation. The organism is always under the influence of complex of factors, which are sometimes «placed» on time very far. Therefore it is sometimes difficult to estimate the priority of this or that factor in infringement of functional reserves of an organism or even in pathology occurrence.

The problem of the combined influence of environment factors on human organism is one of the key problems in biology, medicine and ecology. At the same time it is necessary to recognize, that the importance of the given scientific trend is not understood to the full by the broad audience of scientists. At the same time it is obvious, that the problem of the combined influence of extreme factors exceeds the limits of applied medicine and has now generally biological and wide medical-biologic value. In biology and medicine this problem began to arise from the beginning of 1960th. As well as any other problem, it has theoretical and practical aspects. The theoretical aspect concerns research of mechanisms of reactivity, stability, adaptation, compensatory-adaptive reactions of an organism and the specific reactions caused by the tropism of influencing factor to this or that physiological system, tissue etc. Practical aspect of the problem is connected to normalization of factors, with estimation of efficiency of the means and methods of preventive maintenance, protection, correction and treatment of various disorders, which are intended for use. At the same time the limitation of simple total models in normalization of combined impacts is abundantly clear.

Necessity of strict quantitative approaches at an estimation of the combined impacts has naturally resulted in the circumstance, that the greatest amount of the data on a problem is saved up by radiobiologists and toxicologists, i.e. the experts most widely using approaches «doze—time—effect». The advantage of such method consists in good dosage of radiation and chemical substances, their abilities at doze increase to include in a complex of responses all new and new systems, including central nervous system (CNS). Updating of such quantitative dependencies by other factors will testify first, to biological effect of the concrete factor, and second, about necessity of such combination account for conditions of possible excess of maximum permissible level (MPL). At the same time it is necessary to recognize, that these questions are the least investigated. All stated also has formed the basis for realization of the review — analysis of hypoxic mechanisms of the combined impacts.

Despite of obvious importance of a problem of person adaptation to factors (for example, hypoxia,), it is necessary to ascertain obviously insufficient level of scrutiny and discrepancy in a rating not only thin mechanisms, but even the orientation of adaptive processes, it is especially at the most actual variant — joint influence of various factors. Till now there is an obscure question on an interrelation of adaptive processes and changes breaking adaptation at extreme factors chronic influence.

In this connection I together with S.M. Razinkin carried out the investigation of dependence of hypoxic (HT), thermal (TT) and radiation (RT) tolerance of experimental animals (mice and rats) from duration of hypoxia and overheating chronic influence. Thus the basic attention was given to the study of functional and metabolic changes in CNS — to the system mainly determining an opportunity of purposeful activity of an individual. Screening of various (only 114) regimes (impulsive, ladder-shaped and stationary) of adaptation to hypoxia and heat was carried out on mice. For HT evaluation 3 types of loads were applied: 1) definition of «high-altitude ceiling» (HC) on time of cramps appearance (ΔH); 2) triple (3DH) definition of «high-altitude ceiling» according to the scheme: 0 km — HC_1 — 0 km — HC_2 — 0 km — HC_3 — 0 km; 3) definition of reserve time of cramps appearance at 11 kms height (ΔtH).

Analysis of the received results has allowed making a number of general conclusions. First of all it is necessary to ascertain, that tests on HT have the greatest radiomodificatory features as they had more acute character and consequently, abandoned deeper structurally functional trace in CNS. So, in 1,5 h after the tests significant weakening of radio cerebral syndrome (RCS) manifestations (augmentation of reserve time (RT) parameters) has three times proved to be true. Even in 72 h after the test «tH» it is registered significant ($P < 0,05$) RT_c reduction.

At a comparative study of various regimes of influence it appeared that it is not enough RT significant changes. Concurrence of orientation of HT and reserve time (RT) modification was observed all in 45% of cases that testifies to small interdependency of HT and RT. The received information contradicts a little the experimental facts about positive correlation between reaction of standard metabolism on hypoxic test and mean life duration (MLD) at a cerebral syndrome (Grigor'ev, 1985). However such discrepancy may be explained by various criteria of evaluation of radiation injury and HT.

The basic conclusion is that there is general, though and not always authentic, tendency to RT decrease (within the limits of 10—20%). The above mentioned fact concerns to all terms, except for 7 days after 3 days of hypoxic regimes. It also appeared, that the regime type didn't influence the investigated parameters much — RT decrease was observed with the following frequency: stationary — 70%, ladder-shaped and impulsive — on 63%. Obvious phasal nature of RT fluctuations even after one-day regime is shown at the analysis of two regimes (impulsive and ladder-shaped); RT values on the 3rd and 7th days after hypoxia influence authentically differ among themselves, and on the 7th day (!) even with the control. Thus in the latter case the value of radiation influence dose on CNS is exposed. If at 200 Gr at both regimes RT increase is registered, then at 400 Gr, on the contrary, the decrease is registered. Differently, at stronger influence of radiation there is an original «failure» of the increased background of CNS radiation tolerance.

At thermal regimes of influence the changes had similar character, and the addition of swimming as physical load did not result in modification effect. Such non-specific adaptation has proved to be true in the subsequent experiments on rats.

In the first series of experiments on rats hypoxia was replicated in the altitude chamber by means of daily «rises» on 6 500 m height (rate of rise and descent was 1000 m / min) with stay at the given height within 120 minutes. For thermal adaptation the rats were daily placed in a heat chamber on 180 min at temperature of air and walls +35°, +36° C. In 100 min after craniocaudal irradiation in the dose of 62,5 Gr the material was taken for histological and biochemical researches. This term was determined by us preliminary as maximal, still not accompanying by the significant histochemical changes in brain of not adapted rats. In sections of frontal lobes of the big hemispheres the activity of alkaline phosphatase (AP) and key enzymes of glycolysis and tricarbonic acid cycle — lactate dehydrogenase (LDG) and succinate dehydrogenase (SDG) were found histochemically. In parallel with histochemical researches a status of hydration of CNS 4 departments (frontal and parietal lobes, a cerebellum and a brainstem) were estimated, and hematological and cytochemical researches of a peripheric blood were also carried out (Ushakov etc., 1996).

For the 4th day of adaptation to hypoxia the significant decrease of activity of both investigated dehydrogenases (fig. 1) is observed in frontal lobe cerebral cortex. It may testify to decrease of the metabolic rate developing in the nervous tissue during regeneration (in a day after hypoxia) at not enough adapted animals. In the subsequent relative normalization of enzymes activity takes place, though SDG level is, as a rule, insignificantly increased, and LDG and AP are characterized by a little bit reduced parameters.

A little bit other changes were marked in a peripheric blood (fig. 2). Change of cytochemical parameters during adaptation to hypoxia is caused by rearrangement of the morphological and biochemical device of cellular respiration in various tissues, especially in hemopoietic organs. SDG activity in lymphocytes accrued, except for the 8th day. Apparently it is caused by mobilization of preexisting mitochondria cells system and augmentation of quantity of oxidation substratum, owing to anaerobic glycolysis. The last proves to be true by speed decrease of SDG response. According to A. Lenindzher (1978), the period of mitochondria physiological semirecovery in cells of different organs and at different kinds of animals changes from 7 up to 10 days. At significant functional loads mitochondria destruction increased. Therefore on the 8th day of adaptation it is possible to explain SDG activity decrease by intensifying of mitochondria destruction exceeding in conditions of hypoxia the intensity of their physiological regeneration. The increase of hypoxia tolerance proceeding at this time is provided with maintenance of anaerobic processes at the increased level. It is shown by low values of SDG response rate in lymphocytes, and, according to Z.I.Barbashova (1960), adaptive reactions of the first sort — intensifying of lung ventilation, augmentation of minute volume and oxygen capacity of blood etc. Further, according to the principle of hyperregeneration and overcompensation, regeneration of mitochondria quantity increases, SDG activity begins to rise. Thus anaerobic processes of energy metabolism remain on high compensatory level. These cytochemical changes in lymphocytes correspond to the further augmentation of rats' resistance to hypoxia. Cytochemical changes in blood lymphocytes less correspond to the dynamics of thermal tolerance of animals adapted for hypoxia. It is possible to note, that the increase of thermal tolerance within the first week is connected, apparently, to processes of compensatory redistribution of plastic and energy resources (Viru, 1984) and decrease of heat production.

The hematological researches which have been carried out on rats at adaptation to hypoxia, have shown (fig. 3), that augmentation of lymphocytes quantity and decrease of neutrophils quantity reflect the increase of level of the general and specific resistance.

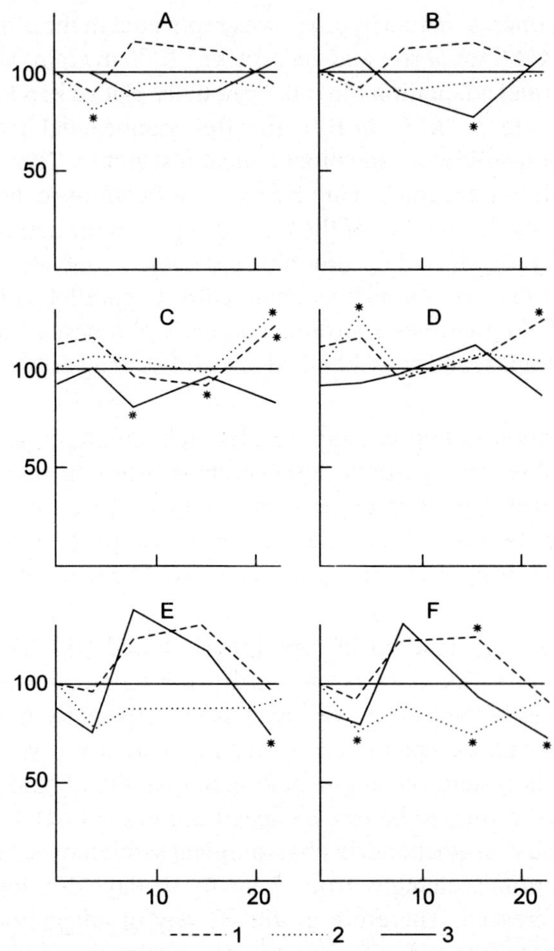

Fig. 1. **The change of SDG(*1*), LDG(*2*), AP(*3*) activity in brain at adaptation to hypoxia (*A, C, E*) and overheating (*B, D, F*), including in 5 h after hypoxic test (*C, D*) and in 100 min after irradiation (*E, F*), conducted on the adaptation background (Razinkin etc., 1989).**
On ordinate axis **— enzymes activity, % to the initial level;** ***on abscissa axis*** **— the term of adaptation, day; *P* < 0,05 in comparison with the control.**

SDG response rate on hypoxic gas mixture (HGM-8) inhalation was significantly reduced at all terms of research.

Cytochemical researches at adaptation to thermal loads were carried out under the same scheme, as at adaptation to hypoxia. Loading test was the same — HGM-8 respiration. The received results (see fig. 2) testify that SDG activity in blood lymphocytes during the whole experiment was close to reference values. SDG response rate on loading test with HGM-8 also changed a little bit and only on the 4th day was statistically significantly reduced ($P < 0{,}05$).

Thus, thermal influences practically do not affect mitochondria apparatus of blood lymphocytes and on the influence on an organism concede to the action of hypoxia that corresponds to the change of

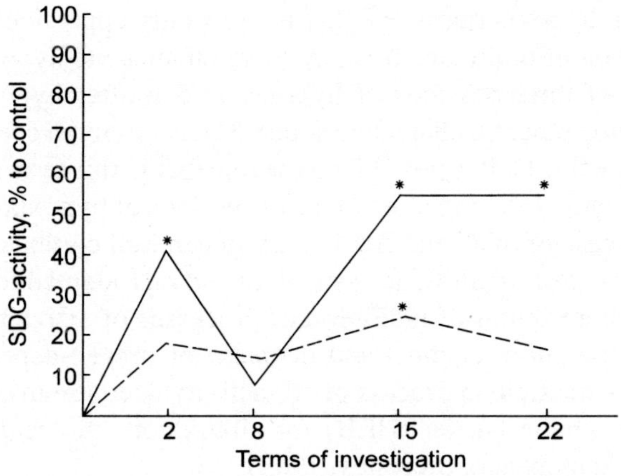

Fig. 2. SDG activity in lymphocytes of rats peripheral blood at adaptation to hypoxia (*1*) *or heat* (*2*); * — *P*<0,05 in comparison with the control.

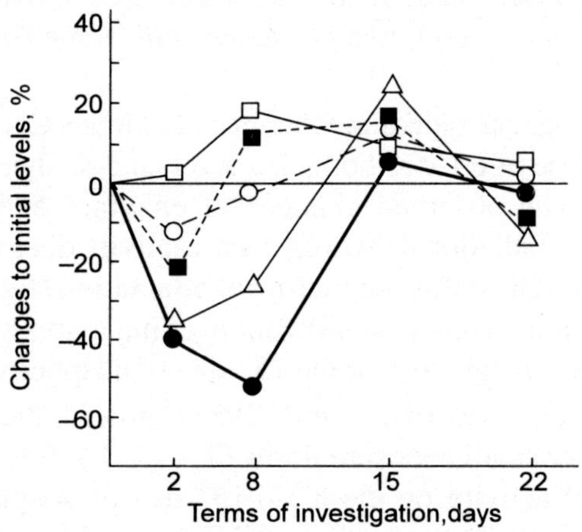

Fig. 3. Hematological indices at rats adaptation to hypoxia: lymphocytes (*1*), neutrophils (*2*); leukocytes (*3*), erythrocytes (*4*), hemoglobin (*5*).

resistance level for hypoxia at rats, which was revealed and appeared insignificant. Thus, the level increase of thermal load acceptability in the first two weeks was more significant, than at the rats adapted for hypoxia. It may be explained by the development of specific mechanisms of adaptation to heat, in particular by rearrangement of thermoregulation processes.

At hematological research the changes in white blood were basically the same, as at adaptation to hypoxia. Differences were revealed for the 14th day that was expressed in the greater degree of an absolute and relative neutrophilia and lymphocytosis at a thermal load. It is principally important, because from L.H.Garkavi's and his co-authors' point of view (1974), adaptive processes should be accompanied in these terms by the decrease of neutrophils level as it was observed at adaptation to hypoxia. Therefore it is possible to speak about specific character of blood changes at thermal adaptation that is accompanied by less substantial increase of nonspecific resistance, than at adaptation to hypoxia. The picture of red blood had the same dynamics as at adaptation to hypoxia.

Adaptation of animals to hypoxia raises HT that is especially appreciable on the 15th day (fig. 4). Thus the character of reaction of brain metabolic systems on an acute hypoxia varies. At not adapted rats and on a background of three sessions of hypoxia in 5 h after hypoxic tests the changes are basically similar and have no authentic character though SDG activity exceeds initial one slightly, and AP parameter is reduced (see fig. 1). It is possible to assume that in this term still there is no high-grade adaptation to the lack of oxygen. Educing after 7 and 14 sessions of hypoxia HT substantial increase is accompanied by sharp decrease of SDG and AP activity in cerebral cortex at the absence of dynamics from LDG in reply to hypoxic test. It allows to assume, that at rats adapted for hypoxia during 5 h after the hypoxic test there educe attributes of inhibition of processes of active transportation through the walls of vessels of microcirculatory channel and decrease of oxigen-dependable oxidation level in brain nervous cells. At the same time in process of AP activity decrease in capillary walls of brain the permeability of hematoencephalic barrier (HEB) for albuminous molecules may be broken in the direction to augmentation (Semchenko, Stepanov, 1982).

On the 22nd day of adaptation to hypoxia the acute hypoxic test is accompanied by significant rising of oxidation-reduction enzymes activity in nervous tissue at conservation of low AP activity in brain vessels. Hence, observable on earlier stages of adaptation decrease of oxidation-reduction processes in reply to hypoxic test in this term is absent, that correlates with some decrease of HT on the 22nd day (see fig. 4).

Adaptation to hypoxia also changes radiation tolerance of animals CNS. However, in contrast to HT it is reduced (fig. 4). The decrease of RT was both on a level, and on dynamics similar at adaptation to hypoxia and to overheating. The observed changes of enzymes activity have completely other dynamics. In 100 minutes after irradiation dehydrogenases activity does not essentially differ from the level, characteristic for brain in the conforming terms of adaptation (fig. 1). At the same time after 7 sessions of hypoxia the irradiation results to significant in comparison with unirradiated adapting rats to rising of AP activity, partly characteristic for the 15th day of adaptation (fig. 1).

Formerly we and A.N. Kordenko (Kordenko etc., 1985) showed, that AP increase in brain in 100 minutes is not observed at rather small exposure doses (2—25 Gr). It is typical only for larger doses. Thus, the augmentation of AP activity on the 8th —15th day of adaptation to hypoxia in reply to irradiation can be regarded as an attribute of radiosensibilization. The intensifying of enzyme activity providing permeability of microcirculatory channel, may result in intensifying of vessels permeability, repeatedly described in the radiobiological literature (Davydov etc., 1991), and is capable to make a neurologic picture harder. Such state of affairs proves to be true at RT research (see fig. 4). On the 22nd day of adaptation to hypoxia AP reaction of endothelium to irradiation undergoes some changes (see fig. 1). Again there is a decrease of indications of active transportation in microcirculatory channel that coincides with some RT CNS regeneration (see fig. 4).

Analyzing TT changes during adaptation to hypoxia, we shall note, that it was a little enlarged from the first 4 days of adaptation and remained at this level in all terms of experiment (see fig. 4). Thus, it was not possible to note connection between changes of enzymes activity during adaptation and TT.

At studying adaptation of animals to overheating the big resemblance in dynamics of enzymes activity in brain attracts attention at the influence of the increased temperature with the results received at adaptation to hypoxia (see fig. 1). The differences concern only the degree of changes manifestation: the decrease of dehydrogenases activity is less important in the first day of adaptation, but the decrease

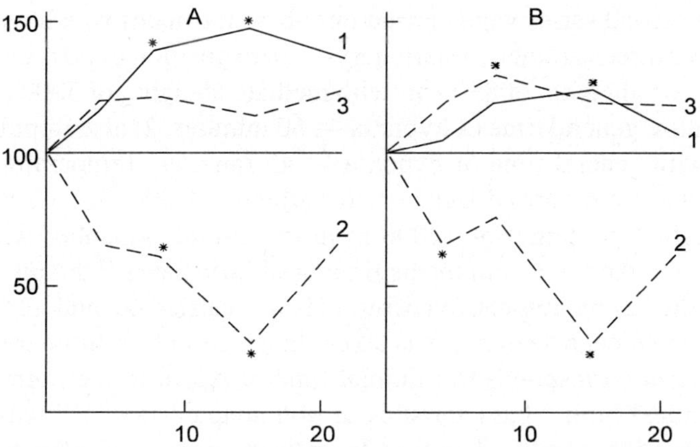

Fig. 4. Changes of hypoxic (*1*), radiation (*2*) and heat (*3*) tolerance at adaptation to hypoxia (*À*) and overheating (*B*) (Razinkin etc., 1989).
***On ordinate axis* — tolerance, % to the initial level; *on abscissa axis* — term of adaptation, days; * — *P* < 0,05 in comparison with the control.**

of AP parameter after 14 sessions of overheating is more expressed. M.S. Usenova and co-authors (1987) ascertained the expressed oppression of AP activity in brain of rats at intensive overheating.

In these experiments the phenomenon of AP activity decrease coincides with similar character of action of both factors on all investigated kinds of tolerance (see fig. 1). RT at long influence of heat also raises, but to a lesser degree, than at specific adaptation to hypoxia. Thus it is not practically observed characteristic on the 8th and 15th days of adaptation to hypoxia of SDG and AP activity decrease in reply to acute hypoxic test.

Almost complete resemblance is observed and in radiomodificatory influence of adaptation to overheating and hypoxia (see fig. 4). Thus, the observed character of changes of all investigated brain enzymes (see fig. 1) coincides basically. Nevertheless it is necessary to note, that rats adapted for overheating at irradiation have more significant and authentic alteration of a metabolic structure in the direction of aerobic processes.

Thus, during adaptation to hypoxia and overheating there is a doubtless rising of hypoxic and thermal tolerance and sharp decrease of radiation tolerance. Similar decrease of radiation resistance after adaptation to moderate (Certkov et al., 1986) and expressed (Amrit etc., 1981) hypoxia was registered even at levels of a hemopoietic syndrome doses (6,75—9,7 Gr) in 14—21 days of training. It was ascertained more often only the rising of tolerance, which had oscillatory character (Grigor'ev, 1982). Some authors managed to chose conditions of training at which by the certain criteria CNS rising tolerance (Sizan, 1979) was achieved. Protecting influence of preliminary hypoxic adaptation on mortality of animals from the acute infringements of blood circulation caused by strong exaltation of brain (Koshelev etc., 1984) was fixed.

Probably, phasal nature of fluctuations, and even biorhythms (Akojev, 1976) of various kinds of stress — tolerance is also the cause of the fact that many authors found out the terms of presence of protective actions of chronic hypoxia in relation to various factors (Krushinskyi etc., 1989) and to physical loads (Doroftein et al., 1987).

Experiments of the second series were carried out on 80 rat-males which were influenced by high-altitude hypoxia in other three variants: à) stationary — an exposition of 60 minutes at «height» of 8500 m; á) impulsive — rise on «height» of 8500 m (with mediate «height» of 3000 m) with the stay on both regimes for 2—3 minutes, general time of hypoxia — 60 minutes; â) also impulsive, but with maximal «height» of 6500 m with general time of hypoxia — 45 minutes. Temperature expositions with the duration of 120 minutes were carried out in two variants: à) 30—32° C, σ) 38—40° C. For HT evaluation rats were lifted on height of 12000 m in the altitude chamber with the rate of 1000 m/ minutes. HT criterion was the time from the beginning of influence till the rats had the second agonal respiration. After that the fast recompression of animals was carried out and, in 5 hours, the material for histochemical and biochemical researches was taken. In a series of preliminary experiments we found out, that exactly this term corresponds to minimal time of return to the norm of the majority of the investigated histochemical brain characteristics at non-adapted rats. TT was determined in a heat chamber at temperature +55°, +56° C. The time from the beginning of influence up to the moment of apnea was the criterion. In connection with the death of rats the material for histological researches was not take. CNS radiation tolerance was evaluated according to the picture of the neurological symptoms, appearing after the craniocaudal g-irradiation from the source ^{60}Ñî in the dose of 62,5 Gr at dose power of 45,8 sGr/s. The integral parameter of tolerance — transient neurological deficiency (TND) — took into account frequency of manifestation and duration of the general tremor, circular movements, hyperkinesias, opisthotonos and cramps, and also their densities — ratio of each symptom effective dose $ED_{0,1\%}$ to tremor effective dose $ED_{0,1\%}$. It turned out that when the adapting influence has an impulsive character (6500 m), which is more effective under the specific factor — hypoxia (Razinkin, Dukhovich, 1986), it already produces the significant RT decrease on the 3rd day of adaptation (tab. 1).

At the increase of force of impulsive hypoxic influence RT decrease was even more expressed. 7-days regenerative interval has removed negative effect of adaptation on RT: TND tended even to decrease (on 30%). RT changes at 3-days stationary hypoxic regime were similar, but less expressed (as well as on HT).

The received regularities were kept and at 7-days regimes: RT decrease was obvious in a day and as a whole was restored in 7 days after the impulsive regime (8500 m) though significant differences on various symptoms (C_3—C_5) nevertheless were kept, i.e. «trace» was deeper, than at 3-days regime. And in this case more «mild» stationary regime produced smaller RT alterations. Repeated influence of heat has not caused the expressed radiomodification.

So, in our experiments evident specificity of adaptable reactions is fixed: adaptation to hypoxia mainly enlarges HT, and adaptation to overheating in the greater degree raises TT.

Thus, in the first three days the main place was occupied with nonspecific reactions of an organism in reply to the extreme factor influence, and since the 7th day the transition to predominance of specific adaptable reactions was planned. It is important to emphasize the certain heterogeneity of reactions not only on terms, but also on systems of an organism. Adaptable influence is accompanied by taking not only «beneficial» qualities (in this case — hypoxic and thermal tolerance increase), but also decrease of CNS radiation tolerance. Separate indicatings on an opportunity of such different reactions are in the published works (Furduj etc., 1985; Jakovlev, 1986; Routh et al., 1984). One more example — on the part of secretory elements of a forward lobe of a pituitary body of rats at irradiation in conditions of high mountains more expressed changes were observed, than at the influence on the background of low mountains (Gabitov etc., 1987). Together with the results which we received on mice, the specified

Table 1. Early transient neurological disorders at rats at craniocaudal ã-irradiation in the dose of 62,5 Gr some time later after preliminary chronic influence of high altitude hypoxia or heat

Adapting factor	Duration, days	Interval till irradiation, days	Frequency of ETND symptoms, ?% to control				TND ±%, to control
			circular movements C_2	hyperkinesias C_3	opisthotonos C_4	cramps C_5	
Hypoxia-impulsive regime (6500 m)	3	1	0	+60*	–80*	0	+87,2*
Hypoxia-impulsive regime (8500 m)	3	1	+40*	+40*	–20	0	+152,0*
Hypoxia-impulsive regime (8500 m)	3	7	–20	+20	0	0	–29,8
Hypoxia- stationary regime (8500 m)	3	1	+40*	+20	–40	0	+107,0*
Hypoxia-stationary regime (8500 m)	3	7	–20	+20	+20	+20	+11,9
Heat (30—32°C)	3	1	0	+20	–40	0	+18,5
Heat (38—40°C)	3	1	0	0	–80*	+20	–29,4
Hypoxia-impulsive regime (6500 m)	7	1	0	+20	+20	+20	+63,6
Hypoxia-impulsive regime (8500 m)	7	1	+20	+60*	+40	+20	+122,3*
Hypoxia-impulsive regime (8500 m)	7	7	0	+40*	–60*	+40*	+20,9
Hypoxia-stationary regime (8500 m)	7	1	0	0	+20	0	+24,9
Hypoxia-stationary regime (8500 m)	7	7	0	+40*	–60	0	+23,9
Heat (30—32°C)	7	1	–40	0	0	0	+10,9
Heat (38—40°C)	7	1	–20	+20	–20	0	+40,0*

* $P < 0{,}05$ according to the control.

reasons confirm, that adaptation to hypoxia is characterized by the compromise (Medvedev, 1982), and its «price» (Medvedev etc., 1985) in our case corresponds to the decrease of CNS RT. The mechanism of the given phenomenon, apparently, has cellular character. An acute excessive swelling (with a loss) brain neurones mitochondrions and decomposition of biological membranes keeping phosphotides, being influenced for a long time by hypoxia (Mezhiborskaya, 1988; Wender et al., 1989), certainly limit CNS reserve opportunities in relation to «unusual», in this case to the radiation stress — factor. Changes of all investigated kinds of tolerance during adaptation in our experiments had phase character. They accrued to the 8th —15th days and were reduced by the 22nd day of adaptation.

The found resemblance in changes of metabolism in brain at adaptation to hypoxia and overheating testifies to presence of some general, nonspecific mechanisms of the adaptation to different environmental factors influence that explains appreciable concurrence in their modifying effect. Identity of hydration-electrolyte brain profile (HEBP) both at tests — loads, and without them at both variants of adaptation also testifies to a generality (nonspecific) reactions to adapting and testing influences (Antipov etc., 1989). The formation of high tolerance to hypoxia during adaptation correlates with development of the reaction directed on the decrease of processes of aerobic oxidation in nervous cells and enzyme-dependable transportation in the endothelium of brain microcirculatory channel.

The received effect of CNS RT decrease is not unexpected if we take into account the decrease of ðÎ$_2$, local cerebral cortex blood flow, and also the metabolic and electrophysiological disorders appearing at adaptation during 3—30 days even to moderate hypoxia (Plehina, 1977; Low et al., 1986). The revealed decrease of CNS radiation tolerance at adaptation to hypoxia and overheating may be connected to observable features of hematoencephalic barrier permeability increase that finds the reflectance in alterations of hydration of cerebral structures. Changes of metabolism in the direction of aerobic process demands further studying.

Thus, any external influence can be surveyed as the second. It means, that at any moment the organism is exposed to external influences and the given researched influence is always realized on their background. The time after the first influence is usually measured in the experiment. Time after the influence, defines the effect of the second one so far as the second one coincides with the certain status of functions (Vlasov, 1994). It is fair as for radiative, so, probably, and for all other influences of ecological factors.

Conclusion

So, hypoxia is the optimal, well-dosed factor (up to extreme levels) for modification of organism of animals and the person tolerance in this or that side. To some extent you can see practically at all factors mechanisms of environment powerful component of tissue hypoxia. Reasonable use of this law allows in the theory and in practice to change tissue resistance or the whole organism in the necessary direction.

Making conclusion, once again it is necessary to note that the problem of the combined influence of environmental factors on person organism is one of the key problems in biology, medicine and ecology though for a long time it was considered a specific problem for aerospace medicine and radiobiology. At the same time it is obvious, that the problem of the combined influence of extreme factors exceeds the limits of these disciplines and has now general biological and wide medical-ecological value.

The fact is very important, that in modifying effect of practically each factor are both negative, and positive sides which should be evaluated from “hypoxic positions”, all depends on the investigated criterion. It is especially obvious at more precise dosed factors, such as the changed gas medium and radiation.

The role of time factor — chronobiology of the combined influences is very important. It is more often the main thing in a cooperative effect and confirms the presence of biooscillatory processes in each critical organism system. It is applying of phases of factors influence, and the importance of influencing factors order. At all «diversity» and complexity the regularities here are the following.

So, in aerospace medicine and as a whole in extreme physiology the phenomenon of so-called two-dimensional increase of organism tolerance to stress — factor influence is well known, especially if they have a powerful lobe of hypoxic component. Therefore at preliminary influence of such factors we can see the rising tolerance in relation to the subsequent influence of the test — factor. At repeated influences including chronic influences of the expressed degrees of hypoxia, motion desease, overloads, heat, electromagnetic radiation, decrease of tolerance to the test — factor is more often recorded. At the subsequent (after the test — factor) influence of the additional extreme factor there is more often an aggravation of damages in the systems of vital importance for an organism.

At the expressed acute (extreme) influences demanding the prompt mobilization of all the reserves of an organism, the most indicative and system creating factors are already mentioned structural-functional effects in hematoencephalic barrier, hydration-electrolyte brain profile (HEBP), and also synapse-architectonics of cerebral structures. As integrating nonspecific mechanisms it is necessary to consider tissue hypoxia and express — aging.

There are no doubts, that the big perspectives are in a quantitative evaluation of hypoxia degree in tissues after this or that influence that will allow predicting more precisely the integral result of any real combination of factors in practice.

References

Akojev I.G. Some results of theoretical analysis of radiative lesion of an organism // Isvestyja of USSR AS. Ser. biol. — 1976. — ¹ 1. — P. 41— 52.

Amrit L.B., Shvydkij V.V., Sumarukov G.V. Barometric training and radioprotection of mice // New Experimental Approaches to Studying Work of Biological Systems. Report MOIP. General biology, 1979. — M., 1981. — P. 39— 40.

Antipov V.V., Davydov B.I., Ushakov I.B., Fyodorov V.P. Influence of space flight factors on the central nervous system. Structurally functional aspects of radiomodificatory influence. — L.: Nauka, 1989. — 328 p.

Barbashova Z.I. Adaptation to hypoxia and its physiological mechanisms. — Ì.; L.: USSR AS Publishing House, 1960. — 216 p.

Viru A.A. // Physiological Problems of Adaptation: Abstracts of All-Union Symposium, Tartu, 1984. — Tartu, 1984. — P. 13—18.

Vlasov V.V. Reaction of an organism to external influences: the general regularities of development and methodical problems of research. — Irkutsk: ISU Publishing House, 1994. — 334 p.

Gabitov V.H., Hamitov B.P., Akmatov B.R. Morphofunctional state of pituitary body at an experimental radial illness in conditions of different mountain heights // Collected Scient. works of Kirg. Med. Institute. — Frunze, 1987. — V. 163. — P. 106—115.

Grigor'ev A.J. Definition of an individual radiosensitiveness at different forms of radial illness: Synopsis of thesis… cand. of biol. sciences. — Ì.: All-Union SII of agricultural radiology, 1985. — 23 p.

Davydov B.I., Ushakov I.B., Fyodorov V.P. Radiative lesion of brain / Edited by academician of USSR APS V.A. Ponomarenko. — Ì.: Energoatomizdat, 1991. — 240 p.

Kordenko A.N., Fyodorov V.P., Ushakov I.B. Morphofunctional state of some components of vascular wall of brain of rats after g-irradiation of head // Radiobiology. — 1985. — V. 25, ¹ 4. — P. 553—556.

Kordenko A.N., Ushakov I.B. Method of forecasting of an individual radiosensitiveness in conditions of hypoxia // Patent for the Invention ¹ 2075078 from March 10, 1997 ã.

Koshelev V.B., Krushinskij A.L., Sotskaja M.N. Protecting influence of hypoxic adaptation on mortality of animals from the acute disorders of blood circulation caused by strong exaltation of brain // Report of USSR AS. — 1984. — V. 276, ¹ 5. — P. 1274—1276.

Krushinskij A.L., Rjasina T.V., Koshelev K.M. Protective influence of different kinds and regimes of adaptation to hypoxia on development of stressful damages at rats of KM line // Physiol. Journal of the USSR. — 1989. — V. 75, ¹ 11. — P. 1576—1584.

Medvedev V.I. Tolerance of physiological and psychologic functions of a person at extreme factors influence. — L.: Nauka, 1982. — 104 p.

Medvedev V.I., Krivoschekov S.G., Jurevich A.Z., etc. Physiological mechanisms of activity optimization. — L.: Nauka, 1985. — 134 p.

Mezhiborskaja N.A. Age features of urgent adaptation energy-producing frames of brain to acute hypoxia // Congress of Geronthologists and Geriatrists USSR, Dnepropetrovsk, Oct.4—6, 1988: Abstracts of dicref. reports. — Kijev, 1988. — P. 160.

Plehina L.V. A status of oxygen exchange of cerebral cortex and a skeletal muscle at the combined influence of high mountains and ionizing radiation // Inform. Scientific Council Bull. on Radiobiol. Problems of USSR AS. — 1977. — ¹ 20. — P. 19— 22.

Razinkin S.M., Duhovich V.M. A relative evaluation of hypoxic express — training regimes in order to increase thermal tolerance of organism // Abstracts to VIII All-Union Conference of Space Biology and Aerospace Medicine, Kaluga, June 25— 27, 1986. — Ì.: Nauka, 1986. — P. 291—292.

Semchenko V.V., Stepanov S.S. Mechanisms of brain plasticity in postresuscitation period // Mechanisms of Brain Plasticity. — Makhachkala, 1982. — P. 98—99.

Sizan E.P. Tolerance increase to radiation of behavioural reactions of rats after adaptation to hypoxia // Radiobiology. — 1979. — ¹ 2. — P. 204—208.

Ushakov I.B. Hydration-electrolitic structure of brain at various variants of influence of environment physical factors / / Works of Voronezh Med. Institute named after N.N. Burdenko. — Voronezh, 1989. — P. 200—205.

Ushakov I.B., Abramov M.M. Radiosensitiveness of an organism at animals irradiation in the changed gas medium: Paravariation of a cerebral set of symptoms at mice by hypoxic hypoxia and hyperoxia during radiation // Radiobiology. — 1984. — V. 24, ¹ 5. — P. 698—699.

Ushakov I.B., Abramov M.M., Hundanov L.L., Zuev V.G. Radioprotectors and hypoxia: mechanisms of the combined protection. — M.: Arms. Policy. Conversion, 1996à. — 152 p.

Ushakov I.B., Gajdamakin A.N. Influence of g-irradiation on enzyme activity of lymphocytes of dogs liquor // Radiobiology. — 1985. — V. 25, ¹ 3. — P. 415—418.

Ushakov I.B., Davydov B.I., Soldatov S.K. Quality of life and ecological risk // Human Ecology. — 1996b. — ¹ 3. — P. 73—76.

Ushakov I.B., Kordenko A.N., Antipov V.V. Tissue basophils and radiomodificatory influence of hypoxic hypoxia // Aerospace and Ecological Medicine. — 1994b. — V. 28, ¹ 3. — P. 40—42.

Ushakov I.B., Razinkin S.M., Antipov V.V., Davydov B.I. Early changes of hypoxic tolerance of gnawers at irregular influences of ionizing radiation // Radiation biology. Radioecology. — 1994c. — V. 34, ed. 4—5. — P. 678—682.

Furduj F.I., Hajdarliu S.H., Mamalyga L.M. The combined influence of extreme factors on an organism. — Kishinev: Shtiintza, 1985. — 140 p.

Jakovlev V.N. Activity of enzymes and the content of metabolites malate shuttle mechanism in cerebral cortex at hyperbaric oxygenous therapy of an acute hemorrhage // Mechanisms of hyperbaric oxygenation. — Voronezh, 1986. — P. 11—14.

Certkov K.S., Musabecov D.T., Evseeva N.K. et al. Verminderung der Radioresistenz und der allgemeinen Wiederstandsfahigkeit bei Ratten in der Initialperiode der postalpinen Readaptation // Radiobiol.-Radiother. — 1986. — Bd. 26, ¹ 6. — S. 807—812.

Doroftein V., Giurgea N., Zirbo V., Glihor E., Rusu V. Effectele expunerii de scurta durata la hipoxie hipoxica asupra rezistentei la effort a sobolanilor // Clujul. Med. — 1987. — Vol. 60, ¹ 4. — 324—329.

Routh A., Kapp J.P., Smith E.E. et al. Oxygen at 2 atmospheres absolute pressure does not increase the radiation sensitivity of normal brain in rats // Intern. J. Radiat. Oncol., Biol., Phys. — 1984. — Vol. 10, ¹ 7. — P. 1063—1065.

Wender V., Adamczewska-Goncrzewicz Z., Zorawski A., Sroczynski E., Grochowalska A. Influence of experimental hypoxia on content and composition of free fatty acids in cerebral white matter // Exp. Pathol. — 1989. — Vol. 36, ¹ 2. — P. 123—127.

Adaptation Biology and Medicine (Volume 4: Current Concepts)
Editors: A. Hargens, N. Takeda and P.K. Singal

17. Role of Renin-Angiotensin System in the Development of Cardiac Hypertrophy and Heart Failure

Weihua Zhang, Vijayan Elimban, Mohinder S. Nijjar, Suresh K. Gupta and Naranjan S. Dhalla

Institute of Cardiovascular Sciences, St. Boniface General Hospital Research Centre,
and Department of Physiology, Faculty of Medicine,
University of Manitoba, Winnipeg, Canada

Abstract

It is now well known that the renin-angiotensin system (RAS) is activated during the development of cardiac hypertrophy and congestive heart failure (CHF). Although both angiotensin converting enzyme (ACE) inhibitors and angiotensin II type 1 (AT_1) receptor antagonists have been shown to exert beneficial actions in reducing cardiac hypertrophy and attenuating the progression of CHF, treatment with these agents neither produce complete prevention nor produce long-lasting effects. In spite of the fact that both types of these drugs deactivate the RAS and produce similar effects in the failing hearts, the mechanisms and sites of their action are different from each other. Furthermore, it is not clear at present whether or not the effects of these two classes of drugs are additive or synergetic. Nonetheless, there is ample evidence which suggests that the activation of RAS and associated signal transduction mechanisms play a crucial role in remodeling various subcellular organelles, as well as myocardium which then may lead to the development of cardiac hypertrophy and progression of CHF.

Introduction

Both cardiac hypertrophy and congestive heart failure (CHF) are common clinical conditions, and in fact CHF is the final outcome of different types of heart diseases. Cardiac hypertrophy occurs in response to various stimuli, including growth hormones, various neuroendocrine factors [endothelin-1 (ET-1), angiotensin II (Ang II), as well as norepinephrine] and the increased mechanical load. Cardiac hypertrophy is characterized by an increase in the mass of cardiomyocytes in the myocardium. This involves alterations in both the cell structure and protein expression that are mediated by changes at the transcriptional and translational levels [1]. In contrast to immature cardiomyocytes, the adult cardiomyocytes undergo hypertrophic growth and do not proliferate. Studies with failing hearts in human and animal models have identified several signaling pathways that play a crucial role in CHF. However, mechanisms that participate in the transition of cardiac hypertrophy to heart failure are not clearly understood. Therefore, studies exploring the functional link between the activation of mediators, their intercellular responses and clinical consequence are of significant importance.

It is pointed out that the renin-angiotensin system (RAS) is one of the critical pathways that contributes to the development of cardiac hypertrophy and heart failure. It is believed that increased activity of the RAS for a prolonged period constitutes one of the important pathways for the progression of CHF and Ang II is the most important effector of the RAS. The blockade of RAS by different types of angiotensin converting enzyme (ACE) inhibitors or Ang II type I receptor (AT_1) blockers, both in patients and animal models with CHF, has been demonstrated to exert beneficial effects in terms of preventing clinical signs, improving heart function and reducing mortality. Therefore, it is the purpose of this article to review the current information regarding the relationship between the RAS and its contribution to the process of cardiac hypertrophy and heart failure.

Development of Heart Hypertrophy and Failure

Cardiac hypertrophy is a complex compensatory mechanism of the heart in order to adapt to excessive workload (pressure or volume overload). In response to various extracellular stimuli such as mechanical stress and growth-promoting factors including Ang II, ET-1 and transforming growth factor-β (TGF-β)?, the myocardium adapts to increased workloads through hypertrophy of terminally differentiated myocytes. Different signaling transduction pathways that link extracellular hypertrophic stimuli to nuclear transcription factors participate in this process. It is generally accepted that cardiac hypertrophy is one of the critical risk factors for heart disease. The process of cardiac hypertrophy can be divided into three stages, (i) the developing hypertrophy phase, (ii) the compensatory hypertrophy stage and (iii) the decompensatory stage which refers to heart failure. Although patients with advanced heart failure can move back and forth, the whole process of clinical heart failure can be viewed as a progression of these three stages of cardiac hypertrophy [2].

Heart failure represents an enormous problem in which cardiac output is not sufficient to meet the metabolic requirements of the body [3]. It is accompanied by increases in venous pressure and molecular defects that cause progressive deterioration of the failing heart and premature death of cardiomyocytes [4]. The available data indicate that heart failure affects approximately 18 million people in North America, and between 5-10 million people in Europe [5]. Therefore, it is a major cause of death, hospitalization and poor quality of life. The mortality from CHF has increased dramatically over the past few decades because of the high incidence and prevalence of CHF, thus becoming a major social and economic burden. More importantly, despite the best available therapy after the onset of symptoms of CHF, survival of the affected individuals is short, averaging less than five years after the first diagnosis [2, 6]; almost all patients with heart failure die within 10 years [7]. Therefore, more attention is being directed towards developing promising therapies to improve the quality of life and to prolong the survival of patients with heart failure.

The RAS

As one of the important pathways that participate in the development of cardiac hypertrophy and heart failure, the RAS not only regulates the blood pressure but also exerts direct effects on the heart, kidneys and blood vessels [8, 9]. The RAS is critically involved in the regulation of the cardiovascular function because its activation results in impaired endothelial cell function, stimulation of growth and development of apoptosis, as well as the occurrence of oxidative stress. It also enhances the paracrine and autocrine production of many factors that induce remodeling and restructuring. These factors include catecholamines, ET-1 and TGF-β [8, 10-13]. Most of the cardiac and vascular responses to mechanical stretch and strain are regulated by cardiac and vascular production of Ang II [14] and thus, Ang II is the most effective factor of the RAS.

a. Biochemistry of the RAS

The RAS includes different components that participate in the regulatory processes. One of the components is renin, which is an enzyme liberated from the juxtaglomerular cells of the afferent arterioles of the kidneys in response to a reduced renal perfusion, low blood volume, low blood pressure or left ventricular (LV) failure. Renin is a glycoproteolytic, single chain aspartyl protease of 37-40-kDa which is highly specific for its substrate, angiotensinogen, a polypeptide [15, 16]. Renin catalyzes the conversion of angiotensinogen, an inactive precursor that contains 14 amino acids, to Ang I in the liver by cleaving a leucine-valine bond in the N-terminal region of angiotensinogen. Ang I is composed of 10 amino acids (decapeptide) and is relatively inactive. However, in circulation it is converted to Ang II by the activated ACE. The ACE is a dipeptidyl carboxypeptidase, a member of the family of zinc metallopeptidases, mainly derived from the capillary bed of the lung and elsewhere in the body. Ang II is an octapeptide, which is a powerful vasoconstrictor [17-19] and exerts a great adaptive response in restoring fluid volume after hemorrhage. This hormone also shows maladaptive response upon long-term exposure causing cardiac hypertrophy and heart failure [20, 21]. Ang II is also generated from Ang I via chymase, a chymotrypsin-like proteinase, which is not affected by ACE inhibition [22].

There are two parallel systems involved in the production of Ang II, the circulating RAS and the tissue RAS (Fig. 1). Ang II production catalyzed by chymase seems to be important in the growth response. However, although chymase has a critical effect on normal formation of Ang II in the human heart, the tissue ACE pathway appears to be more important in the failing heart [23]. Furthermore, Ang II is directly synthesized from angiotensinogen by the proteolytic actions of kallikrein and cathepsin G [22, 24]. Ang II is further metabolized into two active peptides, Ang III (heptapeptide) and IV (hexapeptide), both of which bind to AT_1 and cause vasoconstriction [25-27]. Experimental studies have illustrated that other metabolites of Ang I and Ang II have the ability to cause vasodilation by enhancing the production of bradykinin [28, 29].

b. Biochemistry of Ang II Receptors

Ang II mediates its downstream second messenger pathways through binding to its two different subtypes of receptors, AT_1 and Ang II type 2 (AT_2) receptor (Fig. 2), which link to guanine nucleotide-binding protein [30]. Both of these receptors belong to the seven transmembrane domain receptor family; however, they only share 34% homology to protein sequence and have distinctive functional and pharmacological properties [31]. AT_1 receptors predominate in the adult heart, mediate the vasoconstrictor actions of Ang II and thus are viewed as activator/regulatory receptors [32]. Activation of AT_1 receptors also accounts for the augmentation of myocardial contractility [33-38], the proliferation of the fibrous and blood vessel tissue, the hypertrophic response of cardiac myocytes [39], the enhancement of aldosterone and catecholamine release [40]. AT_1 receptor is composed of 359 amino acids and blocked by its specific antagonist, losartan [30, 41]. In rodents, AT_1 receptor is further identified into two isoforms, designated AT_{1a} and AT_{1b}. In amphibians and in neuroblastoma cell lines, an AT_3 receptor has been recognized and neither losartan nor PD123177 blocked these receptors. AT_4

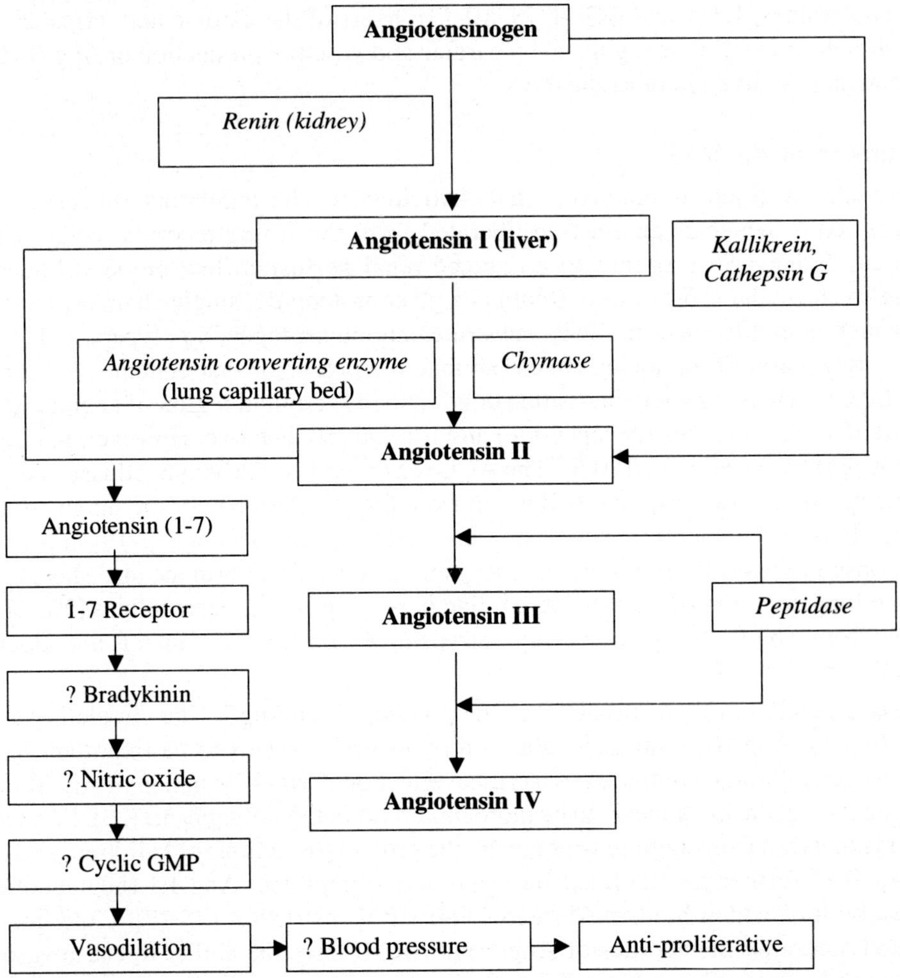

Fig. 1. Renin-angiotensin system.

has been found in vascular smooth muscle cells. The downstream targets of AT_1 receptor include G_q/G_i coupled receptors, phospholipase C (PLC), protein kinase C (PKC), Ca^{2+}, receptor tyrosine kinases, Src family, tyrosine kinases, Janus kinase 2 (JAK2) and mitogen-activated protein kinases (MAPKs). Arachidonic acid and NF-κB are downstream targets for both AT_1 and AT_2 receptors; however, whether or not the shared targets regulate the same cellular functions is unknown [40].

AT_2 receptors exert different effects as compared to AT_1 receptors; AT_2 receptors are encoded by a gene on the X chromosome with the molecular mass of approximately 41,000 kDa [42]. AT_2 downstream targets include G_i-coupled receptors, kinin/NO/cGMP, protein phosphatase, MAPK and ceramide. AT_2 receptors are relatively highly expressed in the fetal hearts which are critical for embryonic heart development and therefore are viewed as a fetal phenotype [43]. Activation of AT_2 receptors generally exerts inhibitory/counter-regulatory effects which include vasodilatation, apoptosis, negative chronotropy, natriuresis and an inhibition of cell growth [40, 44-46]. AT_2 receptors

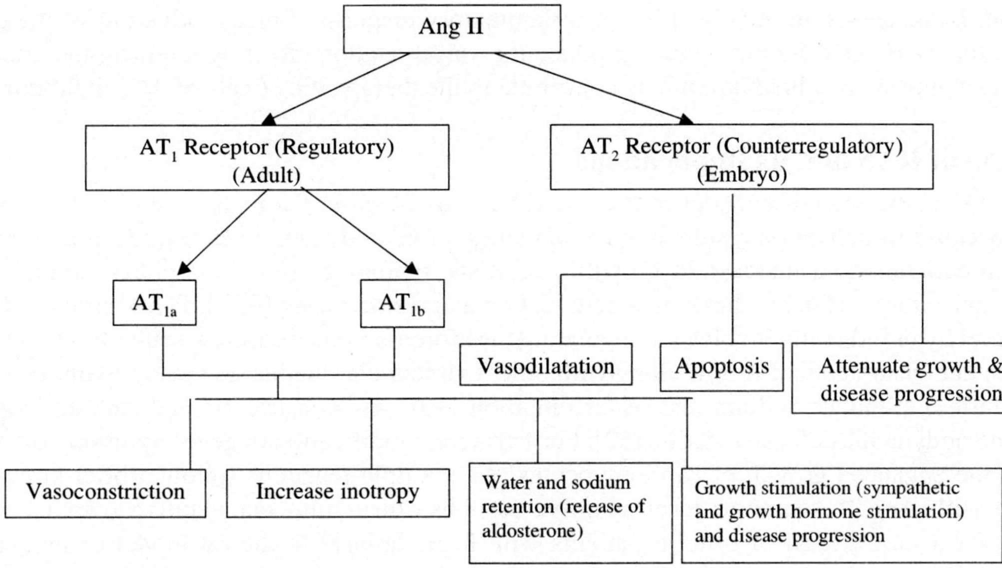

Fig. 2. Two subtypes of angiotensin II receptors exert different functions.

are blocked by PD123177. On its activation AT_2 receptor could amplify the Ang II-induced LV growth response with enhanced PKC translocation to membranes and reduced LV c-GMP content [47]. High density of Ang II receptors is found in the atrioventricular node [48]. The normal ratio of AT_1 and AT_2 in adult human atria is about 2:1. However, because of the reduction of density of AT_1 receptors, the ratio decreases in the failing human hearts [49-51]. Therefore, the relative increase in AT_2 receptors can be viewed as another example of the reversion to the fetal phenotype that accompanies the hypertrophic response in the adult heart [52]. AT_2 receptors exert their inhibitory growth effects either by suppressing cell proliferation and hypertrophy or the stimulation of apoptosis [53-57]. Although the mechanisms of AT_2 signaling transduction cascade remains to be defined, only a handful of investigators have focused their attempts to explore this signal transduction cascade. For example, Horiuchi and colleagues [58] found that the inhibitory effects of the AT_2 receptors are mediated by the activation of phosphotyrosine phosphatase, which inactivates the extracellular signal-regulated kinases (ERK1/2).

c. ACE and Bradykinin

ACE is also known as kinase II and therefore in addition to converting Ang I to Ang II, ACE regulates the degradation of a well-known vasodilator, bradykinin [30]. Bradykinin is an octapeptide and is mainly produced in the plasma. Similar to the actions of Ang II, bradykinin exerts different effects through binding to its receptor subtypes, designated as B_1 and B_2 receptors [59]. The B_2 receptors participate in the circulatory effects and thus mediate the effect of bradykinin for vasodilatation. This action involves the activation of NO generating enzyme, the constitutive nitric oxide synthase [59-61], which catalyzes the formation of vasodilators, prostacyclin and prostaglandin E2, through phospholipase A2 [62] and produces the smooth muscle relaxant effect. Bradykinin may also counter-regulate the maladaptive effects resulting in heart failure via its inhibitory action on growth. On the other hand, B_1 receptors are involved in the inflammatory response. Since bradykinin is one of the substrates for ACE, ACE inhibitors may produce the vasodilatation effect by reducing the arteriolar tone. Thus, it appears that bradykinin may contribute to the therapeutic effects of ACE inhibitors.

Activation of RAS and its Implications

There is compelling scientific evidence that the RAS is involved in the regulation of cardiovascular function because its activation results in the stimulation of hemodynamic defence reaction, impaired endothelial cell function, increase in growth, apoptosis, oxidative stress, and enhancement of the paracrine and autocrine factors that induce remodeling and restructuring [8, 10, 11]. Moreover, Ang II is either directly or indirectly involved in regulating the aforementioned cardiovascular functions [13]. It has been demonstrated that Ang II along with other extracellular mediators (vasopressin, ET-1 and norepinephrine) stimulate sodium and water retention [10], vasoconstriction and cardiac inotropic action in hemodynamic defence reaction [52]. Furthermore, modification of gene expression by Ang II results in the enhanced growth of cardiomyocytes. As multiple reactions follow a brief circulation challenge with Ang II, the short-term adaptive response turns into maladaptive response when sustained for a long period of time in patients with heart failure. In the rat model of myocardial infarction (MI), the mRNA level for AT_{1a} receptors was elevated, whereas that for AT_{1b} receptors did not change [63]. Ang II interacts with AT_1 receptor leading to the activation of PLC which catalyzes the hydrolysis of phosphatidylinosital 4,5-bisphosphate to produce diacylglycerol (DAG) and inositol trisphosphate (IP_3). DAG and IP_3 will further promote the growth of cardiomyocytes through different signaling pathways including the ERK cascade [64]. Mechanical stretch has been demonstrated to be a stimulatory factor for Ang II release, and thus acts as an initial mediator of the hypertrophic response in cardiac myocytes [65]. Since the activation of both peripheral and tissue RAS is considered to contribute to the genesis of cardiac hypertrophy, it is believed that the increased activity of RAS for a prolonged period constitutes one of the important signal transduction pathways in the pathogenesis of CHF.

Experimental studies have illustrated that Ang II, generated either in the circulation or from paracrine and autocrine sources, regulates the activity of MAPKs in the heart [66,67]. However, Ang II generated in the circulating and tissue systems appear to serve different functions. The circulating Ang II is probably the most important factor in regulating the vasomotor tone, whereas Ang II produced in the tissues participates in the signal transduction pathways that regulate gene expression and result in cell proliferation [52]. Many investigators have focused their studies on gene expression and changes in the protein components of the RAS in cardiac tissue in heart failure [63, 68-70]. Ang II plays a major role in the development of volume overload-induced cardiac hypertrophy [68-73]. Extensive studies have provided evidence that blocking Ang II formation inhibits maladaptive cardiac growth [74,75]. Ang II has been demonstrated to regulate the production of ET-1 in patients with heart failure [52, 76-83]. The elevated level of ET-1 in heart failure patients stimulates myocardial contractility, causes vasoconstriction, promotes secretion of aldosterone and retention of sodium and water, and potentiates growth [84-97]. A recent report indicates that blockade of ET-1 receptors improves the survival in a rat heart failure model by inhibiting remodeling. It has also been suggested that inhibition of Ang II will repress the progressive remodeling in the hypertrophic heart [98, 99]. Patients with severe heart failure exhibit the activation of RAS, resulting in the elevation of Ang II in both the circulating and tissue levels, and thus stimulating the release of aldosterone. Aldosterone not only promotes the retention of sodium and water, but also has growth promoting effects, and thus may be involved in the maladaptive hypertrophy and heat failure [53]. Ang II is also directly involved in the maladaptive hypertrophy and heart failure. In cultured adult cardiac fibroblasts, Ang II has been found to induce collagen synthesis, and inhibit the collagenase activity, and therefore may be involved in the pathologic myocardial fibrosis [30, 100]. In addition, Ang II has also been implicated in apoptosis during the onset of diabetes and in response to mechanical deformation [101].

Beneficial Effects of the RAS Blockade

As CHF has become a major social and economic burden due to high prevalence and mortality, the development of potential drug therapy and improved management of patients with heart failure has become a very demanding task. It has been demonstrated that the neuroendocrine stimuli for cardiac function arise from the sympathetic nerves, induce myocardial dysfunction and remodeling. Innovative drug therapy or procedures modulating the signal transduction systems that generate abnormal cardiac phenotypes may therefore make it possible to prevent the transition from adaptive to maladaptive cardiac hypertrophy. Although the cellular mechanisms are still poorly understood, findings from experimental studies and clinical trials in patients with heart failure indicate that the neuroendocrine blockers such as ACE inhibitors, AT_1 receptor antagonists and β-adrenoceptor blockers produce beneficial effects. These drugs partially prevent cardiac remodeling and improve myocytes function in heart failure [102].

a. Beneficial Effects of ACE Inhibitors

ACE inhibitors were initially identified in snake venom and were made available for study as RAS blocking agents. The available ACE inhibitors include captopril, benazepril, enalapril, fosinopril, lisinopril, quinapril, ramipril, perindopril imidapril and trandolapril. Many studies have been carried out regarding the effects of ACE inhibitors on the RAS in either pressure overload or volume overload models. Considerable evidence has demonstrated that this group of drugs provide superior capabilities as compared to other drugs in the control of blood pressure, reduction of proteinuria, and in slowing the progression of renal diseases. These drugs were introduced for treatment of heart failure because of their vasodialatory, antihypertensive and antiproteinuric effects, and their demonstrated ability to delay progression of renal disease in conjunction with their ability to reduce systemic blood pressure. The mechanism by which these drugs improve cardiac function and clinical outcome remains poorly described. However, it is clear that it partially depends on their ability to reduce the plasma Ang II level, increase the plasma bradykinin level, and inhibit the maladaptive cardiac growth [103]. Controversy has nonetheless arisen regarding the ability of ACE inhibitors to produce long-term suppression of Ang II levels. Clinical studies in humans suggest that the inhibition of ACE by most of these drugs might not be sustained throughout the drug-dosing interval because plasma Ang II levels do not fall and in fact, remain at or above the pre-treatment levels [104]. Furthermore, there is growing evidence that an alternative pathway of conversion of Ang I to Ang II (chymase pathway) may restore the circulating or tissue levels of Ang II despite ACE inhibition. In addition, data in some experimental models of ventricular dysfunction suggest that some of the beneficial effects of ACE inhibitors might be mediated by kinin stimulation rather than by Ang II suppression. In this regard, it has been demonstrated that a bradykinin receptor antagonist inhibits the blood pressure-lowering effects of an ACE inhibitor [105].

ACE inhibitors have been shown to improve stroke volume and reduce atrial and ventricular diastolic volume by inducing vasodilatation and arteriolar dilation [30, 106, 107]. Furthermore, ACE inhibitors were found to reduce transmural wall stress and compensatory dilation, increase the end-diastolic and end-systolic volume, as well as decrease mean arterial blood pressure and left ventricular end-diastolic pressure (LVEDP). ACE inhibitors also improve the distribution of coronary flow in surface and transmural areas and depress the LV remodeling process [108]. In addition, experimental studies in the rat model of MI have revealed that long-term treatment with ACE inhibitors decrease the abnormal accumulation of myocardial collagen and fibrosis, which increase the stiffness of myocardium and hasten the remodeling process [30]. Several clinical studies suggest that ACE inhibitors prolong survival in patients with severe heart failure in part by inhibiting apoptosis [109, 110]. Furthermore, treatment with ACE inhibitors can attenuate myosin heavy chain content and the isoform shift in heart failure. Preventative effects of ACE inhibitors on remodeling of sarcoplasmic reticulum and sarcolemmal membrane after MI have also been demonstrated in rats [64].

A vast body of conclusive information has revealed that all members of the class of ACE inhibitors improve long-term prognosis in heart failure [30, 111-114]. Similarly, results of several clinical trials have indicated improved survival rates [115] and reduced hospitalization rates for patients with heart failure in several subgroups based on age, sex, and presumed etiology. These data support the view that ACE inhibitors slow down the progression of heart dysfunction and delay the development of more severe heart failure [116-118]. Clinical trials regarding the usage of enalapril showed the reduction in morbidity and mortality of heart failure patients after MI [107, 119]. It has also been demonstrated that the long-term treatment with ACE inhibitors favourably alters the LV loading conditions, suppresses the progressive remodeling of ventricle and prolongs the survival period [30, 106, 107, 120-124]. In the rat MI model, although the infarct size was not reduced, the use of ACE inhibitors consistently reduced the LV filling pressure and distension, improved ventricular performance and attenuated the dilation of the left ventricule. ACE inhibition in rat heart failure model was associated with improving myofibrillar ATPase activities as well as preventing changes in myosin heavy chain isozyme protein contents and their gene expression [125]. Overall, the mechanism underlying the beneficial effects of the ACE inhibitors is far from clear and their exact site of action on myocardium remains to be identified.

Activation of the RAS is the hallmark of CHF due to MI [126] since it plays an important role in the cardiac remodeling and/or prognosis after MI [127, 128]. The blockade of Ang II production inhibits maladaptive growth [74, 129, 130], which is mediated by the heptahelical receptors that are coupled to $G_{q,}$ and stimulate JAK/STAT-controlled MAPK pathways [66, 67, 131, 132]. Activation of these mitogenic signaling pathways almost all exert worsening effects on the failing heart [133]. Treatment with ACE inhibitors results in significant prevention of cardiac hypertrophy produced in different pressure overload rat models, such as the aortic stenosis and aorta banding or through constriction of abdominal aorta; prolonged survival rate were also observed [75, 134-137]. Moreover, in the volume-overload rat model, ACE inhibitor therapy significantly reduced elevation in the LVEDP suggesting that RAS may exert some protective effects on volume-overload induced cardiac hypertrophy and failure [73, 138-140].

b. Beneficial Effects of AT_1 Receptor Blockers

The blockers of AT_1 receptor appear to act through different mechanisms from the ACE inhibitors and are more specific for the RAS. To date, the available AT_1 receptor blockers include: losartan, valsartan, irbesartan, candesartan cilexetil, telmisartan and eprosartan. These antagonists have no effect on any of the known enzymatic systems that result in formation of Ang II but primarily bind to AT_1 receptors and thus block the binding of Ang II to its high affinity type 1 site. These agents inhibit the vasoconstriction as well as hormone-stimulating, and growth-promoting effects of Ang II. Their antihypertensive and hemodynamic actions appear to be similar to those of the ACE inhibitors. Losartan is an AT_1 receptor blocker that has been shown to be efficacious and safe for the treatment of hypertension. Candesartan, because of its tight and long-lasting binding to the AT_1 receptor, cannot be overcome by high concentration of Ang II, and thus provides pronounced 24h blood pressure control with the effective blockade of all the major negative cardiovascular effects of Ang II [141-147]. There is increasing scientific evidence that if AT_2 receptors were not blocked when the serum level of Ang II was elevated by the AT_1 receptor blockade, counter regulatory effects of AT_2 receptors would be increased. Sophisticated experimental studies indicate that the stimulation of AT_2 receptors results in activation of bradykinin–nitric oxide–cyclic GMP vasodilator cascade, and directly activate kininogenase, leading to enhanced bradykinin production [8, 42, 148-153]. Many studies have suggested that Ang II antagonists show beneficial effect in heart failure induced in different experimental models, such as the volume overload, pressure overload and pacing [137, 138, 154]. It has also been reported that losartan favourably increases the coronary flow in experimental dogs [155]. Losartan is devoid of many side effects including cough, angioedema, renal dysfunction and first-dose hypotension evoked by ACE inhibitors [64, 156, 157] and is considered to be a substitute therapeutic method for patients who cannot tolerate the side effects of ACE inhibitors.

c. Combined Effects of ACE Inhibitors and AT_1 Receptor Blockers

Because of dissimilar mechanisms of actions of ACE inhibitors and AT_1 blockers, their combined effects on blood pressure, reduction in proteinuria and attenuation of glomerulosclerosis as well as tubulointerstitial fibrosis have been studied in different experimental models. However, they both share common features in that they inhibit apoptosis and limit the production of many soluble mediators of fibrosis, including TGF-β and ET-1 [8, 158-164]. These agents produce an equal magnitude of effects in reducing cardiac hypertrophy, restoring minimal coronary vascular resistance in postinfarction reactive hypertrophy, and attenuating the noninfarcted LV myocardial interstitial fibrosis. Schieffer and colleagues [165] have also reported that these agents are probably equally effective in inhibiting the generation of Ang II, and preventing the ventricular remodeling post MI. Similar effects of losartan and enalapril in improving exercise tolerance in patients with heart failure as well as presenting the shift in myosin heavy chain isozymes have also been observed [166]. However, Linz and Scholkens [167] reported that losartan was less effective in preventing cardiac hypertrophy in comparison to ACE inhibition in pressure overload due to aortic banding in rats, whereas Ruzicka and Leenen [71] suggested that AT_1 receptor blockade showed more efficiency than ACE inhibitor in blunting the hypertrophic response in a volume-overload rat model. Theoretically, different mechanisms of action by these two classes of drugs provide an ideal approach to block the RAS more effectively when used together. ACE inhibitors reduce the generation of Ang II, stimulate bradykinin production, and inhibit the degradation of bradykinin. This provides a basis for significant augmentation of the bradykinin-nitric oxide-cyclic GMP signaling cascade, resulting in vasodialation, pressure natriuresis, cytoprotection and attenuation of glomerulosclerosis.

Considerable evidence from both human and experimental animal studies supports the assumption of obtaining the additive effect in kidney protection following combination therapy of these two classes of drugs [168]. In a pig model of heart failure, the reduced densities of L-type Ca^{2+}-channel and sarcoplasmic reticulum Ca^{2+}-pump were restored by a combination therapy with ACE inhibitor benazepril and losartan whereas neither drug produced similar effects independently [169]. In patients with CHF, studies using combination therapy are also underway. Treatment with ACE inhibitors and AT_1 receptor blockers simultaneously reduced the end-diastolic volume in the LV further, and improved exercise tolerance as compared to the treatment with these drugs individually [170, 171]. Hamroff and colleagues [172] reported that combined AT_1 receptor blockade by losartan along with maximal recommended or tolerated doses of ACE inhibitor enhanced the peak exercise capacity and alleviated symptoms in CHF. Measurement of LV dimensions in a clinical trial after the combination treatment of candesartan and enalapril for 43 weeks, revealed attenuation of the ventricular remodeling, which was greater than the treatment with either agent alone [173]. However, not all combination therapies produced similar results. The combination therapy of these two classes of drugs in some experimental models did not show any additive beneficial effects as compared with individual drugs in delaying the progression of renal disease in short treatment period [163, 174]. In view of these data, the benefits of combination drug therapy versus treatment with individual drugs are still not clear, and further in-depth studies are warranted to formulate an effective therapy for treatment of patients with heart failure.

Acknowledgments

The work reported in this article was supported by the Canadian Institute of Health Research (CIHR Group in Experimental Cardiology). NSD holds the CIHR/Pharmaceutical Research and Development Chair in Cardiovascular Research supported by Merck Frosst Canada Ltd. WZ was a trainee supported by the Manitoba Health Research Council. SKG was a visiting professor from the All India Institute of Medical Sciences, New Delhi, India.

References

1. Schluter K.D., Piper H.M. Regulation of growth in the adult cardiomyocytes. FASEB J. 1999; **13 (Suppl)**: S17-S22.
2. Katz, A.M. Maladaptive hypertrophy and the cardiomyopathy of overload: Familial cardiomyopathies. In: A.M. Katz (ed), Heart Failure Pathophysiology, Molecular Biology, and Clinical Management, Lippincott Williams & Wilkins, Philadelphia, 2000; 277-307.
3. Dhalla N.S., Afzal N., Beamish R.E., Naimark B., Takeda N., Nagano M. Pathophysiology of cardiac dysfunction in congestive heart failure. Can J Cardiol. 1993; **9**: 873-887.
4. Katz A.M. Heart Failure. In: A.M. Katz (ed), Physiology of the Heart, Lippincott Williams & Wilkins, Philadelphia; 2001; 658-694.
5. The sixth report of the Joint National Committee on Prevention, Detection, Evaluation, and Treatment of High Blood Pressure. Arch Intern Med. 1997; 157**:** 2413-2446.
6. Ho K K., Anderson K.M., Kannel W.B., Grossman W., Levy D. Survival after the onset of congestive heart failure in Framingham Heart Study subjects. Circulation. 1993; **88**: 107-115.

7. Swedberg K., Kjekshus J., Snapinn S. Long-term survival in severe heart failure in patients treated with enalapril. Ten year follow-up of CONSENSUS. I. Eur Heart J. 1999; **20**: 136-139.
8. Weir M.R., Dzau, V.J. The renin-angiotensin-aldosterone system: a specific target for hypertension management. Am J Hypertens. 1999; **12**: 205S-213S.
9. Sealey J.H., Laragh J.H. The renin-angiotensin-aldosterone system for normal regulation of blood pressure and sodium and potassium homeostasis. In: J.H. Laragh, B.M. Brenner (Eds), Hypertension: Pathophysiology, Diagnosis and Management, Raven Press, New York 1990; 1287-1299.
10. Dzau V.J. Evolving concepts of the renin-angiotensin system. Focus on renal and vascular mechanisms. Am J Hypertens. 1988; **1**: 334S-337S.
11. Gibbons G.H. Autocrine-paracrine factors and vascular remodeling in hypertension. Curr Opin Nephrol Hypertens. 1993; **2**: 291-298.
12. Gibbons G.H., Dzau V.J. The emerging concept of vascular remodeling. N Engl J Med. 1994; **330**: 1431-1438.
13. Griendling K.K., Tsuda T., Berk B.C., Alexander R.W. Angiotensin II stimulation of vascular smooth muscle. J Cardiovasc Pharmacol. 1989; **14 (Suppl 6)**: S27-S33.
14. Ichikawa I. Will angiotensin II receptor antagonists be renoprotective in humans? Kidney Int. 1996; **50**: 684-692.
15. Dzau V.J. Cardiac renin-angiotensin system. Molecular and functional aspects. Am J Med. 1988; **84**: 22-27.
16. Griendling K.K., Murphy T.J., Alexander R.W. Molecular biology of the renin-angiotensin system. Circulation. 1993; **87**: 1816-1828.
17. Braun-Menendez E. Suggested revision of nomenclature-angiotensin. Science. 1958; **127**: 242.
18. Braun-Menendez E., Fasciolo E., Leloir J.C., Munoz J.M. The substance causing renal hypertension. J Physiol (Lond). 1940; **98**: 283-298.
19. Page I.H, Helmer O.M. A crystalline pressor substance (angiotonin) resulting from the reaction between renin and renin activator. J Exp Med. 1940; **71**: 29-32.
20. Dzau V.J., Hollenberg N.K., Williams GH. Neurohumoral mechanisms in heart failure: Role in pathogenesis, therapy, and drug tolerance. Fed Proc. 1983; **42**: 3162-3169.
21. Francis G.S., Goldsmith S.R., Levine TB., Olivari M.T., Cohn J.N. The neurohumoral axis in congestive heart failure. Ann Intern Med. 1984; **101**: 370-377.
22. Urata H, Healy B., Stewart R.W., Bumpus F.M., Husain A. Angiotensin II-forming pathways in normal and failing human hearts. Circ Res. 1990; **66**: 883-890.
23. Urata H., Hoffman S., Ganten D. Tissue angiotensin II system in the human heart. Eur.Heart J. 1994; **15 (Suppl D)**: 68-78.
24. Naveri L. The role of angiotensin receptor subtypes in cerebrovascular regulation in the rat. Acta Physiol Scand. 1995; **630 (Suppl)**: 1-48.
25. Grassi G., Seravalle G., Cattaneo B.M., Lanfranchi A., Vailati S., Giannattasio C., Del Bo A., Sala C., Bolla G.B., Pozzi M. Sympathetic activation and loss of reflex sympathetic control in mild congestive heart failure. Circulation. 1995; **92**: 3206-3211.
26. Li Q., Zhang L., Pfaffendorf M., van Zwieten P.A. Comparative effects of angiotensin II and its degradation products angiotensin III and angiotensin IV in rat aorta. Br J Pharmacol. 1995; **116**: 2963-2970.
27. Li Q., Zhang L., Pfaffendorf M., van Zwieten P.A. Comparative vasoconstrictor effects of angiotensin II, III, and IV in human isolated saphenous vein. J Cardiovasc Pharmacol. 1997; **29**: 451-456.
28. Brosnihan K.B., Li P., Ferrario C.M. Angiotensin-(1-7) dilates canine coronary arteries through kinins and nitric oxide. Hypertension 1996; **27**: 523-528.
29. Ardaillou R., Chansel D. Synthesis and effects of active fragments of angiotensin II. Kidney Int. 1997; **52**: 1458-1468.
30. Pfeffer J.M., Fischer T.A., Pfeffer M.A. Angiotensin-converting enzyme inhibition and ventricular remodeling after myocardial infarction. Annu Rev Physiol. 1995; **57**: 805-826.

31. Antus B., Mucsi I., Rosivall L. Apoptosis induction and inhibition of cellular proliferation by angiotensin II: possible implication and perspectives. Acta Physiol Hung. 2000; **87**: 5-24.
32. Timmermans P.B., Wong P.C., Chiu A.T., Herblin W.F., Benfield P., Carini D.J., Lee R.J., Wexler R.R., Saye J.A., Smith R.D. Angiotensin II receptors and angiotensin II receptor antagonists. Pharmacol Rev. 1993; **45**: 205-251.
33. Ikenouchi, H., Barry W.H., Bridge J.H., Weinberg E.O., Apstein C.S., Lorell B.H. Effects of angiotensin II on intracellular Ca^{2+} and pH in isolated beating rabbit hearts and myocytes loaded with the indicator indo-1. J Physiol (Lond). 1994; **480**: 203-215.
34. Kass R.S., Blair M.L. Effects of angiotensin II on membrane current in cardiac Purkinje fibers. J Mol Cell Cardiol. 1981; **13**: 797-809.
35. Kobayashi M., Furukawa Y., Chiba S. Positive chronotropic and inotropic effects of angiotensin II in the dog heart. Eur J Pharmacol. 1978; **50**: 17-25.
36. Neyses L., Vetter H. Action of atrial natriuretic peptide and angiotensin II on the myocardium: Studies in isolated rat ventricular cardiomyocytes. Biochem Biophys Res Commun. 1989; **163**: 1435-1443.
37. Koch-Weser J. Myocardial actions of angiotensin. Circ Res. 1964; **14**: 337-344.
38. Freer R.S., Pappano A., Peach M.J., Bing K.T., McLean M.J., Vogel S.M., Sprenkle A.B. Mechanism for the positive inotropic effect of angiotensin II on isolated cardiac muscle. Circ Res. 1976; **39**: 178-183.
39. Katz A.M. The hypertrophic response: Programmed cell death. In: A.M. Katz (Ed.), Heart Failure Pathophysiology, Molecular Biology, and Clinical Management, Lippincott Williams & Wilkins, Philadelphia 2000; 173-226.
40. Sadoshima J. Cytokine actions of angiotensin II. Circ Res. 2000; **86**: 1187-1189.
41. Timmermans P.B., Smith R.D. Angiotensin II receptor subtypes: selective antogonists and functional correlates. Eur Heart J. 1994; **15**: 79-87.
42. Carey R.M., Wang Z.Q., Siragy H.M. Role of the angiotensin type 2 receptor in the regulation of blood pressure and renal function. Hypertension. 2000; **35**: 155-163.
43. Zemel S., Millan M.A., Feuillan P., Aguilera G. Characterization and distribution of angiotensin-II receptors in the primate fetus. J Clin Endocrinol Metab. 1990; **71**: 1003-1007.
44. Ichiki T., Labosky P.A., Shiota C., Okuyama S., Imagawa Y., Fogo A., Niimura F., Ichikawa I., Hogan B.L., Inagami T. Effects on blood pressure and exploratory behaviour of mice lacking angiotensin II type-2 receptor. Nature 1995; **377**: 748-750.
45. Stoll M., Steckelings U.M., Paul M., Bottari S.P., Metzger R., Unger T. The angiotensin AT_2-receptor mediates inhibition of cell proliferation in coronary endothelial cells. J Clin Invest. 1995; **95**: 651-657.
46. Hein L., Barsh G.S., Pratt R.E., Dzau V.J., Kobilka B.K. Behavioural and cardiovascular effects of disrupting the angiotensin II type-2 receptor in mice. Nature 1995; **377**: 744-747.
47. Bartunek J., Weinberg E.O., Tajima M., Rohrbach S., and Lorell B.H. Angiotensin II type 2 receptor blockade amplifies the early signals of cardiac growth response to angiotensin II in hypertrophied hearts. Circulation. 1999; **99**: 22-25.
48. Sechi L.A., Griffin C.A., Grady E.F., Kalinyak J.E., Schambelan M. Characterization of angiotensin II receptor subtypes in rat heart. Circ Res. 1992; **71**: 1482-1489.
49. Asano K., Dutcher D.L., Port J.D., Minobe W.A., Tremmel K.D., Roden R.L., Bohlmeyer T.J., Bush E.W., Jenkin M.J., Abraham W.T., Raynolds M.V., Zisman L.S., Perryman M.B., Bristow M.R. Selective downregulation of the angiotensin II AT_1-receptor subtype in failing human ventricular myocardium. Circulation. 1997; **95**: 1193-1200.
50. Haywood G.A., Gullestad L., Katsuya T., Hutchinson H.G., Pratt R.E., Horiuchi M., Fowler M.B. AT_1 and AT_2 angiotensin receptor gene expression in human heart failure. Circulation. 1997; **95**: 1201-1206.
51. Zisman L.S., Asano K., Dutcher D.L., Ferdensi A., Robertson A.D., Jenkin M., Bush E.W., Bohlmeyer T., Perryman M.B., Bristow M.R. Differential regulation of cardiac angiotensin converting enzyme binding sites and AT_1 receptor density in the failing human heart. Circulation. 1998; **98**: 1735-1741.

52. Katz A.M. The hemodynamic defense reaction. In: A.M. Katz (Ed.), Heart Failure Pathophysiology, Molecular Biology, and Clinical Management, Lippincott Williams & Wilkins, Philadelphia, 2000; 109-152.

53. Matsubara H. Pathophysiological role of angiotensin II type 2 receptor in cardiovascular and renal diseases. Circ Res. 1998; **83**: 1182-1191.

54. Horiuchi M., Lehtonen J.Y., Daviet L. Signaling mechanism of the AT_2 angiotensin II receptor: Crosstalk between AT_1 and AT_2 receptors in cell growth. Trends Endocrinol Metab. 1999; **10**: 391-396.

55. Nakajima M., Hutchinson H.G., Fujinaga M., Hayashida W., Morishita R., Zhang L., Horiuchi M., Pratt R.E., Dzau V.J. The angiotensin II type 2 (AT_2) receptor antagonizes the growth effects of the AT1 receptor: Gain-of-function study using gene transfer. Proc Natl Acad Sci USA. 1995; **92**: 10663-10667.

56. Booz G.W., Baker K.M. Role of type 1 and type 2 angiotensin receptors in angiotensin II-induced cardiomyocyte hypertrophy. Hypertension. 1996; **28**: 635-640.

57. Dimmeler S., Rippmann V., Weiland U., Haendeler J., Zeiher A.M. Angiotensin II induces apoptosis of human endothelial cells. Protective effect of nitric oxide. Circ Res. 1997; **81**: 970-976.

58. Horiuchi M., Akishita M., Dzau V.J. Recent progress in angiotensin II type 2 receptor research in the cardiovascular system. Hypertension. 1999;**33**: 613-621.

59. Mombouli J.V., Vanhoutte P.M. Heterogeneity of endothelium-dependent vasodilator effects of angiotensin-converting enzyme inhibitors: Role of bradykinin generation during ACE inhibition. J Cardiovasc Pharmacol. 1992; **20 (Suppl 9)**: S74-S82.

60. Farhy R.D., Carretero O.A., Ho K.L., Scicli A.G. Role of kinins and nitric oxide in the effects of angiotensin converting enzyme inhibitors on neointima formation. Circ Res. 1993; **72**: 1202-1210.

61. Fleming I., Hecker M., Busse R. Intracellular alkalinization induced by bradykinin sustains activation of the constitutive nitric oxide synthase in endothelial cells. Circ Res. 1994; **74**: 1220-1226.

62. Schror K. Role of prostaglandins in the cardiovascular effects of bradykinin and angiotensin-converting enzyme inhibitors. J Cardiovasc Pharmacol. 1992; **20 (Suppl 9)**: S68-S73.

63. Iijima K., Geshi E., Nomizo A., Arata Y., Katagiri T. Alterations in sarcoplasmic reticulum and angiotensin II type 1 receptor gene expression after myocardial infarction in rats. Jpn Circ J. 1998; **62**: 449-454.

64. Shao Q, Panagia V., Beamish R.E., Dhalla N.S. Role of renin-angiotensin system in cardiac hypertrophy and failure. In: N.S. Dhalla, P. Zahradka, I.M.C. Dixon, R.E. Beamish (Eds.), Angiotensin II Receptor Blockade: Physiological and Clinical Implications, Kluwer Academic Publishers, Boston. 1998; 283-310.

65. Sadoshima J., Xu Y., Slayter H.S., Izumo S. Autocrine release of angiotensin II mediates stretch-induced hypertrophy of cardiac myocytes in vitro. Cell. 1993; **75**: 977-984.

66. Marrero M.B., Schieffer B., Paxton W.G., Heerdt L., Berk B.C., Delafontaine P., Bernstein K.E. Direct stimulation of Jak/STAT by the angiotensin II AT_1 receptor. Nature. 1997; **375**: 247-249.

67. Pan J., Fukuda K., Kodama H., Makino S., Takahashi T., Sano M., Hori S., Ogawa S. Role of angiotensin II in activation of the JAK/STAT pathway induced by acute pressure overload in the rat heart. Circ Res.1997; **81**: 611-617.

68. Boer P. H., Ruzicka M., Lear W., Harmsen E., Rosenthal J., Leenen F.H.H. Stretch-mediated activation of cardiac renin gene. Am J Physiol. 1994; **267**: H1630-H1636.

69. Pieruzzi F., Abassi Z.A., Keiser H.R. Expression of renin-angiotensin system components in the heart, kidneys, and lungs of rats with experimental heart failure. Circulation. 1995; **92**: 3105-3112.

70. Iwai N., Shimoike H., Kinoshita M. Cardiac renin-angiotensin system in the hypertrophied heart. Circulation. 1995; **92**: 2690-2696.

71. Ruzicka M., Yuan B., Harmsen E., Leenen F.H.H. The renin-angiotensin system and volume overload-induced cardiac hypertrophy in rats. Effects of angiotensin converting enzyme inhibitor versus angiotensin II receptor blocker. Circulation. 1993; **87**: 921-930.

72. Ruzicka M., Skarda V., Leenen F.H.H. Effects of ACE inhibitors on circulating versus cardiac angiotensin II in volume overload-induced cardiac hypertrophy in rats. Circulation. 1995; **92**: 3568-3573.

73. Ruzicka M., Keeley F.W., Leenen F.H.H. The renin-angiotensin system and volume overload-induced changes in cardiac collagen and elastin. Circulation. 1994; **90**: 1989-1996.
74. Yamazaki T., Komuro I., Kudoh S., Zou Y., Shiojima I., Mizuno T., Takano H., Hiroi Y., Ueki K., Tobe K et al. Angiotensin II partly mediates mechanical stress-induced cardiac hypertrophy. Circ Res. 1995; **77**: 258-265.
75. Linz W., Scholkens B.A., Ganten D. Converting enzyme inhibition specifically prevents the development and induces regression of cardiac hypertrophy in rats. Clin Exp Hypertens. 1989; **11**: 1325-1350.
76. Cody R.J. The potential role of endothelin as a vasoconstrictor substance in congestive heart failure. Eur Heart J. 1992; **13**: 1573-1578.
77. Hiroe M., Hirata Y., Fujita N., Umezawa S., Ito H., Tsujino M., Koike A., Nogami A., Takamoto T., Marumo F. Plasma endothelin-1 levels in idiopathic dilated cardiomyopathy. Am J Cardiol. 1991; **68**: 1114-1115.
78. Kiowski W., Sutsch G., Hunziker P., Muller P., Kim J., Oechslin E., Schmitt R., Jones R., Bertel O. Evidence for endothelin-1-mediated vasoconstriction in severe chronic heart failure. Lancet. 1995; **346**: 732-736.
79. Margulies K.B., Hildebrand Jr. F.L., Lerman A., Perrella M.A., Burnett Jr J.C. Increased endothelin in experimental heart failure. Circulation. 1990; **82**: 2226-2230.
80. McMurray J.J., Ray S.G., Abdullah I., Dargie H.J., Morton J.J. Plasma endothelin in chronic heart failure. Circulation. 1992; **85**: 1374-1379.
81. Ponicke K., Vogelsang M., Heinroth M., Becker K., Zolk O., Bohm M., Zerkowski H.R., Brodde O.E. Endothelin receptors in the failing and nonfailing human heart. Circulation. 1998; **97**: 744-751.
82. Stewart D.J., Cernacek P., Costello K.B., Rouleau J.L. Elevated endothelin-1 in heart failure and loss of normal response to postural change. Circulation. 1992; **85**: 510-517.
83. Wei C.M., Lerman A., Rodeheffer R.J., McGregor C.G., Brandt R.R., Wright S., Heublein D.M., Kao P.C., Edwards W.D., Burnett Jr J.C. Endothelin in human congestive heart failure. Circulation. 1994; **89**: 1580-1586.
84. Brooks D.P. Role of endothelin in renal function and dysfunction. Clin Exp Pharmacol Physiol. 1996; **23**: 345-348.
85. Cavero P.G., Miller W.L., Heublein D.M., Margulies K.B., Burnett Jr J.C. Endothelin in experimental congestive heart failure in the anesthetized dog. Am J Physiol. 1990; **259**: F312-F317.
86. Colucci W.S. Myocardial endothelin. Does it play a role in myocardial failure? Circulation. 1996; **93**: 1069-1072.
87. Cozza E.N., Gomez-Sanchez C.E., Foecking M.F., Chiou S. Endothelin binding to cultured calf adrenal zona glomerulosa cells and stimulation of aldosterone secretion. J Clin Invest. 1989; **84**: 1032-1035.
88. Ichikawa K.I., Hidai C., Okuda C., Kimata S.I., Matsuoka R., Hosoda S., Quertermous T., Kawana M. Endogenous endothelin-1 mediates cardiac hypertrophy and switching of myosin heavy chain gene expression in rat ventricular myocardium. J Am Coll Cardiol. 1996; **27**: 1286-1291.
89. Ishikawa T., Yanagisawa M., Kimura S., Goto K., Masaki T. Positive inotropic action of novel vasoconstrictor peptide endothelin on guinea pig atria. Am J Physiol. 1988; **255**: H970-H973.
90. Ito H., Hiroe M., Hirata Y., Fujisaki H., Adachi S., Akimoto H., Ohta Y., Marumo F. Endothelin ETA receptor antagonist blocks cardiac hypertrophy provoked by hemodynamic overload. Circulation. 1994; **89**: 2198-2203.
91. Ito H., Hirata Y., Hiroe M., Tsujino M., Adachi S., Takamoto T., Nitta M., Taniguchi K., Marumo F. Endothelin-1 induces hypertrophy with enhanced expression of muscle-specific genes in cultured neonatal rat cardiomyocytes. Circ Res. 1991; **69**: 209-215.
92. Karet F.E. Endothelin peptides and receptors in human kidney. Clin Sci (Lond). 1996; **91**: 267-273.
93. Miller W.L., Redfield M.M., Burnett Jr J.C. Integrated cardiac, renal, and endocrine actions of endothelin. J Clin Invest. 1989; **83**: 317-320.
94. Levin E.R. Endothelins. N.Engl.J Med. 1995; **333**: 356-363.

95. Noll G., Wenzel R.R., Luscher T.F. Endothelin and endothelin antagonists: potential role in cardiovascular and renal disease. Mol Cell Biochem. 1996; **157**: 259-267.

96. Shubeita H.E., McDonough P.M., Harris A.N., Knowlton K.U., Glembotski C.C., Brown J.H., Chien K.R. Endothelin induction of inositol phospholipid hydrolysis, sarcomere assembly, and cardiac gene expression in ventricular myocytes. A paracrine mechanism for myocardial cell hypertrophy. J Biol Chem. 1990; **265**: 20555-20562.

97. Suzuki T., Hoshi H., Mitsui Y. Endothelin stimulates hypertrophy and contractility of neonatal rat cardiac myocytes in a serum-free medium. FEBS Lett. 1990; **268**: 149-151.

98. Fraccarollo D., Hu K., Galuppo P., Gaudron P., Ertl G. Chronic endothelin receptor blockade attenuates progressive ventricular dilation and improves cardiac function in rats with myocardial infarction: possible involvement of myocardial endothelin system in ventricular remodeling. Circulation. 1997; **96**: 3963-3973.

99. Mulder P., Richard V., Derumeaux G., Hogie M., Henry J.P., Lallemand F., Compagnon P., Mace B., Comoy E., Letac B., Thuillez C. Role of endogenous endothelin in chronic heart failure: Effect of long-term treatment with an endothelin antagonist on survival, hemodynamics, and cardiac remodeling. Circulation. 1997; **96**: 1976-1982.

100. Crabos M., Roth M., Hahn A.W., Erne P. Characterization of angiotensin II receptors in cultured rat cardiac fibroblasts: Coupling to signaling systems and gene expression. J Clin Invest. 1994; **93**: 2372-2378.

101. Fiordaliso F., Li B., Latini R., Sonnenblick E.H., Anversa P., Leri A., Kajstura J. Myocyte death in streptozotocin-induced diabetes in rats in angiotensin II- dependent. Lab Invest. 2000; **80**: 513-527.

102. Eichhorn E.J., Bristow M.R. Medical therapy can improve the biological properties of the chronically failing heart. A new era in the treatment of heart failure. Circulation. 1996; **94**: 2285-2296.

103. Katz A.M. Therapeutic strategies for managing heart failure. In: A.M. Katz (Ed.), Heart Failure Pathophysiology, Molecular Biology, and Clinical Management, Lippincott Williams & Wilkins, Philadelphia 2000; 309-339.

104. Mooser V., Nussberger J., Juillerat L., Burnier M., Waeber B., Bidiville J., Pauly N., Brunner H.R. Reactive hyperreninemia is a major determinant of plasma angiotensin II during ACE inhibition. J Cardiovasc Pharmacol. 1990; **15**: 276-282.

105. Gainer J.V., Morrow J.D., Loveland A., King D.J., Brown N.J. Effect of bradykinin-receptor blockade on the response to angiotensin-converting-enzyme inhibitor in normotensive and hypertensive subjects. N Engl J Med. 1998; **339**: 1285-1292.

106. Nelson K.M., Yeager B.F. What is the role of angiotensin-converting enzyme inhibitors in congestive heart failure and after myocardial infarction? Ann Pharmacother. 1996; **30**: 986-993.

107. Cody R.J. ACE inhibitors: myocardial infarction and congestive heart failure. Am Fam Physician. 1995; **52**: 1801-1806.

108. Foult J.M., Tavolaro O., Antony I., Nitenberg A. Coronary vasodilation induced by intracoronary enalapril: An argument for the role of a local renin-angiotensin system in patients with dilated cardiomyopathy. Eur Heart J. 1989; **10 (Suppl F)**: 97-100.

109. Kajstura J., Cigola E., Malhotra A., Li P., Cheng W., Meggs L.G., Anversa P. Angiotensin II induces apoptosis of adult ventricular myocytes in vitro. J Mol Cell Cardiol. 1997; **29**: 859-870.

110. Yamada T., Horiuchi M., Dzau V.J. Angiotensin II type 2 receptor mediates programmed cell death. Proc Natl Acad Sci USA. 1996; **93**: 156-160.

111. Shao Q., Takeda N., Temsah R., Dhalla N.S. Prevention of hemodynamic changes due to myocardial infarction by early treatment of rats with imidapril. Cardiovasc Pathobiol. 1996; **1**: 1-7.

112. Pfeffer J.M., Pfeffer M.A., Braunwald E. Influence of chronic captopril therapy on the infarcted left ventricle of the rat. Circ Res. 1985; **57**: 84-95.

113. Sanbe A., Tanonaka K., Kobayasi R., Takeo S. Effects of long-term therapy with ACE inhibitors, captopril, enalapril and trandolapril, on myocardial energy metabolism in rats with heart failure following myocardial infarction. J Mol Cell Cardiol. 1995; **27**: 2209-2222.

114. Takeishi Y., Bhagwat A., Ball N.A., Kirkpatrick D.L., Periasamy M., Walsh R.A. Effect of angiotensin-converting enzyme inhibition on protein kinase C and SR proteins in heart failure. Am J Physiol. 1999; **276**: H53-H62.

115. The CONSENSUS Trial Study Group. Effects of enalapril on mortality in severe congestive heart failure. Results of the Cooperative North Scandinavian Enalapril Survival Study (CONSENSUS). N Engl J Med. 1987; **316**: 1429-1435.

116. Kober L., Torp-Pedersen C., Carlsen J.E., Bagger H., Eliasen P., Lyngborg K., Videbaek J., Cole D. S., Auclert L., Pauly N.C. A clinical trial of the angiotensin-converting-enzyme inhibitor trandolapril in patients with left ventricular dysfunction after myocardial infarction. Trandolapril Cardiac Evaluation (TRACE) Study Group. N Engl J Med. 1995; **333**: 1670-1676.

117. The Acute Infarction Ramipril Efficacy (AIRE) Study Investigators. Effect of ramipril on mortality and morbidity of survivors of acute myocardial infarction with clinical evidence of heart failure. Lancet. 1993; **342**: 821-828.

118. The SOLVD Investigators. Effect of enalapril on mortality and the development of heart failure in asymptomatic patients with reduced left ventricular ejection fraction. N Engl J Med. 1992; **327**: 685-691.

119. Colucci W.S. Molecular and cellular mechanisms of myocardial failure. Am J Cardiol. 1997; **80**: 15L-25L.

120. Mulder P., Devaux B., Richard V., Henry J.P., Wimart M.C., Thibout E., Mace B., Thuillez C. Early versus delayed angiotensin-converting enzyme inhibition in experimental chronic heart failure. Effects on survival, hemodynamics, and cardiovascular remodeling. Circulation. 1997; **95**: 1314-1319.

121. Pfeffer M.A., Braunwald E. Ventricular remodeling after myocardial infarction. Experimental observations and clinical implications. Circulation. 1990; **81**: 1161-1172.

122. Sigurdsson A., Swedberg K. The role of neurohormonal activation in chronic heart failure and postmyocardial infarction. Am Heart J. 1996; **132**: 229-234.

123. Rumberger J.A. Ventricular dilatation and remodeling after myocardial infarction. Mayo Clin Proc. 1994; **69**: 664-674.

124. Pfeffer J.M. Progressive ventricular dilation in experimental myocardial infarction and its attenuation by angiotensin-converting enzyme inhibition. Am J Cardiol. 1991; **68**: 17D-25D.

125. Wang J., Liu X., Ren B., Rupp H., Takeda N., Dhalla N.S. Modification of myosin gene expression by imidapril in failing heart due to myocardial infarction. J Mol Cell Cardiol. 2002; **34**: 847-857.

126. Dhalla N.S., Shao Q., Panagia V. Remodeling of cardiac membranes during the development of congestive heart failure. Heart Fail Rev. 1998; **2**: 261-272.

127. McAlpine H.M., Morton J.J., Leckie B., Rumley A., Gillen G., Dargie H.J. Neuroendocrine activation after acute myocardial infarction. Br Heart J. 1988; **60**: 117-124.

128. Dargie H.J., McAlpine H.M., Morton J.J. Neuroendocrine activation in acute myocardial infarction. J Cardiovasc Pharmacol. 1987; **9 (Suppl 2)**: S21-S24.

129. Katz A.M. Angiotensin II: Hemodynamic regulator or growth factor? J Mol Cell Cardiol. 1990; **22**: 739-747.

130. Sadoshima J., Izumo S. Molecular characterization of angiotensin II—induced hypertrophy of cardiac myocytes and hyperplasia of cardiac fibroblasts. Critical role of the AT_1 receptor subtype. Circ Res. 1993; **73**: 413-423.

131. Dostal D.E., Hunt R.A., Kule C.E., Bhat G.J., Karoor V., McWhinney C.D., Baker K.M. Molecular mechanisms of angiotensin II in modulating cardiac function: Intracardiac effects and signal transduction pathways. J Mol Cell Cardiol. 1997; **29**: 2893-2902.

132. Sadoshima J., Qiu Z., Morgan J.P., Izumo S. Angiotensin II and other hypertrophic stimuli mediated by G protein-coupled receptors activate tyrosine kinase, mitogen-activated protein kinase, and 90-kD S6 kinase in cardiac myocytes. The critical role of Ca^{2+}-dependent signaling. Circ Res. 1995; **76**: 1-15.

133. Katz A.M. The cardiomyopathy of overload: an unnatural growth response in the hypertrophied heart. Ann Intern Med. 1994; **121**: 363-371.

134. Baker K.M., Chernin M.I., Wilson S.K., Aceto J.F. Renin-angiotensin system involvement in pressure-overload cardiac hypertrophy in rats. Am J Physiol. 1990; **259**: H324-H332.
135. Kromer E.P., Riegger G.A. Effects of long-term angiotensin converting enzyme inhibition on myocardial hypertrophy in experimental aortic stenosis in the rat. Am J Cardiol. 1988; **62**: 161-163.
136. Litwin S.E., Katz S. E., Weinberg E.O., Lorell B.H., Aurigemma G.P., Douglas P.S. Serial echocardiographic-Doppler assessment of left ventricular geometry and function in rats with pressure-overload hypertrophy. Chronic angiotensin-converting enzyme inhibition attenuates the transition to heart failure. Circulation. 1995; **91**: 2642-2654.
137. Mohabir R., Young S.D., Strosberg A.M. Role of angiotensin in pressure overload-induced hypertrophy in rats: effects of angiotensin-converting enzyme inhibitors, an AT_1 receptor antagonist, and surgical reversal. J Cardiovasc Pharmacol. 1994; **23**: 291-299.
138. Luttrell L.M., van Biesen T., Hawes B.E., Koch W.J., Krueger K.M., Touhara K., Lefkowitz R.J. G-protein-coupled receptors and their regulation: Activation of the MAP kinase signaling pathway by G-protein-coupled receptors. Adv Second Messenger Phosphoprotein Res. 1997; **31**:263-277.
139. Ruzicka M., Yuan B., Leenen F.H.H. Effects of enalapril versus losartan on regression of volume overload-induced cardiac hypertrophy in rats. Circulation. 1994; **90**: 484-491.
140. Garcia R., Bonhomme M.C., Diebold S. Captopril treatment does not restore either the renal or the ANF release response during volume expansion in moderate to severe high output heart failure. Cardiovasc Res. 1994; **28**: 1533-1539.
141. Ruilope L. Improving prognosis in hypertension: exploring the benefits of angiotensin II type 1 receptor blockade. Blood Press. 2000; **Suppl 1**: 31-35.
142. Ojima M., Inada Y., Shibouta Y., Wada T., Sanada T., Kubo K., Nishikawa K. Candesartan (CV-11974) dissociates slowly from the angiotensin AT_1 receptor. Eur J Pharmacol. 1997; **319**: 137-146.
143. Lacourciere Y., Asmar R. A comparison of the efficacy and duration of action of candesartan cilexetil and losartan as assessed by clinic and ambulatory blood pressure after a missed dose, in truly hypertensive patients: A placebo-controlled, forced titration study. Candesartan/Losartan study investigators. Am J Hypertens. 1999; **12**: 1181-1187.
144. Elmfeldt D., George M., Hubner R., Olofsson B. Candesartan cilexetil, a new generation angiotensin II antagonist, provides dose dependent antihypertensive effect. J Hum Hypertens. 1997; **11 (Suppl 2)**: S49-S53.
145. Heuer H.J., Schondorfer G., Hogemann A.M. Twenty-four hour blood pressure profile of different doses of candesartan cilexetil in patients with mild to moderate hypertension. J Hum Hypertens. 1997; **11 (Suppl 2)**: S55-S56.
146. Arakawa K., Ogihara T., Iimura O., Abe K., Saruta T., Ishii M., et al. Evaluation of clinical usefulness of TCV-116 (candesartan cilexetil) in patients with essential hypertension - a double-blind, parallel group comparison study using enalapril maleate as control drug. J Clin Ther Med. 1996; **12**: 2613-2616.
147. Farsang C., Kawecka-Jaszcz K., Langan J., Maritz F., Zannad F. Antihypertensive effects and tolerability of candesartan cilexetil alone and in combination with amlodipine. Clin Drug Invest. 2001; **2**: 17-23.
148. Dzau V.J., Gibbons G.H., Pratt R.E. Molecular mechanisms of vascular renin-angiotensin system in myointimal hyperplasia. Hypertension. 1991; **18**: II100-II105.
149. Bottari S.P., King I.N., Reichlin S., Dahlstroem I., Lydon N., de Gasparo M. The angiotensin AT_2 receptor stimulates protein tyrosine phosphatase activity and mediates inhibition of particulate guanylate cyclase. Biochem Biophys Res Commun. 1992; **183**: 206-211.
150. Liu Y.H., Yang X.P., Sharov V.G., Nass O., Sabbah H.N., Peterson E., Carretero O.A. Effects of angiotensin-converting enzyme inhibitors and angiotensin II type 1 receptor antagonists in rats with heart failure. Role of kinins and angiotensin II type 2 receptors. J Clin Invest. 1997; **99**: 1926-1935.
151. Nio Y., Matsubara H., Murasawa S., Kanasaki M., Inada M. Regulation of gene transcription of angiotensin II receptor subtypes in myocardial infarction. J Clin Invest. 1995; **95**: 46-54.

152. Gross V., Schunck W.H., Honeck H., Milia A.F., Kargel E., Walther T., Bader M., Inagami T., Schneider W., Luft F.C. Inhibition of pressure natriuresis in mice lacking the AT_2 receptor. Kidney Int. 2000; **57**: 191-202.
153. Tsutsumi Y., Matsubara H., Masaki H., Kurihara H., Murasawa S., Takai S., et al. Angiotensin II type 2 receptor overexpression activates the vascular kinin system and causes vadodilation. J Clin Invest. 1999; **104**: 925-935.
154. Crozier I., Ikram H., Awan N., Cleland J., Stephen N., Dickstein K., Frey M., Young J., Klinger G., Makris L., et al. Losartan in heart failure. Hemodynamic effects and tolerability. Losartan Hemodynamic Study Group. Circulation. 1995; **91**: 691-697.
155. Sudhir K., MacGregor J.S., Gupta M., Barbant S.D., Redberg R., Yock P.G., Chatterjee K. Effect of selective angiotensin II receptor antagonism and angiotensin converting enzyme inhibition on the coronary vasculature in vivo. Intravascular two-dimensional and Doppler ultrasound studies. Circulation. 1993; **87**: 931-938.
156. Israili Z.H., Hall W.D. Cough and angioneurotic edema associated with angiotensin-converting enzyme inhibitor therapy. A review of the literature and pathophysiology. Ann Intern Med. 1992; **117**: 234-242.
157. Sunman W., Sever P.S. Non-angiotensin effects of angiotensin-converting enzyme inhibitors. Clin Sci (Lond). 1993; **85**: 661-670.
158. Klahr S., Ishidoya S., Morrissey J. Role of angiotensin II in the tubulointerstitial fibrosis of obstructive nephropathy. Am J Kidney Dis. 1995; **26**: 141-146.
159. Burdmann E.A., Andoh T.F., Nast C.C., Evan A., Connors B.A., Coffman T.M., Lindsley J., Bennett W.M. Prevention of experimental cyclosporin-induced interstitial fibrosis by losartan and enalapril. Am J Physiol. 1995; **269**: F491-F499.
160. Wu L.L., Cox A., Roe C.J., Dziadek M., Cooper M.E., Gilbert R.E. Transforming growth factor beta 1 and renal injury following subtotal nephrectomy in the rat: Role of the renin-angiotensin system. Kidney Int. 1997; **51**: 1553-1567.
161. Kon V., Fogo A., Ichikawa I. Bradykinin causes selective efferent arteriolar dilation during angiotensin I converting enzyme inhibition. Kidney Int. 1993; **44**: 545-550.
162. Morrissey J.J., Klahr S. Differential effects of ACEI and AT_1 receptor inhibition on chemoattractant and adhesion molecule synthesis. Am J Physiol. 1998; **274**: F580-F586.
163. Ots M., Mackenzie H.S., Troy J.L., Rennke H.G., Brenner B.M. Effects of combination therapy with enalapril and losartan on the rate of progression of renal injury in rats with 5/6 renal mass ablation. J Am Soc Nephrol. 1998; **9**: 224-230.
164. Zoja C., Abbate M., Corna D., Capitanio M., Donadelli R., Bruzzi I., Oldroyd S., Benigni A., Remuzzi G. Pharmacologic control of angiotensin II ameliorates renal disease while reducing renal TGF-beta in experimental mesangioproliferative glomerulonephritis. Am J Kidney Dis. 1998; **31**: 453-463.
165. Schieffer B., Wirger A., Meybrunn M., Seitz S., Holtz J., Riede U.N., Drexler H. Comparative effects of chronic angiotensin-converting enzyme inhibition and angiotensin II type 1 receptor blockade on cardiac remodeling after myocardial infarction in the rat. Circulation. 1994; **89**: 2273-2282.
166. Vescovo G., Dalla L.L., Serafini F., Leprotti C., Facchin L., Volterrani M., Ceconi C., Ambrosio G.B. Improved exercise tolerance after losartan and enalapril in heart failure: Correlation with changes in skeletal muscle myosin heavy chain composition. Circulation. 1998; **98**: 1742-1749.
167. Linz W., Henning R., Scholkens B.A. Role of angiotensin II receptor antagonism and converting enzyme inhibition in the progression and regression of cardiac hypertrophy in rats. J Hypertens. 1991; **9 (Suppl)**: S400-S401.
168. Russo D., Pisani A., Balletta M.M., De Nicola L., Savino F.A., Andreucci M., Minutolo R. Additive antiproteinuric effect of converting enzyme inhibitor and losartan in normotensive patients with IgA nephropathy. Am J Kidney Dis. 1999; **33**: 851-856.
169. Spinale F.G., Mukherjee R., Iannini J.P., Whitebread S., Hebbar L., Clair M.J., Melton D.M., Cox M.H., Thomas P.B., de Gasparo M. Modulation of the renin-angiotensin pathway through enzyme inhibition and specific receptor blockade in pacing-induced heart failure: II. Effects on myocyte contractile processes. Circulation. 1997; **96**: 2397-2406.

170. Willenheimer R., Dahlof B., Rydberg E., Erhardt L. AT_1-receptor blockers in hypertension and heart failure: Clinical experience and future directions. Eur Heart J. 1999; **20**: 997-1008.

171. Tonkon M., Awan N., Niaxi I. Irbesartan combined with conventional therapy, including angiotensin converting enzyme inhibitors, in heart failure. J Am Coll Cardiol. 1998;**31 (Suppl A):** 188A.

172. Hamroff G., Katz S.D., Mancini D., Blaufarb I., Bijou R., Patel R., Jondeau G., Olivari M.T., Thomas S., Le Jemtel T.H. Addition of angiotensin II receptor blockade to maximal angiotensin-converting enzyme inhibition improves exercise capacity in patients with severe congestive heart failure. Circulation. 1999; **99**: 990-992.

173. McKelvie R.S., Yusuf S., Pericak D., Avezum A., Burns R.J., Probstfield J., Tsuyuki R.T., White M., Rouleau J., Latini R., Maggioni A., Young J., Pogue J. Comparison of candesartan, enalapril, and their combination in congestive heart failure: Randomized evaluation of strategies for left ventricular dysfunction (RESOLVD) pilot study. The RESOLVD Pilot Study Investigators. Circulation. 1999; **100**: 1056-1064.

174. Hebert L.A., Falkenhain M.E., Nahman Jr. N.S., Cosio F.G., O'Dorisio T.M. Combination ACE inhibitor and angiotensin II receptor antagonist therapy in diabetic nephropathy. Am J Nephrol. 1999; **19**: 1-6.

Adaptation Biology and Medicine (Volume 4: Current Concepts)
Editors: A. Hargens, N. Takeda and P.K. Singal

18. Spinal Muscle Activation with the Keiser Variable Resistance Device for Space Flight Compared to Standard Earth-Based Weight Devices

Jennifer J. Pedley[1], Richard E. Ballard[1], Toshiaki Ueno[2] and Alan R. Hargens[2]

[1]Life Science Division, NASA Ames Research Center, Moffett Field, CA 94035-1000
and
[2]Department of Orthopaedic Surgery, University of California,
San Diego San Diego, California 92103-8894

Abstract

The objective of this investigation is to compare muscular activation patterns during specific resistive exercises using a variable resistance device Keiser SX-1 (specifically designed for space flight) to similar exercises performed using a standard weight machine and hand-held weights. The standard weight machine and hand-held weights are useless in space because of the weightlessness environment. To investigate paraspinal muscle activation, five men and four women performed eight exercises: four on the SX-1, three on the standard weight machine, and one exercise using hand-held weights (dumbbells). Bilateral electromyographic (EMG) activity was recorded from the trapezius, latissimus dorsi, and erector spinae muscles. For each exercise device (Keiser SX-1 compared to standard weight machine or dumbbells), volunteers performed two sets of five repetitions of the following exercises: anterior pull down, posterior pull down, row, and shoulder press. Keiser SX-1 exercises were performed in the supine and prone positions, whereas the "standard" exercises were performed in sitting or standing posture. Overall, the activation maxima were very similar for the Keiser and standard weight machine. However, EMG activity in the erector spinae was significantly greater with the Keiser than the standard weight machine during the pull-down posterior exercise. On the other hand, the dumbbell shoulder press yielded higher EMG activity of the trapezius compared to the Keiser. Despite these two differences, the Keiser SX-1 machine provides high levels of spine and shoulder muscle activation and thus, should be considered a prime candidate for exercise during long-duration space flight.

Introduction

Muscle atrophy and decreased bone density are serious consequences of extended exposure to microgravity. The absence of normal 1g loads on the musculoskeletal system is thought to cause these adverse physiological changes. Thus, astronauts must exercise during long-duration space flight to reduce these detrimental effects. However, recent calculations and Earth-based studies suggest that most exercise in space lacks sufficient loads to maintain preflight muscle mass and bone density, including the density of vertebral bodies (12, 14). Also, the reduction or absence of normal gravitational loads and alteration of muscle forces on spinal structures increases body height 4 cm or more in microgravity (9). Due to lack of spinal loading, sixty-eight percent of astronauts report back pain during exposure to microgravity (16). Back pain may be caused by a stretching of muscles and ligaments, nerve roots, and/or the spinal cord (13).

In collaboration with NASA Ames Research Center and Palo Alto Veterans Administration Rehabilitation Research and Development Center, the Keiser SX-1 variable resistance exercise device (Keiser Sports Health Equipment, Fresno, CA) was developed to prevent muscle atrophy and bone weakness during long-duration space flight. In addition to other exercises, the SX-l provides axial loading exercises such as anterior and posterior pull down, row, and shoulder press. A space-related benefit of the Keiser SX-1 is the potential to load the spine and paraspinal muscles of the vertebral column, thus maintaining bone and muscle strength within the spine. This paper extends previous studies of leg musculature using the Keiser SX-1 device (1).

The purpose of this evaluation is to compare the magnitude of activation of three back muscles (erector spinae, latissimus dorsi, and trapezius) during exercises performed on the Keiser SX-1 with equivalent exercises performed on a standard resistance device designed for 1-g. We hypothesized that muscle activation using the SX-1 is equivalent to a standard resistive exercise device when performing exercises that load the spine. Of course, standard, weight-based equipment is useless in space.

Methods and Materials

Subjects

Five healthy males and four healthy females (ages 23-53) volunteered to participate in the evaluation conducted in the Gravitational Research Branch at NASA Ames Research Center. All subjects provided written, informed consent.

Standard resistance device

A standard weight machine (Gold's Gym, CSA, Inc., South Easton, MA) and dumbbells (Ivanko Barbell Co., San Pedro, CA) were used as standards to which the SX-1 was compared. The standard weight machine was composed of pulleys and cables connected to a weight stack for resistance training to increase muscle strength and size. Of course, this hardware will not load muscles in space due to the microgravity environment.

Keiser SX-1

Two pneumatic pistons provided variable and high resistance for the lower body exercises whereas a single piston allowed resistance exercises for the upper body and spine (Figure 1). The Keiser device also provided concentric and eccentric actions. When performing an exercise, the user was secured into a harness to provide proper positioning for the upper body. When loading the spine or activating the leg muscles, the user's feet were secured into separate foot-holds. The device included an

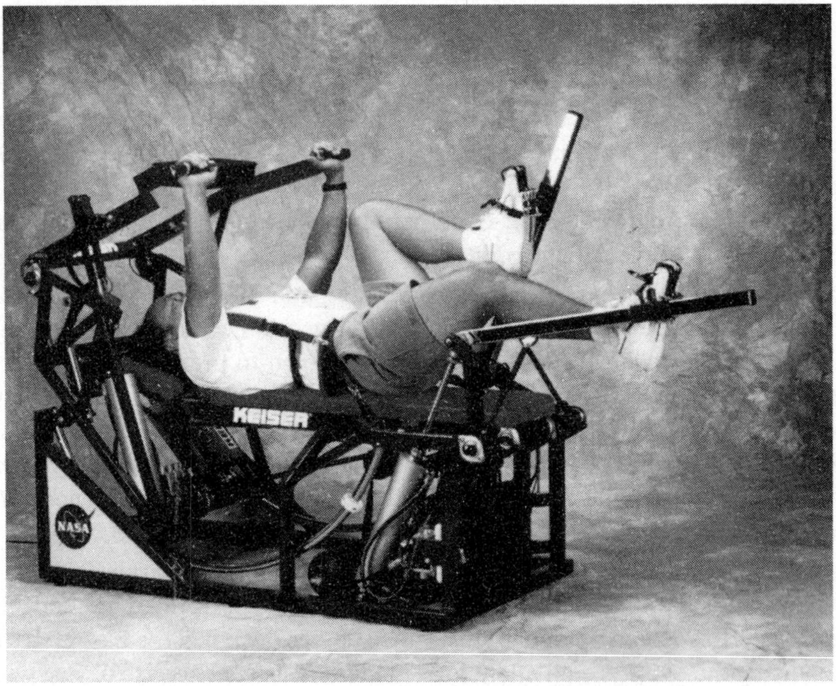

Fig. 1. Keiser SX-1 prototype for ground-based studies relevant to long-duration space flight.

adjustable monitor providing feedback such as force, work, and power. Other features included strength and cardiovascular modes represented on the monitor. In the strength mode, the monitor displayed the number of repetitions and the angle of the upper-body exercise levers. The cardiovascular mode conveyed repetitions per minute, total time of the exercise for upper and lower body, and graphic indicators to represent the range of motion. The Keiser SX-1 was designed to fit into a standard Space Station rack. The total weight of the prototype was 120 kg but can be substantially reduced using aluminum or other composite materials.

All exercises were performed in one or two positions by using the four buttons located on the handgrips. Two thumb buttons on each handgrip adjusted: 1) amount of resistance to the upper and lower extremities, 2) linkage from a pulling to pushing exercise (i.e. pull down to a chest press), and 3) range of motion for arms from 0-70 degrees (i.e. row to shoulder press exercise). Minimum and maximum resistance values for the lower body ranged from 100 to 1,500 Newtons and for the upper body from 50 to 1,000 Newtons.

A user can perform resistive exercises from supine and prone positions on Earth. These exercises included the following: 1) bilateral chest press for strengthening the pectoralis major, anterior deltoids, and triceps; 2) bilateral row for strengthening the latissimus dorsi, rhomboids, and biceps; 3) bilateral shoulder press, supine or prone position for strengthening the deltoids and triceps; 4) bilateral latissimus pull-down, supine or prone position for strengthening the latissimus dorsi and biceps; 5) bilateral or unilateral leg press for strengthening the gluteals, quadriceps, hamstrings, calf muscles, and lower back postural muscles; and 6) bilateral or unilateral hip flexion. Many of the above exercises loaded spinal musculature in order to prevent spinal muscle and bone loss associated with long-term exposure to microgravity.

Equipment set-up

Surface electromyographic (EMG) signals (Therapeutics Unlimited, Iowa City, IA) were collected, amplified, and processed to produce root mean square values by a 8 channel EMG system (model 7400, Cadwell, Kennewick, WA). All data were collected and displayed on an eight channel strip chart recorder (Astro-Med, Inc., West Warwick, RI). At the same time, all data were acquired by an IBM Pentium-based computer with use of Windaq software (DATAQ Instruments, Akron OH) at a sampling rate of 100 Hz/channel. A goniometer (Penny & Giles, United Kingdom) was also employed to detect eccentric and concentric phases of the exercises. Saline-based Redux creme (Medical Products Group, Waltham, MA) was used to improve electrical contact between the EMG electrodes and skin. Surgical tape stabilized the electrodes to prevent sliding over the muscle and changing the specific position.

Surface EMG electrodes were placed bilaterally at six sites on the muscle belly over the erector spinae of the low back (L3 region), latissimus dorsi of the middle back (T10-12 region), and trapezius of the upper back (T2 region). The reference electrode was placed over the tibia. Skin resistance was reduced by cleaning with rubbing alcohol.

Protocol

Prior to the evaluation, nine volunteers were familiarized with the eight exercises. At this time, volunteers determined their one repetition maximum for each exercise on the Keiser, the standard exercise device, and hand free weights after warming up and stretching. The one repetition maximum is the greatest amount of resistance each subject was able to lift on one occasion. Seven days later, each subject performed all resistance exercises wearing the EMG electrodes and goniometer.

The exercises performed for the evaluation were as follows: anterior pull down, posterior pull down, shoulder press, and row. Exercises on the Keiser were compared to comparable exercises on the standard weight machine and hand-held weights with similar joint action. During the anterior pull down, shoulder press, and row exercises, the volunteer was in a supine position (lying face up) on the SX-1. The volunteer performed the Keiser SX-1 posterior pull down in a prone position (lying face down). The "standard" dumbbell shoulder press was performed in the standing position to simulate a shoulder press on the Keiser SX-1, which requires subjects to lie supine with the legs extended. For the Keiser shoulder press, not only was resistance placed on the upper body but also on the lower body. The objective of this method was to provide axial loading of the spinal column. The remaining exercises on the Keiser SX-1 did not include the legs. Furthermore, the exercises on the standard weight machine were performed seated.

So that all exercises were achievable by our sample of volunteers, subjects performed two sets of five repetitions at 70% of their one repetition maximum for the shoulder press exercise and at 80% of their one rep-maximum for the remaining exercises (Table 1). The order of the exercises was randomized for each volunteer. The rate of contraction was standardized by completion of each repetition within approximately 3 seconds (15 seconds per set). Subjects rested 2 to 3 minutes between sets. All exercises on all equipment were performed in one day to eliminate errors associated with multiple EMG electrode applications.

Table 1. Ranges of resistance used to compare the Keiser SX-1 and standard weight machine or dumbbell exercises. Values were determined by 70% of one repetition maximum for the shoulder press exercise and 80% of one repetition maximum for the remaining exercises. * Denotes dumbbell shoulder press exercise

	Keiser SX-1 (N)	Standard 1-g Exercise (N)
Pull-down Posterior	152 - 424	222 - 534
Pull-down Anterior	200 - 458	200 - 489
Row	224 - 576	222 - 445
Shoulder Press	126 - 350	58 - 146 *

Statistical analyses

For each muscle group during each type of exercise, differences in EMG activity between the exercise devices were assessed with paired t-tests. EMG data were normalized to represent percent of the maximum observed value for each muscle group. Data are presented as means ± standard error (SE) for all 9 subjects. Statistical significance was set at $p < 0.05$.

Results

With only two exceptions, peak EMG amplitudes were not significantly different between the Keiser and standard devices. Overall, the magnitudes tended to be higher with the Keiser SX-1. The exceptions are discussed later.

Pull-down posterior exercise

The Keiser SX-1 generated greater activity of the erector spinae during pull-down posterior exercise (p=0.0002) (Figure 2). The trapezius and latissimus dorsi were not significantly different in EMG activity comparing the Keiser and standard weight machine.

Pull-down anterior exercise

This exercise had no significant differences in peak EMG activity comparing the Keiser and the standard weight machine for the trapezius (p=0.16), latissimus dorsi (p=0.67), and erector spinae (p=0.13). The Keiser and the standard weight machine were not significantly different in EMG activity during the pull-down anterior exercise (Figure 3).

Row exercise

There were no significant differences for the row exercise (Figure 4) comparing the Keiser and the standard weight machine for peak EMG activity of the trapezius (p=0.38), erector spinae (p=0.65), and latissimus dorsi (p=0.52).

Shoulder press exercise

The dumbbell standing shoulder press exercise produced greater peak EMG values (79%) than the Keiser shoulder press exercise (57%; p=0.04) for the trapezius (Figure 5). The latissimus dorsi and erector spinae displayed no significant differences between the Keiser and hand-held weights .

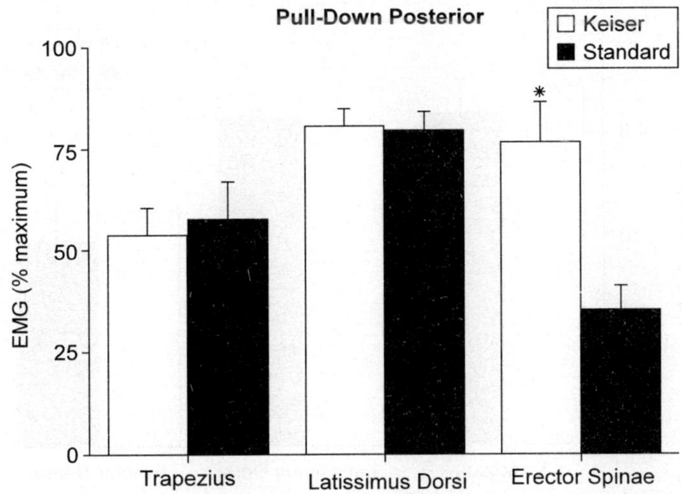

Fig. 2. Average EMG activity during the pull-down posterior exercise for three muscle groups expressed as a percentage of maximum EMG activity in all 9 subjects (mean ± SE). * Denotes significant difference between the Keiser and Standard weight machine.

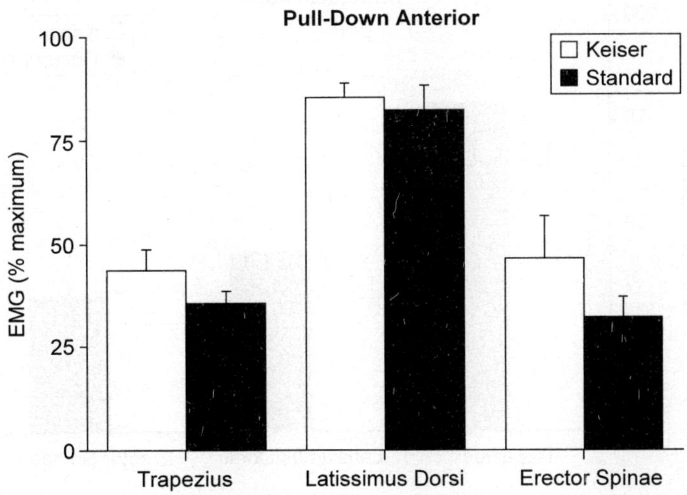

Fig. 3. Average EMG activity during the pull-down anterior exercise for three muscle groups expressed as a percentage of maximum EMG activity in all 9 subjects (mean ± SE). * Denotes significant difference between the Keiser and Standard weight machine.

Discussion

The Keiser SX-1 produces very similar levels of muscle activation compared to the "standard" weight devices when performing the anterior and posterior pull down, row, and shoulder press exercises. These exercises require multi-joint actions of the shoulder and elbow joints, involving the trapezius, latissimus dorsi, and erector spinae. The trapezius functions to elevate the scapula and clavicle, adduct, retract, depress, and upward rotate the scapula. The latissimus dorsi functions to adduct, extend, and

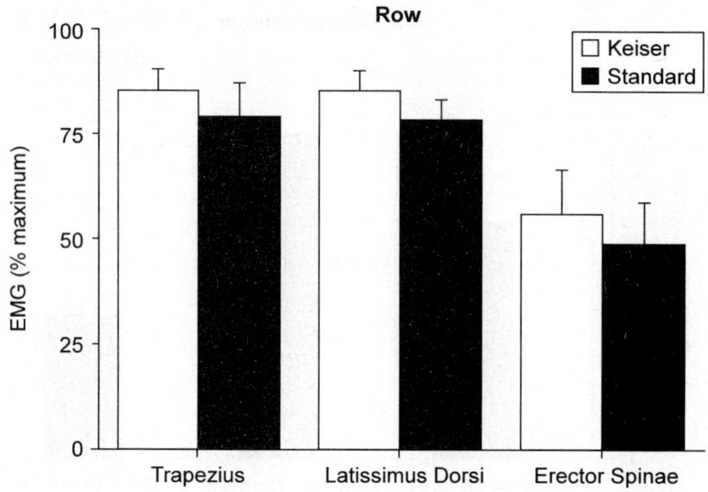

Fig. 4. Average EMG activity during the row exercise for three muscle groups expressed as a percentage of maximum EMG activity in all 9 subjects (mean ± SE). * Denotes significant difference between the Keiser and Standard weight machine.

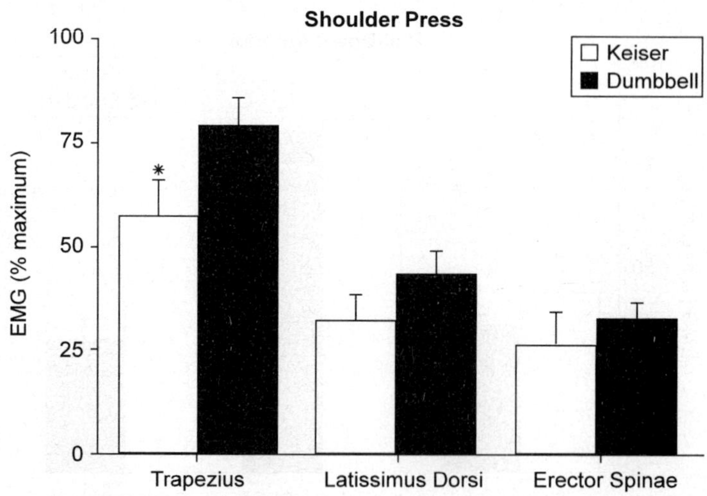

Fig. 5. Average EMG activity during the shoulder press exercise for three muscle groups expressed as a percentage of maximum EMG activity in all 9 subjects (mean ± SE). * Denotes significant difference between the Keiser and hand-held dumbbells.

hyperextend the humerus. The erector spinae functions to extend and stabilize the vertebral column (11). Because no specific back extensions were performed in this study, erector spinae EMG activity detected during the investigation is due primarily to spinal stabilization.

During the pull-down posterior exercise, the trapezius and latissimus dorsi show no significant differences between the Keiser and standard weight machine, but the erector spinae have greater EMG activity using the Keiser. This higher muscle activity is probably caused by the volunteers lifting their head and chest against the shoulder straps and the force of gravity while lying face down or prone, thus extending the spine during the concentric phase of the exercise. For the pull-down anterior exercise, both resistance devices, Keiser and standard weight machine, have similar EMG averages for all three back muscles. Joint action is equivalent in both devices giving comparable averages. The mean of EMG peak values of each volunteer performing the row exercise on the Keiser tends to be greater than that for the standard weight machine. However, there are no significant differences between the trapezius, latissimus dorsi, and erector spinae.

The Keiser SX-1 is compared to the dumbbells during the shoulder press exercise because this shoulder press exercise is similar in movement to the Keiser SX-1. The Keiser has equal resistive forces on the extended legs and upper body. Shoulder press or squat-type exercise is performed using the Keiser to provide high resistance axial loading of the spine, which may be effective for increasing bone mineral density of vertebral bodies (10). The only muscle group with a significant difference in EMG amplitude is the trapezius. The dumbbells produce greater EMG activation of the trapezius than the Keiser. Volunteers probably activated the trapezius more to control their joint action using dumbbells. Also, the majority of the back muscles assist to keep the torso upright during the lift. Using the Keiser, the volunteer lies supine on the bench and thus, the erector spinae are not required to stabilize the torso. Most subjects reported that the resistance used for the Keiser shoulder press felt easier than the dumbbell press. Therefore, an increase in resistance on the Keiser may have promoted greater activation.

Resistance training is probably required for astronauts exposed to long-term microgravity to reduce muscle and bone atrophy. However, exercise protocols and equipment for astronauts in space are unresolved (4,7), although recent calculations suggest that most exercise in space lacks sufficient loads to maintain preflight bone mass (12). To maintain muscle fiber mass and protein phenotype, resistance training is strongly recommended as an effective countermeasure (2). The loss of mass and strength in slow- and fast-twitch muscle fibers requires endurance and resistive exercises to sustain skeletal muscle during long space flights (5). Resistive exercise training stresses the musculoskeletal system and therefore, high impact eccentric exercise is recommended as a means of maintaining muscle and bone strength during space flight (3,6,8). Bone atrophy occurs at rates between 0.5 and 2.0% per month depending on gender and site (15). A mechanical factor that influences bone loss is the magnitude of the muscle force acting at the insertion site, particularly in the lower spine (15).

To improve muscle and bone strength, resistive exercises should stress the musculoskeletal system at very large levels of load. We found that the Keiser SX-1, a variable resistance device based on pneumatic compression and designed for microgravity, exhibits no differences in peak EMG activity compared to the 1-g "standard" devices. The standard devices maintain muscle strength by utilizing "weights" or "weight stacks" which are useless in a microgravity environment. The Keiser SX-1 utilizes compression pistons in order to adjust resistance levels. Exercises on the Keiser SX-1 provide high resistance and axial loading which may be important to strengthen paraspinal muscles and increase bone density. The Keiser SX-1 incorporates both concentric and eccentric contractions for all exercises in this study. Therefore, this device may be beneficial for maintaining muscle and bone strength during long-term space flight. Our study documents that the Keiser SX-1, a variable resistance device, provides high levels of spine and shoulder muscle activation and thus, may be an efficacious countermeasure device for long-duration space flight.

Acknowledgements

The authors thank the subjects for their participation. This research was supported by NASA Grant 199-80-02-05 and NAG 9-1425.

References

1. Artino, AR. Physiological evaluation of the Keiser SX-1 variable-resistance exercise machine. Colorado State University, Colorado: Thesis, 1996; 1-112.
2. Baldwin KM. Effect of spaceflight on the functional, biochemical, and metabolic properties of skeletal muscle. Med. Sci. Sports Exerc. 1996: 28:983-987.
3. Cavanagh PR, Davis BL, Miller TA. A biomechanical perspective on exercise countermeasures for long-term spaceflight. Aviat. Space Environ. Med. 1992; 63:482-5.
4. Convertino VA. Physiological adaptations to weightlessness: effects on exercise and work performance. Exer. Sport Sci. Rev. 1990; 18:119-66.
5. Convertino VA. Exercise as a countermeasure for physiological adaptation to prolonged spaceflight. Med. Sci. Sports Exerc. 1996; 28:999-1014.
6. Dudley GA, Tesch PA, Miller BJ, Buchanan P. Importance of eccentric actions in performance adaptations to resistance training. Aviat. Space Environ. Med. 1991; 62:543-50.
7. Greenleaf JE, Bulbulian R, Bernauer EM, Haskell WL, Moore T. Exercise training protocols for astronauts in microgravity. J. Appl. Physiol. 1989; 67: 2191-204.
8. Hargens AR, Parazynski S, Aratow M, Friden. Muscle changes with eccentric exercise: Implications on Earth and in Space. Adv. Myochem. 1989; 2:299-312.
9. Hargens AR, KJ Hutchinson, RE Ballard and G Murthy. "Intervertebral Disc: Loaded on Earth and Unloaded in Space." In: Connective Tissue Biology: Integration and Reductionism, edited by R Reed and K Rubin. London: Portland Press, Ltd, 1998, pp. 125-133.
10. McCarthy JP, Bamman MM, LeBlanc AD, Rowe R, Spector E, Fortney SM, Greenisen MC. Heavy resistance training increases vertebral bone mineral density and thigh muscle volume. Med. Sci. Sports Exerc. 1995; 27: S180; Abstract 1014.
11. Moore KL. Clinically Oriented Anatomy. Maryland: Williams & Wilkins, Chapt. 4,6, 1992; 3:353,530.
12. Morey-Holton ER, Whalen RT, Arnaud SB, Van der Meulen MC. The skeleton and its adaptation to gravity. In: Handbook of Physiology: Section 4, Environmental Physiology, edited by Fregly MJ and Blatteis CM. III: The gravitational envionment, volume1: Microgravity. New York: Oxford University Press, Chapt. 31, 1996; 691-719.
13. Styf JR, Ballard RE, Fechner K, Watenpaugh DE, Kahan NJ, Hargens AR. Height increase, neuromuscular function, and back pain during 6 degree head-down tilt with traction. Aviat Space Environ. Med. 1997; 68:24-9.
14. Schneider SM, Amonette WE, Blazine K, Bentley J, Lee SM, Loehr JA, Moore AD Jr, Rapley M, Mulder ER, Smith SM. Training with the International Space Station interim resistive exercise device. Med. Sci. Sports Exerc. 2003, 35:1935-1945.
15. Tipton CM, Hargens AR. Physiological adaptations and countermeasures associated with long-duration spaceflights. Med. Sci. Sports Exerc. 1996; 28:974-976.
16. Wing PC, Tsang IKY, Susak L, Gagnon R, Potts JE,. Back pain and spinal changes in microgravity. Orthop. Clin. North Am. 1991;22:255-62.

Adaptation Biology and Medicine (Volume 4: Current Concepts)
Editors: A. Hargens, N. Takeda and P.K. Singal

19. Induction of the Heat Shock Protein in Rat Lungs Following Intermittent Hypoxic Training

Kodo Okuyama[1], Jingtao Jiang[2]

[1]Clinical Research Laboratory of IHT
2-21-15 Shimouma Setagaya-ku Tokyo JAPAN

[2]Central Institute for Electron Microscopic Researches,
Nippon Medical School, Sendagi, Bunkyo-ku, Tokyo, Japan.

Abstract

In the previous study we showed, ultrastructurely IHT is characterized by hyperplasia of alveolar type = II cells, which may have enabled them to more rapidly repair damage resulting from hypoxia and may represent a key mechanism in the IHT.

In order to demonstrate the mechanism of intermittent hypoxic training (IHT)*, we studied the expression of HSP70 by immunohistochemistry using the Streptavidin Biotin Peroxidase Complex(SABC) Method on alveolar type I , type II epithelial cells, macrophages from rats with IHT. The expression of HSP70 in IHT in comparison with control was significantly increased on alveolar type I, type II epithelial cells, macrophages and was significantly correlated with the duration of IHT. This study demonstrates that expression of HSP70 may be a mechanism of adaptation of hypoxia by IHT.

Introduction

Intermittent hypoxic training (IHT), with repeated short-term inhalation of hypoxic mixtures, has been used to treat and prevent certain diseases and a very favorable effect for the exercise of athletes [1,2]. Investigations of IHT have showed that increased hypoxic ventilatory response (HVR)[3,4] is important physiological response. Recent studies have displayed that IHT inhibits the free radical production, which gives harmful effect to the cells and tissues, and raise the metabolic rate as a result of sympathetic nervous system activation[5,6]. Rats trained to intermittent normobaric hypoxia developed an increase of the glycogen contents in the heart and liver parenchymatous cells and offered as many beneficial effects in protecting against myocardial injuries [7,8]. Antioxidant enzymes and stress proteins may be part of the mechanisms contributing to the cardioprotection of the intermittent hypoxic adaptation[7].

Heat shock causes intracellular expression of a specific group of proteins called heat shock proteins (HSPs) that have broad cytoprotective properties[9,10]. The first demonstration of HSP- mediated cytoprotection involved the phenomenon of thermotolerance, whereby a brief heat shock conferred protection against subsequent exposure to otherwise lethal hyperthermia [11]. Subsequent studies demonstrated that induction of HSPs also protected cells and whole organs against nonthermal cytotoxic agents such as oxidants, nitric oxide, tumor necrosis factor-alpha, and endotoxin [12,14]. Previous studies also demonstrated that induction of HSPs protected against in vitro and in vivo models of acute lung injury and may have therapeutic value for attenuating acute lung injury. HSP 70 has been shown to be protective following ischemic injury. Similarly, a member of the small heat shock family, HSP27 has been shown to play a role in cellular repair and mechanisms of protection against cell stress. In this study, we are used monoclonal antibody to heat shock protein 70 to investigate whether IHT induces the expression of HSP70 in lungs.

Materials and Methods

1. Animals

A total of 18 male Wistar rats, aged 12 weeks were used: three animals for control and rest for the experimental groups. They were allowed free access to food and water during intermittent hypoxic training.

2. Intermittent hypoxic training

Hypoxia was induced by exposure to 10% oxygen with machine. The rats were sustained hypoxia for 15min one time a day for 3, 7 or 21 consecutive days, respectively. Control rats exposured to room air.

3. Light and electron microscopy

At 3D, 7D and 21 Days after intermittent hypoxic training (IHT), the animals were anesthetized with pentobarbital sodium (50mg/kg) and lungs were removed. For light microscopic examination, the tissues were fixed with 10% formalin in phosphate buffer solution, and embedded in paraffin.

Then paraffin sections of 2 mkm in thickness were prepared and stained with hematoxylin and eosin. For electron microscopic examination, rat lung specimens were cut into $2mm^3$ blocks, fixed 2.5% glutaraldehyde in 0.1M phosphate buffer and postfixed with 1% osmium tetroxide, dehydrated in a graded alcohol series and embedded in Epon 812. Semithin sections stained with toluidine blue were used for high light microscopy and selection of areas for thin sectioning. Thin sections were cut with 5000 Ultrotome, stained with uranyl acetate and lead citrate. The sections were examined under a JEM-1010 transmission electron microscope.

4. Immunohistochemistry

The Streptavidin Biotin Peroxidase Complex (SABC) Method was employed for immunohistochemistry for heat shock protein (HSF70). Briefly, deparaffinized sections were treated for 30 min with 0.3% H_2O_2 to block endogenous peroxidase and rinsed again 3-5 min in PBS. Sections were then incubated for 30 min with block nonspecific reactive sites by applying 1 : 20 normal goat serum and incubated with Monoclonal anti-HSP antibody (NOVO) diluted 1:40 in PBS for 60 min. After washing in PBS, they were incubated with goat anti-mouse immunoglobulins for 10 min and then incubated with a mixture of streptavidin and biotinylated horseradish peroxidase for 5 min. After washing in PBS, reacted with 0.05% 3 - 3' diaminobenzidine (DAB) containing 0.01 %H_2O_2.

Results

Light microscopic observations

The morphological observations in the control group were normal from 3 days to 21 days. After three days IHT, the remarkable interstitial edema, increased thickness of the alveolar septa, marked capillary dilatation, proliferation of interstitial cells, the collapse of alveoli and dilatation of the alveolar ducts were observed compared with controls (Fig. 1A). After 7 days IHT, those pathologic changes decreased than 3 days (Fig.1B). After 21 days of IHT, the nearly normal structure of lungs was observed (Fig.1C).

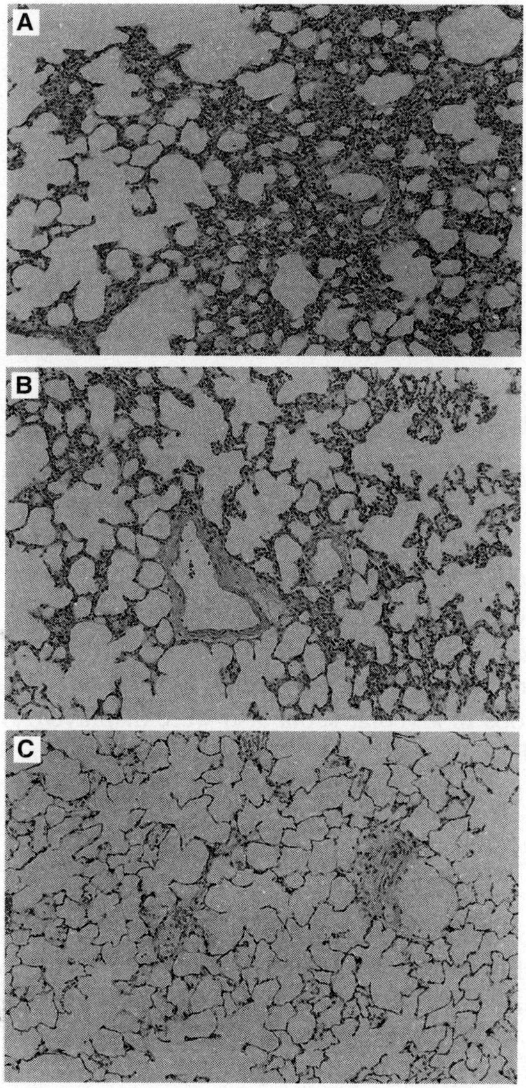

Fig. 1. Change of light microscope in IHT rat lungs. A: 3 days IHT. B:7days IHT. C: 21 days IHT.

Immunohistochemical observation

The heat shock protein 70 monoclonal antibody was used to stain the lung tissue from the control and IHT rats immunohistochemically. In control lungs, there are weak positive staining for HSP70 observed in the bronchial epithelial cells as well as in some alveolar type II epithelial cells.

After 3 days IHT, HSP70 was moderately expressed in alveolar type I ,type II epithelial cells, macrophages and bronchial epithelial cells. HSP70 expressed in cytoplasm and nuclei (Fig.2A). After 7 days IHT, expression of HSP70 was same as 3 days IHT (Fig.2B). After 21 days IHT, there was strong expression of HSP70 in alveolar type I, type II epithelial cells, macrophages and bronchial epithelial cells (Fig.2C).

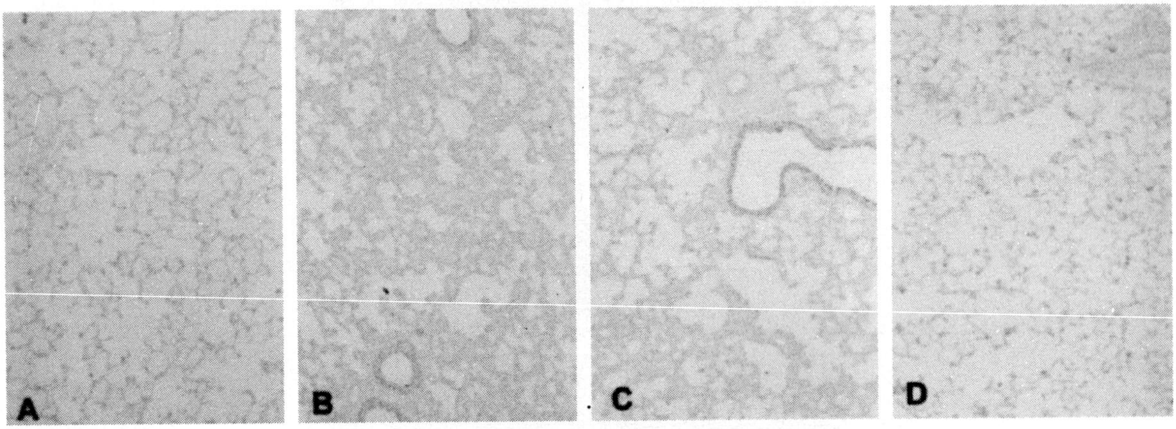

Fig. 2. Immunohistochemical staining of rat lung with anti-HSP70 after IHT. A: 3 days IHT. B: 7 days IHT. C: 21 days IHT.

Transmission electron microscopic observations

Electron microscopic observation revealed that lungs after 3 days IHT displayed marked capillary dilatation, widening of alveolar septa, interstitial cell proliferation, and type I cells hypertrophy (Fig.3A). Degenerated osmiophilic lamellar body, dense proteinous exudate and red cells were seen in the alveolar space. Lipid drops in alveolar septa also were displayed. By 7 days, the congestion of capillary, type II cell proliferation, and lipid drops in alveolar septa were observed. By 21 days, congestion of capillary, increased capillary endothelial volume, lipid drops in the alveolar septa and proliferation of alveolar type II cells were noted (Fig.3B).

Discussion

The principle of intermittent hypoxic training (IHT), with repeated short-term inhalation of hypoxic mixtures had been proposed by S. Strelkov and his associates in the early of 1980's based on their obstetrical practice. Intermittent hypoxic training (IHT) has showed promise for prevention and treatment of some diseases and efficiently produces great advancement in athletic training [1,2]. The mechanism of IHT remains unidentified. A number of mechanisms have been postulated including optimizing both hypothalamic-pituitary-adrenal axis functioning and free radical-mediated process

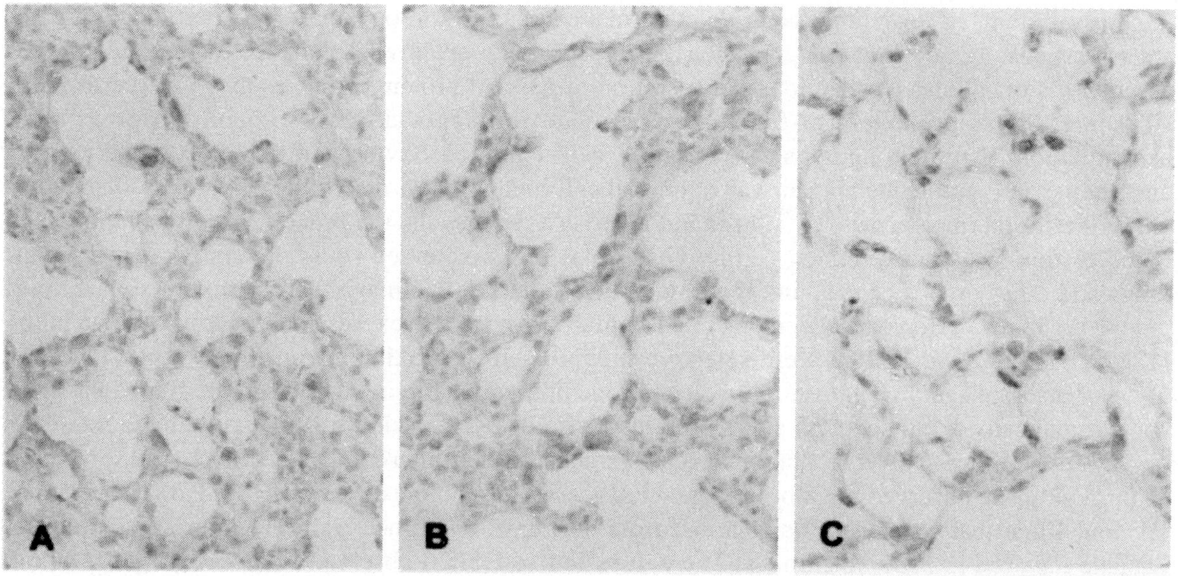

Fig. 3. Ultrastructural changes of lung in IHT: A: 3 days IHT. B: 21 days IHT

control [5], increase of the quantity and secretory activity of peptidergic neurons of the paraventricular hypothalamic nucleus (PHN) [16],enhancement of neurotransmission in the carotid body (CB) as well as in central structures through NADPH oxidase stimulation [17], increase in ventilatory response under repeating hypoxia, changes in suprapontine facilitation of respiratory activity and changes in monoamine metabolism or release [18], and raise the metabolic rate as a result of sympathetic nervous system activation [6].

In our clinical practice, we found that IHT could release the stress in some patients. In this study, we found that IHT induced the expression of HSP70. The response of cells or organisms to stress such as exposure to heat or chemicals is associated with the induction of heat shock proteins (HSPs). Heat shock proteins (HSPs) are an evolutionarily conserved group of proteins that are highly inducible by a wide variety of stressors. HSPs are grouped by molecular weight and amino acid sequence similarity into five main families: The high molecular weight 100-110kDa family; the 83-90kDa family; the 70kDa family ranging from 66 to 78kDa and containing the highly inducible HSP 70; the 60kDa family present in bacteria, mitochondria, and chloroplasts; and a diverse group of small HSPs ranging from 15 to 30kDa. Of great interest are observations demonstrating that once a heat shock response has been induced, the cells or organs can show remarkable resistance to subsequent metabolic stress. Heat shock protein 70 (HSP70) has been shown to have a protective role in ischemic disease, inflammation, infection and a potential role in antigen processing as well as a possible regulatory role in cytokine biosynthesis [13,14]. HSP70 exists in the cell in equilibrium between its free state, in the cytoplasm, and its bound state, protecting proteins in the nucleolus, perhaps either by helping refold some of the unfolded ribosomal proteins or by solubilising the denatured ribosomal proteins to facilitate their turnover. During release from heat shock and as the nucleoli begin to recover their normal activities, most of the HSP 70 returns to the cytoplasm.

Stress proteins have an important role in normal cellular physiology apart from participation in the stress response. Under normal conditions, stress proteins are involved in the successful folding, assembly, intracellular localization, and secretion of nascent protein chains as they emerge from the ribosome. Stress proteins also function to regulate the degradation of proteins to prevent the accumulation of protein aggregates within the cell. Cultured bovine and ovine pulmonary artery endothelial cells and guinea pig airway epithelial cells and alveolar macrophages expressed abundant HSP 70 after thermal stress [14,19,20]. In rabbit alveolar type II cells, the process of cell isolation itself induced stress protein expression [21]. In vivo thermal stress increased stress protein expression in the lungs and other organs of rats, and the time courses and relative magnitudes of expression differed among organs [22,23]. Bonay et al demonstrated limited stress protein expression in normal human lungs. HSP90, HSP 70 and HSP63 were selectively expressed in proximal bronchiolar epithelium and alveolar macrophage. In contrast, more distal bronchiolar epithelium, type I and type II alveolar cells, and stromal cells did not express stress proteins [24]. HSP 70 expression was substantially increased in airway epithelium and alveolar macrophages of patients with asthma compared with control subjects [25]. In this study, we observed the morphologic changes of lungs and expression of HSP70 after rat IHT. We found that that pulmonary damage occurred at 3 days IHT, one week IHT later, the pulmonary damage repaired in hypoxic animals. The expression of HSP70 observed in alveolar type I, type II epithelial cells, macrophages and bronchial epithelial cells after 3 days IHT, and continually expressed until 2l days IHT. Expression of HSP 70 in 21 days IHT was stronger than 3 days IHT. This revealed that IHT could induce HSP70 in alveolar type I, type II epithelial cells, macrophages and bronchial epithelial cells, and was significantly correlated with the duration of IHT.

The stress response is a highly conserved cellular defense mechanism defined by the rapid and specific expression of stress proteins. The stress proteins mediate cellular and tissue protection against diverse cytotoxic stimuli. Some studies confirmed that stress protein induction protected against nonthermal cytotoxic agents, such as tumor necrosis factor, inflammation, ultraviolet radiation and ischemia [26,27,28]. Villar et al demonstrated a cytoprotective effect of stress protein induction in a rat model of acute lung injury caused by intratracheal administration of phospholipase A1 and systemic administration of endotoxin [22,23].

This study is the first to demonstrate an expression of HSP 70 in alveolar type I, type II epithelial cells, macrophages and bronchial epithelial cells after IHT. HSP70 expressed after 3 days IHT, and continued to 21 days IHT. Although the exact significance of these data is still unresolved, it is proposed expression of HSP may be a mechanism of adaptation of hypoxia with IHT.

Reference

* Kodo Okuyama, Jingtao Jiang, Kaoru Aihara.

An Ultrastructural Observation of Lungs Treated by the Hypoxic Therapy: An Assessment of Its Therapeutic Efficacy as One of the Impulse Therapy. Adaptation Biology and Medicine (Vol.3). 328-336, 2002 Narosa Publishing House

1. Serebrovskaya T, Swanson R, Karaban IN, Serebrovskaya Z, Kolesnikova EE. Intermittent hypoxia alters hypoxic ventilatory responses. Fiziol Zh. 45(5): 9-18, l999
2. Serebrovskaya T, Swanson R, Mankovskaya I, Serebrovskaya Z, Moshchich V, and Oberenko 0. Training with Intermittent hypoxia influence free radical processes and glutathione antioxidant system enzymes in bronchial asthma patients. Allerg. Immunol. 27: 266, 1995

3. Howard LS, Robbins PA. Alterations in respiratory control during 8 h of isocapnic and poikilocapnic hypoxia in humans. J Appl Physiol. 78: 1098-107,1995
4. Schoene RB, Roach RC, Hackett PH, Sutton JR, Cymerman A, Houston CS, Operation Everest II: ventilatory adaptation during gradual decompression to extreme altitude. Med Sci Sports & Exercise. 22:804-10,1990
5. Adiiatulin AI, Piliavskaia AN, Takchuk EN, Guliaeva NV, [Various mechanisms of protective action of interval hypoxic training during preparation for abdominal delivery]. [Russian] Patol Fiziol Eksp Ter.(3):26-9, 1997
6. Cao KY, Zwillich CW, Berthon-Jones M, Sullivan CE. Increased normoxic ventilation induced by repetitive hypoxia inconscious dogs. J Appl Physiol. 73:2083.8, 1992
7. Zhuang J, Zhou Z. Protective effects of intermittent hypoxic adaptation on myocardium and its mechanisms. Biol Sinals Recept. 8:316-22,1999.Review.
8. Lebkova NP, Chizhov AI, Bobkov II. The adaptational intracellular mechanism regulating energy homeostasis during intermittent normobaric hypoxia. Ross Fiziol Zh lm I M Sechenova. 85:403-11, 1999
9. Minowada G, Welch WJ: Clinical implications of the stress response. J Clin. Invest. 95:3-12, 1995
10. Wang HR, Eispe JR: The stress response and the lung. Am J Physiol 273: L1-9, 1997
11. Gerner EW, Schneider MJ: Induced thermal resistance in Hela cells. Nature 256:500-2, 1975
12. Meerson FZ, Malyshev I Yu, Zamotrinsky AV. Differences in adaptive stabilization of structures in response to stress and hypoxia relate with the accumulation of hsp 70 isoforms. Mol Cell Biochem. 111:87-95, 1992
13. Koh Y, Lim CM, Kim MJ, Shin TS, Lee SD, Kim WS, Kim DS, Kim WD. Heat shock response decrease endotoxin-induced acute lung injury in rats. Respirology.4:325-30, 1999
14. Wong HR, R.J Mannix, J.M. Rusnak, A. Boota, H. Zar, S. C. Watkins, J.S. Lazo, B.R. Pitt. The heat shock response attenuates lipopolysaccharide-mediated apoptosis in cultured sheep pulmonary artery endothelial cells. Am. J. Respir. Cell Mol. Biol. 15:745-51, 1996
15. Wong HR, Ryan M, Menedez IY, Denenberg A and Wispe JR. Heat shock protein induction protects human respiratory epithelium against nitric oxide-mediated cytotoxicity. Shock 8: 213-18, 1997
16. Abramov AV. [Effect of the intermittent hypoxic training on the functioning of peptidergic neurons of the paraventrieular hypothalamic nucleus and brain stem neurons in rats]. [Russian] Ross Fiziol Zh lm I. M. Sechenova. 84(3): 173-81, 1998
17. 0lano M, Song D, Murphy S, Wilson DF, Pastuszko A. Relationships of dopamine, cortical oxygen pressure, and hydroxyl radicals in brain of newborn piglets during hypoxia and posthypoxic recovery. J Neurochem. 65(3):1205-12, 1995
18. Soto-Arape I, Burton MD, Kazemi H. Central amino acid neurotransmitters and the hypoxic ventilatory response. American J Respir Crit Care Med. 151(4):1113-20, 1995
19. Rinaldo J. E, M. Gorry R, Stricter H, Cowan R, Abdolrasulnia V. Shepard. Effect of endotoxin-induced cell injury on 70-kD heat shock proteins in bovine lung endothelial cells. Am. J. Respir. Cell Mol. Biol. 3:207-16, 1990
20. Cohen D.S, E. Palmer WJ, Welch, D. Sheppard. The response of guinea pig airway epithelial cells and alveolar macrophages to environmental stress. Am. J. Respir. Cell Mol. Biol. 5:133-43, 1991
21. Brandes M. E, J. N Finkelstein. Induction of the stress response by isolation of rabbit type II pneumocytes. Exp. Lung.Res. 15: 93-111, 1989.
22. Villar J, J. D. Edelson, M. Post, B. Mullen, A. S. Slutsky. Induction of heat Stress proteins is associated with decreased mortality in an animal model of acute lung injury. Am. Rev. Respir. Dis. 147:177-81, 1993.
23. Villar J., S. P. Ribeiro, J. B. M. Mullen, M. Kuliszewski, M. Post, A. S. Slutsky. Induction of the heat shock response reduces mortality rate and organ damage in a sepsis-induced acute lung injury model. Crit. Care Med. 22:914-22, 1994.

24. Bonay M, P. Soler M. Riquet, J. P. Battesti A. J. Hance, A. Tazi. Expression of heat shock proteins in human lung and lung cancers. Am. J. Respir. Cell Mol. Biol. 10:453-61, 1994
25. Vignola A. M, P. Chanez B. S. Polla, P. Vie, P. Godard, J. Bousquet. Increased expression of heat shock protein 70 on airway cells in asthma and chronic bronchitis. Am. J. Respir. Cell'Mol. Biol. 13:683-91, 1995.
26. Jaatela M, D. Wissing, P. A. Bauer, G. C. Li. Major heat shock protein hsp70 protects tumor cells from tumor necrosis factor cytotoxicity. EMBO J. 11:3507-12, 1992
27. Yoo, C.G., Lee S., Lee C. T., Rim Y. W., Ham S. K., and Shin Y. S. Anti-inflammatory effect of heat shock protein induction is related to stabilization of I-kappa B-alpha through preventing I-kappa B kinase activation in respiratory epithelial cells. J. Immunol 164:5416-23, 2000
28. Simon M. M, A. Reikerstolfer, A. Schwarz, C. Kronis, T. G. Lunger, M. Jaatela, T. Schwarz. Heat shock protein 70 overexpression affects the response to ultraviolet light in murine fibroblast. J. Clin. Invest. 95:926-933,1995.

Adaptation Biology and Medicine (Volume 4: Current Concepts)
Editors: A. Hargens, N. Takeda and P.K. Singal

20. Role of Oxidative Stress in Enhanced Expression of Giα Proteins and Adenylyl Cyclase Signalling in Hypertension*

Georgios Lappas[#] and Madhu B. Anand-Srivastava[**]

Department of Physiology and Groupe de recherche sur le système nerveux autonome, Faculty of Medicine University of Montreal, Montreal, Québec, Canada

Abstract

We have previously shown an enhanced expression of Giα proteins and their mRNA from hearts and aorta from spontaneously hypertensive rats (SHR). This enhanced expression of Gia proteins precedes the development of hypertension. Since oxidative stress has been shown to be increased in SHR, the present studies were undertaken to examine the role of oxidative stress in enhanced expression of Gia proteins in SHR. Vascular smooth muscle cells (VSMC) from 12 week-old SHR and their age-matched Wistar-Kyoto rats (WKY) were used for the present studies. VSMC from SHR exhibited enhanced expression of $G_{i\alpha}$-2 and $G_{i\alpha}$-3 proteins as compared to age-matched WKY, however the levels of Gs_a were not different between the two groups. Treatment of VSMC with N-acetylcysteine (NAC) or diphenyleneiodonium (DPI) for 24 hours decreased the enhanced expression of $G_{i\alpha}$-2 and $G_{i\alpha}$-3 proteins by 45% and 55% respectively in VSMC from SHR treated with NAC and by 50% and 60% respectively in VSMC from SHR treated with DPI as determined by immunoblotting. In addition, VSMC from SHR showed an enhanced inhibition of forskolin (FSK)-stimulated adenylyl cyclase activity by GTPγS as compared to VSMC from WKY which was restored to WKY levels by NAC or DPI. Furthermore, angiotensin-II (AngII) and C-ANP$_{4-23}$ (a ring deleted analog of atrial natriuretic peptide) inhibited adenylyl cyclase activity to a greater extent in VSMC from SHR as compared to WKY and NAC or DPI were able to restore the enhanced inhibition of adenylyl cyclase to WKY levels. These results suggest that enhanced Gi and associated functions in SHR may be attributed to the enhanced oxidative stress present in hypertension.

Introduction

Guanine nucleotide regulatory proteins (G proteins) are a family of GTP-binding proteins that play an important role in the regulation of a variety of signal transduction systems, including the adenylyl cyclase/cAMP system. This system is composed of three components: receptor, catalytic subunit, stimulatory (G_s) and inhibitory (G_i) guanine nucleotide regulatory proteins (1,2). The stimulation and inhibition of adenylyl cyclase by hormones are mediated by these two distinct G proteins (G_s and G_i),

*This study was supported by a grant from the Canadian Institutes of Health Research (MOP 53074)
**To whom correspondence should be addressed.
#GL is a recipient of the GRSNA masters scholarship award.

which couple the receptor to the catalytic subunit. G proteins are heterotrimeric and are composed of α, β and γ subunits. The α subunit is responsible for binding and hydrolyzing GTP and confers specificity in receptor and effector interaction. Molecular cloning has revealed four different forms of $G_{s\alpha}$ resulting from the differential splicing of a single gene (3,4) and three distinct forms of $G_{i\alpha}$ ($G_{i\alpha}$-1, $G_{i\alpha}$-2, $G_{i\alpha}$-3) encoded by three distinct genes (5). All three forms of $G_{i\alpha}$ are implicated in adenylyl cyclase inhibition (5) and in activation of atrial K^+ channels (6).

G_i protein and associated adenylyl cyclase signalling has been shown to be implicated in a variety of cellular functions such as vascular permeability (7), salt and water transport (8) and cathecholamine release (9), all of which play an important role in the regulation of blood pressure. Alterations of the levels of G_i proteins that result in the impaired cellular functions lead to various pathological states such as hypertension. These abnormalities have been reported in cardiovascular tissues from genetic models (spontaneously hypertensive rats) and different models of experimentally induced hypertensive rats (10-12). An increased expression of G_i proteins and G_i protein mRNA in hearts and aortas from SHR and in hearts from deoxycorticosterone acetate (DOCA)-salt hypertensive rats with established hypertension has been reported (10-12). On the other hand, the levels of $G_{s\alpha}$ were shown to be unaltered in SHR (10,12). The increased expression of $G_{i\alpha}$ proteins precedes the development of hypertension in SHR (13). It has also been reported that pertussis toxin attenuates the development of high blood pressure in SHR by inactivating G_i proteins (14), suggesting that the enhanced levels of G_i proteins that result in the decreased levels of cAMP and associated cellular functions may be the contributing factors in the pathogenesis of hypertension.

The levels of various vasoactive peptides including angiotensin II (AngII) that have been shown to be enhanced in hypertension may be responsible for the enhanced expression of $G_{i\alpha}$ proteins. This was supported by studies showing that treatment of SHR with captopril, an antihypertensive drug that acts by blocking the angiotensin I converting enzyme decreased blood pressure and enhanced G_i protein levels (15). Furthermore, AngII has been shown to increase the levels of Gi proteins in A10 smooth muscle cells (16) which was attenuated by losartan treatment (17). Ang II also increases oxidative stress by activating NADPH oxidase (18). An increased oxidative stress has also been reported in SHR (19) and other diseases such as diabetes and atherosclerosis (20, 21).

Taken together, it may be possible that increased oxidative stress in SHR may be a contributing factor in enhanced expression of G_i proteins and thereby hypertension. To examine this possibility, the present studies were undertaken to determine the effect of antioxidant treatment on the expression of G_i proteins and adenylyl cyclase activity in vascular smooth muscle cells from SHR and their age-matched control Wistar-Kyoto (WKY) rats.

Materials and Methods

Materials

3-Isobutyl-1-methylxanthine (IBMX) was purchased from Aldrich Chemical Corporation (Milwaukee, WI). N-acetyl-L-cysteine (NAC) was purchased from BDH inc. (Toronto, Ontario, Canada). [α-^{32}P]ATP was from Amersham Corp. (Oakville, Ontario, Canada) and antibodies AS/7 and EC/2 and RM/1 were from Santa Cruz Biotechnology (Santa Cruz, CA). Myokinase (EC 2.7.4.3) and all other chemicals used in these experiments were purchased from Sigma Chemical Co. (St-Louis, MO).

Methods

Cell culture and incubation

Vascular smooth muscle cells from 12-weeks old SHR and their age-matched WKY were cultured from aortas as described previously (22) and were plated in 75 cm^2 flasks and incubated at 37 °C in 95% air and 5% CO_2 humidified atmosphere in Dulbecco's modified Eagle's medium (DMEM) (with glucose, L-glutamine, pyridoxine hydrochloride and 110 mg/L sodium pyruvate) containing antibiotics and 10% heat-inactivated bovine serum (FBS). The cells were passaged upon reaching confluence with 0.5% trypsin containing 0.2% EDTA and utilized between passages 4 and 12. Confluent cell cultures were starved by incubation for 3 hours in DMEM without FBS at 37°C. These cells were then incubated with either NAC (20 mM) or diphenyleneiodonium chloride (DPI) (10 μM) for 24 hours. After incubation, cells were washed with ice-cold homogenizing buffer (TE buffer (10 mM Tris-HCl, 1 mM EDTA, pH 7.5)). The vascular smooth muscle cells were scraped in ice-cold homogenizing buffer with a rubber policeman and collected in a homogenizing tube. Cells were homogenized with a potter (10 strokes) and membranes were collected by centrifugation at 4°C for 10 minutes at 2800 RPM and resuspended in TE buffer. Homogenates were used for immunoblotting and adenylyl cyclase assay.

Adenylyl cyclase activity determination

Adenylyl cyclase activity was determined by measuring [^{32}P]cAMP formation from [α-^{32}P]ATP, as described previously (10,11). Briefly, the assay medium contained 50 mM glycylglycine, pH 7.5, 0.5 mM MgATP, [α-^{32}P]ATP (1.5 × 10^6 cpm), 5 mM $MgCl_2$ (in excess of ATP concentration), 100 mM NaCl, 0.5 mM cAMP, 1mM IBMX, 2 mM phosphocreatine (CRP), 0.1 mM EGTA, 10 μM guanosine 5'-O-(3-thiotriphosphate) (GTPγS) and an adenosine triphosphate (ATP)-regenerating system consisting of 0.1 mg creatine phosphokinase/ml and 0.1 mg of myokinase/ml in a final volume of 200 μL. Incubations were initiated by the addition of the membrane preparations (20-30 μg) to the reaction mixture, which had been thermally equilibrated for 2 minutes at 37°C. The reactions conducted in triplicate for 10 minutes at 37°C were terminated by the addition of 0.6 ml of 120 mM zinc acetate. cAMP was purified by coprecipitation of other nucleotides with $ZnCO_3$ by addition of 0.5 ml of 144 mM Na_2CO_3 and subsequent chromatography by the double column system as previously described (23). Under the assay conditions used, adenylyl cyclase activity was linear with respect to protein concentrations and time of incubation. Protein concentration was determined using the Lowry method (24) with bovine serum albumin as standard.

Immunoblotting

Immunoblotting of G proteins was performed as described previously (11). After SDS-PAGE, the separated proteins were electrophoretically transferred to nitrocellulose paper (Sigma) with a semidry transblot apparatus (Bio-Rad) at 15 V for 45 minutes. After transfer, the membranes were washed with phosphate-buffered saline (PBS) and were incubated in PBS containing 2% bovine serum albumin overnight. The following day, the blots were washed in PBS containing 0.2% Tween 20 for 10 minutes and were incubated after with antisera (Santa Cruz) against $G_{i\alpha}$-2 and $G_{i\alpha}$-3 proteins in PBS containing 0.2% Tween 20 at room temperature for 90 minutes. The blots were washed three times with PBS containing 0.2% Tween 20. After, the antibody-antigen complexes were detected by incubating the blots with goat anti-rabbit IgG (Bio-Rad) conjugated with horseradish peroxidase for 90 minutes at room temperature. The blots were washed three times with PBS containing 0.2% Tween 20 before reaction with enhanced chemiluminescence (ECL) Western blotting detection reagents from Santa Cruz. Quantitative analysis of the Gi proteins was performed by densitometric scanning of the autoradiographs employing the enhanced laser densitometer (LKB Ultroscan XL) and quantified using the gel scan evaluation software (version 2.1) form Pharmacia (Quebec, Canada).

Statistical analysis

Results are expressed as mean ± S.E.M. Comparisons between groups were made with ANOVA in conjunction with the Newman-Keuls test. Results were considered significant at a value of $P < 0.05$.

Results

We have previously shown an increased expression of $G_{i\alpha}$-2 and $G_{i\alpha}$-3 proteins in hearts and aortas of SHR compared to WKY while the levels of Gs_{α} were unchanged (10,12). In order to investigate if VSMC from aorta from SHR also exhibited enhanced expression of $G_{i\alpha}$ proteins as compared to WKY rats, the levels of $G_{i\alpha}$ proteins were determined by immunoblotting techniques using specific antibodies against $G_{i\alpha}$ proteins. As shown in figure 1, antibody AS/7 detected a single protein of 40 kDa corresponding to $G_{i\alpha}$-2 and antibody EC/2 detected a single protein of 41 kDa corresponding to $G_{i\alpha}$-3 in VSMC from both SHR and WKY rats, however, the levels of immunodetectable $G_{i\alpha}$-2 and $G_{i\alpha}$-3 in VSMC from SHR were significantly enhanced by about 30% as compared to VSMC from WKY as determined by densitometric scanning. On the other hand, antibody RM/1 against Gs_{α} recognized three protein bands at 45, 47 and 52 kDa corresponding to three different isoforms of α subunits of Gs in both VSCM from SHR and WKY rats, however, no significant difference in the levels of Gs_{α} were observed between the two groups.

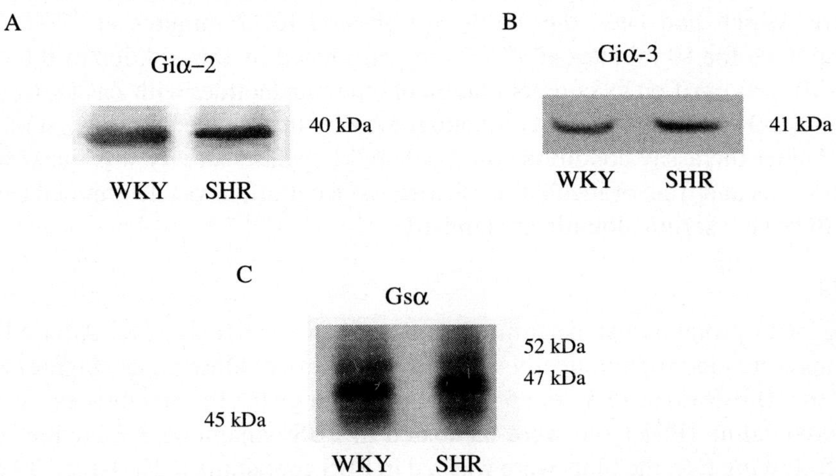

Fig. 1. Representative autoradiogram of $G_{i\alpha}$-2 (A), $G_{i\alpha}$-3 (B) and (C) $G_{s\alpha}$ protein expression in VSMC from 12 weeks-old WKY and SHR. Membrane proteins (30 µg) from SHR and WKY were separated and transferred to nitrocellulose, which was immunoblotted with specific antibodies against $G_{i\alpha}$-2 , $G_{i\alpha}$-3 and $G_{s\alpha}$ as described in 'Methods'. The autoradiogram is representative of three separate experiments. Detection of a-subunits was performed with chemiluminescence Western blotting detection reagents.

Effect of antioxidants on $G_{i\alpha}$ Protein Expression

In order to investigate if the enhanced expression of G_{ia} proteins in VSMC from SHR is attributed to increased oxidative stress, the effect of antioxidant treatment on $G_{i\alpha}$ protein expression was examined. VSMC from SHR exhibited enhanced expression of $G_{i\alpha}$-2 and $G_{i\alpha}$-3 proteins as compared to VSMC from WKY by about 30% as shown in figure 2. NAC, at 20 mM, restored the enhanced expression of $G_{i\alpha}$-2 and $G_{i\alpha}$-3 proteins to control levels. In addition, DPI at 10 μM was also able to restore the enhanced expression of $G_{i\alpha}$-2 and $G_{i\alpha}$-3 towards control levels (fig 3). However NAC and DPI did not have any effect on the $G_{i\alpha}$ levels in VSMC from WKY rats (data not shown).

Effect of antioxidants on Gi functions

We have previously shown that enhanced expression of $G_{i\alpha}$-2 and $G_{i\alpha}$-3 proteins in hearts and aortas of SHR compared to WKY is responsible for enhanced Gi functions (10). In order to examine if the enhanced levels of $G_{i\alpha}$-2 and $G_{i\alpha}$-3 proteins observed in VSCM from SHR is also reflected in enhanced Gi functions, receptor-independent and-dependant functions of $G_{i\alpha}$ proteins were investigated. The receptor-independent functions of Gi were investigated by studying the effect of GTPγS on forskolin (FSK)-stimulated adenylyl cyclase activity, whereas, receptor-dependant functions were studied by examining the hormonal inhibitions of adenylyl cyclase activity.

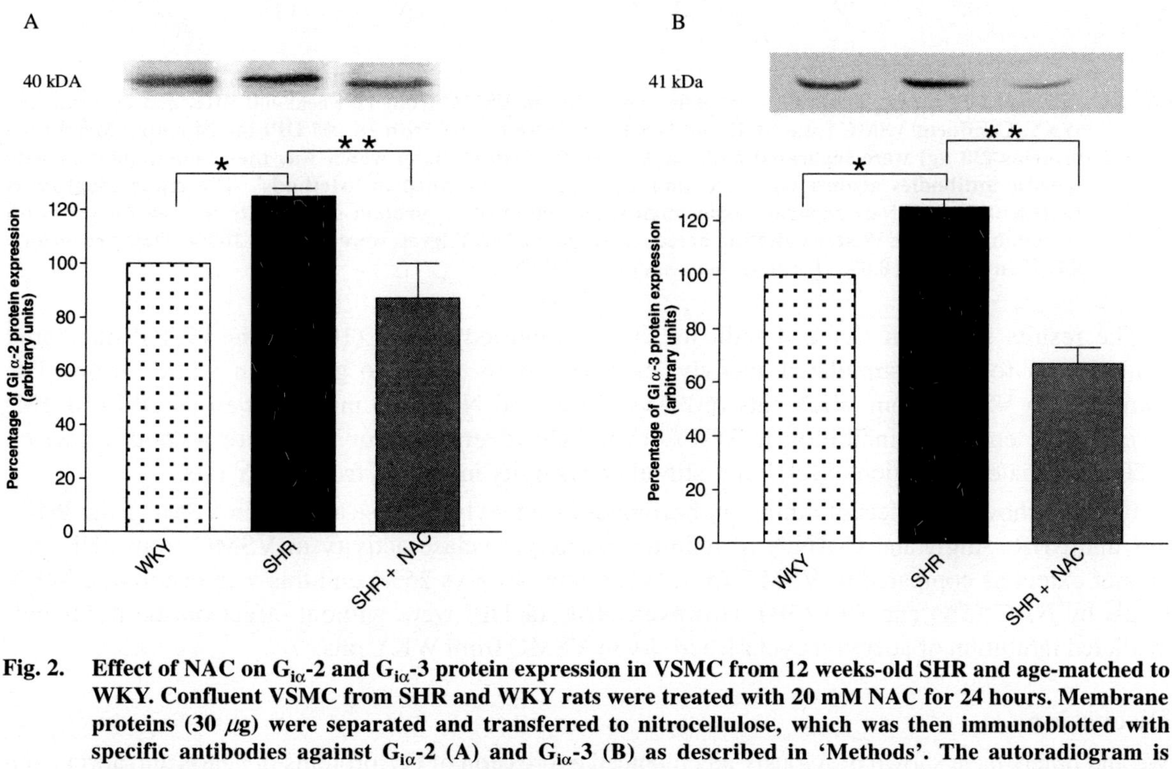

Fig. 2. Effect of NAC on $G_{i\alpha}$-2 and $G_{i\alpha}$-3 protein expression in VSMC from 12 weeks-old SHR and age-matched to WKY. Confluent VSMC from SHR and WKY rats were treated with 20 mM NAC for 24 hours. Membrane proteins (30 μg) were separated and transferred to nitrocellulose, which was then immunoblotted with specific antibodies against $G_{i\alpha}$-2 (A) and $G_{i\alpha}$-3 (B) as described in 'Methods'. The autoradiogram is representative of five separate experiments. Detection of G_i protein α-subunits was performed with chemiluminescence Western blotting detection reagents. WKY levels were taken as 100%. Data are mean ± S.E.M (n = 5). $^*P < 0.05$, $^{**}P < 0.01$ between indicated bars.

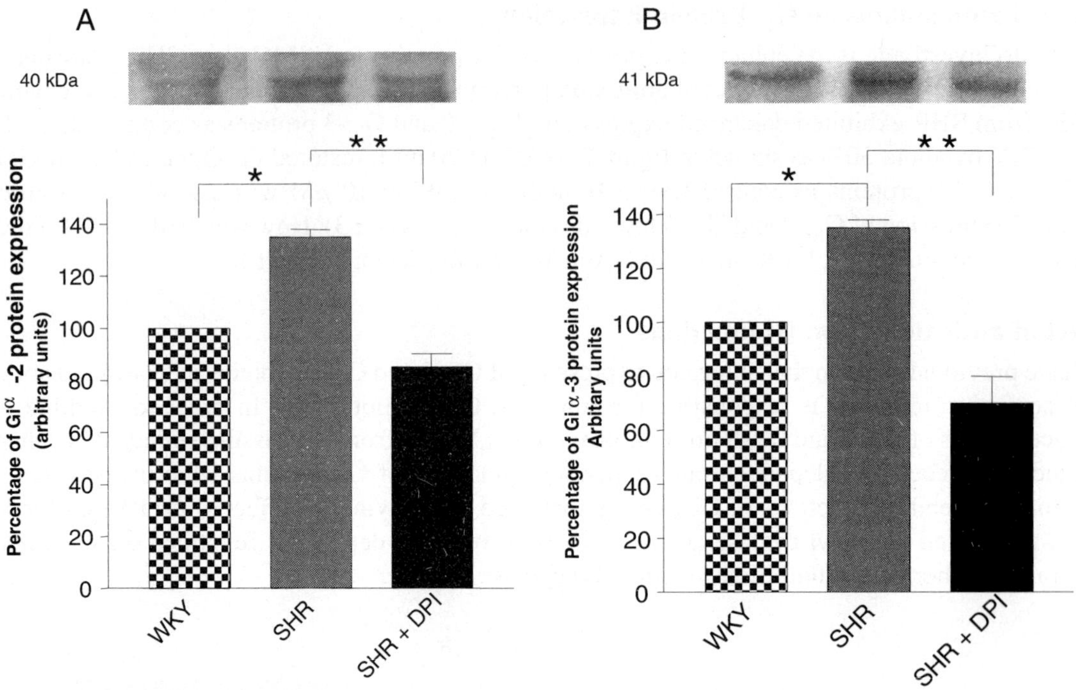

Fig. 3. Effect of DPI on $G_{i\alpha}$-2 and $G_{i\alpha}$-3 protein expression in VSMC from 12 weeks-old SHR and age-matched WKY. Confluent VSMC from SHR and WKY rats were treated with 10 μM DPI for 24 hours. Membrane proteins (30 μg) were separated and transferred to nitrocellulose, which was then immunoblotted with specific antibodies against $G_{i\alpha}$-2 (A) and $G_{i\alpha}$-3 (B) as described in 'Methods'. The autoradiogram is representative of four separate experiments. Detection of G_i protein α-subunits was performed with chemiluminescence Western blotting detection reagents. WKY levels were taken as 100%. Data are mean ± S.E.M (n = 5). $^*P < 0.05$, $^{**}P < 0.01$, between indicated bars.

The results shown in figure 4 indicate that as reported earlier (10,14), the GTPγS-mediated inhibition of forskolin-stimulated adenylyl cyclase activity was also greater in VSMC from SHR compared to VSMC from WKY rats (60% vs. 25%) and NAC (20 mM) as well as DPI (10 μM) reversed the enhanced inhibition to WKY levels. However, NAC or DPI were without effect on GTP*g*S-mediated inhibition of forskolin-stimulated activity in VSMC from WKY rats.

Figure 5 shows the effect of inhibitory hormones on adenylyl cyclase activity in VSMC from WKY rats and SHR. AngII and C-ANP_{4-23} inhibited adenylyl cyclase activity in VSMC from SHR to a greater extent as compared to VSMC from WKY rats (40% vs 25%) and this was restored to WKY levels by NAC (5A) and DPI (5B). However, NAC or DPI were without effect on the hormonal-mediated inhibition of adenylyl cyclase activity in VSMC from WKY rats.

Discussion

We and others have shown previously an enhanced expression of $G_{i\alpha}$ proteins in hearts and aorta from SHR (10, 12) and experimentally induced hypertensive rat (HR) models, including DOCA-salt and 1K1C HR (11, 25). The enhanced expression of $G_{i\alpha}$ proteins occurs before the onset of hypertension

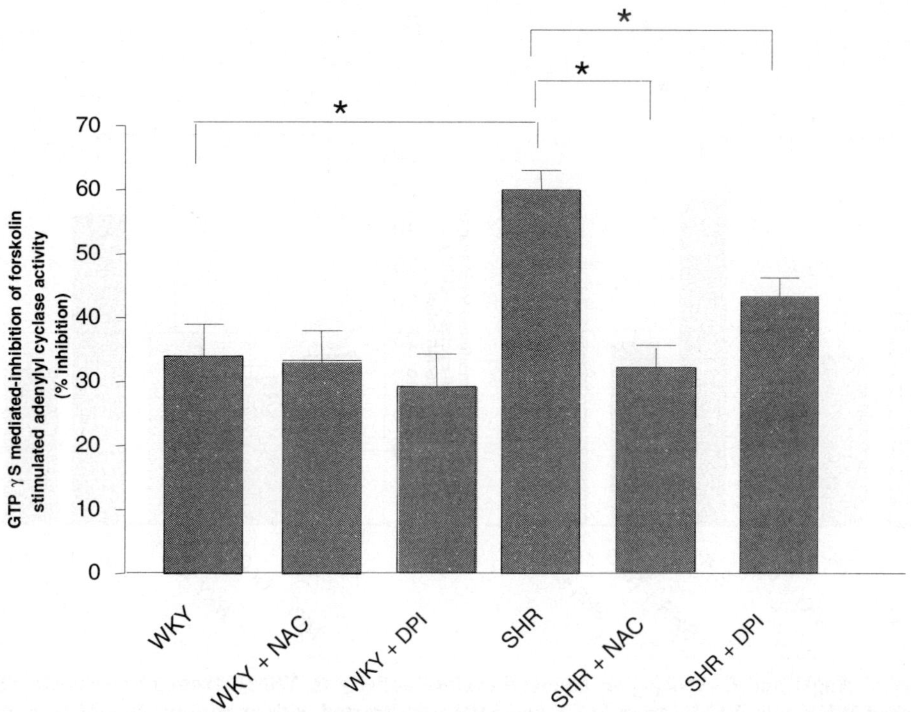

Fig. 4. Effect of GTPγS on forskolin-stimulated adenylyl cyclase activity in VSMC from 12 weeks-old WKY and SHR. VSMC from SHR and WKY were treated with or without 20 mM NAC or 10 μM DPI for 24 hours. Adenylyl cyclase activity in the membranes prepared from these cells was determined as described in 'Methods' in the presence of 100 μM forskolin alone, taken as 100% and in the presence of 10 μmol/L GTPgS. Adenylyl cyclase activities in the absence of presence of 100 *m*M forskolin in WKY were 177.28 ± 12.34 and 14 212.18 ± 1202.63 and in SHR were 154.67 ± 9.67 and 26 534 ± 2343.76 (pmol cAMP/mg protein per 10 minutes). Values are mean ± S.E.M of four separate experiments. *P < 0.05 between indicated bars.

(13, 26) and suggests that the enhanced expression of $G_{i\alpha}$ proteins may be one of the contributing factors in the pathogenesis of hypertension. This was further confirmed by our recent studies showing that inactivation of enhanced expression of $G_{i\alpha}$ proteins, by intraperitoneal injection of pertussis toxin into 2-week-old prehypertensive SHR, attenuated the development of high blood pressure in SHR (14), and suggesting that the enhanced levels of G_i proteins that result in the decreased levels of cAMP and impaired cellular functions may be the contributing factor in the pathogenesis of hypertension (14).

In the present studies, we report that VSMC from SHR also exhibited enhanced expression of $G_{i\alpha}$-2 and $G_{i\alpha}$-3 proteins as compared to control WKY rats, and the fact that antioxidant treatment restored the enhanced levels of $G_{i\alpha}$ proteins to control WKY levels suggests the implication of oxidative stress in enhanced expression of $G_{i\alpha}$ proteins in SHR. We have previously shown that captopril treatment of SHR as well as of one kidney-one clip (1K1C) hypertensive rats that also exhibited enhanced levels of $G_{i\alpha}$ proteins attenuated the blood pressure and enhanced levels of $G_{i\alpha}$ proteins toward control levels (15, 25), suggesting the implication of AngII in augmented levels of $G_{i\alpha}$ proteins, which have been shown to be responsible for the pathogenesis of hypertension (15, 25). Furthermore, AngII has been shown to increase the levels of $G_{i\alpha}$ proteins in A10 VSMC which was restored to control levels by

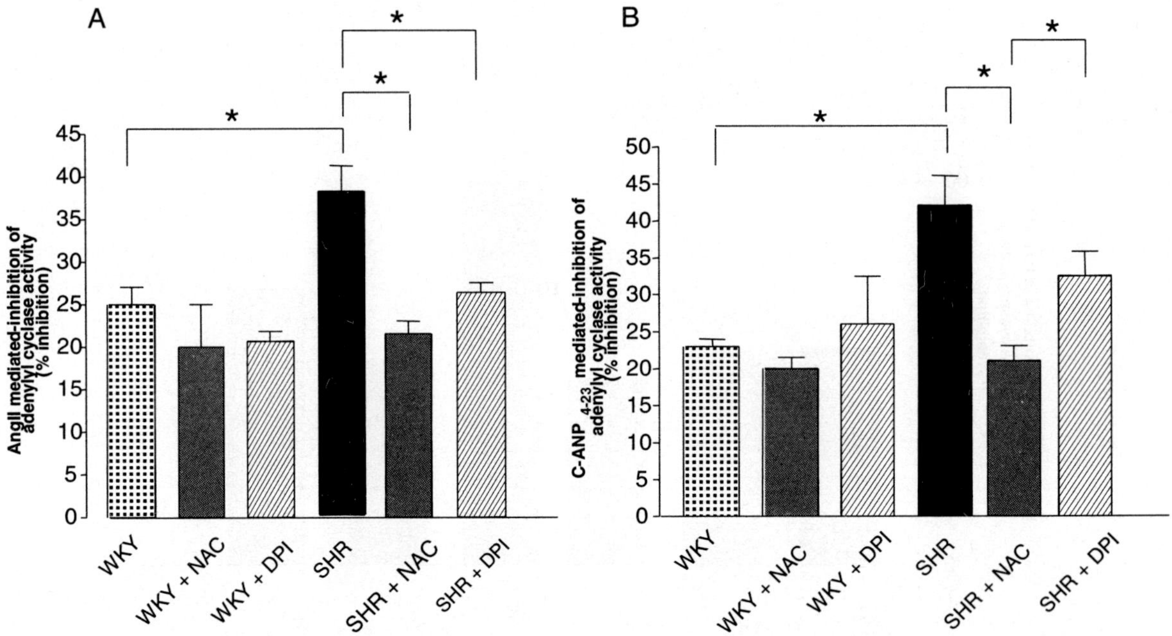

Fig. 5. Effect of AngII and C-ANP$_{4\text{-}23}$ on adenylyl cyclase activity in VSMC from 12 weeks-old SHR and age-matched WKY rats. VSMC from WKY and SHR were treated with or without 20 mM NAC or 10 μM DPI for 24 hours. Adenylyl cyclase activity in the membranes prepared from these cells was determined as described in 'Methods' in the presence of 10 *m*mol/L GTPγS alone (basal), taken as 100% and in the presence of 10^{-5} M AngII (A) or 10^{-6} M C-ANP$_{4\text{-}23}$ (B). Basal activities in the presence of 10 μmol/L GTPγS alone in WKY and SHR were 3722.65 ± 183.45 and 6319.85 ± 565.98 respectively (pmol cAMP/mg protein per 10 minutes). Values are mean ± S.E.M of six separate experiments. $^{*}P < 0.05$ between indicated bars.

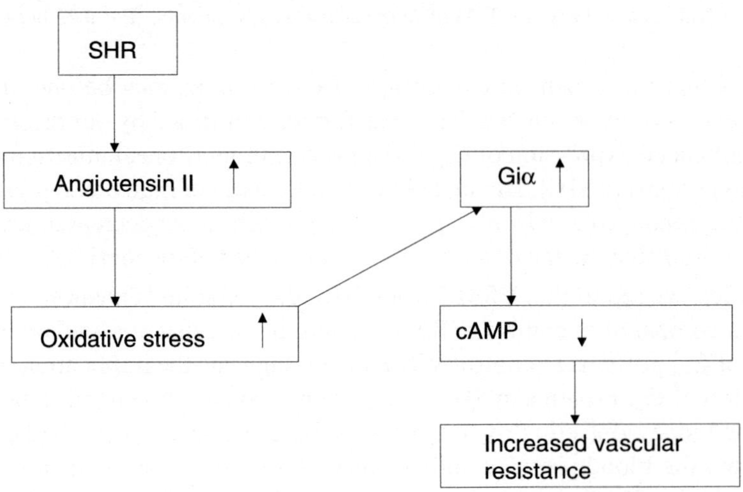

Fig. 6. Possible mechanism involving Angiotensin II and oxidative stress on enhanced expression of G_i protein expression in hypertension.

losartan treatment (16, 17). In addition, we have also shown that AngII-induced increased expression of G_{ia} proteins in VSMC was attenuated by antioxidant treatment (unpublished data) which suggest the implication of oxidative stress in AngII-induced enhanced levels of $G_{i\alpha}$ proteins. Taken together, it may be possible that the enhanced oxidative stress observed in VSMC from SHR may be attributed to the enhanced levels of AngII. In this regard, AngII has been shown to increase oxidative stress (27). We have also shown an enhanced production of superoxide anion in VSMC from SHR as compared to age-matched WKY rats (unpublished observation), however, the role of AngII in enhanced oxidative stress in VSMC from SHR needs to be investigated.

The enhanced levels of $G_{i\alpha}$ proteins in VSMC from SHR as compared to WKY rats was also reflected in enhanced Gi functions, as demonstrated by increased inhibition of FSK-stimulated adenylyl cyclase activity by a low concentration of GTPγS and enhanced inhibition by AngII and C-ANP$_{4\text{-}23}$. Antioxidants NAC or DPI that result in the restoration of enhanced levels $G_{i\alpha}$ proteins to control levels also restored the C-ANP$_{4\text{-}23}$ and AngII-mediated enhanced inhibition of adenylyl cyclase activity and enhanced inhibition of FSK-stimulated adenylyl cyclase activity by GTPγS. Our results are in agreement with the previous studies showing that captopril or losartan treatment of 1K1C or L-NAME hypertensive rats that restored the enhanced levels of $G_{i\alpha}$ proteins also restored the enhanced Gi functions to control levels (25, 28). Furthermore, pertussis toxin treatment of SHR, which inactivated and decreased the enhanced levels of $G_{i\alpha}$ proteins has been shown to result in decreased Gi functions and therefore increased formation of cAMP, which contributes to the attenuation of hypertension.

The generation of reactive oxygen species (ROS) that increase oxidative stress has been implicated in the pathogenesis of vascular diseases such as hypertension, diabetes, atherosclerosis and vascular remodelling by several investigators (20, 21, 29). The treatment of hypertensive rats with antioxidants have been shown to decrease the blood pressure (36). Wu et al. have shown that treatment of SHR with aspirin (100 g/kg/day) for 12 days decreased blood pressure and superoxide anion production (31). However, the mechanism by which antioxidants decrease blood pressure has not been fully understood.

In the present studies, we provide the first evidence showing that antioxidant treatment of VSMC from SHR decreased the enhanced levels of $G_{i\alpha}$ proteins and associated signalling that results in the enhanced levels of cAMP. The resultant increased levels of cAMP may contribute to the attenuation of blood pressure (fig 6). However, further studies have to be undertaken in order to investigate whether increased oxidative stress is the cause or effect of enhanced $G_{i\alpha}$ protein expression in SHR.

References

1. Neer EJ. Heterotrimeric G proteins: organizers of transmembrane signals. *Cell.* 1995; 80:249- 257.
2. Rodbell M, Krans HM, Pohl SL, Birnbaumer L. The glucagon-sensitive adenylyl cyclase system in plasma membranes of rat liver. IV. Effects of guanylnucleotides on binding ^{125}I-glucagon. *J Biol Chem.* 1971; 246: 1872-1876.
3. Bray P, Carter A, Simons C, Guo V, Puckett C, Kamholz J, Spiegel A, Nirenberg M. Human cDNA clones for four species of G_{sa} signal transduction protein. *Proc Natl Acad Sci USA.* 1986; 83; 8893-8897.
4. Robishaw JD, Smigel MD, Gilman AG. Molecular Basis for two forms of the G protein that stimulates adenylate cyclase. *J Biol Chem.* 1986; 261:9587-9590.

5. Itoh H, Toyama R, Kozasa T, Tsukamoto T, Matsuoka M, Kaziro Y. Presence of three distinct molecular species of Gi protein a subunit: structure of rat cDNAs and human genomics DNAs. *J Biol Chem.* 1988; 263:6656-6664.
6. Yatani A, Mattera R, Codina J, Graf R, Okabe K, Padrell E, Iyengar R, Brown AM, Birnbaumer L. The G protein-gated atrial K^+ channel is stimulated by three distinct Gi a-subunits. *Nature.* 1988; 336:680-682.
7. Noll T, Hempel A, Piper NM. Neuropeptide Y reduces macromolecule permeability of coronary endothelial monolayers. *Am J Physiol.* 1996; 271: H1878-H1-1883.
8. Feraille E, Doucet A. Sodium-potassium adenosine triphosphatase-dependant sodium transport in the kidney : hormonal control. *Physiol Rev.* 2001; 81:345-418.
9. Tsuda K, Tsuda S, Nishio I, Goldstein M, Masuyama Y. Modulation of [^{3}H]dopamine release by neuropep^tide Y in rat striatal slices. *Eur J Pharmacol.* 1997; 321 :5-11.
10. Anand-Srivastava MB. Enhanced expression of inhibitory guanine nucleotide regulatory protein in spontaneously hypertensive rats: relationship to adenylyl cyclase inhibition. *Biochem J.* 1992; 288:79-85.
11. Anand-Srivastava MB, de Champlain J, Thibault C. DOCA-salt hypertensive rat hearts exhibit altered expression of G-proteins. *Am J Hypertens.* 1993; 6: 72-75.
12. Thibault C, Anand-Srivastava MB. Altered expression of G-protein mRNA in spontaneously hypertensive rats. *FEBS Lett.* 1992; 313:160-164.
13. Marcil J, Thibault C, Anand-Srivastava MB. Enhanced expression of Gi-protein precedes the development of blood pressure in spontaneously hypertensive rats. *J Mol Cell Cardiol.* 1997; 29:1009-1022.
14. Li Y, Anand-Srivastava MB. Inactivation of enhanced expression of Gi proteins by pertussis toxin attenuates the development of high blood pressure in spontaneously hypertensive rats. *Circ Res.* 2002; 91:247-254.
15. Pandey SK, Anand-Srivastava MB. Modulation of G-protein expression by the angiotensin converting enzyme inhibitor captopril in hearts from spontaneously hypertensive rats: Relationship with adenylyl cyclase. *Am J Hyper.* 1996; 9:833-837.
16. Palaparti A, Ge C, Anand-Srivastava MB. Angiotensin II enhances the expression of Gia in A10 cells (smooth muscle): Relationship with adenylyl cyclase activity. *Arch Biochem Bioph.* 1999; 365:113-122.
17. Anand-Srivastava MB, Palaparti A. Angiotensin-II-induced enhanced expression of Gi proteins is attenuated by losartan in A10 vascular smooth muscle cells: role of AT1 receptors. *Can J Physiol Pharmacol.* 2003; 81: 150-158.
18. Cai H, Harrison DG. Endothelial dysfunction in cardiovascular diseases: The role of oxidative stress. *Circ Res.* 2000; 87: 840-844.
19. Wu R, Millette E, Wu L, de Champlain J. Enhanced superoxide anion formation in vascular tissues from spontaneously hypertensive and desoxyxorticosterone acetate-salt hypertensive rats. *J Hyper.* 2001; 19 :741-748.
20. Baynes JW. Role of oxidative stress in development of complications in diabetes. *Diabetes.* 1991; 40: 405-412.
21. Jun T, Ke-yan F, Catalano M. Increased superoxide anion production in humans : a possible mechanism for the pathogenesis of hypertension. *J Hum Hypertens.* 1996; 10: 305-309.
22. Anand-Srinastava MB, Franks DJ, Cantin M and Genest J. Presence of "RA" and "P"-site receptors for adenosine coupled to adenylyl cyclase in cultured vascular smooth muscle cells. *Biochem. Biophys. Res. Comm.* 1982; 108: 213-219.
23. Salomon Y, Londos C, Rodbell M. A highly sensitive adenylate cyclase assay. *Anal Biochem.* 1974; 58:541-548.
24. Lowry OH, Rosebrough NJ, Farr AL, Randall RJ. Protein measurement with the folin phenol reagent. *J Biol Chem.* 1951; 193:265-275.
25. Ge C, Garcia R, Anand-Srivastava MB. Altered expression of Gi-protein and adenylyl cyclase activity in hearts from one kidney one clip hypertensive rats: effect of captopril. *J Hypertens.* 1999; 17:1617-1626.

26. Marcil J, de Champlain J, Anand-Srivastava MB. Overexpression of Gi-proteins precedes the development of DOCA-salt-induced hypertension : relationship with adenylyl cyclase. *Cardiovasc Res.* 1998; 39:492-505.
27. Laplante MA, Wu R, El Midaoui A, de Champlain J. NAD(P)H oxidase activation by angiotensin II is dependent on p42/44 ERK-MAPK pathway activation in rat's vascular smooth muscle cells. *J Hypertens.* 2003; 21:927-936.
28. Hashim S, Anand-Srivastava MB. Losartan-induced attenuation of blood pressure in L-NAME hypertensive rats is associated with reversal of the enhanced expression of Gia proteins. *J Hypertens.* 2003; 222: article in press.
29. Friedman J, Peleg, E, Kagan T, Shnizer S, Rosenthal T. Oxidative stress in hypertensive, diabetic and diabetic hypertensive rats. *Am. J Hypertens.* 2003; 16:1049-1052.
30. Midaoui AE, Elimadi A, Wu L, Haddad PS, de Champlain J. Lipoic acid prevents hypertension, hyperglycemia, and the increase in heart mitochondrial superoxide production. *Am. J Hypertens.* 2003; 16: 173-179.
31. Wu R, Lamontagne D, de Champlain J. Antioxidative properties of acetylsalicylic Acid on vascular tissues from normotensive and spontaneously hypertensive rats. *Circulation.* 2002; 105: 387- 392.
32. Wong YH, Conklin BB, Bourne HR. Gz-mediated hormonal inhibition of cyclic AMP accumulation. *Science.* 1992; 255:339-342.
33. Suzuki H, Swei A, Zweifach BW, Schmid-Schnobein GW. In vivo evidence for microvascular oxidative stress in spontaneously hypertensive rats. Hydroethidine microfluorography. *Hypertension.* 1995; 25: 1083-1089.
34. McCord JM, Fridovich I. Superoxide dismutase: the first twenty years (1968-1988). *Free Radic Biol Med.* 1988;5:363-369.
35. Fridovich I. Biological effects of the superoxide radical. *Arch Biochem Biop.* 1986; 247: 1-11.

Adaptation Biology and Medicine (Volume 4: Current Concepts)
Editors: A. Hargens, N. Takeda and P.K. Singal

21. Resistance to Glucose-induced Apoptosis: Possible Mechanisms

Craig Ricci[1], Viktoriya Solodushko[1], Mahmood Mozzaffari[2], and Stephen W. Schaffer[1]

[1]University of South Alabama, College of Medicine Department of Pharmacology Mobile, Alabama
and
[2]Department of Oral Biology and Maxillofacial Pathology, Medical College of Georgia
School of Dentistry, Augusta, Georgia

Introduction

Recently it has been shown that oxidative stress may underlie many of the adverse complications associated with diabetes and hyperglycemia. This is thought to be due to the interplay of three seemingly independent biochemical pathways: glucose-induced activation of protein kinase C isoforms; increased formation of glucose-derived advanced glycosylation end-products; and increased glucose flux through the aldose reductase pathway (2,11). These pathways appear to be a consequence of hyperglycemia-induced overproduction of superoxide by the mitochondrial electron-transport chain (2,11). Superoxide is generated during normal functioning of the electron transport chain. Although the mitochondria normally contain sufficient levels of superoxide dismutase to neutralize these reactive oxygen species, the balance between free radical formation and degradation can be disrupted by specific metabolic conditions that lead to the excessive accumulation of reducing equivalents. The inability of the electron transport chain to adequately oxidize these reducing equivalents results in the diversion of electrons from the electron transport chain to oxygen, forming superoxide. Because the pathological accumulation of reactive oxygen species can trigger cytochrome c release and activate the caspase cascade, they are recognized initiators of mitochondria-mediated apoptosis

In adult ventricular cardiomyocytes, high glucose-induced activation of the renin-angiotensin II system may also serve as a major source of free radicals through activation of NADPH oxidase (6). According to Fiordaliso et al. (6), p53 is glycosylated in response to elevated glucose levels, leading to the upregulation of the renin angiotensin II system. Upregulation of angiotensin II promotes apoptosis through a cascade of events involving the activation of both NADPH oxidase and nitric oxide synthase, major sources of reactive oxygen and nitrogen species (8). One mechanism by which these reactive species may induce apoptosis is through their ability to cause p53 to be phosphorylated. In its activated phosphorylated state, p53 promotes cell death by suppressing the expression of anti-apoptotic genes, such as bcl-2, while simultaneously enhancing the expression of pro-apoptotic genes, such as Bax (6).

Notably, in the study by Fiordaliso et al. (6), it was shown that activation of the renin angiotensin II system by high glucose results in the phosphorylation and activation of p53.

Hyperglycemia-induced oxidative stress has also been shown to result in p53-mediated apoptosis through mechanisms independent of the renin angiotensin II system (1,5,7). Free radicals can activate p38 MAP kinase and Jun kinase, enzymes capable of directly phosphorylating p53. Free radicals can also cause DNA damage, which results in the activation of additional protein kinases capable of phosphorylating p53. In each case, phosphorylated p53 acts to drive the expression of the pro-apoptotic gene, Bax, thereby promoting apoptosis.

Despite evidence that hyperglycemia initiates apoptosis in many cells (1,3,5,6,7,10), some cells are resistant to hyperglycemia-induced apoptosis (9,13,14). Hall et al. (9) demonstrated that high glucose-induced activation of protein kinase C inhibits apoptosis in vascular smooth muscle cells. Sakuma et al. (13) found that high glucose similarly inhibits apoptosis in human coronary artery smooth muscle cells by the upregulation of anti-apoptotic bcl-2 family members, bcl-xl and bfl-1/A1. Our lab has previously reported that chronic hyperglycemia preconditions rat neonatal cardiomyocytes against hypoxia-induced apoptosis through the upregulation of bcl-2 (14). However, the mechanism by which hyperglycemia confers resistance to apoptosis in some cells, but not others, is unclear. Therefore, the aim of the present study was to further examine the mechanisms involved in the resistance of neonatal cardiomyocytes to hyperglycemia-induced apoptosis.

Methods

Cardiomyocyte preparation and incubation conditions

All care and treatment of animals were in accordance with the guidelines of the National Institute of Health and subjected to prior approval by the Institutional Care and Use Committee of the University of South Alabama. Rat neonatal cardiomyocytes were prepared as described previously (14). The cells were suspended in minimal essential medium containing 10% newborn calf serum and 0.1 mM 5'-bromo 2'-deoxyuridine and allowed to plate on either glass coverslips or polystyrene treated Petri dishes (Corning #430167) at a density of ~10 X 10^6 cells/dish (10 cm diameter). They were then placed in serum-free medium containing minimal essential medium and supplemented with either no addition (Control) or 25 mM Glucose (Glucose) for 3 days. After 2 days, some cells were incubated with either Chelerythrine (0.2, 1.0, 3.5, or 10 1 ìM) or 1nM Angiotensin II for the remaining 24 hours. To induce the hypoxic insult, some of the cells were transferred to medium lacking glucose but containing 10 mM deoxyglucose and 3 mM amobarbital (Amytal). At the appropriate time, the cells were either used for analysis of apoptosis or Western blot analysis.

TdT-mediated dUTP nick end labeling procedure

The cell specimens were fixed in 4% formaldehyde (in 1x PBS) for 15 minutes at room temperature and resuspended in TBS for 15 minutes. The Klenow-FragEL DNA Fragmention Detection Kit was then used to assess DNA breaks in apoptotic nuclei. Specimens were rehydrated in TBS and incubated with 20 ìg/ml proteinase K for 20 minutes. Following rehydration in TBS, the specimens were incubated with 3% H_20_2 for 5 minutes to inactivate endogenous peroxidases, and rehydrated again in TBS. Specimens were then incubated with 1X Klenow Equilibration Buffer for approximately 20 minutes. After removing the Klenow Equilibration Buffer, specimens were incubated at 37°C with

Klenow Labeling Reaction Mixture for 90 minutes. The labeling reaction was terminated by rehydrating the specimens in TBS and then incubating with Stop Solution for 5 minutes. Specimens were rehydrated in TBS and incubated with Blocking Buffer for 10 minutes at room temperature. After removing the Blocking Buffer, specimens were incubated at 37°C with 1X peroxidase-streptavidin conjugate for 30 minutes. Specimens were rehydrated in TBS and incubated with 3,3-diaminobenzidine and 0.6 mg of H_2O_2–urea solution for 15 minutes at room temperature and rinsed with dH_20. Specimens were counterstained with methyl green counterstain for 3 minutes. Color was fixed by immersing the specimens in 100% ethanol and then xylene. Five separate fields in the light microscope were examined for dark brown (apoptotic) and green (normal) nuclei.

Western blot analyses

Cellular content of Bcl-2, Bax, and p53 (phosphorylated serine 20) were determined by Western blot analysis using a modification of methods described previously (14). To dislodge the cells from the bottom of Petri dishes, the cells were incubated for 5-7 min with medium containing trypsin. They were then centrifuged at 500g for 5 min. After washing the cells with PBS, they were suspended in lysis buffer [62.5 mM Tris, pH 6.8, containing 2% w/v SDS and 10% glycerol, to which was added 1 mM orthovanadate, 0.1 mg PMSF and 1/100 dilution of protease inhibitor cocktail (Calbiochem)]. The cells were disrupted by drawing them into a pipette and then discharging them several times. The samples were then heated to 95-100°C for 5 min and placed on ice for 15 min. The samples were subjected to SDS-polyacrylamide gel electrophoresis (12% for Bcl-2 and Bax; 8% for the phosphorylated form of p53). The proteins were then transferred to nitrocellulose membranes, where they were blocked. After incubation with the appropriate antibody (purchased from Santa Cruz and Cell Signaling), the membranes were washed and then incubated with a secondary antibody, goat anti-rabbit IgG. The Western blots were detected by the enhanced chemiluminescence reaction. All data were analyzed by densitometry using ChemiImage ^{TM}4400 (Alpha Innotech Corp).

Statistical analysis

The statistical significance of the data was determined using the Student's t-test for comparison with groups and analysis of variance (ANOVA) combined with Tukey's post hoc test for comparison between groups. Values of $p < 0.05$ were considered statistically significant.

Results

Schaffer et al. (14) have reported that incubation of rat neonatal cardiomyocytes with medium containing 25 mM glucose preconditions the cells against hypoxia-mediated apoptosis. This effect has been attributed to the upregulation of bcl-2 and the inhibition of the Na^+/H^+ exchanger. Figure 1 shows that the cardioprotective effect of glucose is blocked by the protein kinase C inhibitor, chelerythrine. The protein kinase C inhibitor also blocks the glucose-mediated upregulation of the anti-apoptotic factor, bcl-2, but has no effect on the expression of the pro-apoptotic factor, Bax (Figure 2).

Figure 3 shows that the cardioprotective effect of high glucose is also blocked by addition of 1 nM angiotensin II to the incubation medium. Since angiotensin II initiates apoptosis in rat neonatal cardiomyocytes, the reversal of the cardioprotective action of high glucose is not surprising. Nonetheless, the results suggest that the endogenous renin-angiotensin II system is able to overcome preconditioning by high glucose in the adult cardiomyocytes, but not the neonatal cardiomyocytes. Figure 4 reveals that high glucose does not promote the phosphorylation of p53 in the neonatal cardiomyocyte as it does in the adult cardiomyocyte. Moreover, removal of insulin from the medium containing 25 mM glucose further reduced the phospho-p53 (serine 20) content by 35%. Therefore, the p53-dependent apoptotic pathway is not activated by high glucose in the neonatal cardiomyocyte.

Discussion

High concentrations of glucose are toxic to most cell types. According to Brownlee (2), mitochondrial superoxide production is a common element for hyperglycemia-induced vascular damage. Reactive oxygen species have also been implicated in glucose-induced apoptosis in human endothelial cells (5), SV40-transformed murine glomerular mesangial cells (1), rat Schwann cells (4), cardiac myoblast H9c2 cells (3), and adult ventricular cardiomyocytes (6). However, in some cells, high glucose protects against oxidative-mediated apoptosis (9,13,14). The status of the endogenous renin-angiotensin II system, p53 and the bcl-2 family of proteins appear to be major players in determining the outcome of a glucose challenge. Keim et al. (10) found that murine preimplantation embryos exposed to medium containing 52 mM glucose overexpressed the pro-apoptotic factor, Bax, and underwent apoptosis.

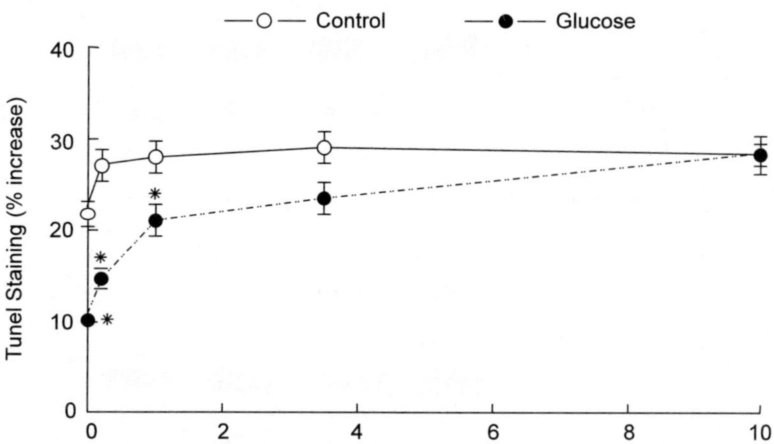

Fig. 1. ***Effect of chelerythrine on hyperglycemia-induced protection from hypoxia-induced apoptosis*. Neonatal rat cardiomyocytes were incubated for 3 days with medium containing either 5 mM (control) or 25 mM glucose (glucose-treated). After 2 days, cells from each group were exposed to 0, 0.2, 1.0, 3.5, or10 μM chelerythrine for the remaining 24 hours. One hour prior to TUNEL analysis, cells were then exposed to normal medium or to medium lacking glucose but containing 10 mM deoxyglucose and 3 mM amytal (chemical hypoxia). In total, 4 groups of cells were analyzed: *Control group 1*, control cells treated with 0, 0.2, 1.0, 3.5, or 10 μM chelerythrine and exposed to 1 hour normal medium; *control group 2*, control cells treated with 0, 0.2, 1.0, 3.5, or 10 μM chelerythrine and exposed to 1 hour chemical hypoxia; *glucose group 1*, glucose-treated cells exposed to 0, 0.2, 1.0, 3.5, or 10 μM chelerythrine and exposed to 1 hour normal medium; *glucose group 2*, glucose-treated cells exposed to 0, 0.2, 1.0, 3.5, or 10 μM chelerythrine and exposed to 1 hour chemical hypoxia. For each group, the extent of apoptosis was assessed from the number of cells exhibiting positive TUNEL staining. To calculate percent increase in TUNEL staining, the baseline level of apoptotic control or glucose-treated cells exposed to 1 hour of normal medium were subtracted from the level of apoptotic control or glucose-treated cells exposed to 1 hour of chemical hypoxia for each concentration of chelerythrine.**

However, blastocytes from p53 null mice cultured in 52 mM glucose neither underwent apoptosis nor exhibited enhanced Bax expression. Since p53 is known to upregulate Bax, it is significant that glucose-mediated apoptosis in SV40-transformed murine glomerular mesangial cells was associated with an upregulation of the bax/bcl-2 ratio (1). Fiordaliso et al. (6) have attributed glucose-mediated apoptosis in adult ventricular cardiomyocytes to the glycosylation of p53, which leads to angiotensin II formation followed by p53 phosphorylation. The activation of p53 was associated with a decrease in bcl-2 expression and an elevation in Bax content, effects that are blocked by the angiotensin II inhibitor, losartan. Indeed, Grishko et al. (8) found that the phosphorylation of p53 is a likely step in angiotensin II-mediated apoptosis.

The absence of glucose-mediated apoptosis in neonatal cardiomyocytes exposed to medium containing 25 mM glucose can be attributed to the failure of hyperglycemia to activate p53. Although several mechanisms can contribute to the activation of p53, three of the common mechanisms involve post-translational modifications, enhanced expression and mdm2-linked degradation (12). According to Fiordaliso et al. (6), significant increases in the cellular levels of both unphosphorylated and phosphorylated p53 are observed in glucose treated adult cardiomyocytes. Since the effects of

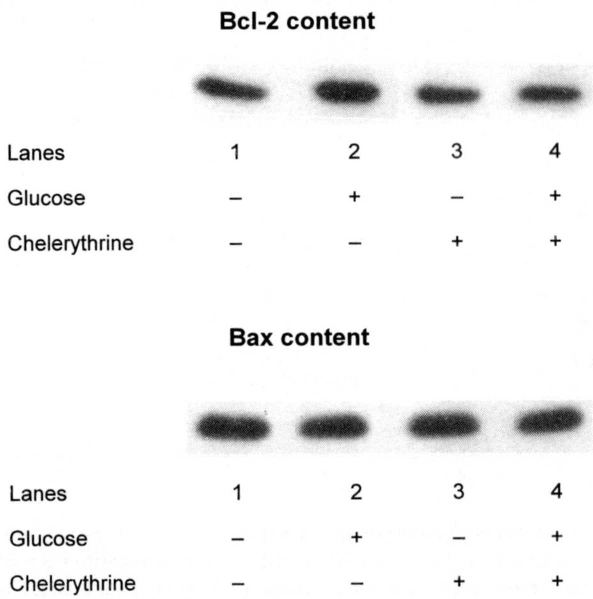

Fig. 2. ***Effect of chelerythrine on hyperglycemia-induced regulation of Bcl-2 and Bax levels*. Neonatal rat cardiomyocytes were incubated for 3 days with medium containing either 5 mM (Control) or 25 mM glucose (Glucose). After 2 days, some cells from each group were exposed to 1.0 μM chelerythrine for the remaining 24 hours. Cells were then lysed, and lysate was subjected to SDS-PAGE. After transfer to nitrocellulose membranes, samples were incubated with antibodies directed against Bcl-2 or Bax. A: Western blots detected by enhanced chemiluminescence reaction after exposure to goat anti-rabbit IgG. *Lane 1*, bcl-2 in control cells; *lane 2*, bcl-2 in glucose-treated cells; *lane 3*, bcl-2 in control cells exposed to chelerythrine; *lane 4*, bcl-2 in glucose-treated cells exposed to chelerythrine. B: Western blots detected by enhanced chemiluminescence reaction after exposure to goat anti-rabbit IgG. *Lane 1*, Bax in control cells; *lane 2*, Bax in glucose-treated cells; *lane 3*, Bax in control cells exposed to chelerythrine; *lane 4*, Bax in glucose-treated cells exposed to chelerythrine.**

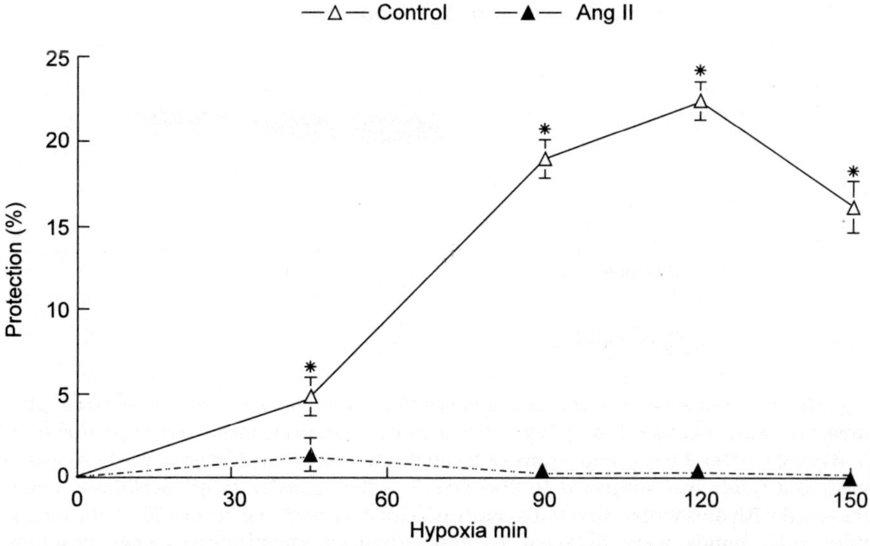

Fig. 3. ***Effect of angiotensin II on hyperglycemia-induced protection from hypoxia-induced apoptosis*. Neonatal rat cardiomyocytes were incubated for 3 days with medium containing either 5 mM (control) or 25 mM glucose (glucose-treated). After 2 days, some cells from the glucose-treated group were exposed to 1 nM angiotensin II for the remaining 24 hours. Prior to analysis by TUNEL staining, cells were then exposed to medium lacking glucose but containing 10 mM deoxyglucose and 3 mM amytal (chemical hypoxia) for 0, 45, 90, 120, or 150 minutes. In total, 3 groups were analyzed: *group 1*, control cells treated with 0 nM angiotensin and exposed to chemical hypoxia (0-150 minutes); *group 2*, glucose-treated cells incubated with 0 nM angiotensin II and exposed to chemical hypoxia (0 - 150 minutes); and *group 3*, glucose-treated cells incubated with 1 nM angiotensin II and exposed to chemical hypoxia (0 - 150 minutes). For each group, the extent of apoptosis was assessed from the number of cells exhibiting positive TUNEL staining. To calculate protection (control), the percentage of surviving control cells (group 1) was subtracted from the percentage of surviving glucose-treated cells (group 2); to calculate protection following treatment with angiotensin II (Ang II), the percentage of surviving control cells (group 1) was subtracted from the percentage of surviving glucose-treated cells incubated with 1 nM angiotensin II (group 3).**

hyperglycemia were blocked by the angiotensin II inhibitor, losartan, angiotensin II-mediated activation of NADPH oxidase may play a role in the regulation of p53. NADPH oxidase-mediated free radical generation may activate protein kinases that phosphorylate p53. Among these enzymes are p38 MAP kinase and Jun kinase, which are activated in the diabetic heart. Yet, the phosphorylation state of p53 remains unaltered in the glucose treated neonatal cardiomyocyte.

The missing component appears to be the activation of the endogenous renin-angiotensin II system. However, another possibility for the difference between adult and neonatal cardiomyocytes could reside in the translocation and activation of an angiotensin II-sensitive protein kinase C isoform. Once activated, this isoform is thought to activate NADPH oxidase, causing the generation of toxic reactive oxygen species (8). Although PKC_d and PKC_e translocate to the particulate fraction in response to angiotensin II treatment, it is unclear which isoform contributes to angiotensin II-mediated apoptosis. Both isoforms are affected by hyperglycemia and are logical candidates for the difference between the adult and neonatal cardiomyocyte.

$p53_{ser\ 20}$ content

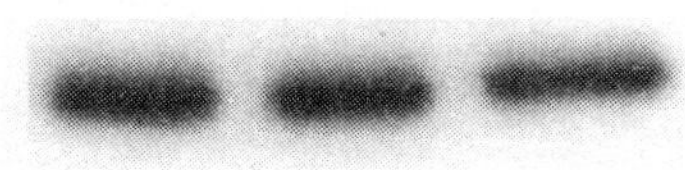

Lanes	1	2	3
Glucose	–	+	+
Chelerythrine	+	+	–

Fig. 4. ***Effect of glucose treatment on the phosphorylation state of p53 (phosphoserine 20).*** **Neonatal rat cardiomyocytes were incubated for 3 days with medium containing either 5 mM (control) or 25 mM glucose (glucose-treated). After 2 days, some glucose-treated cells were transferred to medium lacking insulin. Cells were lysed, and lysate was subjected to SDS-PAGE. After transfer to nitrocellulose membranes, samples were incubated with antibodies directed against p53 (phosphorylated serine 20). Following exposure to goat anti-rabbit IgG, bands were detected by the enhanced chemiluminescence reaction.** ***Lane 1,*** **p53 (phosphorylated serine 20) in control cells;** ***lane 2,*** **p53 (phosphorylated serine 20) in glucose-treated cells;** ***lane 3,*** **p53 (phosphorylated serine 20) glucose-treated cells without insulin.**

References

1. Barinder K, Frencher S, Reddy V, Kessler A, Malhotra A, Meggs LG. High glucose promotes mesangial cell apoptosis by oxidant-dependent mechanism. *Am J Physiol Renal Physiol* 2002; 284: F455-F466.
2. Brownlee M. Biochemistry and molecular cell biology of diabetic complications. *Nature* 2001; 414: 813-820.
3. Cai L, Li W, Wang G, Guo L, Jiang Y, Kang Y. Hyperglycemia-induced apoptosis in mouse myocardium: mitochondrial cytochrome c-mediated caspase-3 activation pathway. *Diabetes* 2002; 51: 1938-1948.
4. Delaney CL, Russell JW, Cheng HL, Feldman EL. Insulin-like growth factor-1 and over-expression of bcl-xl prevent glucose-mediated apoptosis in schwann cells. *Journal of Neuropathology and Experimental Neurology* 2001; 60(2): 147-160.
5. Du XL, Stockklauser-Farber K, Rosen P. Generation of reactive oxygen intermediates, activation of NF-êB, and induction of apoptosis in human endothelial cells by glucose: role of nitric oxide synthase? *Free Radical Biology and Medicine* 1999; 27 (7/8): 752-763.
6. Fiordaliso F, Leri A, Cesselli D, Limana F, Safai B, Nadal-Ginard B, Anversa P, Kajstura J. Hyperglycemia activates p53 and p53-regulated genes leading to myocyte cell death. *Diabetes* 2001; 50:2363-2375.
7. Greene DA, Stevens MJ, Obrosova I, Feldman EL. Glucose-induced oxidative stress and programmed cell death in diabetic neuropathy. *European Journal of Pharmacology* 1999; 375: 217-223.
8 Grishko V, Pastukh V, Solodushko V, Gillespie M, Azuma J, Schaffer SW. Apoptotic cascade initiated by angiotensin II in neonatal cardiomyocytes: role of DNA damage. *Am J Physiol Heart Circ Physiol* 2003;
9. Hall JL, Matter CM, Wang X, Gibbons GH. Hyperglycemia inhibits vascular smooth muscle cell apoptosis through a protein kinase-c dependent pathway. *Circ Res* 2000; 87: 574-580.
10. Keim AL, Chi MMY, Moley KH. Hyperglycemia-induced apoptotic cell death in the mouse blastocyst is dependent on the expression of p53. *Mol Reprod Dev* 2001; 60: 214-224.

11. Nishikawa T, Edelstein D, Du XL, Yamagishi S, Matsumura T, Kaneda Y, Yorek MA, Beebe D, Oates PJ, Hammes HP, Giardino I, Brownlee M. Normalizing mitochondrial superoxide production blocks three pathways of hyperglycaemic damage. *Nature* 2000; 404: 787-790.
12. Prives C, Hall P. The p53 pathway. *J Pathol* 1999; 187: 112-126.
13. Sakuma H, Yamamoto M, Okumura M, Kojima T, Maruyama T, Yasuda K. High glucose inhibits apoptosis in the human coronary artery smooth muscle cells by increasing bcl-xl and bfl-1/A1. *Am J Physiol Cell Physiol* 2001; 283: C422-C428.
14. Schaffer SW, Croft CB, Solodushko V. Cardioprotective effect of chronic hyperglycemia: effect on hypoxia-induced apoptosis and necrosis. *Am J Physiol Heart Circ Physiol* 2000; 278(6): H1948-H1954.

Adaptation Biology and Medicine (Volume 4: Current Concepts)
Editors: A. Hargens, N. Takeda and P.K. Singal

22. Enhancing Myocardial Ischemic Tolerance Via Adaptation to Acute Systemic Hypoxia: Pivotal Role of iNOS as the Trigger and Mediator

Lei Xi and Rakesh C. Kukreja

Division of Cardiology, Department of Internal Medicine, Virginia Commonwealth University, Richmond, VA 23298-0281, USA

Introduction and Historical Survey

Systemic hypoxia (SH) represents a common pathophysiological condition that may be caused by environmental factors (such as high altitude) or by a number of cardiopulmonary and hematological diseases (such as heart failure, apnea, and anemia). These factors may interfere or disrupt any stage(s) of the oxygen supply, transport, and utilization process, resulting in tissue oxygen deficiency and impairment of the normal cellular function fueled mainly by ATP generated through oxidative phosphorylation. In contrast, SH may also elicit a complex physiological response that leads to adaptation at system, organ, and tissue levels, in order to compensate the lower availability of oxygen. In 1960, a Peruvian physician named Hurtado first described an interesting phenomenon in his paper [1], which showed that human residents on high altitude had extremely low incidence of myocardial infarction and hypertension. He also stated that these high altitude populations from various ethnic groups also possessed greater vascularity and vasodilatation in the major organs. Subsequently, as summarized in Table 1, several laboratories in Eastern Europe, Russia, and USA had confirmed this striking clinical observation in various animal models. All of the earlier studies had demonstrated a paradoxical enhancement in myocardial ischemic tolerance after chronic exposure to either continuous or intermittent SH in adult mammals [2,3,4]. Thus, the discovery of SH-induced myocardial protection well preceded the first description of another cardioprotective phenomenon termed as "Ischemic Preconditioning" in 1986 [5], which has been overwhelmingly investigated around the world during the past two decades. Meerson and his associates have already demonstrated the wide-spectrum of beneficial effects gaining from adaptation to intermittent SH in human subjects using hypobaric chamber [6].

Chronic continuous SH was also shown to induce cardioprotection in adult rats [7] and neonatal rabbits [8,9]. Most recently the acute SH-induced cardioprotective effects in adult rodents have been demonstrated independently by our laboratory [10] and two other groups [11,12]. These new advances

Table 1. Representative Studies on Systemic Hypoxia-Induced Cardioprotection

Authors & Pub. Year	Species	Types of Hypoxia & Cardioprotection	Signaling Mechanisms	Ref. #
Hurtado 1960	Human	ALH (3370-4540m, years to life long) infarction ↓ hypertension↓	/	[1]
Poupa *et al.* 1968	Rat	ALH (5000-7000m, 24h+24hRO, 6 weeks) cardiac necrosis↓ function↑	/	[2]
McGrath *et al.* 1968	Rat	ALH (7500m, 20h+4hRO for 15 days) function↑	Glycolysis	[3]
Meerson *et al.* 1973	Rat	ALH (6000m, 5h/day for 40 days) infarct size↓ function- mortality↓	/	[4]
Meerson 1991	Human	ALH (5000m, 5h/day for 40 days) arrhythmia↓ hypertension↓	/	[6]
Tajima *et al.* 1994	Rat	HH (10%O_2, 21 days) function↑	Lactate	[7]
Baker *et al.* 1997	Rabbit	HH (12%O_2, from birth to 7-10 days) function↑	K_{ATP}, Lactate	[8]
Arkhipenko *et al.* 1997	Rat	HH (10%O_2, 11x5min/3minRO,23 days) arrhythmia↓ function↑	Antioxidant enzymes	[15]
Baker *et al.* 1998	Rabbit	HH (12%O_2, from birth to 7-10 days) function↑	NOS3	[9]
Asemu *et al.* 1999	Rat	ALH (5000m, 4h/day for 21 days) arrhythmia↓	mito-K_{ATP}	[17]
Eells *et al.* 2000	Rabbit	HH (12%O_2, from birth to 7-10 days) function↑	mito-K_{ATP}, ATP	[18]
Sasaki *et al.* 2001	Rat	HH (10%O_2, 4h+24hRO) function↑ angiogenesis- apoptosis↓	VEGF, NFkB	[11]
Xi *et al.* 2002	Mouse	HH (10%O_2, 2 x 4h+24hRO) infarct size↓ CF- function →	NOS2, NOS3, COX-2	[10]
Cai *et al.* 2003	Mouse	HH (6%O_2, 5 x 6min/6minRO+24hRO) infarct size↓ function↑	HIF-1, EPO	[12]

Abbreviations: ALH – high altitude hypoxia; HH – hypoxic hypoxia; RO – reoxygenation CF – coronary flow; mito-K_{ATP} – mitochondrial ATP-sensitive potassium channel HIF – hypoxia-inducible factor; EPO – erythropoietin; VEGF – vascular endothelial growth factor; NFkB – nuclear factor kappa B; ↓ decreased; ↑ increased; → unchanged

have revitalized this important field of research. The cardioprotection elicited by *acute* SH is of great clinical interest, because the adverse effects of *chronic* SH, such as pulmonary hypertension and right ventricular hypertrophy [13] may be effectively avoided in this modality of adaptation.

Mechanistic Concerns and Rationale for Our Studies in SH-induced Cardioprotection

The mechanism of SH-induced cardioprotection is not fully understood. Several studies have attempted to establish a temporal profile of the myocardial enzymes that regulate antioxidant defense [14] and energy metabolism [15] in the adult rats exposed to chronic hypobaric hypoxia. There is mounting evidence suggesting the role of sarcolemmal and/or mitochondrial ATP-sensitive potassium channels (K_{ATP}) in SH-induced cardioprotection in immature or adult mammals [8,17,18]. An increase in nitric oxide (NO) production after exposure to chronic SH was also reported [9,19,20]. In the immature rabbit model of chronic SH, Baker and colleagues reported upregulation of endothelial NO synthase (eNOS or NOS3) rather than inducible NO synthase (iNOS or NOS2) in the hypoxic hearts [9,20]. In contrast, several studies in adult rodents demonstrated that SH enhances iNOS expression in various organs and tissues [21,22,23] and chronic SH may actually downregulate eNOS expression *in vivo* [24]. We and others have previously demonstrated that iNOS is an essential mediator for delayed pharmacological or ischemic preconditioning [25,26,27,28,29,30,31]. Similar to the heart, a NO-dependent mechanism has been proposed in acute SH-induced neuronal protection against ischemic injury in the brain [32]. In addition, it has been recently shown that cyclooxygenase 2 (COX-2) also plays a critical role in the late phase of ischemic preconditioning in rabbits [33] and mice [34]. However, no data are available to show the effect of SH on myocardial COX-2 expression, although this protein is induced by hypoxia in lungs [35]. Therefore, in order to further understand the signaling mechanisms underlying the SH-induced cardioprotection, we designed a study targeted on the following three specific goals: 1) to determine if moderate acute SH induces delayed cardioprotection in mouse; 2) to elucidate the role of NOS2 as potential trigger or mediator of the SH-induced cadioprotection; 3) to determine the possible involvement of COX-2 in delayed protection induced by acute SH.

The Mouse Model of SH-induced Cardioprotection

The recent advances in molecular biology and genetic engineering techniques have provided some new research tools such as gene knockout mice. In order to take advantage of these new developments, we have established a mouse model of acute SH-induced cardioprotection.

1. Source of animals and chemicals

Adult male outbred ICR mice were supplied by Harlan Sprague Dawley (Indianapolis, IN). Adult male homozygous (–/–) iNOS gene knockout mice were purchased from The Jackson Laboratory (Bar Harbor, ME). Chemicals for preparing the heart perfusion buffer as well as the selective inhibitors of NOS2 (S-methylisothiourea sulfate, SMT) or COX-2 (NS398) were purchased from Sigma-Aldrich (St. Louis, MO).

2. Systemic hypoxia pretreatment

A cage containing 3 to 4 conscious, unrestrained mice was placed in a normobaric Plexiglas chamber ($100 \times 60 \times 50$ cm; see Figure 1) with 10% inspiratory oxygen fraction (*i.e.* 0.10 F_IO_2) by introducing pure N_2 into the chamber. The oxygen concentration was continuously monitored with a Beckman oxygen analyzer and precisely maintained at 10% by adjusting influx flow of N_2. Normoxia control experiments were conducted in identical way, except that compressed air, instead of N_2, was introduced into the chamber for maintaining a condition of 21% inspiratory oxygen fraction. A thermo-hygrometer (Fisher Scientific) was placed inside the chamber for continuously monitoring the temperature and humidity.

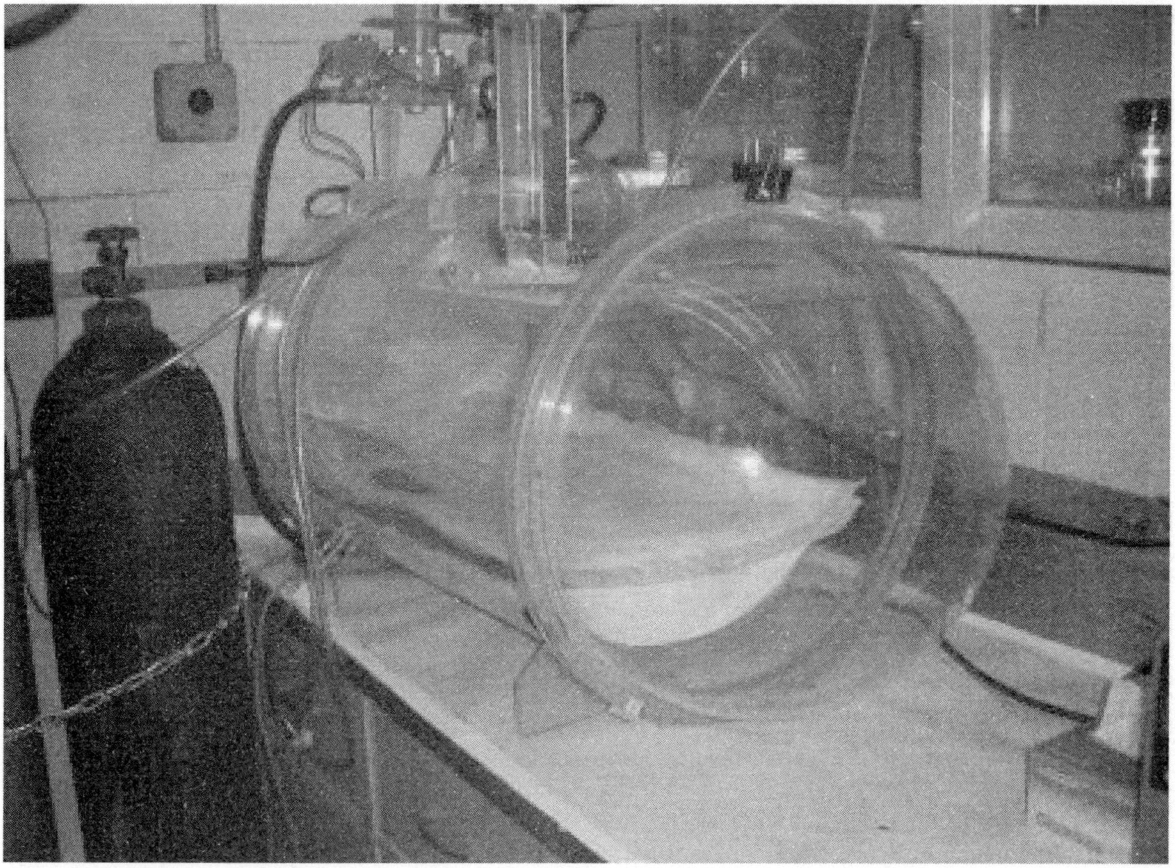

Fig. 1. Systemic hypoxia chamber. With this system, a normobaric hypoxia environment can be rapidly created by introducing pure nitrogen gas into the chamber and stably maintained at any chosen level of inspired oxygen fraction. Up to 8 conscious, unrestrained adult mice can be simultaneously treated for any given time duration.

3. Langendorff heart model of global ischemia-reperfusion

The methodology of Langendorff isolated buffer-perfused mouse heart preparation was previously described in detail [27,28,36]. Ventricular contractile function was measured periodically during the 20 min of no-flow global ischemia and 30 min of reperfusion (I/R) with a force-displacement transducer (Grass, Model FT03) attached to the apex through a No. 5 surgical thread and a metal hook. The resting tension was initially adjusted to ~0.30 g and kept at this level without readjustment thereafter. Ventricular developed force was recorded with a Beckman R-511A polygraph connected to the force transducer. The coronary flow rate was calculated by timed collection of the efflux perfusate and expressed as ml/min/g wet weight of the heart. At the end of I/R experiment, heart was removed from the Langendorff apparatus, weighed and immediately stored in a –20°C freezer. The frozen heart was cut from apex to base into 7 transverse slices of equal thickness (~ 1 mm) and the slices were incubated in 10% triphenyl tetrazolium chloride (TTC) in phosphate buffer at room temperature for 30 minutes. The TTC buffer was then replaced by 10% formaldehyde and the heart slices were fixed for 4 to 6 hours before the measurement of areas of infarct tissue by computer morphometry (Bioquant 98). The risk area was the sum of total ventricular area minus cavities. The infarct size was measured in each slice of both left and right ventricular myocardium and presented as % of risk area.

4. Experimental groups

Mice were randomized into the following 12 experimental groups (n=6-8/each): *Normoxia* – ICR mice were kept in the chamber under normoxic condition for 4 hrs followed by 24 hrs interval before I/R; *H30min & H4h* – ICR mice pretreated with hypoxia for 30 min or 4 hrs followed by 24 hrs reoxygenation before I/R; *H2hx2 & H4hx2* – ICR mice pretreated with two cycles of either 2 or 4 hrs hypoxia followed by 24 hrs reoxygenation before I/R; *SMT+H4hx2 & H4hx2+SMT* – SMT was given (3 mg/kg, *i.p.*) either 30 min before 2 cycles of 4 hrs hypoxia followed by 24 hrs reoxygenation or 30 min prior to I/R following SH pretreatment in ICR mice; *iNOS-KO+H4hx2* – NOS2 knockout mice pretreated with the repetitive SH before I/R; *NS398+H4hx2 & H4hx2+NS398* – NS398 was given (10 mg/kg, *i.p.*) either 30 min before the repetitive SH or 30 min before I/R following SH pretreatment in ICR mice; *Normoxia+ NS398 & Normoxia+SMT* – ICR mice pretreated under normoxia and received NS398 or SMT 30 min before I/R. In addition, we chose to use our previously reported data [37] for serving as the iNOS-KO normoxic control group, in order to avoid unnecessary redundant experiments under the identical experimental settings and protocol in these gene knockout mice.

5. Western blot analysis for protein expression

In parallel series of experiments, ventricular tissue samples (n=3-8/group) were collected following various pretreatments (see *Experimental Groups*). Tissue samples were ground under liquid nitrogen and homogenized with Polytron at 4°C in 1 ml PBS (pH 7.4). The homogenate was then centrifuged at 12,000 g for 10 min and the supernatant was recovered. For measurement of COX-2 expression in sub-cellular compartments, cytosolic and membranous fractions were prepared by the method of Shinmura *et al.* [33]. In brief, the heart tissue was homogenized in ice-cold lysis buffer using glass pestle and single burst of 5 sec with a Polytron homogenizer. Under 4°C, the homogenate was centrifuged at 45,000 g for 1 hour and the supernatant was recovered as the cytosolic samples. The pellets were then incubated in lysis buffer+1% Triton X-100 for one hour, re-homogenized and centrifuged at 45,000 g for 1 hour, as described above. The supernatant representing the membranous samples was finally recovered. Either 40 μg (for COX-2) or 60 μg (for iNOS and eNOS) of protein from each sample was separated by SDS/PAGE on 10% acrylamide gels. Proteins were then transferred to a nitrocellulose membrane and blocked with 5% non-fat dry milk in Tris Buffer Saline. The membrane was subsequently incubated with a rabbit polyclonal antibody reacting specifically to iNOS or eNOS (Santa Cruz; dilution 1:500 for iNOS and eNOS), or with a goat polyclonal antibody reacting specifically to COX-2 (Santa Cruz, 1:100 dilution). The secondary antibody was a horseradish peroxidase-conjugated anti-rabbit or anti-goat IgG (Amersham, 1:1000 or 2000 dilution). The membranes were developed using enhanced chemiluminescence and exposed to x-ray film. Optical density for each Western blot band was determined with a scanner/densitometer system (Molecular Dynamics 4.0) and normalized against background density for each gel.

Salient Findings

1. Acute SH induces significant reduction in infarct size and mild improvement in post-ischemic ventricular function

In spite of the large body of evidence on chronic continuous or intermittent SH-induced cardioprotection in several mammalian species including humans [1,2,3,4,5,6,7,15,17], it remains unclear if acute or sub-acute SH could also produce similar protection. Our results [10] showed that acute SH induced delayed protection in a duration-sensitive manner (Figure 2). Pretreatment with 4 hrs of SH resulted in a significant reduction in infarct size 24 hrs after SH (i.e. *H4h* group, 21.4±2.2%), as compared to *Normoxia* (29.7±2.6%; *P*<0.05; Figure 1). Two cycles of the SH further reduced infarct size to 16.0±3.1% (*H4hx2*; *P*<0.05). Shorter durations of SH (30 min or 2 hrs) were insufficient to reduce infarct size (*H30min* - 27.5±6.0%; *H2hx2* - 29.0±4.2%; *P*>0.05 *vs. Normoxia*). Only mild improvement in ventricular contractile function during reperfusion was observed following SH (*P*>0.05 *vs. Normoxia*). Such a disassociation between functional improvement and infarct reduction has been reported previously by us [36] and others [38] following classic ischemic preconditioning or delayed pharmacological preconditioning [27,28]. On the other hand, a good association between infarct reduction and functional improvement was observed with other preconditioning modalities, including whole body hyperthermia in mice [39]. There was no significant difference in pre-ischemic cardiac function among the groups. Following 20 min of global ischemia, ventricular developed force and rate-force product during the reperfusion period were depressed in all the groups, whereas heart

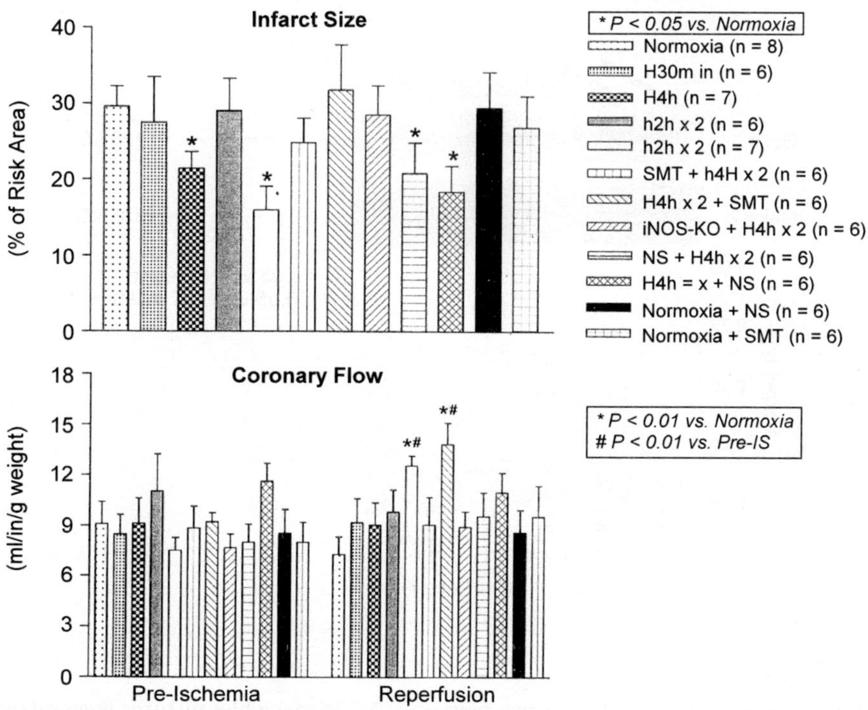

Fig. 2. Effect of acute systemic hypoxia on myocardial infarct size (*Top*) and coronary flow (*Bottom*). Values are means±SEM. Adopted from [10].

rate remained reasonably constant and was comparable to the pre-ischemic values. The only exception was *H4hx2+SMT* group, which possessed both positive inotropic and chronotropic effects especially during the early stage of reperfusion. The pre-ischemic coronary flow was not different among the groups (Figure 2; $P>0.05$). However, post-ischemic coronary flow was generally higher in all SH-treated groups as compared to *Normoxia*.

2. Acute SH-induced infarct-limiting effect is triggered and mediated by iNOS

One of the most important observations in our present study is that iNOS served as the trigger and mediator of SH-induced late cardioprotection. The role of iNOS in the protective process was supported by the following three pieces of evidence obtained from our experiments. First, the infarct limiting effect of SH in *H4hx2* group was abolished by SMT – the iNOS inhibitor, given either before or after SH (*SMT+H4hx2* - 24.8±3.3%; *H4hx2+SMT* - 31.8±5.9%; $P>0.05$ *vs. Normoxia*; Figure 2). SMT alone had no significant effect on infarct size in normoxic hearts (*Normoxia+SMT* - 26.8±4.2%). Second, SH exposure resulted in consistent upregulation in iNOS protein expression in all the hypoxic groups as compared with *Normoxia* (n=4-8/group; Figure 3). The densitometric analysis indicated significant increase in iNOS in *H4h, H2hx2*, and *H4hx2* ($P<0.05$ *vs. Normoxia*), but not in *H30min* group. Despite the general trend of iNOS upregulation in all SH-treated hearts no significant linear correlation was observed between iNOS protein content and myocardial infarct size. Administration of SMT before SH completely abolished the induction of iNOS by SH (see *SMT+H4hx2*). Third, the absence of SH-induced delayed cardioprotection in iNOS gene knockout mice, *i.e.* no difference in

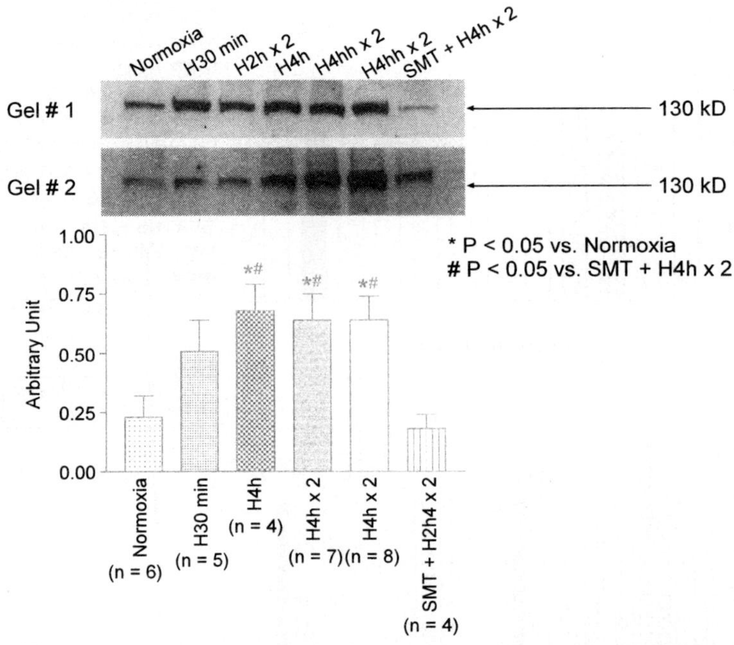

Fig. 3. iNOS expression in mouse heart. *Top*: two representative Western blot pictures demonstrate iNOS protein expression in mouse heart following various pretreatments. *Bottom*: densitometric quantification of iNOS expression. Adopted from [10].

infarct size was found between *iNOS-KO+ H4hx2* group (28.5±3.8%; Figure 2) and the control iNOS-KO group (23.5±3.8%; n=10; P>0.05; from [37]).

As proposed previously [25,27], upregulation of iNOS may increase myocardial NO level that could open mitochondrial K_{ATP} channel [41], which indeed has been considered as the potential end-effector for SH-induced cardioprotection [17,18]. Inhibition of iNOS may block the signaling pathway via iNOS-generated superoxide and/or peroxynitrite [42], which are well-known triggers of preconditioning. Previous studies have argued against the triggering role of iNOS in delayed ischemic preconditioning in rabbits [43]. Since iNOS was constitutively expressed in normal mouse hearts (Figure 3 and [30]), such a role of this enzyme may be species-specific. On the other hand, the lack of linear correlation between reduction in infarct size and the level of iNOS expression following shorter duration of SH, *i.e. H2hx2* (Figure 2 and 3) could suggest that longer duration of SH (*i.e.* 4 hours) may activate certain unknown cofactor(s) that may potentially control the post-translational modifications of iNOS, which in turn regulate its activity. Furthermore, inhibition of iNOS with SMT did not reverse the improvement of post-ischemic coronary flow in *H4hx2* (Figure 2). These results indicate that SH could improve vascular endothelial function independent of iNOS. It is also conceptually consistent with the previous findings of ours [27] and others [40] on monophosphoryl lipid A-induced cardioprotection.

3. eNOS plays a negligible role in the acute SH-induced cardioprotection

It is suggested that eNOS plays an important role in the chronic SH-induced cardioprotection in immature rabbits [9,20]. In the present study, we found that eNOS was constitutively expressed in both normoxic and hypoxic mouse hearts (Figure 4). Acute SH of various durations caused slight decrease in eNOS protein expression in the heart (*P*>0.05 *vs. Normoxia*). SMT treatment had no effect on the expression of eNOS. Since eNOS expression was not increased following SH pretreatment (Figure 4), it was suggested that this protein is unlikely to be involved in acute SH-induced delayed cardioprotection. These differences may be attributed to the species (rabbit *vs.* mouse), age (immature *vs.* adult), and duration of hypoxia (chronic *vs.* acute). However, the triggering role of eNOS in the SH-induced protection cannot be ruled out completely in the present study. This is because the blockade of SH-induced infarct size reduction was relatively partial when SMT was given before SH (*SMT+H4hx2* - 24.8±3.3% *vs. Normoxia* - 29.7±2.6%; Figure 2) as compared with the complete blockade when SMT was given before I/R (*H4hx2+SMT* - 31.8±5.9%). The questions concerning the role of eNOS in acute SH-induced late cardioprotection need to be addressed in the future investigations that would include the use of eNOS-KO mice.

4. Lack of role for COX-2 in the acute SH-induced protection

Recent studies proposed that COX-2 could serve as a critical mediator of delayed ischemic preconditioning in rabbits [33] and mice [34]. However, our results have indicated a lack of the role for this enzyme because NS398, a selective inhibitor of COX-2 did not block SH-induced cardioprotection, regardless of the timings of its administration, *i.e.* before or after hypoxia pretreatment (Figure 2; *NS398+H4hx2* - 20.8±4.0%; *H4hx2+NS398* - 18.4±3.4%; *P*<0.05 *vs. Normoxia*). NS398 *per se* had no effect on infarct size in normoxic controls (*Normoxia+NS398* - 29.4±4.7%). The improvement in coronary flow was partially blocked in the NS398-treated groups.

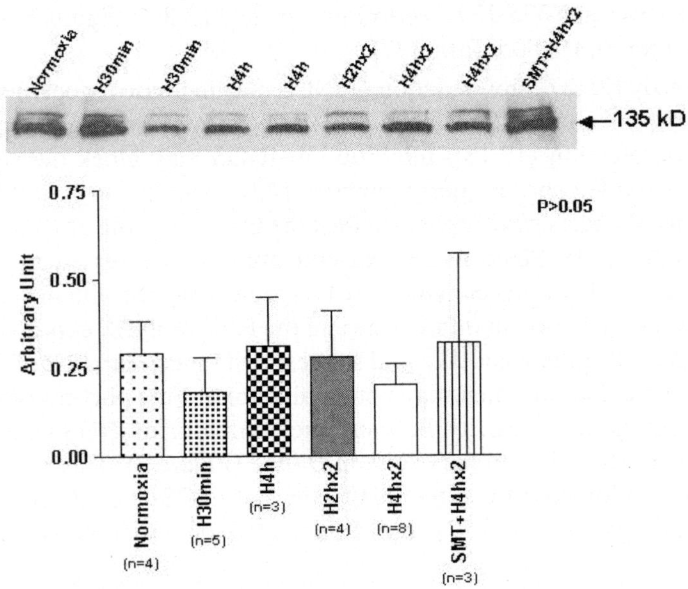

Fig. 4. **eNOS expression in mouse heart. *Top*: Representative Western blot picture demonstrate eNOS protein expression in mouse heart following various pretreatments. *Bottom*: densitometric quantification of eNOS expression. Adopted from [10].**

COX-2 was preferentially expressed in the membranous fraction (Figure 5), similar to the previously described rabbit study [33]. However, no increase in the membranous COX-2 protein expression was found in the preconditioned hearts (*H4hx2*) as compared with *Normoxia* (Figure 5). The densitometric results indicated a rather slight non-significant downregulation of COX-2 expression in the membranous fraction of *H4hx2* hearts. These results suggest that COX-2 may not have any role in SH-induced cardioprotection. The possible explanation for the discrepancy between this study and the rabbit study could be that the moderate SH stimulus (0.10 F_IO_2) may not be powerful enough to activate the COX-2 dependent pro-inflammatory pathways triggered with multiple cycles of coronary occlusion-reperfusion [33,34]. Thus, unlike the essential role of NOS2 in delayed cardioprotection with pharmacologic [25,27,28,30,31], ischemic [26,29], or hypoxic preconditioning in our recent study ([10]; Figure 2 and 3), the involvement of COX-2 may be dependent on the type of preconditioning stimulus. In support of this hypothesis, a recent study has also demonstrated that COX-2 did not mediate the delayed pharmacological preconditioning induced by adenosine A_1 or A_3 receptor agonists in rabbit heart [44].

Clinical Relevance

SH is a clinically relevant condition with potential importance in cardiovascular pathophysiology. For example, the anti-ischemic and anti-hypertensive beneficial effects have been observed in the human subjects adapted to SH under the simulated high altitude environment [1]. Furthermore, recent studies demonstrated that the gene expression and enzyme activity of iNOS was upregulated, whereas eNOS activity and gene expression were downregulated in the right atrial tissues in children with cyanotic

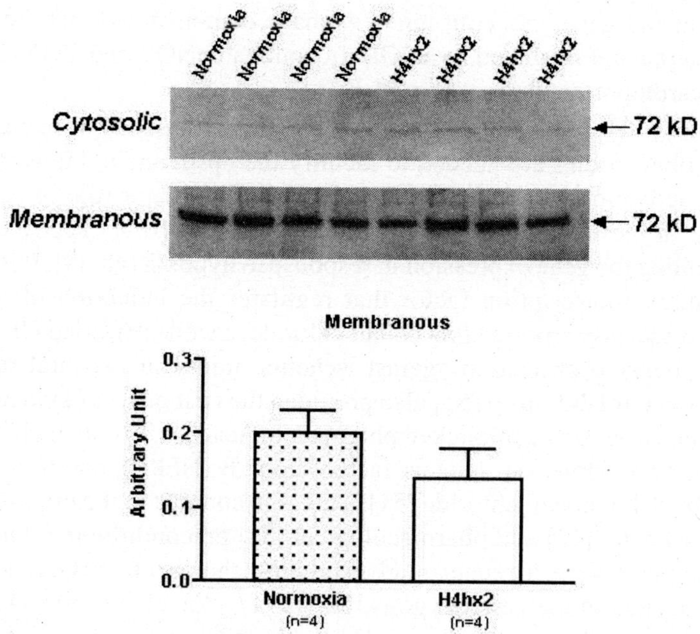

Fig. 5. COX-2 expression in mouse heart. *Top*: Western blots of COX-2 protein expression in cytosolic and membranous fraction of the heart tissue following normoxic or hypoxic (H4hx2) pretreatment. *Bottom*: densitometric quantification of COX-2 expression. Adopted from [10].

congenital heart defects [45]. The iNOS upregulation may represent an adaptive response to the condition of SH persisting in the sick children. These clinical observations further support the importance of an iNOS-dependent adaptive mechanism in SH. The recent findings from us [10] and others [11,12] on delayed cardioprotection induced by *acute* exposure of SH are quite exciting, since it indicates that SH-induced cardioprotection can be achieved without bearing the adverse effects of *chronic* SH, such as pulmonary hypertension and right ventricular hypertrophy [13]. In addition, pretreatment of neonatal rats with acute SH rendered protection against cerebral ischemic injury [32,46]. Therefore, one could expect that an adequate degree and duration of SH may induce protective effect in multiple organs, which may be more advantageous than ischemic preconditioning where the remote protection has not been consistently demonstrated. For example, a brief ischemia in kidneys or skeletal muscle could reduce myocardial infarct size caused by a subsequent coronary occlusion, a transient cerebral ischemia failed to produce the similar cardioprotection [47]. This unique feature of SH-induced multi-organ protection and the relatively non-invasive and practicable nature of using low oxygen gas mixtures or hypobaric chamber would encourage the eventual clinical application of "Hypoxia Therapy", which has already been explored in humans [6].

Summary and Future Perspectives

In summary, we have demonstrated that pretreatment with moderate acute SH can induce delayed protection against myocardial infarction in mice. The length of SH exposure influenced the degree of cardioprotection, with repetition of the exposure conferring more significant protection. Using pharmacological inhibition and gene knockout mice, we have demonstrated that the infarct-limiting effect of acute SH is triggered and mediated by iNOS. In contrast, eNOS and COX-2 may only have insignificant roles in the cardioprotection in this model.

As illustrated in Figure 6, SH may activate a complex signaling cascade, in which iNOS plays a pivotal role. However, further studies are needed to identify the upstream and downstream signaling cascade that leads to the activation of iNOS, which in turn plays a major role in acute SH-induced delayed cardioprotection. In particular, hypoxia inducible factor 1 (HIF-1) appears to be a critical transcription factor controlling the gene expression in response to hypoxia [48,49]. It is likely that HIF-1 also serves as the primary transcription factor that regulates the induction of iNOS following exposure to SH [23]. It was recently reported that cobalt chloride, a well-identified HIF-1 enhancer can mimic acute SH-induced delayed protection against ischemic injury in neonatal rat brain [50]. In addition, a recent study from our laboratory [51] also provided the first piece of evidence showing that SH-induced late cardioprotection can be mimicked pharmacologically with cobalt chloride (30 mg/kg) via activation of HIF-1 in mice. However, nuclear factor kappa B (NFkB), another key transcription factor, was not activated by SH or cobalt chloride [51]. This is in contrast to the proposed essential role of NFkB in the delayed ischemic [52] and pharmacological [31] preconditioning. On the other hand, our findings are in agreement with a recent study showing that acute SH-induced late cardiac preconditioning was diminished in the heterozygous HIF-1a (+/-) knockout mice [12]. Furthermore, endogenous substances such as adenosine and catecholamine [53] may be released during hypoxia,

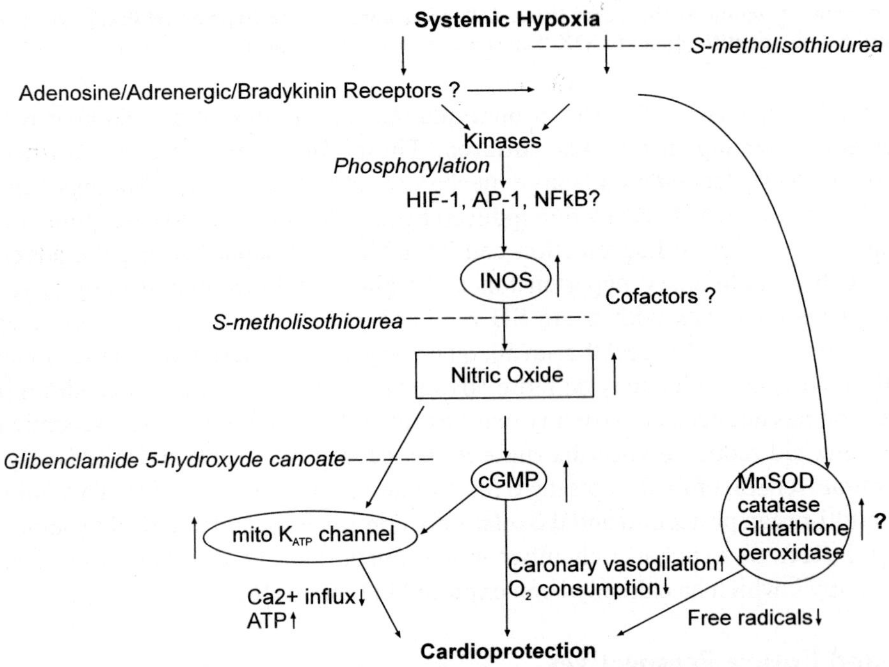

Fig. 6. Current understanding of the signaling mechanisms for SH-induced delayed cardioprotection. *Abbreviations:* reactive oxygen species (ROS); hypoxia-inducible factor 1 (HIF-1); activator protein 1 (AP-1); nuclear factor kappa B (NFkB); manganese superoxide dismutase (MnSOD); mitochondrial ATP-sensitive potassium channel (mitoK_{ATP}).

which could also play a role in the upstream signal transduction pathways. Similarly, hypoxia is known to be able to activate a broad array of protein kinases [54,55,56]. The role of these kinases in acute SH-induced cardioprotection remains to be further determined. Recent interests have also focused on the downstream target genes that are regulated by hypoxia and HIF-1, for example vascular endothelial growth factor (VEGF) [57,58] and erythropoietin [12,59]. Taken together, these new advances in understanding the SH-induced cardioprotection have just opened a new frontier in the approaches of protecting ischemic myocardium via endogenous adaptation mechanisms.

Acknowledgement

The authors' original studies as well as this review article were supported by the grants from National Institutes of Health (HL51045 and HL59469 to R.C. Kukreja) and American Heart Association, Mid-Atlantic Affiliate (9804811U and 0060289U to L. Xi). We are indebted to all of our colleagues - D. Tekin, E. Gursoy, F. Salloum, M. Taher and J.E. Levasseur for their important contributions to the original mouse experiments that are discussed in this chapter.

References

1. Hurtado A. Some clinical aspects of life at high altitudes. *Ann Intern Med* 53: 247-258, 1960.
2. Poupa O, Krofta K, Prochazka J, and Turek Z. Acclimation to simulated high altitude and acute cardiac necrosis. *Federation Proc* 25: 1243-1246, 1968.
3. McGrath JJ and Bullard RW. Altered myocardial performance in response to anoxia after high-altitude exposure. *J Appl Physiol* 25: 761-764, 1968.
4. Meerson FZ, Gomzakov OA, and Shimkovich MV. Adaptation to high altitude hypoxia as a factor preventing development of myocardial ischemic necrosis. *Am J Cardiol* 31: 30-34, 1973.
5. Murry CE, Jennings RB, and Reimer KA. Preconditioning with ischemia: a delay of lethal cell injury in ischemic myocardium. *Circulation* 74: 1124-1136, 1986.
6. Meerson FZ. *Adaptive Protection of the Heart: Protecting against Stress and Ischemic Damage.* CRC Press Inc. Boca Raton, Florida, 1991.
7. Tajima M, Katayose D, Bessho M, and Isoyama S. Acute ischemic preconditioning and chronic hypoxia independently increase myocardial tolerance to ischemia. *Cardiovasc Res* 28: 312-319, 1994.
8. Baker JE, Curry BD, Olinger GN, and Gross GJ. Increased tolerance of chronically hypoxic immature heart to ischemia. Contribution of the K_{ATP} channel. *Circulation* 95: 1278-1285, 1997.
9. Baker JE, Holman P, Kalyanaraman B, and Pritchard KA Jr. Adaptation of hearts to chronic hypoxia increases tolerance to subsequent ischemia by increased nitric oxide production. *Adv Exp Med Biol* 454: 203-217, 1998.
10. Xi L, Tekin D, Gursoy E, Salloum F, Levasseur JE, and Kukreja RC. Evidence that NOS2 acts as a trigger and mediator of late preconditioning induced by acute systemic hypoxia. *Am J Physiol* 283: H5-H12, 2002.
11. Sasaki H, Ray PS, Zhu L, Otani H, Asahara T, and Maulik N. Hypoxia/reoxygenation promotes myocardial angiogenesis via an NF kappa B-dependent mechanism in a rat model of chronic myocardial infarction. *J Mol Cell Cardiol* 33: 283-294, 2001.
12. Cai Z, Manalo DJ, Wei G, Rodriguez ER, Fox-Talbot K, Lu H, Zweier JL, and Semenza GL. Hearts from rodents exposed to intermittent hypoxia or erythropoietin are protected against ischemia-reperfusion injury. *Circulation* 108: 79-85, 2003.
13. Ostadal B, Ostadalova I, and Dhalla NS. Development of cardiac sensitivity to oxygen deficiency: Comparative and ontogenetic aspects. *Physiol Rev* 79: 635-659, 1999.

14. Nakanishi K, Tajima F, Nakamura A, Yagura S, Ookawara T, Yamashita H, Suzuki K, Taniguchi N, and Ohno H. Effects of hypobaric hypoxia on antioxidant enzymes in rats. *J Physiol (London)* 489: 869-876, 1995.

15. Arkhipenko YuV, Sazontova TG, Tkatchouk EN, and Meerson FZ. Adaptation to continuous and intermittent hypoxia: Role of the active oxygen-dependent system. In: Sharma BK et al. (ed): *Adaptation Biology and Medicine* (Vol. 1), pp251-259, Narosa Publishing House, New Delhi, 1997.

16. Novel-Chate V, Mateo P, Saks VA, Hoerter JA, and Rossi A. Chronic exposure of rats to hypoxic environment alters the mechanism of energy transfer in myocardium. *J Mol Cell Cardiol.* 30: 1295-1303, 1998.

17. Asemu G, Papousek F, Ostadal B, and Kolar F. Adaptation to high altitude hypoxia protects the rat heart against ischemia-induced arrhythmias. Involvement of mitochondrial K_{ATP} channel. *J Mol Cell Cardiol* 31: 1821-1831, 1999.

18. Eells JT, Henry MM, Gross GJ, and Baker JE. Increased mitochondrial K_{ATP} channel activity during chronic myocardial hypoxia: Is cardioprotection mediated by improved bioenergetics? *Circ Res* 87: 915-921, 2000.

19. Malyshev IY, Zenina TA, Golubeva LY, Saltykova VA, Manukhina EB, Mikoyan VD, Kubrina LN, and Vanin AF. NO-dependent mechanisms of adaptation to hypoxia. *Nitric Oxide* 3: 105-113, 1999.

20. Shi Y, Pritchard KA, Holman P, Rafiee P, Griffith OW, Kalyanaraman B, and Baker JE. Chronic myocardial hypoxia increases nitric oxide synthase and decrease caveolin-3. *Free Radical Biol Med* 29: 695-703, 2000.

21. Gess B, Schricker K, Pfeifer M, and Kurtz A. Acute hypoxia upregulates NOS gene expression in rats. *Am J Physiol* 273: R905-R910, 1997.

22. Rouet-Benzineb P, Eddahibi S, Raffestin B, Laplace M, Depond S, Adnot S, and Crozatier B. Induction of cardiac nitric oxide synthase 2 in rats exposed to chronic hypoxia. *J Mol Cell Cardiol* 31: 1697-1708, 1999.

23. Jung F, Palmer LA, Zhou N, and Johns RA. Hypoxic regulation of inducible nitric oxide synthase via hypoxia inducible factor-1 in cardiac myocytes. *Circ Res* 86: 319-325, 2000.

24. Toporsian M, Govindararu K, Nagi M, Eidelman D, Thibault G, and Ward ME. Downregulation of endothelial nitric oxide synthase in rat aorta after prolonged hypoxia in vivo. *Circ Res* 86: 671-675, 2000.

25. Zhao L, Weber PA, Smith JR, Comerford ML, Elliott GT. Role of inducible nitric oxide synthase in pharmacological "preconditioning" with monophosphoryl lipid A. *J Mol Cell Cardiol.* 1997;29:1567-1576.

26. Guo Y, Jones WK, Xuan YT, Tang XL, Bao W, Wu WJ, Han H, Laubach VE, Ping P, Yang Z, Qiu Y, and Bolli R. The late phase of ischemic preconditioning is abrogated by targeted disruption of the inducible NO synthase gene. *Proc Natl Acad Sci USA* 96: 11507-11512, 1999.

27. Xi L, Jarrett NC, Hess ML, and Kukreja RC. Essential role of inducible nitric oxide synthase in monophosphoryl lipid A-induced late cardioprotection: evidence from pharmacological inhibition and gene knockout mice. *Circulation* 99: 2157-2163, 1999.

28. Xi L, Salloum F, Tekin D, Jarrett NC, and Kukreja RC. Glycolipid RC552 induces delayed preconditioning-like effect via iNOS-dependent pathway in mice. *Am J Physiol* 277: H2418-H2424, 1999.

29. Imagawa J, Yellon DM, and Baxter GF. Pharmacological evidence that inducible nitric oxide synthase is a mediator of delayed preconditioning. *Br J Pharmacol* 126: 701-708, 1999.

30. Zhao T, Xi L, Chelliah J, Levasseur JE, and Kukreja RC. Inducible nitric oxide synthase mediates delayed myocardial protection induced by activation of adenosine A_1 receptors: evidence from gene-knockout mice. *Circulation* 102: 902-907, 2000.

31. Zhao TC, Taher MM, Valerie KC, and Kukreja RC. p38 triggers late preconditioning elicited by anisomycin in heart: Involvement of NF-kB and iNOS. *Circ Res* 89: 915-922, 2001.

32. Gidday JM, Shah AR, Maceren RG, Wang Q, Pelligrino DA, Holtzman DM, and Park TS. Nitric oxide mediates cerebral ischemic tolerance in a neonatal rat model of hypoxic preconditioning. *J Cereb Blood Flow Metab* 19: 331-340, 1999.

33. Shinmura K, Tang X-L, Wang Y, Xuan Y-T, Liu S-Q, Takano H, Bhatnagar A, and Bolli R. Cyclooxygenase-2 mediates the cardioprotective effects of the late phase of ischemic preconditioning in conscious rabbits. *Proc Natl Acad Sci USA* 97: 10197-10202, 2000.

34. Guo Y, Bao W, Wu WJ, Shinmura K, Tang XL, and Bolli R. Evidence for an essential role of cyclo-oxygenase-2 as a mediator of the late phase of ischemic preconditioning in mice. *Basic Res Cardiol* 95: 479-484, 2000.
35. Chida M and Voelkel NF. Effects of acute and chronic hypoxia on rat lung cyclooxygenase. *Am J Physiol* 270: L872-L878, 1996.
36. Xi L, Hess ML, and Kukreja RC. Ischemic preconditioning in isolated perfused mouse heart: reduction in infarct size without improvement of post-ischemic ventricular function. *Mol Cell Biochem* 186: 69-77, 1998.
37. Xi L, Jarrett NC, Hess ML, and Kukreja RC. Myocardial ischemia/reperfusion injury in the inducible nitric oxide synthase knockout mice. *Life Sci* 65: 935-945, 1999.
38. Cohen MV, Yang XM, and Downey JM. Smaller infarct after preconditioning does not predict extent of early functional improvement of reperfused heart. *Am J Physiol* 277: H1754-H1761, 1999.
39. Tekin D, Xi L, Zhao T, Tejero-Taldo MI, Atluri S, and Kukreja RC. Mitogen-activated protein kinases mediate heat shock-induced delayed protection in mouse heart. *Am J Physiol* 281: H523-H532, 2001.
40. Laude K, Richard V, Henry J-P, Lallemand F, and Thuillez C. Evidence against a role of inducible nitric oxide synthase in the endothelial protective effects of delayed preconditioning. *Br J Pharmacol* 130: 1547-1552, 2000.
41. Sasaki N, Sato T, Ohler A, O'Rourke B, and Marban E. Activation of mitochondrial ATP-dependent potassium channels by nitric oxide. *Circulation* 101: 439-445, 2000.
42. Xia Y and Zweier JL. Superoxide and peroxynitrite generation from inducible nitric oxide synthase in macrophages. *Proc Natl Acad Sci USA* 94: 6954-6958, 1997.
43. Xuan Y-T, Tang X-L, Qiu Y, Banerjee S, Takano H, Han H, and Bolli R. Biphasic response of cardiac NO synthase isoforms to ischemic preconditioning in conscious rabbits. *Am J Physiol* 279: H2360-H2371, 2000.
44. Kodani E, Shinmura K, Xuan Y-T, Takano H, Auchampach JA, Tang X-L, and Bolli R. Cyclooxygenase-2 does not mediate late preconditioning induced by activation of adenosine A_1 or A_3 receptors. *Am J Physiol* 281: H959-H968, 2001.
45. Ferreiro CR, Chagas ACP, Carvalho MHC, Dantas AP, Jatene MB, de Souza LCB, and da Luz PL. Influence of hypoxia on nitric oxide synthase activity and gene expression in children with congenital heart disease: a novel pathophysiological adaptive mechanism. *Circulation* 103: 2272-2276, 2001.
46. Gorgias N, Maidatsi P, Tsolaki M, Alvanou A, Kiriazis G, Kaidoglou K, and Giala M. Hypoxic pretreatment protects against neuronal damage of the rat hippocampus induced by severe hypoxia. *Brain Res* 714: 215-225, 1996.
47. de Zeeuw S, Lameris TW, Duncker DJ, Hasan D, Boomsma F, van den Meiracker AH, and Verdouw PD. Cardioprotection in pigs by exogenous norepinephrine but not by cerebral ischemia-induced release of endogenous norepinephrine. *Stroke* 32: 767-774, 2001.
48. Semenza GL, and Wang GL. A nuclear factor induced by hypoxia via de novo protein synthesis binds to the human erythropoietin gene enhancer at a site required for transcriptional activation. *Mol Cell Biol* 12: 5447-5454, 1992.
49. Jones NM, and Bergeron M. Hypoxic preconditioning induces changes in HIF-1 target genes in neonatal rat brain. *J Cereb Blood Flow Metab* 21: 1105-1114, 2001.
50. Bergeron M, Gidday JM, Yu AY, Semenza GL, Ferriero DM, and Sharp FR. Role of hypoxia-inducible factor-1 in hypoxia-induced ischemic tolerance in neonatal rat brain. *Ann Neurol* 48: 285-296, 2000.
51. Xi L, Taher M, Salloum F, and Kukreja RC. Cobalt chloride induces delayed preconditioning in mouse heart: Role of hypoxia-inducible factor 1alpha and inducible nitric oxide synthase. *Circulation (suppl.)* 2003 (In Press).
52. Xuan Y-T, Tang X-L, Banerjee S, Takano H, Li RCX, Han H, Qiu Y, Li J-J, and Bolli R. Nuclear factor-kB plays an essential role in the late phase of ischemic preconditioning in conscious rabbits. *Circ Res* 84: 1095-1109, 1999.

53. Cohen MV, Walsh RS, Goto M, and Downey JM. Hypoxia preconditions rabbit myocardium via adenosine and catecholamine release. *J Mol Cell Cardiol* 27: 1527-1534, 1995.
54. Seko Y, Tobe K, Ueki K, Kadowaki T, and Yazaki Y. Hypoxia and hypoxia/reoxygenation activate Raf-1, mitogen-activated protein kinase kinase, mitogen-activated protein kinases, and S6 kinase in cultured rat cardiac myocytes. *Circ Res* 78: 82-90, 1996.
55. Goldberg M, Zhang HL, and Steinberg SF. Hypoxia alters the subcellular distribution of protein kinase C isoforms in neonatal rat ventricular myocytes. *J Clin Invest* 99: 55-61, 1997.
56. Laderoute KR, and Webster KA. Hypoxia/reoxygenation stimulates Jun kinase activity through redox signaling in cardiac myocytes. *Circ Res* 80: 336-344, 1997.
57. Minchenko A, Bauer T, Salceda S, and Caro J. Hypoxic stimulation of vascular endothelial growth factor expression in vitro and in vivo. *Lab Invest* 71: 374-379, 1994.
58. Shweiki D, Itin A, Soffer D, and Keshet E. Vascular endothelial growth factor induced by hypoxia may mediate hypoxia-initiated angiogenesis. *Nature* 359: 843-845, 1992.
59. Calvillo L, Latini R, Kajstura J, Leri A, Anversa P, Ghezzi P, Salio M, Cerami A, Brines M. Recombinant human erythropoietin protects the myocardium from ischemia-reperfusion injury and promotes beneficial remodeling. *Proc Natl Acad Sci USA* 100: 4802-4806, 2003.

Adaptation Biology and Medicine (Volume 4: Current Concepts)
Editors: A. Hargens, N. Takeda and P.K. Singal

23. Changes in the Electroretinogram during Ischemia-reperfusion in Young and Aged Rats under Normothermic and Hypothermic Conditions

H. Katano[1] and Y. Kawai[2]

[1]Division of Ophthalmology and Visual Science,
[2]Division of Adaptation Physiology, Faculty of Medicine, Tottori University, Yonago 683-8503, Japan

Introduction

Ischemia-reperfusion has been extensively investigated in the brain, heart and many other organs, including the eye. A number of studies have demonstrated histological [9, 11], electrophysiological [4, 5], and hemodynamic changes [15, 23] in the eye tissues exposed to ischemia-reperfusion. Since an ischemic disease occurs more often in old patients than in young, it is important to know the difference in the ischemia-induced changes between young and aged animals. We have previously shown that there were age-dependent differences of hemodynamic and histological changes in rat eyes during reperfusion after exposure to ischemia induced by increasing intraocular pressure (IOP) [10].

Electrophysiological function of retina is known to correlate with ischemic damage. The b-wave of flash-elicited electroretinogram (ERG) is generated in the bipolar or Muller cells [2, 17, 27]. Exposure to ischemia reduces the amplitude of b-waves in rabbits [4, 5, 26], cats [20, 21], and rats [6, 7, 8]. The damages of retinal function in ischemia-reperfusion are different between young and aged rats. Recently, we demonstrated the effects of aging on the ERG during ischemia-reperfusion in rats [12], showing that the recovery of ERG waves during reperfusion was prolonged in aged rats as compared with young rats.

Medical treatment for retinal ischemia has drawn considerable amount of interest. The application of hypothermia in cardiac surgery [14] and neurosurgery [16] has been proven to be beneficial for preventing ischemia-induced tissue damages. It was reported that local hypothermia during vitrectomy in ischemic eyes decreased retinal damage [25]. Thus, the present study was undertaken to investigate 1) the effect of hypothermia on b-wave of ERG during ischemia-reperfusion, and 2) the difference in the efficacy of hypothermia between young and aged rats.

Materials and Methods

Animal preparation

Forty-seven male Wistar rats, 4 months old (n = 24) and over 18 months old (n = 23), were used in this study. The rats were divided into 6 groups (Groups 1-3: young rats and Groups 4-6: aged rats) (Table 1). The animals were anesthetized with ketamine hydrochloride (3 to 8 mg/kg/h, i.v.) and artificially ventilated with room air, following paralysis with pancronium bromide to eliminate saccadic eye movements. Then, the rats were fixed in a stereotaxic frame for measurement of choroidal blood flow. Body temperature was monitored by a thermistor inserted into the rectum. During experiments, mean arterial pressure was 100-130 mmHg, PaO_2 was 100-140 mmHg, and pH was 7.34-7.43. There were no significant differences in these parameters between young and aged rats. Animals in which these parameters changed significantly during the experiment were excluded from the present study.

Ischemia-reperfusion protocol

A 27-gauge needle was inserted into the left anterior chamber through the cornea and connected to a bottle filled with artificial aqueous humor. The intraocular pressure (IOP) of the left eye was altered by changing the height of the bottle to produce a certain level of ischemia. After recording the baseline value of choroidal blood flow and ERG, the IOP was elevated from 15 mmHg to 80 mmHg to produce ischemia in the eye tissues for 120 min (Groups 2, 3 and 5, 6), and then returned to 15 mmHg to allow reperfusion for 6 h. In the control animals (Groups 1 and 4), the IOP was maintained at 15 mmHg throughout the experiment.

Measurement of ChBF

The choroidal blood flow (ChBF) was measured continuously by means of a laser Doppler flowmeter in the left eye. Although this method does not yield measurements of absolute value, it provides valuable relative measurements of blood flow [22]. Blood flow can be calculated as the product of blood flow velocity and blood volume. The procedures have been described in detail previously [15]. Briefly, a small part of the bulbar conjunctiva, approximately 2-3 mm posterior to the upper limbs of the left eye, was removed. A laser probe, which operated in the infrared region at 780 nm, was placed on the exposed sclera using a micromanipulator.

Table 1. Animal groups and their experimental conditions.

Group	*n*	Age	Ischemic period	Body temperature
1	8	4 months	(control)	Normothermia
2	8	4 months	120 min	Normothermia
3	8	4 months	120 min	Hypothermia
4	8	> 18 months	(control)	Normothermia
5	8	> 18 months	120 min	Normothermia
6	7	> 18 months	120 min	Hypothermia

n : number of animals.

The output of ChBF recording was averaged for 30 s before (baseline value), during (at 1 min, 59 min, and 119 min in Groups 2, 3 and 5, 6), and after ischemia (at 1 min, 9 min, 29 min, and every hour for 6 h after the end of ischemia). In the control rats (Groups 1 and 4), data were collected at the corresponding time periods. Relative ChBF was expressed as a percentage of the baseline value in each rat. ERG recordings were performed right after each data collection for ChBF.

ERG recordings

The ERGs were recorded to provide the assessment of the retinal function prior to and following the ocular ischemia. The pupil of both eyes was fully dilated with a mixed solution of 0.5% tropicamide and 0.5% phenylephrine hydrochloride. Active Ag/AgCl electrodes were placed in contact with the cornea, and reference and ground electrodes were placed on the nose and on the right leg, respectively. A photostimulator was held at a distance of 20 cm in front of both eyes. Then the room was kept dark throughout the experiment. After dark adaptation for at least 30 min, ERG responses to single white light flashes (20 joules) were recorded in both eyes. The flash-elicited ERG b-waves were amplified with a biophysical amplifier. The waveforms captured on a memory oscilloscope were recorded by means of a data acquisition system connected to a computer. The frequency of band-pass filter was set between 0.5 and 1,000 Hz. The amplitude of b-wave was measured from the trough of a-wave to the peak of b-wave (Fig. 1). In order to eliminate individual variation, the amplitude of ERG was expressed as a percentage of baseline value, i.e., $100 \times (iA/iA_{pre})$ where iA_{pre} and iA are the amplitude of each wave in ischemic eye before and during (or after) ischemia, respectively. Since ERG amplitude shows time-to-time variation [7, 13, 24], the percentage was further corrected by a time index which was niA/niA_{pre}, where niA_{pre} and niA are the amplitude of each wave in non-ischemic control eye before and during (or after) ischemia, respectively. Thus, the change in amplitude of ERG waves is calculated as :

$$\text{Normalized amplitude (\%)} = 100 \times (iA/iA_{pre})/(niA/niA_{pre}).$$

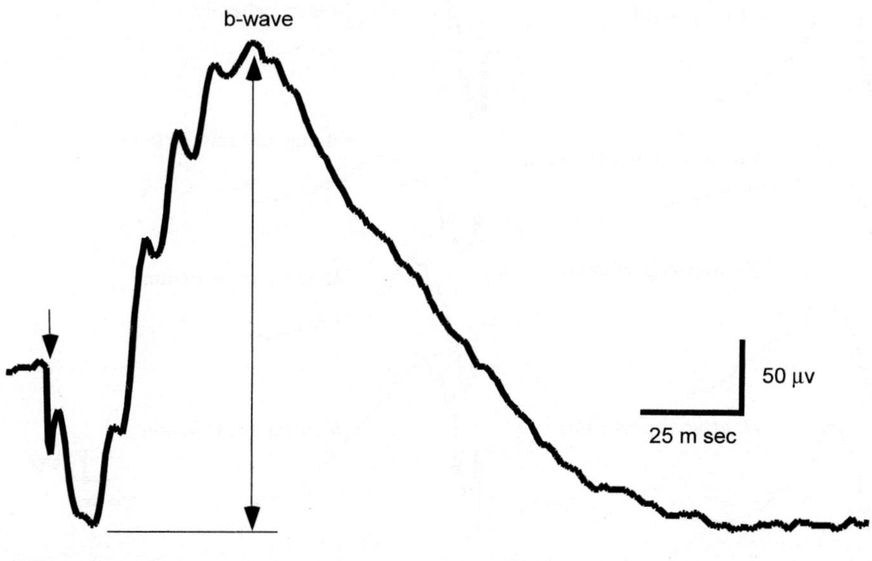

Fig. 1. Typical ERG waveform recorded in a young rat. The left downward arrows show the onset of a light flash. (Fig. 1:modified from Ref. 12)

Results and Discussion

Changes in ChBF

In the control rats of both young (Group 1) and aged (Group 4) groups, ChBF did not change significantly throughout the experiments. On the other hand, ChBF decreased to 40 – 60% of the baseline value during ischemia in Groups 2, 3, 5, and 6 (Table 2). There were no significant differences in the level of ischemia between any two groups.

Table 2. Choroidal blood flow during ischemia.

	n	during ischemia (% of baseline flow)
Group 2 : young, 120-min ischemia, normothermia	8	49.0 ± 2.3
Group 3 : young, 120-min ischemia, hypothermia	8	48.9 ± 2.9
Group 5 : aged, 120-min ischemia, normothermia	8	45.5 ± 3.4
Group 6 : aged, 120-min ischemia, hypothermia	7	45.0 ± 3.4

Values are means ± SEM. n : number of animals. No significant differences were noted between any two groups.

Changes of ERG b-wave amplitude in normothermic and hypothermic conditions

The b-wave amplitude of ERG were recorded under normothermic and hypothermic conditions (Fig. 2 and Fig. 3). The rectal temperature was maintained at 38-39°C using a heating pad in normothermia groups. On the other hand, it was decreased to 30.0-33.0°C by using a domestic cooling pad during ischemia in hypothermia groups.

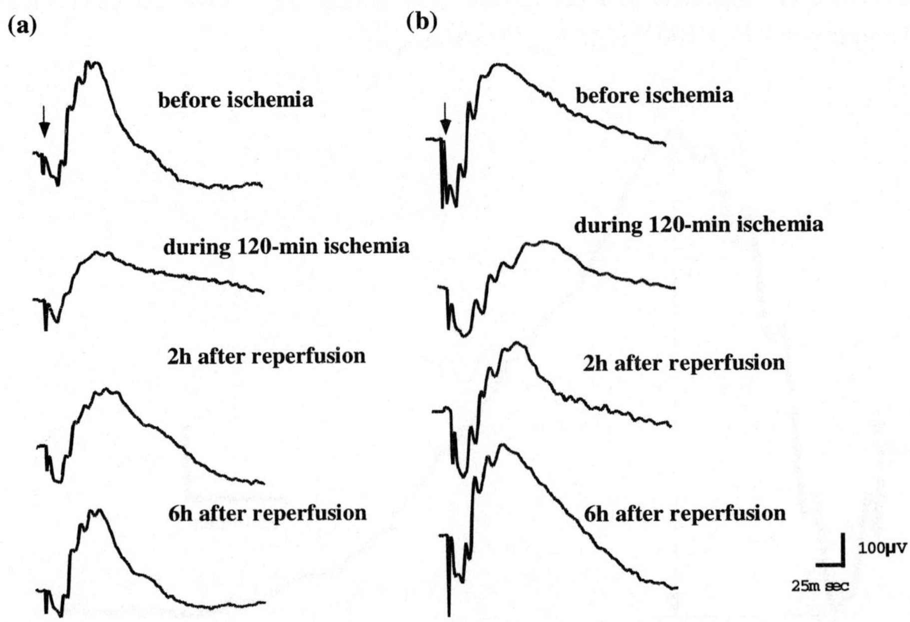

Fig. 2. Changes in ERG waveforms during and after 120-min ischemia in a young rat under normothermia (a) and hypothermia (b). The downward arrows show the onset of a light flash. (Fig. 2a:modified from Ref. 12)

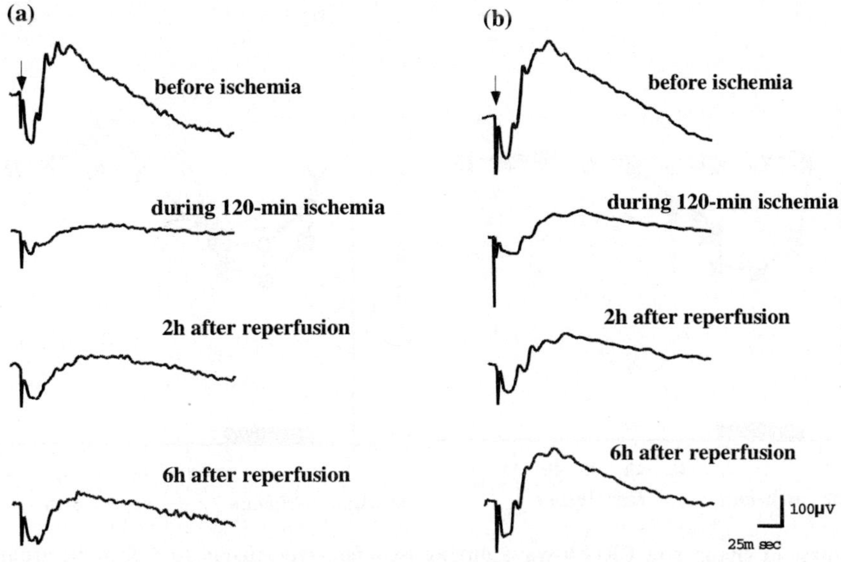

Fig. 3. Changes in ERG waveforms during and after 120-min ischemia in an aged rat under normothermia (a) and hypothermia (b). The downward arrows show the onset of a light flash. (Fig. 3a:modified from Ref. 12)

In the young rats, the normalized amplitude of b-wave decreased during ischemia to 60.6±3.0% of the baseline value under normothermic condition [12] and to 70.8±5.3% under hypothermic condition. During reperfusion, the amplitude of the b-wave recovered to the baseline level by 2 hours under normothermic condition [12], and by 1 hour under hypothermic condition (Fig. 4a and Fig. 4b).

In the aged rats, exposure to ischemia decreased the amplitude of b-wave to 38.9±5.0% under normothermic condition [12] and to 55.3 ± 7.1% under hypothermic condition. In the aged rats, it did not recover to the baseline level within 6 hours during reperfusion under normothermic condition [12], while it recovered by 5 hours under hypothermic condition (Fig. 5a and Fig. 5b).

These results suggest that hypothermic condition accelerates recovery from electrophysiological deterioration of retinal function after ischemia-reperfusion in both young and aged rats. A morphological study showed that hypothermia protects the retina significantly from ischemic injury [3]. Adachi and coworkers demonstrated that ischemia-induced cell loss in the ganglion cell layer was markedly reduced by lowering body temperature to 33°C, suggesting that the process of neurodegeneration after retinal ischemia is dependent on body temperature [1]. Hypothermia is likely to protect retinal cells by inhibiting the action of enzymes and neurotransmitters like glutamate.

We previously showed that the electrophysiological function of the retina was less tolerable against ischemia-reperfuison in aged animals than in young ones [12]. Although aged rats are more susceptible compared to young ones, electrophysiological damage after retinal ischemic episode can be rescued by hypothermic therapy even in aged rats. Ooboshi and coworkers reported that brain hypothermia protects against ischemic neuronal damages even in the aged animals, and the protection is associated with inhibition of excessive effluxes of both excitatory and inhibitory amino acids [19]. Free radicals and excitatory amino acids are generated as a consequence of events occurring during the period of

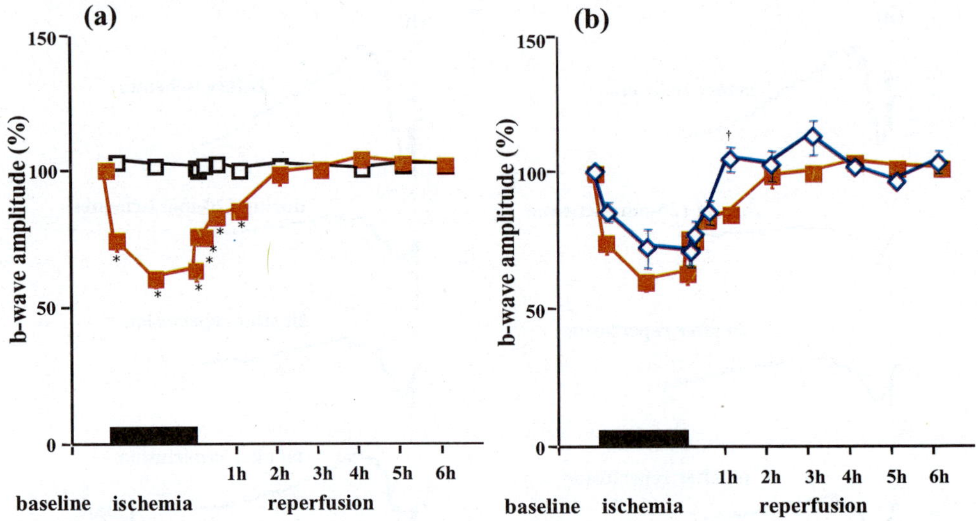

Fig. 4. **Time course of changes in ERG b-wave during ischemia-reperfusion (n = 8 in all groups). (a) Group 1 (young control rats, □-□) and Group 2 (young normothermic rats with 120-min ischemia, ■-■). *$p<0.05$ vs corresponding value in the control group; (b) Group 2 (young normothermic rats with 120-min ischemia, ■-■) and Group 3 (young hypothermic rats with 120-min ischemia, ◇-◇). †$p<0.05$ vs corresponding value in the normothermia group. (Fig. 4a:modified from Ref. 12)**

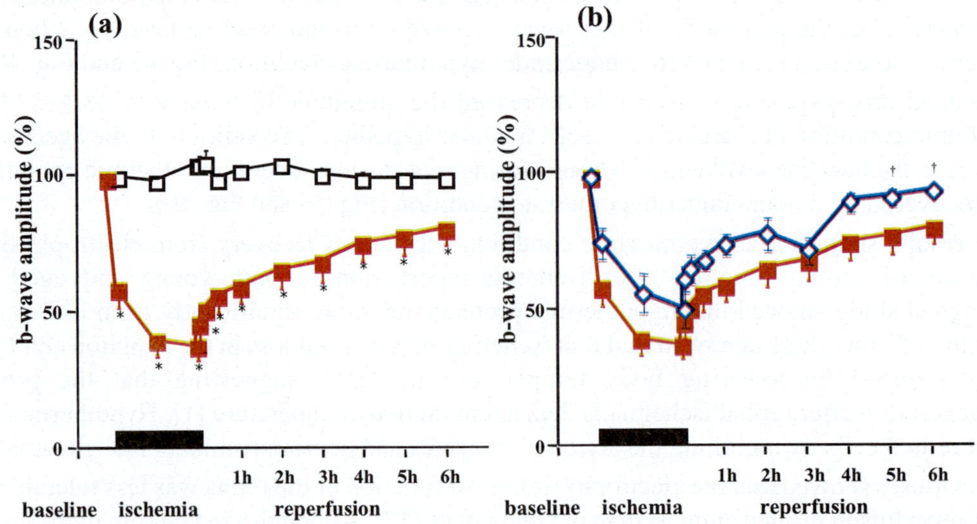

Fig. 5. **Time course of changes in ERG b-wave during ischemia-reperfusion (n = 8 in groups 4 and 5, n = 7 in group 6). (a) Group 4 (aged control rats, □-□) and Group 5 (aged normothermic rats with 120-min ischemia, ■-■). *$p<0.05$ vs corresponding value in the control group; (b) Group 5 (aged normothermic rats with 120-min ischemia, ■-■) and Group 6 (aged hypothermic rats with 120-min ischemia, ◇-◇). †$p<0.05$ vs corresponding value in the normothermia group. (Fig. 5a:modified from Ref. 12)**

ischemia and at the onset of reperfusion. Hypothermia may protect the retina by decreasing adenosine formation, reducing glutamate release, inhibiting protease activation, and decreasing hydroxyl radical production. Further study is needed to obtain the direct evidence.

Tamai and coworkers reported that local application of hypothermia during vitrectomy in ischemic eyes decreased retinal damage [25]. There are another reports that even mild cooling greatly enhanced post-ischemic ERG recovery [18]. Further research is needed to determine whether human's eye can be protected similarly from injury by local hypothermia in clinical situation and what temperature is the best in elderly persons to protect the retina from ischemia-reperfusion injury.

In conclusion, we investigated the effect of hypothermia on b-wave of ERG during ischemia-reperfusion, and the difference in the efficacy of hypothermia between young and aged rats. Hypothermia plays a beneficial role in protecting the retinal function during ischemia-reperfusion even in aged rats. These findings will provide important information for the treatment of elderly patients with retinal ischemic disease.

Acknowledgements

The authors thank Professor A. Tamai, Division of Ophthalmology and Visual Science, Faculty of Medicine, Tottori University, for his critical reading of the manuscript. This research was supported in part by a Grants-in-Aid for Scientific Research (08670051) from the Japanese Ministry of Education, Science, Sports and Culture.

References

1. Adachi, K., Y. Fujita, C. Morizane, A. Akaike, M. Ueda, M. Satoh, H. Masai, S. Kashii and Y. Honda. Inhibition of NMDA receptor and nitric oxide synthese reduces ischemic injury of the reitna. *Eur. J. Pharmacol.* 1998;350: 53-57.
2. Brown, KT. The Electroretinogram: its components and their origins. *Vision Res.* 1968; 8: 633-677.
3. Faberowski, N., E. Stefansson, and R.C. Davidson. Local hypothermia protects the retina from ischemia. *Invest. Ophthalmol. Vis. Sci.* 1989;30: 2309-2313.
4. Feghali, J.G., J.-C. Jin and J.V. Odom. Effect of short-term intraocular pressure elevation on the rabbit electroretinogram. *Invest. Ophthalmol. Vis. Sci.* 1991;32: 2184-2189.
5. Foulds, W.S. and N.F. Johnson. Rabbit electroretinogram during recovery from induced ischaemia. *Trans. Ophthal. So.c U.K.* 1974; 94: 383-393.
6. Hangai, M., K. Miyamoto, K. Hiroi, A. Tujikawa, Y. Ogura, Y. Honda and N. Yoshimura. Roles of constitutive nitric oxide synthase in postischemic rat retina. *Invest. Ophthalmol. Vis. Sci.* 1999;40: 450-458.
7. Hangai, M., N. Yoshimura, K. Hiroi, M. Mandai and Y. Honda. Inducible nitric oxide synthase in retinal ischemia-reperfusion injury. *Exp. Eye Res.* 1996;63: 501-509.
8. Hangai, M., Y. Yoshimura, K. Hiroi, M. Mandai and Y. Honda. Role of nitric oxide during the initial phase of reperfusion after retinal ischemia in the rat. *Ophthalmic. Res.* 1999;31: 16-23.
9. Hughes, W.F. Quantitation of ischemic damage in the rat retina. *Exp. Eye Res.* 1991;53: 573-582.
10. Ishihara, M., T. Nakano, E. Ohama and Y. Kawai. Postischemic reperfusion in the eyes of young and aged rats. *Jpn. J. Physiol.* 2000;50: 125-132.
11. Johnson, N.F. Effects of acute ischaemia on the structure of the rabbit retina. *Trans. Ophthal. Soc. UK* 1974; 94: 394-405.

12. Katano, H., M. Ishihara, Y. Shiraishi and Y. Kawai. Effects of aging on the electrorerinogram during ischemia-reperfusion in rats. *Jpn. J. Physiol.* 2001;51:89 –97.
13. Lawwill, T. Practical rabbit electroretinography. *Am. J. Ophthalmol.* 1972;74: 135-41.
14. Lewis, F.J., M. Traufic and M. Minn. Closure of arterial septal defects with the aid of hypothermia; Experimental accomplishment and the report of one of successful case. *Surgery* 1953; 33: 52-59.
15. Matsuura, K. and Y. Kawai. Effects of hypothermia and aging on postischemic reperfusion in rat eyes. *Jpn. J. Physiol.* 1998;48: 9-15.
16. McDowall, D.G. The current usage of hypothermia in British neurosurgery. *Br. J. Anaesth.* 1971;43:1083-1087.
17. Miller, R.F. and J.E. Dowling. Intracellular responses of the Muller (glial) cells of mudpuppy retina: their relation to b-wave of the erectroretinogram. *J. Neurophysiol.* 1970;33: 323-341.
18. Nayak, M.S. and M.F. Marmor. Post-ischemia ERG recovery is influenced by temperature. *Curr. Eye Res.* 1995;14: 81-85.
19. Ooboshi, H., S. Ibayashi, K. Takano, S. Sadoshima, A. Kondo, H. Uchimura and M. Fujishima. Hypothermia inhibits ischemia-induced efflux of amino acids and neuronal damage in the hippocampus of aged rats. *Brain Res.* 2000;884: 23-30.
20. Ostwald, P., I.M. Goldstein, A. Pachnanda and S. Roth. Effect of nitric oxide synthase inhibition on blood flow after retinal ischemia in cats. *Invest. Ophthalmol. Vis. Sci.* 1995;36: 2396-2403.
21. Ostwald, P., S.S. Park, A.Y. Toledano and S. Roth. Adenosine receptor blockade and nitric oxide synthase inhibition in the retina: impact upon post-ischemic hyperemia and the electroretinogram. *Vision Res.* 1997;37: 3453-3461.
22. Riva, C.E., S.D. Cranstoun, R.M. Mann and G.E. Barnes. Local choroidal blood flow in the cat by laser Doppler flowmetry. *Invest. Ophthalmol. Vis. Sci.* 1994;35: 608-618.
23. Roth, S. and Z. Pietrzyk. Blood flow after retinal ischemia in cats. *Invest. Ophthalmol. Vis. Sci.* 1994;35: 3209-3217.
24. Spivey, B.E. and J.T. Pearlman. Day-to-day variation in the ERG of humans and rabbits. *Am. J. Ophthalmol.* 1963;55: 1013-20.
25. Tamai, K. and E. Toumoto. Effect of local hypotheremia on ischmic eyes in vitrectomy. *Jpn. J. Ophthalmol.* 1996;40: 220-228.
26. Veriac, S., G. Tissie and C. Bonne. Oxygen free radicals adversely affect the regulation of vascular tone by nitric oxide in the rabbit retina under high intraocular pressure. *Exp. Eye Res.* 1993;56: 85-88.
27. Yonemura, D. and K. Kawasaki. Electrophysiological study on activities of neuronal and non-neuronal retinal elements in man with reference to its clinical application. *Jpn. J. Ophthalmol.* 1978;22: 195-213.

Adaptation Biology and Medicine (Volume 4: Current Concepts)
Editors: A. Hargens, N. Takeda and P.K. Singal

24. Simultaneous Measurements of Cerebral and Muscle Oxygenation and Blood Volume Responses in Healthy Men during Exposure to Seated Whole-body Vibration (WBV)

Rammohan V. Maikala[1], Yagesh N. Bhambhani[2]

[1]Liberty Mutual Research Institute for Safety, Hopkinton, MA 01748, USA,
email: rammohan.maikala@libertymutual.com, FAX: 508-435-0482
[2]Faculty of Rehabilitation Medicine, University of Alberta, Edmonton, T6G 2P6, CANADA

Abstract

Aim: To evaluate the changes in cerebral and erector spinae oxygenation and blood volume measured by near infrared spectroscopy during rhythmic handgrip contractions while subjects were exposed to whole body vibration (WBV). **Methods:** Thirteen healthy males were randomly exposed to three doses (3, 4.5, and 6 Hz at approximately $0.9g_{r.m.s}$ in the vertical direction) of WBV on a seated vibrating base with backrest support. Each independent session included 6 min baseline period without WBV, 8 min of WBV exposure including 1 min of right hand maximal voluntary intermittent rhythmic handgrip contractions, and 4 min recovery. One NIRS sensor was placed on the right frontal lobe and another was placed on the right lumbar erector spinae muscle at the L3 level. **Results:** Systematic increases were observed in the cerebral oxygenation and blood volume responses at each dose compared to the seated resting condition, implying increased blood perfusion and neuronal activity during WBV to the pre-frontal cortex. Concomitantly, muscle oxygenation and blood volume decreased during WBV compared to the initial baseline, suggesting a reduction in muscle venous oxygen saturation due to vibration. Statistical analysis revealed that changes in cerebral and muscle oxygenation and blood volume responses were similar during all doses of WBV. Addition of the handgrip contractions during WBV elicited further increases in the cerebral responses, suggesting an increase in cerebral activity resulting from functional motor simulation. As well, there was a greater decrease in erector spinae oxygenation without a significant change in blood volume, suggesting greater oxygen extraction in the muscle. **Conclusions:** These acute changes in tissue oxygenation and blood volume during exposure to WBV indicate that there is a heterogeneity of perfusion and oxygen delivery in cerebral and muscle tissue. These alterations may be one of the reasons why exposure to WBV is implicated in occupational low-back pain.

Introduction

Whole-body vibration (WBV) is vibration transmitted to the entire human body from a vibrating surface such as the seat in a heavy equipment vehicle, truck, bus or aircraft. The most dominant frequency dose identified in motorized vehicles ranges from 3 to 6 Hz (Wilder et al. 1982), with the transfer of maximum mechanical energy to the spine resulting at about 4.5 to 5 Hz (Panjabi et al. 1986, Pope et al. 1998, Wilder et al. 1982). It has been demonstrated that the transmissibility of vibration from the buttocks to the head in a seated posture increases in an exponential manner (Wilder et al. 1982). Electromyographic WBV studies of the paraspinal muscles in the low-back demonstrated the development of localized muscular fatigue in a variety of postural positions and vibration doses (Hansson et al. 1991, Pope et al. 1998, Wilder et al. 1982). It was suggested that this localized fatigue could be due to compromised blood flow, resulting in reduced oxygenation and availability of nutrients to these muscles (Hansson et al. 1991, Pope et al. 1990; Zimmerman et al. 1993). This hypothesis, however, has yet to be objectively tested. Compared to exposure to WBV alone, physical factors such as handling controls, static work, prolonged sitting, attention, mental stress, in association with environmental factors such as noise, light, temperature, etc. might have additive or variable effects on WBV exposed populations (Manninen 1988, Seidel et al. 1988). However, the role of physical work (e.g., handgrip) on cerebral and muscle activity during WBV, and its influence on human performance has not been investigated.

Near infra-red spectroscopy (NIRS) is a non-invasive optical technique capable of measuring changes in oxygenation and blood volume in the near infra-red region (700 to 1000 nm) in the skeletal muscle and brain (Chance et al. 1988, Mancini et al. 1994, Villringer et al. 1994). Tissue oxygenation, defined as the relative saturation of oxyhemoglobin, depends on the balance between oxygen delivery and localized metabolic rate (Mancini et al. 1994, Simonson and Piantadosi 1996). NIRS indicates the relative change in tissue oxygenation within the illuminated area by measuring the difference in tissue absorbency between the oxygenated and deoxygenated states of hemoglobin in the near infra-red range. Sum of these two states of hemoglobin reflects the changes in the cerebral blood volume of the illuminated region of the tissue. The validity of NIRS in evaluating changes in cerebral and muscle oxygenation and blood volume has been well established in humans (Hamoka et al. 2000, Mancini et al. 1994, Pollard et al. 1996, Quaresima et al. 2000, Sako et al. 2001). The reliability of this technique in evaluating cerebral and erector spinae muscle oxygenation and blood volume was reported recently (Bhambhani et al. 2000, Maikala et al. 2000).

To date, cerebral functional activity research using NIRS has been limited to cognitive demand, motor activation, and visual stimulation studies (Colier et al. 1999, Fallgatter and Strik 1998, Hock et al. 1997, Hoshi and Tamura 1993, Obrig et al. 1996, Obrig and Villringer 1997, Villringer et al. 1994). These studies demonstrate an increase in cerebral oxygenation and blood volume during psychomotor tasks, implying greater neruronal activation under these conditions. Similarly, erector spinae oxygenation and blood volume changes using NIRS have been limited to sub-maximal and maximal isometric contractions (Jensen et al. 1999, McGill et al. 2000, Maikala et al. 2000, Yoshitake et al. 2001). No studies, however have evaluated the oxygenation and blood volume trends in both cerebral and skeletal muscle regions during exposure to WBV.

The purposes of this study were to examine the effects of 3 Hz, 4.5 Hz, and 6 Hz WBV doses on the relative changes in oxygenation and blood volume, simultaneously both in the prefrontal cortex region and lumbar erector spinae muscle, in healthy men during with and without handgrip exercise. It was hypothesized that: (1) cerebral and lumbar erector spinae muscle oxygenation and blood volume responses will differ significantly during exposure to WBV but would be independent of the dose, and (2) the changes in cerebral and muscle oxygenation and blood volume would not be effected by the addition of handgrip exercise during WBV.

Materials and Methods

Written informed consent was obtained from thirteen healthy men (age 24.7 ± 3.9 yrs, mass 70.8 ± 12.1 kg, height 1.71 ± 0.07 m, right hand grip strength 34.2 ± 9.1 kg). Subjects were undergraduate and graduate students recruited from the university population, and all subjects were right hand dominant. They all completed the Revised Physical Activity Readiness Questionnaire (Canadian Society for Exercise Physiology, 1994) to identify contraindications for exercise. The test protocols utilized were approved by the Human Ethics Review Board at the University of Alberta.

Vibrating base

A steel vibrating base that housed an electro-mechanical motor connected to a cam mechanism (Advanced Therapy Products, Inc., VA, USA) was modified with an external DC speed control device. Varying the speed of this motor from 0 to 100% corresponded to vibrating frequencies of 0 Hz to 6.2 Hz. These frequencies were verified with an oscilloscope (Hitachi Digital Oscilloscope VC-6050, JAPAN). The vibrating base was also attached with a displacement transducer (Intertechnology, Inc., ON, CANADA) to measure the cam linear displacement during vibration. The average linear displacement with a subject sitting on the base during vibration was 6.1 mm at 3 Hz, 6.4 mm at 4.5 Hz and 6.6 mm at 6 Hz. The vibrating base was fitted with a seat that had an internal spring-suspension system with a weight-adjustable knob. This seat was adjustable to accommodate a maximum sitting weight capacity of 300 lbs. Acceleration of the vibrating base was measured by a tri-axial micro-machined accelerometer (Crossbow, Inc., CA, USA), and was found to be approximately $0.9g_{r.m.s}$ in the vertical direction.

Test protocols

Each subject was exposed to three WBV tests with each dose (3 Hz, 4.5 Hz, and 6 Hz) administered on a separate day in randomized order. The test protocol on each day lasted 18 minutes, and included initial six-minute rest without vibration, eight-minute vibration, and four-minute recovery from vibration. Throughout the test, subjects sat in the vibrating chair against the backrest support with the eyes open. A footrest was provided for subjects to place their feet at a comfortable level.

Before the vibration session, right hand grip size was adjusted on the dynamometer (JAMAR, CA, USA) to a position that was comfortable for each subject. During the fifth minute of each vibration condition, the subject performed rhythmic maximal contractions for one minute at a contraction rate of one every five seconds. Contractions were performed with the right hand with the forearm in a horizontal position and the elbow at an angle of 180°. The accuracy of the handgrip dynamometer was verified by calibrating it against known weights, according to the procedure described by Schmidt and Toews (1970).

Oxygenation and blood volume measurements

Two continuous dual wave NIRS units (MicroRunman, NIM Inc., PA, USA) were used to evaluate relative changes in cerebral and muscle oxygenation and blood volume during the vibration tests. Each unit consists of: a superficial sensor consisting of a tungsten lamp placed at a distance of 4 cm from two silicone diodes which absorb light at 760 nm and 850 nm and a display unit that amplifies the absorbency signal generated. Before calibration, one sensor was placed on the anterior right frontal lobe approximately 2-4 cm from the mid-line of the forehead and 2 cm above the supra-orbital ridge (Fallgatter and Strik 1998, Obrig et al. 1996). Using a linear scale, the sensor placement on each subject's head was measured and was used for all the vibration sessions. For muscle NIRS measurements, the second NIRS sensor was placed at the 3rd Lumbar region and 3 cm from the mid line of the spine. Placement of the sensor was noted to the nearest millimeter, thus ensuring its correct placement on each subject for all the testing sessions. A piece of clear plastic was wrapped around the sensor to prevent sweat from distorting the absorbency signal. Further, a dark elastic bandage was wrapped around each sensor to secure it in place and minimize any loss of light.

As per the manufacturer's specifications, each sensor was calibrated at 760 nm and 850 nm wavelengths before the test for each subject. The vertical penetration depth of light was set to 4 cm. The difference in absorbency between these two wavelengths indicated the change in oxygenation saturation and the sum of these absorbencies indicated the change in total blood volume. Both oxygenation and blood volume responses were measured in terms of optical density, which is defined as the logarithmic ratio of intensity of light calibrated at each wavelength to the intensity of measured light at the same wavelength (MicroRunman User Manual, NIM Inc., PA, USA, 1999). Real time data were recorded using the NIRCOM software provided by the manufacturer.

NIRS Data Analysis

The real time NIRS optical density values were averaged every 20 seconds using a customized Microsoft Excel software program specially designed for this study. Baseline oxygenation and blood volume values were monitored during initial rest from each vibration dose.

Cerebral changes

Maximum optical density values for cerebral region were identified for each dose during vibration with and without rhythmic handgrip contractions. The change (delta) in cerebral oxygenation and blood volume for each vibration dose (3Hz, 4.5 Hz, and 6 Hz) and workload (vibration alone and vibration combined with rhythmic handgrip contractions), was calculated as the difference between the maximum and baseline optical density values identified for each phase of the test session. Oxygenation and blood volume responses 20 seconds before the beginning of each WBV session were identified as baseline values, and were used to calculate delta values.

Lumbar erector spinae muscle changes

Minimum optical density values for muscle were recorded for each dose during vibration with and without rhythmic handgrip contractions. Delta values for both oxygenation and blood volume responses for each condition of vibration dose and workload were calculated as the difference between the baseline and minimum values. Similar to the cerebral region, oxygenation and blood volume values 20 seconds before the beginning of each WBV session were identified as baseline values, and were used to calculate delta values.

Statistical Analysis

All statistical analyses were performed using the delta values calculated for each test session. A two-way analysis of variance, using two repeated measures factors (dose and workload) with a fully crossed design was used to evaluate the differences in the oxygenation and blood volume responses. To minimize the violation of the assumption of homogeneity of variance, the 'Greenhouse-Geiser' adjustment was used. Since multiple comparisons were made for each dependent variable in the present study, the Bonferroni adjustment for a P value of 0.05 was applied to minimize Type 1 error. The Bonferroni adjustment was calculated as the ratio of 0.05 and number of statistical comparisons. Thus, statistical significance was considered at $P < 0.01$. Significant F ratios were further analyzed with the Scheffe post hoc multiple comparison test. The Statistical Package for Social Sciences SPSS (version 10) was used for all statistical analyses (SPSS Inc., Chicago, USA).

Results

NIRS trends during different doses of whole body vibration

Cerebral region

A typical profile of the cerebral oxygenation and blood volume trends at 4.5 Hz dose for one subject is shown in Figures 1a and 1b respectively. It is evident that as soon as the vibration started, cerebral oxygenation and blood volume increased from the baseline (resting) value during the 4 minute period. During vibration combined with rhythmic handgrip contractions for 1 minute, both these variables increased to higher levels compared to vibration alone. As soon as the rhythmic handgrip contractions stopped, cerebral oxygenation and blood volume dropped to the initial vibration level. During recovery from WBV, the values dropped further towards the baseline levels (Figures 1a and 1b).

No significant differences were observed in the mean oxygenation and blood volume values for all doses ($P > 0.01$). However, mean oxygenation and blood volume values were significantly higher during vibration combined with rhythmic handgrip contractions than during vibration alone (Figures 2a and 2b respectively).

Lumbar erector spinae muscle

A typical profile of the lumbar erector spinae oxygenation and blood volume trends at a dose of 4.5 Hz is shown in Figures 1a and 1b respectively. It is evident from both figures that as soon as the vibration started, oxygenation and blood volume responses increased slightly for about 20-30 seconds, and then decreased from the baseline (resting) value during the four-minute period. During vibration combined with rhythmic handgrip contractions, oxygenation values decreased to a lower level than vibration alone. As soon as the rhythmic handgrip contractions stopped during vibration, oxygenation (Figure 1a) and blood volume (Figure 1b) trends returned to the initial vibration level. In the recovery phase, oxygenation and blood volume responses increased towards the baseline values.

No significant differences were observed in mean oxygenation ($P = 0.636$) and blood volume ($P = 0.405$) values for all doses. However, mean oxygenation and blood volume values were significantly higher during vibration combined with rhythmic handgrip contractions than vibration alone (Figures 3a and 3b respectively).

Discussion

Occupations which involve exposure to WBV are often associated with factors such as awkward (and often prolonged) posture, constant attention during driving, operating various controls and hand-held

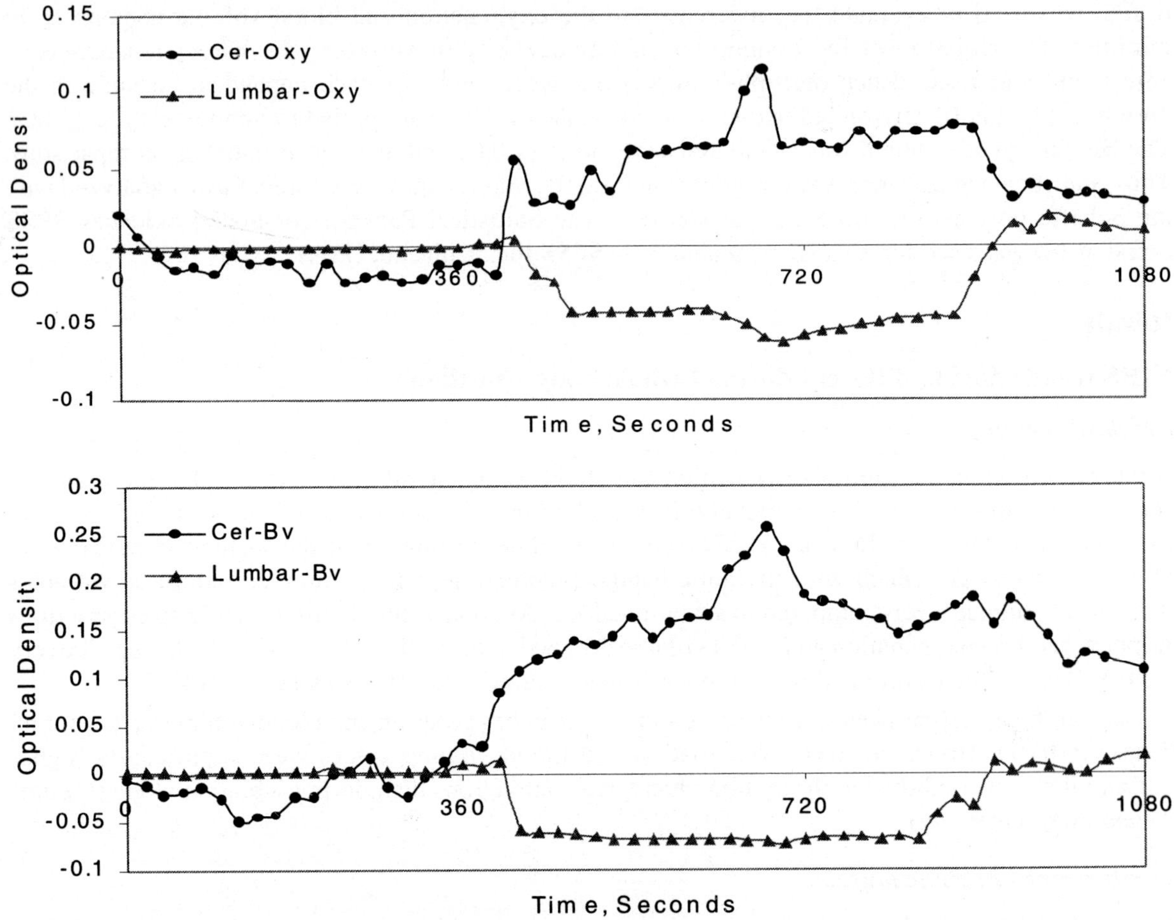

Fig. 1. **a. Oxygenation Trends during Vibration @ 4.5 Hz [$0.9g_{rms}$]**
b. Blood Volume Trends during Vibration @ 4.5 Hz [$0.9g_{rms}$]

levers, etc. These activities combined with WBV can be both physically demanding and mentally challenging. Such combined exposures have been implicated in both low-back disorders (Pope et al. 1998), and development of neck pain leading to headaches (Scutter et al. 1997). Hence, it is important to understand the energetics of specific tissues, in particular the 'focal' changes in cerebral and muscle regions that may be recruited simultaneously during exposure to WBV.

In this study, NIRS was used to examine the acute changes in oxygenation and blood volume simultaneously in the lumbar erector spinae muscle (as an indirect measure of evaluating physical workload) and pre-frontal cortex region (as an indirect measure of evaluating psychological workload) during exposure to 3 Hz, 4.5 Hz and 6 Hz WBV in healthy men and women. The subjects were asked to perform a motor task (maximal rhythmic handgrip contractions for a period of one minute) during WBV. Exposure to WBV elicited an increase in cerebral oxygenation and blood volume with a concomitant decrease in these variables in the lumbar erector spinae muscle. These changes were not dependent upon the WBV dose. Addition of handgrip work elicited an increase in cerebral activation

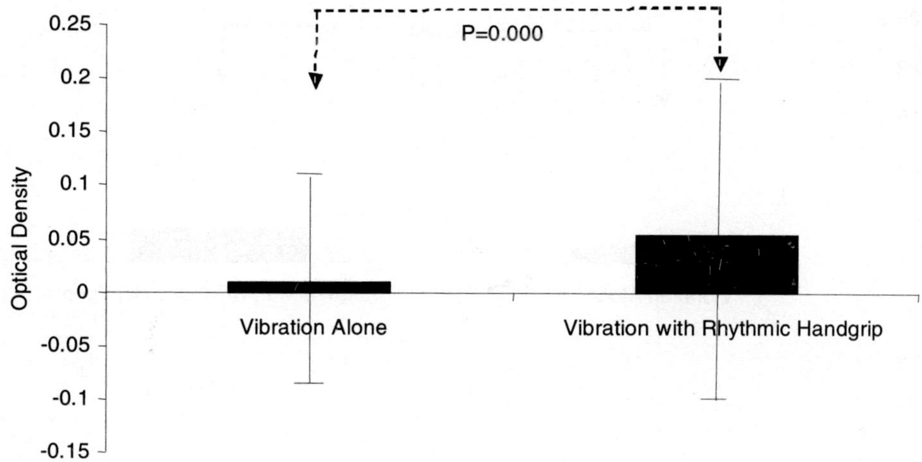

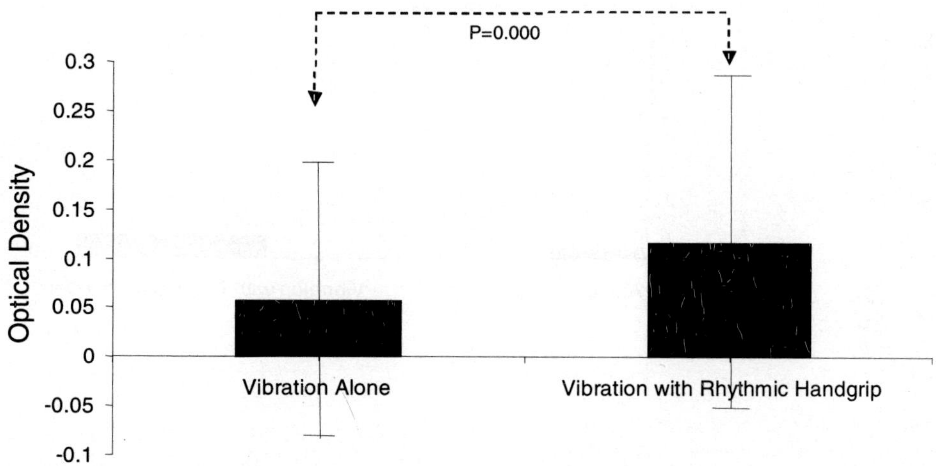

Fig. 2. **a. Effect of Handgrip Contractions - Oxygenation Chanages (Means ± SD)**
b. Effect of Handgrip Contractions - Blood Volume Changes (Mean ± SD)

(indicated by increases in both cerebral oxygenation and blood volume responses) with a concomitant decrease in the lumbar erector spinae muscle oxygenation (and blood volume responses in majority of subjects).

These observations raise several interesting questions. Why is an increase in cerebral oxygenation and blood volume associated with a concomitant decrease in lumbar erector spinae oxygenation and blood volume during WBV, and vice versa? Why does such an inverse relationship exist between these two tissues? Does an increase in cerebral activation observed in the right prefrontal cortex in the present study demonstrate a physiological pathway from the muscle to the brain during WBV?

During WBV, a decrease in substance P [in the dorsal root ganglion, a major output structure of the frontal cortex and considered as the 'brain' of the functional spinal unit (Weinstein 1991)] has been considered to be an indication of increased axonal transport in the brain. Based on animal studies, several authors reported an increase of axonal transport in the frontal cortex during WBV, thus

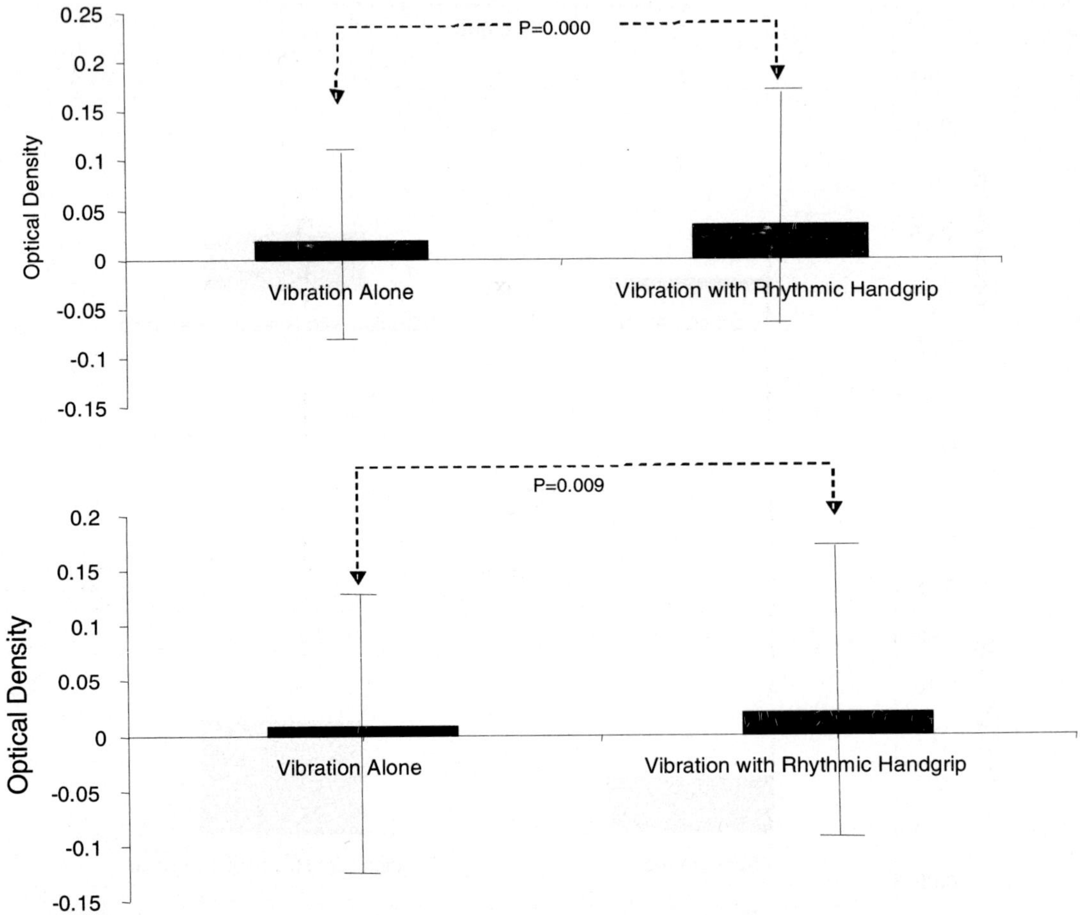

Fig. 3. **a. Effect of Handgrip Contractions - Oxygenation Changes (Mean ± SD)**
b. Effect of Handgrip Contractions - Blood Volume Changes (Mean ± SD)

affecting the neuropeptides (e.g. substance P) present in the sensory parts of the nervous system (Nakamura et al. 1988 and 1994, Weinstein 1991, Weinstein et al. 1988). The present findings demonstrated that there was an increase in the 'focal' cerebral oxygenation and blood volume in the prefrontal cortex during all conditions of WBV (compared to rest without WBV or post-WBV period), suggesting an increase in neuronal activity with a subsequent increase in perfusion to the prefrontal cortex (Villringer and Chance 1997). This indirect evidence suggests a possible afferent feedback to the cerebral cortex during exposure to WBV in humans. It appears, therefore, that the increase in synaptic activity resulting from exposure to WBV elicits an increase in cerebral oxygenation and blood volume in the pre-frontal cortex which can be monitored non-invasively using NIRS.

Spinal reflex studies have demonstrated a decrease in human sensorimotor performance during WBV, suggesting a possible feedback mechanism induced by vibration via the proprioceptive and central nervous systems (Gauthier et al. 1981, Martin et al. 1984, Roll et al. 1980). Martin et al. (1984) regarded the role of WBV as a combination of synchronous vibration applied 'locally' and simultaneously to several muscle tendons. The current observations in the specific paraspinal muscle suggest that WBV induces a 'localized vasoconstrictor stimulus' in the regions of the lumbar erector spinae muscle. Consequently, the reduction in blood flow would result in a lower blood volume and greater deoxygenation in this area monitored by NIRS. Based on electromyographic investigations, Hansson et al. (1991) hypothesized that there was a lack of blood flow to the back muscles during exposure to WBV. Kauppila and Tallroth (1993) investigated postmortem lumbar arteriorgrams of subjects with and without low-back pain in the lumbar and middle sacral arteries, and demonstrated that "insufficient arterial blood flow may be an underlying factor for low-back symptoms". Thus, the current evidence, demonstrates that the decrease in oxygenation may be the result of a compromised blood flow to the paraspinal muscles during WBV, and supports the use of NIRS in evaluating these changes.

It has been shown that 'localized' vibration (e.g. hand-arm vibration during a drilling task in 'construction' occupations) results in vasoconstriction of blood vessels in the hand thereby enhancing peripheral circulatory disturbances. This condition is termed "Vibration-induced White Finger" or "Raynaud Phenomenon" (Griffin 1990). Martin and Park (1997) showed that such localized vibration triggers the tonic vibration reflex in active muscles. However, to date there are no studies that have demonstrated the tonic vibration reflex in the trunk muscles during WBV. It could be argued that since exposure to WBV is a 'cumulative' of local vibrations being transmitted from the seat, floor, backrest, body segments, etc., a mechanism similar to the 'Raynaud Phenomenon' might occur 'locally' at the paraspinal muscles during prolonged exposure to WBV, thus resulting in a decrease in muscle oxygenation and blood volume in this area.

Several authors have demonstrated an increase in the erector spinae muscle activity during cycling or repetitive loading due to WBV results in a greater recruitment of motor units in this muscle group (Pope et al. 1998, Seroussi et al. 1989, Wilder et al. 1982). Based on the current investigations, this increase in muscular activity might lead to increased cortical activation. It can be argued that in contrast to the vasoconstrictor stimulus observed in the lumbar erector spinae muscle (demonstrated through decrease in oxygenation and blood volume), WBV elicits a cerebral 'vasodilator stimulus' as a result of increased vibration transmission to the head.

Another factor that should be considered is the cerebral oxygen extraction factor. Based on human positron emission tomography studies of somatosensory and visual stimulation, Fox and Raichle (1984) and Fox et al. (1988) demonstrated a greater proportion of increase in cerebral blood flow and cerebral glucose utilization, but a very small increase in the cerebral oxygen uptake. Such an imbalance in these variables suggests that less oxygen is being removed from the blood; i.e., a low cerebral oxygen extraction factor. This phenomenon might result in vasodilation and opening of precapillaries (thus maintaining autoregulation), accompanied by an increase in both cerebral blood volume and oxygenation trends. In contrast, based on the trunk muscle NIRS trends, it could be argued that the oxygen extraction in the muscle is considerably greater than that occurring simultaneously in the brain during WBV. This could be the result of vasoconstriction in the 'focal' muscle during this period, which would compromise blood flow and therefore result in reduced blood volume and oxygenation. Along these lines, Jorgensen (1997) stated that: "muscle contraction may increase the intramuscular pressure and thereby cause restriction of the blood flow which limits the rate of energy supply". The reverse cerebral and muscle trends observed concomitantly during exposure to WBV may suggest a redistribution of blood [the 'stealing' phenomenon as addressed by McAllister (1997)] to the brain to match the needs of neuronal activity due to WBV. Similarly, Schumacker and Cain (1987) proposed that *optimization of blood flow* occurs in such a way that the regional redistribution in the tissues matches its metabolic activity, thereby minimizing the possibility of overperfusing some organs. Moreover, Sibbald et al. (2000) suggested a positive correlation between perfusion heterogeneity and heterogeneous tissue metabolic demand.

It is conceivable, therefore, that during WBV a differential outflow of blood to these two regions in need (i.e., cerebral and lumbar erector spinae muscle) at the same time might have resulted in the contrasting trends observed in the oxygenation and blood volume responses. If such an argument is tenable, such a dual and out-of-phase phenomenon suggests that the human body is trying to maintain homeostasis while matching the needs of oxygen demand at the 'focal' lumbar erector spinae muscle region to the oxygen delivery to the brain at the same time.

Although these acute responses provide useful information, it is essential to study the effects of chronic WBV exposure (hours per shift to days and years of exposure) to determine the long term effects on these tissues. These results will help health professionals develop dose-response guidelines for populations exposed to WBV in various industries, information that is currently lacking in the widely used Human WBV Standards document (ISO 2631/part 1, 1997). Furthermore, many of the occupations in which individuals are exposed to WBV necessitate manual work such as the operation of controls, gripping tools, etc. Based on the present findings, the addition of rhythmic isometric work significantly elevated cerebral oxygenation and blood volume responses and simultaneously reduced muscle oxygenation and blood volume responses to a greater extent, compared to the absence of such physical work. Such work-related factors should also be considered in designing workstations and seats in motorized vehicles and in recommending non-vibration hand-operated controls to be used by the exposed populations, in order to minimize undue fatigue and reduce the risk of musculoskeletal injuries in the workplace.

Conclusions

The results of this study indicated that exposure to eight minutes of seated WBV between 3Hz to 6Hz elicits significant increases in cerebral oxygenation and blood volume suggesting increased neuronal activation. As well, such exposures also elicit significant decreases in erector spinae oxygenation and blood volume, implying greater oxygen utilization. The addition of a handgrip exercise increased the changes in the cerebral and muscle oxygenation responses, indicating further cerebral activation and enhanced metabolic demand. All these responses were independent of the WBV dose administered to the subjects.

References

1. Bhambhani Y, Maikala R, Farag M, and Ting W (2000) Reliability of cerebral oxygenation measurements during rhythmic handgrip contractions using near infra-red spectroscopy (Abstract). Canadian Society of Exercise Physiology Annual Scientific Conference, October 25-28, Canmore, CANADA
2. Chance B, Leigh JS, Miyake H, Smith DS, Nioka S, Greenfeld R, Finander M, Kaufmann K, Levy W, Young M, Cohen P, Yoshioka H, and Boretsky R (1988) Comparison of time-resolved and –unresolved measurements of deoxyhemoglobin in brain. *Proc Natl Acad Sci USA* 85: 4971-4975
3. Colier WNJM, Quaresima V, Oeseburg B, and Ferrari M (1999) Human motor-cortex oxygenation changes induced by cyclic coupled movements of hand and foot. *Exp Brain Res* 129: 457-461

4. Fallgatter AJ and Strik WK (1998) Frontal brain activation during the Wisconsin card sorting test assessed with two-channel near-infrared spectroscopy. *Eur Arch Psychiatry Clin Neurosci* 248: 245-249
5. Fox PT and Raichle ME (1984) Stimulus rate determines regional brain blood flow in straite cortex. *Ann Neurol* 17: 303-305
6. Fox PT, Raichle ME, Mintun MA, and Dence C (1988) Nonoxidative glucose consumption during focal physiologic neural activity. *Science* 241: 462-464
7. Gauthier GM, Roll JP, Martin B, and Harlay F (1981) Effects of whole-body vibrations on sensory motor system performance in man. *Aviat Space Envi Med* 52(8): 473-479
8. Giller CA, Giller AM, Cooper CR, and Hatab MR (2000) Evaluation of the cerebral hemodynamic response to rhythmic handgrip. *J Appl Physiol* 88: 2205-2213
9. Griffin MJ (1990) Vibration and discomfort. In: *Handbook of Human Vibration.* New York, Academic Press, pp 43-123
10. Hamoka T, Katsumura T, Murase N, Nishio S, Osada T, Sako T, Higuchi H, Kurosawa Y, Shimomitsu T, Miwa M, and Chance B (2000) Quantifiation of ischemic muscle deoxygenation by near infrared time-resolved spectroscopy. *J Biomed optics* 5(1): 102-105
11. Hansson T, Magnusson M, and Broman H (1991) Back muscle fatigue and seated whole-body vibrations: an experimental study in man. *Clin Biomech* 6(3): 173-178
12. Hock C, Villringer K, Heekeren H, Hofmann M, Wenzel R, Villringer A, and Muller-Spahn F (1997) A role for near infrared spectroscopy in psychiatry? *Adv Exp Med Biol* 413: 105-23
13. Hoshi Y and Tamura M (1993) Detection of dynamic changes in cerebral oxygenation coupled to neuronal function during mental work in man. *Neurosci Lett* 150: 5-8
14. International Organization for Standardization 2631 Part 1 (1997) Mechanical vibration and shock - Evaluation of human exposure to whole-body vibration – Part 1: General Requirements. ISO 2631/1-1997 (E)
15. Jensen BR, Jorgensen K, Hargens AR, Nielsen PK, and Nicolaisen T (1999) Physiological response to submaximal isometric contractions of the paravetebral muscles. *Spine* 24(22): 2332-2338
16. Jorgensen K (1997) Human trunk extensor muscles physiology and ergonomics. *Acta Physiol Scand Suppl* 160: 1-58
17. Kauppila LI and Tallroth K (1993) Postmortem angiographic findings for arteries supplying the lumbar spine: Their relationship to low-back symptoms. *J Spinal Disord* 6(2): 124-129
18. McAllister RM (1997) Adaptations in control of blood flow with training: splanchnic and renal blood flows. *Med Sci Sports Exerc* 30(3): 375-381
19. McGill SM, Hughson RL, and Parks K (2000) Lumbar erector spinae oxygenation during prolonged contractions: implications for prolonged work. *Ergonomics* 43(4): 486-493
20. Maikala R, Farag M, and Bhambhani Y (2000) Low-back muscle oxygenation trends during simple postural variations – Intersession reliability using NIRS. Proceedings of International Ergonomics Conference, San Diego, USA: pp 5.9-5.12
21. Mancini DM, Bolinger L, Kendrick K, Chance B, and Wilson J (1994) Validation of NIRS in humans. *J Appl Physiol* 77: 2740-2747
22. Manninen O (1988) Changes in hearing, cardiovascular functions, haemodynamics, upright body sway, urinary catecholamines and their correlates after prolonged successive exposures to complex environmental conditions. *Int Arch Occup Environ Health* 60: 249-272
23. Martin BJ, Roll JP, and Gauthier GM (1984) Spinal reflex alterations as a function of intensity and frequency of vibration applied to the feet of seated subjects. *Aviat Space Envi Med* 55(1): 8-12
24. Martin BJ and Park H (1997) Analysis of the tonic vibration reflex: influence of vibration variables on motor unit synchronization and fatigue. *Eur J Appl Physiol* 75: 504-511
25. Nakamura H, Moroji T, Nagase H, Okazawa T, and Okada A (1994) Changes of cerebral vasoactive intestinal polypeptide and somatostatin-like immunoreactivity induced by noise and whole-body vibration in the rat. *Eur J Appl Phyisiol* 68: 62-67

26. Nakamura H, Okada A, Nohara S, and Nakamura H (1988) The effect of whole body vibration on the cerebral metabolites in rats. Aerospace Science – Proceedings of the 1st Nihon University International Symposium on Aerospace Medicine, Nihon University Press, Japan, pp 153-156
27. Obrig H, Hirth C, Junge-Hulbsing JG, Doge C, Wolf T, Dirnagl U, and Villringer A (1996) Cerebral oxygenation changes in response to motor stimulation. *J Appl Physiol* 81(3): 1174-1183
28. Obrig H and Villringer A (1997) Near-infrared spectroscopy in functional activation studies. *Adv Exp Med Biol* 413: 113-127
29. Panjabi MM, Andersson GBJ, Jorneus L, Hult E, and Mattsson L (1986) In vivo measurement of spinal column vibrations. *J Bone Joint Surg* 68A(5): 695-703
30. Pollard V, Prough DS, DeMelo E, Deyo DJ, Uchida T, and Stoddart HF (1996) Validation in volunteers of a near-infrared spectroscope for monitoring brain oxygenation in vivo. *Anesth Analg* 82: 269-277
31. Pope MH, Magnusson M, and Wilder D (1998) Kappa Delta Award - Low back pain and whole-body vibration. *Clin Orthop Research* 354: 241-248
32. Pope MH, Magnusson M, Lindell V, Svensson M, Andersson GBJ (1990). The measurement of oxygen uptake under whole-body vibration. *Iowa Orthop* J 10: 85-88
33. Quaresima V, Sacco S, Totaro R, and Ferrari M (2000) Noninvasive measurement of cerebral hemoglobin oxygen saturation using two near infrared spectroscopy approaches. *J Biomed Optics* 5: 201-205
34. Roll JP, Martin B, Gauthier GM, and Ivaldi FM (1980) Effects of whole-body vibration on spinal reflexes in man. *Aviat. Space Environ Med* 51: 1227-1233
35. Sako T, Hamaoka T, Higuchi H, Kurosawa Y, and Katsumura T (2001) Validity of NIRS spectroscopy for quantitatively measuring muscle oxidative metabolic rate in exercise. *J Appl Physiol* 90: 338-344
36. Schmidt RT and Toews JV (1970) Grip strength as measured by the Jamar dynamometer. *Arch Phys Med Rehab* 51: 321-327
37. Schumacker PT and Cain SM (1987) The concept of a critical oxygen delivery. *Int Care Med* 13: 223-229
38. Scutter S, Turker KS, and Hall R (1997) Headaches and neck pain in farmers. *Aust J Rural Health* 5(1): 2-5
39. Seidel H, Harazin B, Pavlas K, Sroka C, Richter J, Bluthner R, Erdmann U, Grzesik J, Hinz B, and Rothe R (1988) Isolated and combined effects of prolonged exposures to noise and whole-body vibration on hearing, vision and strain. *Int Arch Occup Environ Health* 61: 95-106
40. Seroussi RE, Wilder DG, and Pope MH (1989) Trunk Muscle Electromyography and Whole Body Vibration. *J. Biomech* 22: 219-229
41. Sibbald WJ, Messmer K, and Fink MP (2000) Roundtable conference on tissue oxygenation in acute medicine, Brussels, Belgium, 14-16 March 1998. *Int Care Med* 26: 780-791
42. Simonson SG, and Piantadosi CA (1996) NIRS: Clinical Applications. *Crit Care Clin* 12(4): 1019-1029
43. Villringer A and Chance B (1997) Non-invasive optical spectroscopy and imaging of human brain function. *Trends Neurosci* 20:435-441
44. Villringer A, Planck J, Stodieck S, Botzel K, Schleinskofer L, and Dirnagl U (1994) Noninvasive assessment of cerebral hemodynamics and tissue oxygenation during activation of brain cell function in human adults using near infrared spectroscopy. *Adv Exp Med Biol* 345: 559-565
45. Weinstein J, Pope M, Schmidt R, and Seroussi R (1988) Neuropharmacologic effects of vibration on the dorsal root ganglion – An Animal Model. *Spine* 13(5): 521-525
46. Weinstein J (1991) Neurogenic and nonneurogenic pain and inflammatory mediators. *Orthopedic Clinics of North America* 22: 235-244
47. Wilder D, Woodworth BB, Frymoyer JW, and Pope MH (1982) Vibration and the human spine. *Spine* 7(3): 243-254
48. Yoshitake Y, Ue H, Miyazaki M, and Moritani T (2001) Assessment of lower-back muscle fatigue using electromyography, mechanomyography, and near-infrared spectroscopy. *Eur J Appl Physiol* 84: 174-179
49. Zimmerman CL, Cook TM, and Goel VK (1993) Effects of seated posture on erector spinae EMG activity during whole body vibration. *Ergonomics* 36(6): 667-675

Adaptation Biology and Medicine (Volume 4: Current Concepts)
Editors: A. Hargens, N. Takeda and P.K. Singal

25. Vascular Adaptation to Microgravity: Role and Implications of Local Vascular Renin-Angiotensin System

Li-Fan Zhang and Jun-Xiang Bao

Department of Aerospace Physiology, Fourth Military Medical University, Xi'an 710032, P.R.China

Vascular Adaptation to Microgravity

Animals have adapted Earth's gravity of I G over millions of years. Humans and other terrestrial species have evolved unique structural and functional adaptations to gravity in their vascular systems. Exposure to microgravity undoubtedly results in a redistribution of transmural pressures and blood flows across and within the arterial vasculature due to the removal of hydrostatic gradients. Therefore, blood vessels in dependent body regions are chronically exposed to lower than their normal upright 1-G blood pressure during spaceflight. While vessels in upper body regions are exposed to higher than normal 1-G blood pressure. In the early 1980s, Hargens and coworkers (16, 30) first predicted that these chronic changes in local hemodynamic stresses may differentially alter the structure and function of the vessels in different body regions during extended exposure to microgravity. They further stressed that the vascular adaptation may be more important during and after prolonged existence in microgravity (16, 30).

In the past decade, there has been an increased interest in studies on vascular adaptation in ground-based animal studies using the tail-suspended hindlimb-unloaded rat model to mimic the vascular effect of microgravity. Our previous work has revealed that simulated microgravity may induce upward and downward regulations in the structure, function, and innervation state of the cerebral and hindquarter vessels. Likewise, work from other laboratories has demonstrated that differential adaptations in structure and function also occur in resistance vessels (for review, see 32). These findings not only substantiate in general the prediction made by Hargens and coworkers, but are also on the whole consistent with findings from recent human studies. Evidence from bedrest and postflight human studies indicates that the inability to adequately elevate the peripheral resistance and the enhanced cerebral vasoreactivity are important factors in postflight orthostatic intolerance (32,33).

Despite the progress in the last decade, several issues will have to be addressed in the coming years before we can fully appreciate the contribution of the autoregulation in vessels and cardiac muscle in the occurrence of postflight cardiovascular dysfunction. These studies may also provide us the scientific rationale for the development of multisystem countermeasures. An important issue, which has not been addressed to the full extent, is the prevailing local hemodynamic conditions in special circulation, particularly the cerebral circulation, during prolonged existence in the microgravity environment. Hypothetically, during microgravity exposure, removal of hydrostatic pressure gradients would induce pressure changes of similar magnitudes in both cerebro-vascular and cerebrospinal fluid (CSF) pressures. Thus, the increase in transmural pressure across the cerebral vasculature would be greatly compromised. However, the nature of the adaptational changes in cerebral vessels during simulated microgravity strongly suggests a sustained elevation of transmural pressure in cerebral vessels (32). Addressing these issues in full detail will provide further insight into the local hemodynamic changes that may initiate differential adaptation of vessels in microgravity environment. Another important issue is to understand the differential adaptation process in vessels of different regions at cellular and molecular levels. Given the complexity of the process of mechanotransduction, mediators, intracellular signaling pathways, and nuclear events involved, it is likely of success to fully use the achievements in modern vascular biomedicine, in particular the pathophysiology of vessels as reference, to design new experiments. For reasons listed below, the aim of our current work was to explore whether vascular local renin-angiotensin system plays a pivotal role in differential vascular adaptation to microgravity. The third important issue that needs to be addressed in the future is to understand vascular adaptation to microgravity as a whole. This should be a systems approach. It needs not only the detailed data regarding the autoregulation of various kinds of small resistance vessels and vascular beds in special circulation, but also integrative experimental studies coupled with modeling and digital simulation studies as well. Systems approach allows us to ascertain the true mechanism of postflight cardiovascular dysfunction and to assess whether and to what extent the autoregulatory mechanism intrinsic in the vascular wall tissue contribute to it. Finally, it is also important to extend the observation with primates and humans using innovative noninvasive techniques in future ground-based and International Space Station researches to fill the gaps in our knowledge (32).

In the present article, we review up-to-date evidence indicating the existence of local RAS in the vascular wall tissue and its role in vascular adaptation in cardiovascular diseases as well as during microgravity exposure.

Vascular Local Renin-Angiotensin System

In 1898, Tigerstedt and Bergmann discovered renin, one of the key enzymes of the renin-angiotensin system (RAS). In the following decades, other enzymes and effector peptides of the RAS were discovered (important steps were made by Page et al, 1940; Braun-Menendez et al, 1940; and Skeggs et al, 1958). Classically, the RAS has been described in terms of the systemic blood-borne system (23,26). Renin is a proteolytic enzyme secreted into the blood stream by the juxtaglomerular cells of the kidney. It cleaves a plasma protein substrate, angiotensinogen (AGT) produced by the liver, to yield the decapeptide angiotensin I (Ang I). Two amino acids from the carboxyl terminus of this peptide are cleaved by angiotensin-converting enzyme (ACE) to produce the active octapeptide angiotensin II (Ang II). Recently, shorter angiotensin fragments, including Ang III (2-8), Ang IV (3-8) and Ang (1-7) have been described. However, it is generally thought that Ang II is of the greatest biological significance (27-29). Ang II binds to a family of receptors including Ang II type 1 receptor (AT_1R, 60 kDa) and type 2 receptor (AT_2R, 60 kDa). Both receptors play a role in VSMC growth, but with different effects: AT_1R being associated with proliferation, hypertrophy, and antiapoptotic effect, whereas the AT_2R is associated with pro- apoptotic effect. Both receptors are seven-transmembrane domain receptors (3, 17, 27-29).

Over the last two decades, it has been well established that angiotensin can be generated not only in the systemic circulation, but also in multiple tissue sites. Currently, there is a great deal of evidence indicating the existence of local RASs in heart, vessels, kidney, brain, adrenal, pituitary, adipose tissue, and reproductive organs (5, 6, 7-9, 13-15, 24, 27-29, 34). These local systems act in both autocrine and paracrine fashion to elicit responses which may be concerned with tissue growth and repair, or with other highly specific functions which are not necessarily related to the functions of the circulatory RAS. For example, in reproductive system, Ang II has been suggested as an important paracrine agent with significant roles in several functions of reproductive system (28,29). In brain, Ang II is concerned with drinking behavior, blood pressure regulation, vasopressin as well as catecholamine release (24, 27). Whereas the role of adrenal angiotensin is probably to regulate aldosterone biosynthesis (29). Hence, Ang II has the overall significance as a universal organizer and regulator of functions of various tissues. The generation of Ang II locally in proximity to its receptors may ensure that tissue-specific functions are precisely regulated (5,29). However, precise data regarding the cellular localization of the sites of local synthesis of components of local RASs, the relationship between local synthesis and uptake of certain components from the circulation, the precise localization and regulation of local Ang II generation, their relationship to the sites of Ang II action, and highly specific manners of responses of paracrine target cells to locally generated Ang II in different tissues are still lacking in most cases (5, 7-9, 28, 29). Recently, evidence is emerging to indicate that Ang II can perform a variety of physiologically relevant intracrine actions, including influencing cardiac conduction and contractility (10).

The existence of a local RAS in vascular tissue is supported by multiple lines of evidence obtained in experimental as well as in clinical studies. The introduction of molecular biology technique has provided direct measures to identify the presence of principal RAS components in the vessel wall tissue. Gene and protein expressions for angiotensinogen (AGT), renin, angiotensin converting enzyme (ACE), and AT_1R and AT_2R receptors have been demonstrated in large and small arteries by in-situ hybridization histochemistry, immunohistochemistry, and RT-PCR, Northern blotting, and Western blotting. However, the origin of renin in vascular tissue has been debated and there is evidence for both uptake from the circulating blood and local synthesis. The existence of vascular local RAS has been further verified by in vitro studies using cultured VSMCs and endothelial cells, cultured aortic organs, isolated perfused vascular segments and vascular beds, and in vivo studies with intact animals and humans both under normal and pathological conditions. However, the precise mechanisms underlying local generation of Ang II and its regulation in the vascular tissue remain to be further addressed. With respect to methodological challenges, the mRNA and protein expression levels for some RAS components in vessel wall tissues are very low for ordinary methods. Development of techniques able to detect minute quantities of Ang I and II at the "local receptor level" is also in need (5). Special pretreatment of samples to prevent the ex vivo generation and breakdown of vascular angiotensins and to make appropriate corrections for any losses of intact Ang I and II during extraction and assay merit further attention (7, 9).

It has been postulated that the principal function of the circulating RAS is to provide short-term blood pressure and volume homeostasis. It is subjected to feedback regulation and is activated in response to hypotension, hypovolemia, hemorrhage, and severe heart failure (13, 14). On the other hand, vascular local RAS plays an important role both in local regulation of vascular tone and growth. Its function is to provide long-term regulation by sustained activation of local RAS and the secondary structural changes. Convincing evidence also comes from the clinical and pharmacological studies. The development of oral ACE inhibitors and the demonstration of their wide clinical efficacy have been regarded as " intellectual triumphs of the past half-century" (1). Animal studies have demonstrated that an increase in local production of vascular angiotensin may result in net vasoconstriction and possibly hypertension. For example, in the SHR, systemic blood pressure correlates closely with aortic renin concentration but not with plasma renin activity. In the 2K1C rat model, whose plasma renin activity is suppressed, hypertension is associated with an increase in aortic ACE activity. Administration of ACE inhibitor lowers blood pressure in both animal models of hypertension (cited from 14). However, the beneficial effects of these drugs are not yet fully understood.

It is now clear that the differential adaptation of vessels from different body regions to microgravity is primarily a structural adaptation of vessels to prevailing hemodynamic conditions, due to the removal of gravity (30,32). Thus, what we faced is a growth-regulating problem for vessels, notably due to the regional differential changes in transmural pressures. Studies with a model of cultured rabbit aorta have provided further evidence demonstrating the crucial role of mechanical stresses in the maintenance of differentiated phenotype of the VSMCs and the homeostasis of the vessels. Aortic organ culture experiments also demonstrated that augmented local angiotensin levels mediate the enhanced total protein and fibronectin synthesis induced by high intraluminal pressure (2,18). Although a multitude of growth factors, or mitogenic agonists are certainly implicated in the process of differential adaptation (12, 22), we speculated that differential changes in local vascular RAS activity of different vessels in response to changes in local prevailing stresses may play a pivotal role among them. Ang II has been reported to stimulate hyperplasia, hypertrophy, and both proapoptotic and antiapoptotic effects on VSMCs. Stretch due to increased transmural pressure may act on unknown stretch receptors to stimulate the RAS, leading to the production of Ang II (18). This acts on the G-protein coupled AT1 receptor through phospholipase C, activating protein kinase C and raising the cytoplasmic calcium. Protein kinase C activation leads to activation of the Ras-Raf pathway and thus ERK1/2 activation, which leads through activation of transcription factors to activation of protooncogenes like *c-fos* and *c-myc* and protein synthesis (22). Recently, Berk (3) summarized that Ang II regulates VSMC growth via at least four different growth pathways. They are: 1) direct effects of the AT1 receptor, 2) transactivation of EGF-R and PDGF-R, 3) increased reactive oxygen species (ROS) generation, and 4) induction of other growth factors including PDGF-A and PDGF-B, ET-1, FGF, epiregulin, IL-6, IGF-I, TGF-β, HBEGF, and activin.

Given the complexity of the vascular local RAS, one of the challenges is to obtain a clearer insight into the mechanisms and regulation of local Ang II production in vivo. Studies on changes in gene and protein expressions of principal RAS components in different vascular tissues during the process of adaptation to simulated microgravity will assist in this endeavor.

Differential Changes in Expressions of L-RAS Components of Different Vessels Due to Simulated Microgravity

Gene and Protein Expressions of Angiotensinogen Although many different enzymes in the vascular wall are able to cleave angiotensinogen (AGT) to release angiotensins, AGT is the only known precursor of the angiotensin peptides. Thus, the presence of gene and protein expression has been

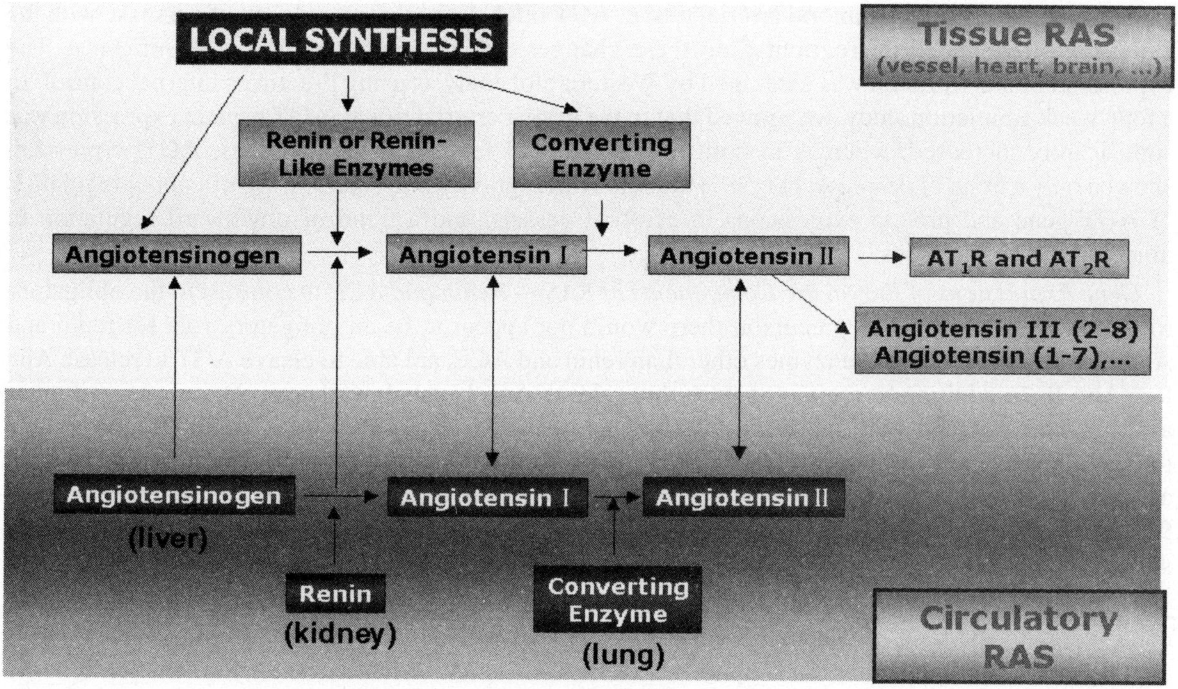

Fig. 1. Diagram showing circulatory vs. local renin-angiotensin systems

regarded as the definitive evidence suggesting the existence of independent tissue RAS (5, 6). In systemic RAS, liver is the established site of AGT synthesis. With respect to vessels, the synthesis of AGT has been documented for VSMCs in cell culture; and for the aortic media and adventitia, and fatty tissue surrounding the blood vessels (6,14,15, 24). In addition, vascular AGT may also be derived from the circulating blood (14). The importance of AGT synthesis can be fully appreciated from the following facts. In the circulating RAS, it has been found that the AGT concentration is rate-limiting for the maximal velocity of Ang I formation. Physiological observations support that there is a critical relationship between AGT synthesis and the RAS tone (4).

To determine whether AGT expression is differentially regulated in cerebral and hindquarter arteries during simulated microgravity, we examined the gene and protein expressions of AGT in different vascular tissues of 2-, 4-, as well as 8-week tail-suspended hindlimb-unloaded rats and compared with these of simultaneous control rats (21). AGT mRNA hybridization signals were detected in basilar, common carotid, femoral arterial and abdominal aortic tissues. They were also found in the media, adventitia and even in the perivascular fatty cells. Polyclonal antiserum against rat AGT was specially prepared to examine AGT protein expression (20). Immunohistochemical staining demonstrated the presence of AGT in the rat basilar arterial and liver tissues. Expression of AGT gene was further examined by RT-PCR with GAPDH as the internal control. This study has demonstrated that simulated microgravity leads to upward and downward regulation of AGT gene expression in cerebral and hindquarter arterial tissues. In basilar arterial tissue, the AGT mRNA level began to show an increasing tendency after two weeks, reached a significantly high level after four weeks, and remained at a higher level after eight weeks. In femoral arterial tissue, AGT mRNA showed a tendency of decrease with the extension of simulated microgravity, but these changes did not reach the level of significance. The expression of AGT protein was examined by Western blot analysis using β-actin as internal control. In a four-week simulation study, we showed that in the basilar arterial tissue, AGT protein expression was significantly increased; whereas in both mesenteric and femoral arterial tissues, AGT expression showed only a trend of decrease. In brief, simulated microgravity may lead to a significant upregulation of AGT gene and protein expressions in cerebral vessels, and a trend of downward regulation in hindquater arterial tissues.

Gene Expressions of Enzymatic Components of RAS — Renin and ACE In contrast to the obligatory role of AGT as angiotensin precursor, there would not appear to be an obligatory role for renin and ACE in local RAS, because enzymes other than renin and ACE, are able to cleave AGT to release Ang I or Ang II. In addition to renin, enzymes that release Ang I include cathepsin D, pepsin, and other aspartyl proteases, and renin-like enzymes. Enzymes that cleave AGT to release Ang II directly include tonin, cathepsin G, trypsin, and kallikrein (5). Ang II can also be formed from Ang I by the action of another pathway, in particular, by another enzyme, chymase, which is a potent and specific Ang II-forming serine protease (7, 28). Nevertheless, the detection of mRNAs for renin and ACE is still a strong evidence for the existence of local RAS.

Renin is a glycoproteolytic enzyme responsible for the first step in the formation of Ang II. One controversy in the field of vascular local RAS has been the source of vascular renin. Now there is evidence for both uptake and local synthesis (8, 9, 14, 31). ACE is an ectoenzyme anchored in the membrane of the endothelial cells. The localization of ACE in the vessel wall has been demonstrated by enzyme activity assay, immunohistochemistry, and autoradiography using radioactively labeled ACE inhibitors. ACE is found in the endothelium, and, at a lower density, in the adventitia (15). Some data suggest that it may also exist in VSMCs (14).

To determine whether the gene expressions for renin, ACE, and chymase are also differentially regulated in different vascular tissues, we designed experiments to examine the mRNAs of the three enzymatic components in basilar and femoral arterial tissues of one- and four-week simulated microgravity rats. Because of the difficulties associated with the detection of the vascular renin mRNA at a very low level, a semi-nested PCR was used specifically to examine the gene expression of renin. After one week of simulated microgravity, significant changes were observed in different vascular tissues: in basilar arterial tissue, renin mRNA was significantly increased; whereas in femoral arterial tissue, ACE mRNA was significantly decreased. After four weeks of simulated microgravity, mRNA expression for both ACE and chymase showed differential trends of increase and decrease, respectively, in cerebral and femoral arterial tissues, but these changes were not significant. In brief, our results suggest that significant differential changes in gene expression of enzymatic components appear to be an early, acute adaptive response during initial stage of microgravity exposure.

Gene and Protein Expression of Ang II Receptors — AT1R Two main subtypes of angiotensin receptors have been classified as AT1 and AT2 receptors according to their sensitivity to the Ang II antagonists (17, 29). In rats and mice, the AT1 receptor subtype has two isoforms, AT1a and AT1b, which have 94% of homology with regard to amino acid sequence, and have similar pharmacological properties and tissue distribution patterns (17, 27). All the classic well-known effects of Ang II appear to be mediated via the AT1 receptor, which is widely distributed in peripheral tissues. In the vasculature, the AT1 receptor is particularly prominent on the luminal surface of the endothelium (29).

The AT_2 receptor is expressed abundantly and transiently in fetal tissue, and in the adult, its expression is limited in the uterus, ovary, certain brain nuclei, heart and adrenal (17, 27). The role of AT2 receptor in vascular tissues remains to be clarified. Evidence from in vitro studies suggests that AT1 and AT2 receptors may counteract each other in their growth-modulating action (17). Thus, the local expression of Ang II receptors is another obligatory requirement for an independent tissue RAS.

Our results demonstrated differential change in the expression of AT1 receptor in cerebral and hindquarter arterial tissues and its time course during simulated microgravity for four weeks. After one week of simulated microgravity, no significant changes in mRNA expression for AT1 receptor were noted, although there were differential trends of increase and decrease, respectively, for cerebral and femoral arterial tissues. However, after four weeks of simulated microgravity, the differential changes in mRNA of AT1 receptor were significant : in basilar arterial tissue, mRNA expression of two isoforms of AT1 receptor — AT1a and AT1b, was significantly increased; whereas in femoral arterial tissue, mRNA expression of AT1a was significantly decreased. The protein expression of AT1 receptor was examined by Western blot analysis using β-actin as internal control. In a four-week simulation study, we showed that in the basilar arterial tissue, the protein expression of AT1 receptor was significantly increased; whereas in both mesenteric and femoral arterial tissues, the protein expression of AT1 receptor was significantly decreased. In brief, a mid-term simulated microgravity may induce upward and downward regulations in gene and protein expressions of AT_1 receptor in cerebral and hindquarter arterial tissues.

Mechanisms and Implications

Mechanisms Table 1 summarizes our results. As can be seen, the gene and protein expressions of AGT and AT1 receptor showed significant differential changes in cerebral and hindquarter arterial tissues after four weeks of simulated microgravity, whereas the mRNA expressions of renin and ACE showed differential changes only after one week of simulated microgravity. The enhanced and depressed

Table 1. Differential expression of L-RAS components in different arterial tissues

		AGT	renin	ACE	chymase	AT_1
				mRNA expression		
1 wk SUS	Hindquarter artary	—	—	↓	↓	—
	Cerebral artary	—	↑	—	—	—
4 wk SUS	Hindquarter artary	↓	—	↓	↓	↓
	Cerebral artary	↑	—	↑	↑	↑
				Protein expression		
1 wk SUS	Hindquarter artary	/	/	/	/	/
	Cerebral artary	/	/	/	/	/
4 wk SUS	Hindquarter artary	↓	/	/	/	↓
	Cerebral artary	↑	/	/	/	↑

Notes: ↑ significantly increased; ↓ significantly decreased;
↑ tendency of increase; ↓ tendency of decrease;
— no obvious changes; / not examined.

vascular local RAS tone in different vascular tissues are apparently elicited by the local hypertension and hypotension in cerebral and hindquarter arteries during simulated microgravity. Our results strongly support that vascular local renin-angiotensin system may play a pivotal role in differential vascular adaptation to microgravity. The significance of vascular RAS is particularly related to the rapid progress in our understanding of the action of Ang II, including the understanding from the conventional signaling pathways toward signal transduction involving specific tyrosine kinases and its actions of inducing not only vasoconstriction but also proto-oncogene expression, protein synthesis, hypertrophy, and growth. The significance of the studies aimed at elucidating the pivotal role of vascular RAS in vascular adaptation is also closely associated with the issues regarding the important role of interaction of and balance between local RAS and NO systems in vascular homeostasis (25).

In addition to the RAS of vessels, other RASs, at least, in heart, kidney, brain, and adipose tissue also merit attention in addressing issues such as mechanism of cardiac adaptation to microgravity and postflight cardiovascular deconditioning and mechanism of fluid and electrolyte homeostasis during adaptation to microgravity. It is of interest to point out that the brain RAS plays a role in the drinking behavior of rats, as well as a role in central osmoregulation (24,27,29). Furthermore, the role played by the interaction between circulatory and various tissue RASs in adaptation to microgravity is also of interest. These studies will also lead to a better understanding of the RAS by integrating data from in vitro with in vivo studies.

Implications In our present work, of particular interest is the observation that the time course of both the upward and downward regulations of AGT expression in different vascular tissues during simulated microgravity for eight weeks parallels with that of the differential changes in the structure of different vessels (32). Given that there is a positive correlation between local AGT and Ang II concentrations, the local Ang II in the cerebral arterial wall tissue would be in a sustained high level, which is the principal factor that mediates and maintains the hypertrophy and hyperreactivity of the cerebral vessels. This may protect the microcirculation in the brain to prevent cerebral congestion and edema. However, this sustained elevated local RAS tone during vascular adaptation may also lead to an adverse effect on the cerebral vasculature, particularly during a prolonged existence in microgravity. Recent discoveries have provided a deeper understanding of the role of Ang II in initiation and amplification of the pathologic events in cardiovascular diseases. Evidence indicates that Ang II has a significant proinflammatory action in the vascular wall, including the production of reactive oxygen species (ROS), and activation of ancient inflammatory mechanisms. Through these actions, Ang II augments vascular inflammation, induces endothelial dysfunction, and enhances the atherogenic process. The activation of a pivotal transcription factor, NF-κB, and related genes is involved in this process (4, 11, 19). Recently, end-organ damage due to increased activities of RAS has been studied with a double-transgenic rat model overexpressing human AGT and human renin genes, which has facilitated the studies on blood pressure-independent Ang II-related effects (19). Although the pathogenesis of atherosclerosis is undoubtedly a multifactorial and slowly progressed process, the possibility of the existence of a new kind of adverse effects due to microgravity exposure — vascular damage — merits further attention. One point should not be overlooked is that the Earth-like distribution of transmural pressures across the cerebral vasculature can not be restored and maintained by conventional exercise-based countermeasures. It seems also not by some additional proposals. For example, the "exercise within LBNP" proposed by Hargens and co-workers (16, 30) can provide an Earth-like distribution of transmural pressures across the blood vessels of the lower body during microgravity exposure; but for the cerebral vessels, it seems not (32).

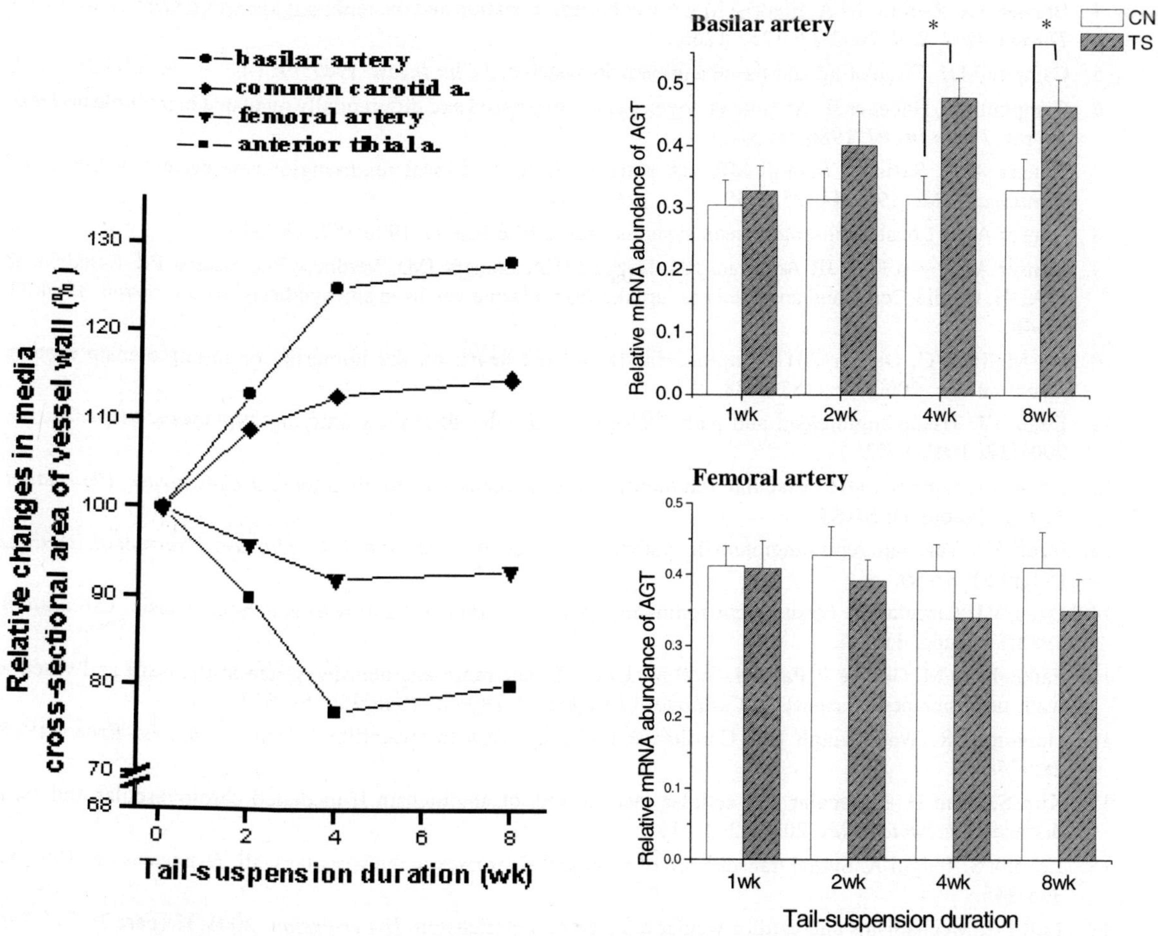

Fig. 2. Comparison between differential changes in wall media CSA (modified from [32]) and arterial AGT mRNA expression in different arteries during simulated microgravity up to 8 weeks

Acknowledgements

This research was supported by the National Natural Science Foundation of China (No.30171032) and the Defense Medical Fund (No.01MB122). The monoclonal antibody for the AT1 receptor was a generous gift from Professor GP Vinson (Queen Mary & Westfield College, London, UK).

References

1. Alexander RW, Dzau VJ. Vascular biology: the past 50 years. *Circulation.* 2000;102: IV-112 - IV-116.
2. Bardy N, Merval R, Benessiano J, Samuel JL, Tedgui A. Pressure and angiotensin II synergistically induce aortic fibronectin expression in organ culture model of rabbit aorta: evidence for a pressure-induced tissue renin-angiotensin system. *Circ Res.* 1996;79: 70-78.
3. Berk BC. Vascular smooth muscle growth: autocrine growth mechanisms. *Physiol Rev.* 2001;81: 999-1030.

4. Brasier AR, Recinos III A, Eledrisi MS. Vascular inflammation and the renin-angiotensin system. *Arterioscler Thromb Vasc Biol.* 2002;22: 1257-1266.
5. Campbell DJ. Circulating and tissue angiotensin systems. *J Clin Invest.* 1987;79: 1-6.
6. Campbell DJ, Habener JF. Angiotensinogen gene is expressed and differentially regulated in multiple tssues of the rat. *J Clin Invest.* 1986;78: 31-39.
7. Danser AHJ, Saris JJ, Schuijt MP, van Kats JP. Is there a local renin-angiotensin system in the heart? *Cardiovasc Res.* 1999;44: 252-265.
8. Danser AHJ. Local renin-angiotensin systems. *Mol Cell Biochem.* 1996;157: 211-216.
9. Danser AHJ, van Kats JP, Admiraal PJJ, Derkx FHM, Lamers JMJ, Verdouw PD, Saxena PR, Schalekamp MADH. Cardiac renin and angiotensins: uptake from plasma versus in situ synthesis. *Hypertension.* 1994;24: 37-48.
10. De Mello WC, Danser AHJ. Angiotensin II and the heart: on the intracrine renin-angiotensin system. *Hypertension.* 2000;35: 1183-1188.
11. Dzau VJ. Tissue angiotensin and pathobiology of vascular disease: a unifying hypothesis. *Hypertension.* 2001;37: 1047-1052.
12. Dzau VJ, Gibbons GH. Vascular remodeling: mechanisms and implications. *J Cardiovasc Pharmacol.* 1993;21(Suppl 1): S1-S5.
13. Dzau VJ. Vascular renin-angiotensin system and vascular protection. *J Cardiovasc Pharmacol.* 1993;22 (Suppl 5): S1-S9.
14. Dzau VJ. Circulating versus local renin–angiotensin system in cardiovascular homeostasis. *Circulation.* 1988;77 (Suppl 1): 1-4.
15. Falkenhahn M, Gohlke P, Paul M, Stoll M, Unger T. The renin-angiotensin system in the heart and vascular wall: new therapeutic aspects. *J Cardiovasc Pharmacol.* 1994;24 (Suppl 2): S6-S13.
16. Hargens AR, Watenpaugh DE. Cardiovascular adaptation to spaceflight. *Med Sci Sports Exerc.* 1996; 28:977-982.
17. Kim S, Iwao H. Molecular and cellular mechanisms of angiotensin II-mediated cardiovascular and renal diseases. *Pharmacol Rev.* 2000;52: 11-34.
18. Lehoux S, Tedgui A. Signal transduction of mechanical stresses in the vascular wall. *Hypertension.* 1998;32: 338-345.
19. Luft FC. Mechanisms and cardiovascular damage in hypertension. *Hypertension.* 2001;37 (part 2): 594-598.
20. Meng QJ, Li J, Zhang WH, Zhang LN, Zhang LF. Preparation and identification of polyclonal antiserum against angiotensinogen. *Acta Physiol Sinica.* 2003; 55: 110-113.
21. Meng QJ, Zhang LF, Zhang LN, Ma J. Changes of angiotensinogen expression in arteries of tail-suspended rats. *J Gravit Physiol.* 2002; 9 (1): P-87 – P-88.
22. Mulvany MJ. Small artery remodeling and significance in the development of hypertension. *News Physiol Sci.* 2002;17: 105-109.
23. Peach MJ. Renin-angiotensin system: biochemistry and mechanisms of action. *Physiol Rev.* 1977; 57: 313-370.
24. Phillips MI, Speakman EA, Kimura B. Levels of angiotensin and molecular biology of the tissue renin angiotensin systems. *Regulatory Peptides.* 1993;43: 1-20.
25. Raij L. Hypertension and cardiovascular risk factors: role of the angiotensin II-nitric oxide interaction. *Hypertension.* 2001;37 (part 2): 767-773.
26. Reid IA, Morris BJ, Ganong WG. The renin-angiotensin system. *Annu Rev Physiol.* 1978;40:377-410.
27. Stroth U, Unger T. The renin-angiotensin system and its receptors. *J Cardiovasc Pharmacol.* 1999;33 (Suppl 1): S21-S28.
28. Vinson GP, Saridogan E, Puddefoot JR, Djahanbakhch O. Tissue renin-angiotensin systems and reproduction. *Human Reproduction.* 1997;12: 651-662.

29. Vinson GP, Ho MM, Puddefoot JR. The distribution of angiotensin II type 1 receptors, and the tissue renin-angiotensin systems. *Molecular Medicine Today.* 1995; 35-39.
30. Watenpaugh DE, Hargens AR. The cardiovascular system in microgravity. In: *Handbook of Physiology. Environmental Physiology*. Bethesda MD: Am. Physiol. Soc., 1996, Sect. 4, vol. I Chapt.29, p. 631-674.
31. Xiao F, Puddefoot JR, Vinson GP. The expression of renin and the formation of angiotensin II in bovine aortic endothelial cells. *J Endocrinol.* 2000;164: 207-214.
32. Zhang LF. Vascular adaptation to microgravity: what have we learned? *J Appl physiol.* 2001;91: 2415-2430.
33. Zhang LF, Yu ZB, Ma J, Mao QW. Peripheral effector mechanism hypothesis of postflight cardiovascular dysfunction. *Aviat Space Environ med.* 2001;72: 567-575.
34. Engeli S, Negrel R, Sharma AM. Physiology and pathophysiology of the adipose tissue renin-angiotensin system. Hypertension. 35:1270-1277

Index